Practical Gastroenterology and Hepatology:
Small and Large Intestine and Pancreas

Companion website

This book has a companion website:

practicalgastrohep.com

with:

- Videos demonstrating procedures

- The videos are all referenced in the text where you see this symbol:

Practical Gastroenterology and Hepatology

Small and Large Intestine and Pancreas

EDITOR-IN-CHIEF

Nicholas J. Talley, MD, PhD

Pro Vice Chancellor and Professor of Medicine Faculty of Health
University of Newcastle, NSW, Australia;
Adjunct Professor of Medicine
College of Medicine
Mayo Clinic
Rochester, MN, and Jacksonville, FL, USA;
Foreign Adjunct Professor of Gastroenterology
Karolinska Institute
Stockholm, Sweden;
Adjunct Professor
University of North Carolina
USA

EDITORS

Sunanda V. Kane, MD, MSPH

Professor of Medicine
College of Medicine, Mayo Clinic
Consultant, Miles and Shirley Fitterman Division of Gastroenterology and Hepatology
Mayo Clinic
Rochester, MN, USA

Michael B. Wallace, MD, MPH

Professor and Chair, Division of Gastroenterology and Hepatology
College of Medicine, Mayo Clinic
Consultant, Division of Gastroenterology and Hepatology
Mayo Clinic
Jacksonville, FL, USA

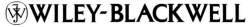

WILEY-BLACKWELL

A John Wiley & Sons, Ltd., Publication

Contents

A companion website for this book is available at:
practicalgastrohep.com

Contributors

Faten N. Aberra, MD, MSCE
Assistant Professor of Medicine
Division of Gastroenterology
Hospital of the University of Pennsylvania
Philadelphia, PA, USA

Reza Y. Akhtar, MD
Fellow in Gastroenterology
Henry D. Janowitz Division of Gastroenterology
Mount Sinai School of Medicine
New York, NY, USA

Nadir Arber, MD, MSc, MHA
Professor of Medicine and Gastroenterology
Yechiel and Helen Lieber Professor for Cancer Research
Head of The Integrated Cancer Prevention Center
Tel-Aviv Sourasky Medical Center
Sackler Faculty of Medicine
Tel-Aviv University
Tel Aviv, Israel

Fernando Azpiroz, MD
Professor of Medicine
Chair, Department of Gastroenterology
University Hospital Vall d'Hebron
Barcelona, Spain

Nison Badalov, MD
Assistant Director
Brooklyn Gastroenterology and Endoscopy Associates
Maimonides Medical Center
State University of New York — Health Sciences Center
New York, NY, USA

Peter A. Banks, MD
Professor of Medicine
Division of Gastroenterology
Center for Pancreatic Disease
Harvard Medical School
Brigham and Women's Hospital
Boston, MA, USA

English F. Barbour, RD, LD, CNSD
Dietitian
Digestive Disease Center
Medical University of South Carolina
Charleston, SC, USA

Todd H. Baron, MD
Professor of Medicine
Division of Gastroenterology and Hepatology
Director of Pancreaticobiliary Endoscopy
Mayo Clinic
Rochester, MN, USA

Adil E. Bharucha, MBBS, MD
Professor of Medicine
Clinical Enteric Neuroscience Translational and
Epidemiological Research Program
Division of Gastroenterology and Hepatology
Mayo Clinic
Rochester, MN, USA

Ernest P. Bouras, MD
Assistant Professor of Medicine
Division of Gastroenterology and Hepatology
Mayo Clinic
Jacksonville, FL, USA

Stacy A. Brethauer, MD
Staff Surgeon
Bariatric and Metabolic Institute
Cleveland Clinic
Cleveland, OH, USA

William R. Brugge, MD
Director, Gastrointestinal Endoscopy
Gastrointestinal Unit
Massachusetts General Hospital
Professor of Medicine
Harvard Medical School
Boston, MA, USA

Alan L. Buchman, MD, MSPH
Professor of Medicine and Surgery
Division of Gastroenterology
Feinberg School of Medicine
Northwestern University
Chicago, IL, USA

Anna M. Buchner, MD, PhD
Instructor of Medicine
Fellow in Advanced Endoscopy
Department of Gastroenterology
University of Pennsylvania
Philadelphia, PA, USA

John R. Cangemi, MD
Assistant Professor
Division of Gastroenterology and Hepatology
Department of Internal Medicine
Mayo Clinic
Jacksonville, FL, USA

John M. Carethers, MD
John G. Searle Professor and Chair
Department of Internal Medicine
University of Michigan
Ann Arbor, MI, USA

Natasha Chandok, MD
Instructor of Medicine
Division of Gastroenterology and Hepatology
University of Western Ontario
London, ON, Canada

Lin Chang, MD
Professor of Medicine
Center for Neurobiology of Stress
Division of Digestive Diseases
David Geffen School of Medicine at UCLA
VA Greater Los Angeles Healthcare System
Los Angeles, CA, USA

Louis Chaptini, MD
Assistant Professor of Medicine
Division of Gastroenterology and Liver Diseases
Cooper University Hospital
Robert Wood Johnson Medical School
University of Medicine and Dentistry of New Jersey
Camden, NJ, USA

Disaya Chavalitdhamrong, MD
Research Fellow
Division of Digestive Diseases
David Geffen School of Medicine at UCLA
Los Angeles, CA, USA

Gary C. Chen, MD
Clinical Fellow
Division of Digestive Diseases
David Geffen School of Medicine at UCLA
Los Angeles, CA, USA

William D. Chey, MD
Professor of Medicine
Director, GI Physiology Laboratory
University of Michigan Health System
Ann Arbor, MI, USA

Robert R. Cima, MD, MA
Associate Professor of Surgery
Department of Surgery
Mayo Clinic
Rochester, MN, USA

Michael Cox, MB BS, MS
Professor of Surgery
Department of Surgery
University of Sydney
Nepean Hospital
Penrith, NSW, Australia

Sheila E. Crowe, MD
Professor of Medicine
Division of Gastroenterology and Hepatology
Department of Medicine
University of Virginia
Charlottesville, VA, USA

G. Anton Decker, MB BCh, MRCP
Associate Professor of Medicine
Director of the Pancreas Clinic
Division of Gastroenterology
Mayo Clinic
Scottsdale, AZ, USA

Christopher Deitch, MD
Assistant Professor of Medicine
Division of Gastroenterology and Liver Diseases
Cooper University Hospital
Robert Wood Johnson Medical School
University of Medicine and Dentistry of New Jersey
Camden, NJ, USA

Mark DeLegge, MD
Professor of Medicine
Director, Digestive Disease Center
Medical University of South Carolina
Charleston, SC, USA

Douglas A. Drossman, MD
Co-Director, UNC Center for Functional GI and
Motility Disorders
Division of Gastroenterology and Hepatology
University of North Carolina
Chapel Hill, NC, USA

Steven J. Esses, BA
Research Fellow
Division of Gastroenterology
Mount Sinai School of Medicine
New York, NY, USA

George T. Fantry, MD
Associate Professor of Medicine
Director, Heartburn and Dyspepsia Program
Division of Gastroenterology
University of Maryland School of Medicine
Baltimore, MD, USA

Nielsen Q. Fernandez-Becker,
MD, PhD
Instructor of Medicine
Division of Gastroenterology and Hepatology
Stanford University School of Medicine
Stanford, CA, USA

Christopher E. Forsmark, MD
Professor of Medicine
Chief, Division of Gastroenterology, Hepatology, and Nutrition
University of Florida
Gainesville, FL, USA

Amy E. Foxx-Orenstein, DO
Associate Professor of Medicine
Division of Gastroenterology and Hepatology
Miles and Shirley Fiterman Center for Digestive Diseases
Mayo Clinic
Rochester, MN, USA

Martin L. Freeman, MD
Professor of Medicine
Interim Director, Division of Gastroenterology, Hepatology
and Nutrition
Director, Pancreaticobiliary Endoscopy Fellowship
Codirector, Minnesota Pancreas and Liver Center
University of Minnesota
Minneapolis, MN, USA

Jonathan P. Fryer, MD
Associate Professor of Surgery
Division of Transplantation
Department of Surgery
Feinberg School of Medicine
Northwestern University
Chicago, IL, USA

Katherine S. Garman, MD
Assistant Professor of Medicine
Division of Gastroenterology and Institute for Genome
Sciences and Policy
Veterans Affairs Medical Center
Duke University
Durham, NC, USA

Patrick Gatmaitan, MD
Fellow in Advanced Laparoscopic and Bariatric Surgery
Bariatric and Metabolic Institute
Cleveland Clinic
Cleveland, OH, USA

Kanwar Rupinder S. Gill, MD
Staff Gastroenterologist
Department of Gastroenterology
Sutter Gould Medical Foundation
Modesto, CA, USA

Madhusudan Grover, MD
Fellow in Gastroenterology
Division of Gastroenterology and Hepatology
Mayo Clinic
Rochester, MN, USA

Nalini M. Guda, MD
Clinical Associate Professor of Medicine
University of Wisconsin School of Medicine and Public Health
Pancreatobiliary Services
St. Luke's Medical Center
Milwaukee, WI, USA

Stephen B. Hanauer, MD
Professor of Medicine and Clinical Pharmacology
Chief, Section of Gastroenterology, Hepatology and Nutrition
University of Chicago Medical Center
Chicago, IL, USA

Richard Hodin, MD
Professor of Surgery
Department of Surgery
Harvard Medical School
Massachusetts General Hospital
Boston, MA, USA

Laura Hwang, BA
Medical Student
GI Motility Program
Cedars-Sinai Medical Center
Los Angeles, CA, USA

Ana Ignjatovic, BA, BMBCh, MRCP
Research Fellow in Endoscopy
Wolfson Unit for Endoscopy
St Mark's Hospital
Harrow, UK

Rome Jutabha, MD
Associate Professor of Medicine
Director, UCLA Center for Small Bowel Diseases
Division of Digestive Diseases
David Geffen School of Medicine at UCLA
Los Angeles, CA, USA

Bobby Kalb, MD
Assistant Professor
Body MRI Applied Research Program
Department of Radiology
Emory University School of Medicine
Atlanta, GA, USA

Nithin Karanth, MD
Fellow in Gastroenterology
Department of Gastroenterology
Drexel University College of Medicine
Philadelphia, PA, USA

John B. Kisiel, MD
Instructor of Medicine
Division of Gastroenterology and Hepatology
Mayo Clinic
Rochester, MN, USA

Saravanan Krishnamoorthy, MD
Assistant Professor
Department of Diagnostic Radiology
Yale University
New Haven, CT, USA

John Thomas LaMont, MD
Chief of Gastroenterology
Division of Gastroenterology
Beth Israel Deaconess Medical Center
Professor of Medicine
Harvard Medical School
Boston, MA, USA

Jonathan A. Leighton, MD
Professor of Medicine
Chair, Division of Gastroenterology
Mayo Clinic
Scottsdale, AZ, USA

Blair S. Lewis, MD
Clinical Professor of Medicine
Henry D. Janowitz Division of Gastroenterology
Mount Sinai School of Medicine
New York, NY, USA

Gary R. Lichtenstein, MD
Professor of Medicine
Division of Gastroenterology
Hospital of the University of Pennsylvania
Philadelphia, PA, USA

John G. Lieb II, MD
Instructor of Medicine
Division of Gastroenterology
University of Pennsylvania
Philadelphia, PA, USA

Paul J. Limburg, MD, MPH
Professor of Medicine
Division of Gastroenterology and Hepatology
Mayo Clinic
Rochester, MN, USA

Vera P. Luther, MD
Assistant Professor of Medicine
Section on Infectious Diseases
Department of Internal Medicine
Wake Forest University School of Medicine
Winston-Salem, NC, USA

Sumit R. Majumdar, MD, MPH
Associate Professor
Department of Medicine
University of Alberta
Edmonton, AB, Canada

Advitya Malhotra, MD, MS
Fellow in Gastroenterology
Department of Gastroenterology and Hepatology
University of Texas Medical Branch (UTMB)
Galveston, TX, USA

Brad E. Maltz, MD
Fellow in Gastroenterology
Division of Gastroenterology
Vanderbilt University
Nashville, TN, USA

Monthira Maneerattanaporn, MD
Research Fellow in Gastroenterology
University of Michigan
Ann Arbor, MI, USA;
Clinical Lecturer, Department of Medicine
Siriraj Hospital
Mahidol University
Bangkok, Thailand

Diego R. Martin, MD, PhD
Professor of Radiology
Department of Radiology
Emory University School of Medicine
Atlanta, GA, USA

Lloyd Mayer, MD
Professor of Immunology and Medicine
Divisions of Clinical Immunology and Gastroenterology
Mount Sinai Medical Center
New York, NY, USA

Koenraad J. Mortele, MD
Associate Professor of Radiology
Harvard Medical School;
Associate Director, Division of Abdominal Imaging and Intervention
Director of Abdminal and Pelvic MRI
Department of Radiology
Brigham and Women's Hospital
Boston, MA, USA

Menachem Moshkowitz, MD
Assistant Professor of Medicine
Integrated Cancer Prevention Center
Tel-Aviv Sourasky Medical Center
Sackler Faculty of Medicine
Tel-Aviv University
Tel-Aviv, Israel

Alan C. Moss, MD
Assistant Professor of Medicine
Harvard Medical School
Director of Translational Research
Center for Inflammatory Bowel Disease
Division of Gastroenterology
Beth Israel Deaconess Medical Center
Boston, MA, USA

Joseph A. Murray, MD
Professor of Medicine and Immunology
Division of Gastroenterology and Hepatology
Mayo Clinic
Rochester, MN, USA

Timothy T. Nostrant, MD
Professor of Medicine
Department of Internal Medicine
University of Michigan
Ann Arbor, MI, USA

David J. Owens, MD
Clinical Instructor
Division of Gastroenterology
University of California, San Diego
San Diego, CA, USA

Darrell S. Pardi, MD
Associate Professor of Medicine
Inflammatory Bowel Disease Clinic
Division of Gastroenterology and Hepatology
Mayo Clinic
Rochester, MN, USA

P. Samuel Pegram, MD
Professor of Medicine with Tenure
Department of Internal Medicine
Wake Forest University School of Medicine
Winston-Salem, NC, USA

Steven Peikin, MD
Professor of Medicine
Division of Gastroenterology and Liver Diseases
Cooper University Hospital
Robert Wood Johnson Medical School
University of Medicine and Dentistry of New Jersey
Camden, NJ, USA

Robert M. Penner, MD, MSc
Assistant Clinical Professor
Department of Medicine
University of Alberta
Edmonton, AB, Canada;
Department of Medicine
University of British Columbia
Vancouver, BC, Canada

Mark Pimentel, MD
Director, GI Motility Program
Cedars-Sinai Medical Center
Los Angeles, CA, USA

Charlene M. Prather, MD, MPH
Associate Professor of Internal Medicine
Program Director, Gastroenterology Fellowship Program
Department of Medicine
Saint Louis University School of Medicine
St. Louis, MO, USA

Dawn Provenzale, MD, MS
Professor of Medicine
Veterans Affairs Medical Center
Division of Gastroenterology
Duke University Medical Center
Durham, NC, USA

Eamonn M.M. Quigley, MD
Professor of Medicine and Human Physiology
Department of Medicine
Alimentary Pharmabiotic Centre
University College Cork
Cork, Ireland

Karthik Ravi, MD
Fellow
Clinical Enteric Neuroscience Translational and
Epidemiological Research Program
Division of Gastroenterology and Hepatology
Mayo Clinic
Rochester, MN, USA

Douglas K. Rex, MD
Distinguished Professor of Medicine
Indiana University School of Medicine
Director of Endoscopy
Indiana University Hospital
Indianapolis, IN, USA

James C. Reynolds, MD
June F. Klinghoffer Distinguished Professor
Chair, Department of Medicine
Drexel University College of Medicine
Philadelphia, PA, USA

Erica N. Roberson, MD
Fellow in Women's Health—Women's Veteran Health Program
Instructor in Medicine
Section of Gastroenterology and Hepatology
University of Wisconsin School of Medicine and Public Health
Madison, WI, USA

Juan P. Rocca, MD
Assistant Professor of Surgery
Mount Sinai School of Medicine
Transplant Surgeon
Recanati/Miller Transplant Institute
New York, NY, USA

Suzanne Rose, MD, MSEd
Professor of Medical Education and Medicine
Associate Dean for Academic and Student Affairs
Associate Dean for Continuing Medical Education
Department of Medical Education and Department of
Medicine
Division of Gastroenterology
Mount Sinai School of Medicine
New York, NY, USA

Alberto Rubio-Tapia, MD
Assistant Professor of Medicine
Division of Gastroenterology and Hepatology
Mayo Clinic
Rochester, MN, USA

Sonali Sakaria, MD
Fellow
Department of Medicine
Division of Digestive Diseases
Emory University School of Medicine
Atlanta, GA, USA

Brian Saunders MD, FRCP
Consultant Gastroenterologist
Reader in Endoscopy
Imperial College London
Director of Wolfson Unit for Endoscopy
St Mark's Hospital
Harrow, UK

Michael D. Saunders, MD
Clinical Associate Professor of Medicine
Division of Gastroenterology
Director of Digestive Disease Center
University of Washington Medical Center
Seattle, WA, USA

Thomas J. Savides, MD
Professor of Clinical Medicine
Division of Gastroenterology
University of California, San Diego
San Diego, CA, USA

Samantha A. Scanlon, MD
Medical Resident
Department of Internal Medicine
Mayo Clinic
Rochester, MN, USA

Philip R. Schauer, MD
Director, Bariatric and Metabolic Institute
Cleveland Clinic
Cleveland, OH, USA

Lawrence R. Schiller, MD
Program Director, Gastroenterology Fellowship
Division of Gastroenterology
Baylor University Medical Center
Dallas, TX, USA

David A. Schwartz, MD
Associate Professor of Medicine
Director, IBD Center
Division of Gastroenterology
Vanderbilt University
Nashville, TN, USA

Lauren K. Schwartz, MD
Assistant Professor of Medicine
Division of Gastroenterology
Mount Sinai Hospital
New York, NY, USA

James S. Scolapio, MD
Professor of Medicine
Director of Nutrition
Division of Gastroenterology and Hepatology
Mayo Clinic
Jacksonville, FL, USA

Joseph H. Sellin, MD
Professor of Medicine
Division of Gastroenterology
Baylor College of Medicine
Houston, TX, USA

Carol E. Semrad, MD
Associate Professor of Medicine
Gastroenterology Section
The University of Chicago
Chicago, IL, USA

Sheryl A. Serbowicz
Medical Student
Department of Medical Education
Mount Sinai School of Medicine
New York, NY, USA

David M. Shapiro, MD
Fellow in Gastroenterology and Hepatology
Division of Gastroenterology
Feinberg School of Medicine
Northwestern University
Chicago, IL, USA

Shanthi V. Sitaraman, MD, PhD
Professor
Department of Medicine
Division of Digestive Diseases
Emory University School of Medicine
Atlanta, GA, USA

Nib Soehendra, MD
Endoscopy Practice am Glockengiesserwall
Hamburg, Germany

Ronald L. Stone, RD
Assistant Professor of Nutrition
Department of Dietetics
Mayo Clinic
Jacksonville, FL, USA

Lisa L. Strate, MD, MPH
Assistant Professor of Medicine
Division of Gastroenterology
University of Washington School of Medicine
Harborview Medical Center
Seattle, WA, USA

Chee-Chee H. Stucky, MD
Resident, General Surgery Residency Program
Department of General Surgery
Mayo Clinic
Scottsdale, AZ, USA

Patricia Sylla, MD
Instructor in Surgery
Harvard Medical School
Assistant in Surgery
Division of Colorectal Surgery
Department of Surgery
Massachusetts General Hospital
Boston, MA, USA

Scott Tenner, MD, MPH
Associate Professor of Medicine
Division of Gastroenterology
Department of Medicine
Maimonides Medical Center
State University of New York—Health Sciences Center
New York, NY, USA

Elizabeth J. Videlock, MD
Medical Resident
Beth Israel Deaconess Medical Center
Boston, MA, USA

Arnold Wald, MD
Professor of Medicine
Section of Gastroenterology and Hepatology
University of Wisconsin School of Medicine and Public Health
Madison, WI, USA

Kymberly D.S. Watt, MD
Assistant Professor of Medicine
Division of Gastroenterology and Hepatology
William J. von Liebig Transplant Center
Mayo Clinic
Rochester, MN, USA

Field F. Willingham MD, MPH
Clinical and Research Fellow in Medicine
Harvard Medical School
Gastrointestinal Unit
Massachusetts General Hospital
Boston, MA, USA

Jacqueline L. Wolf, MD
Associate Professor of Medicine
Harvard Medical School
Division of Gastroenterology
Beth Israel Deaconess Medical Center
Boston, MA, USA

Tonia M. Young-Fadok, MD, MS
Professor of Surgery
Chair, Division of Colorectal Surgery
Mayo Clinic
Scottsdale, AZ, USA

Yan Zhong, MD
Endoscopy Practice am Glockengiesserwall
Hamburg, Germany

Timothy L. Zisman, MD, MPH
Assistant Professor of Medicine
Division of Gastroenterology
University of Washington Medical Center
Seattle, WA, USA

Preface

Welcome to *Practical Gastroenterology and Hepatology*, a new comprehensive three volume resource for everyone training in gastroenterology and for those certifying (or recertifying) in the subspecialty. We have aimed to create three modern, easy to read and digest stand-alone textbooks. The entire set covers the waterfront, from clinical evaluation to advanced endoscopy to common and rare diseases every gastroenterologist must know.

Volume two specifically deals with disorders of the small and large intestine, and pancreas. Each chapter highlights, where appropriate, a clinical case which demonstrates a common clinical situation, its approach, and management. Simple easy to follow clinical algorithms are demonstrated throughout the relevant chapters. Endoscopy chapters provide excellent video examples, all available electronically.

Each chapter has been written by the best of the best in the field, and carefully peer reviewed and edited for accuracy and relevance. We have guided the writing of this textbook to help ensure experienced gastroenterologists, fellows, residents, medical students, internists, primary care physicians, as well as surgeons all will find something of interest and relevance.

Each volume and every chapter has followed a standard template structure. All chapters focus on key knowledge, and the most important clinical facts are highlighted in an introductory abstract and summary box at the end; irrelevant or unimportant information is omitted. The chapters are deliberately brief and readable; we want our readers to retain the material, and immediately be able to apply what they learn in practice. The chapters are illustrated in color, enhanced by a very pleasant layout. A Web based version has been created to complement the textbook including endoscopy images and movies.

In this volume, section one addresses the pathobiology of the intestine and pancreas, providing a scientific basis for disease. The emphasis here is, as in all volumes, on the practical and clinically relevant, as opposed to the esoteric. Section two deals with endoscopy issues including colonoscopy, ERCP and endoscopic ultrasound. Section three covers endoscopic, radiologic and physiologic testing of the small intestine and pancreas, including capsule endoscopy and balloon assisted enteroscopy. Section four approaches disorders from a problem or symptom based standpoint with a simple, clear guide to diagnosis and management strategies. Section five covers important diseases of the small intestine including malabsorptive diseases, Crohn's disease, and tumors of the small intestine. Section six addresses diseases of the colon and rectum including inflammatory bowel disease, polyps, colon cancer and diverticulitis. The section on diseases of the pancreas covers both acute and chronic pancreatitis as well as pancreatic cancer and cystic neoplasms. Endoscopic palliation of malignant obstruction including related obstruction of the small intestine is reviewed. Section eight covers functional gastrointestinal disorders including irritable bowel syndrome, constipation, abdominal pain and bloating. Section nine deals with transplantation of gastrointestinal organs with specific attention to indications and postoperative management. Finally, section ten covers diseases of the peritoneum, and hernias.

We have been thrilled to work with a terrific team in the creation of this work, and very much hope you will enjoy reading this volume as much as we have enjoyed developing it for you.

Nicholas J. Talley
Michael Wallace
Sunanda Kane

Foreword

This book is impressive for its breadth and depth, and serves an important niche for the broad readership. As leaders in the broad field of gastroenterology, the Editors, Doctors Nicholas J. Talley, Sunanda V. Kane, and Michael B. Wallace, are to be commended for undertaking this task. Covering diverse topics, the team of recruited authors is recognized for their individual and collective experience and expertise in their respective fields. The chapters are integrated through cross-referencing, annotated with key points for the readership, well illustrated, and referenced in a current fashion. In an era when one is challenged to obtain information through a variety of options, this book certainly serves that need. In that context, the book will appeal to gastroenterologists, hepatologists, pancreatologists, fellows, residents, students, and allied health care personnel, and be a requirement for institutional libraries.

Anil K. Rustgi, MD
T. Grier Miller Professor of Medicine
Chief of Gastroenterology
University of Pennsylvania

PART 1

Pathobiology of the Intestine and Pancreas

1

CHAPTER 1
Clinical Anatomy, Embryology, and Congenital Anomalies

Advitya Malhotra[1] and Joseph H. Sellin[2]

[1] Department of Gastroenterology and Hepatology, University of Texas Medical Branch (UTMB), Galveston, TX, USA

[2] Division of Gastroenterology, Baylor College of Medicine, Houston, TX, USA

Summary

As clinicians and educators we update ourselves routinely with various aspects of our practicing field. Mainly, the focus is centered on the pathogenesis, diagnosis, and management aspects of the clinical problem. Rarely, we delve in to the anatomy of the organ system responsible for the presentation. However, some embryological anomalies can present in later decades of life and present unexpected and difficult challenges in both diagnosis and management. Hence, a practical working knowledge on this subject is critical for the clinical gastroenterologist.

We have compiled a chapter that deals succinctly with the clinical anatomy, embryology, and congenital anomalies of the gastrointestinal tract. The main body of the chapter is in line with the evolving division of the gastrointestinal tract of the embryo into foregut, midgut, and the hindgut. We briefly cover the anatomy, embryogenesis, and the congenital anomalies of each derivative of the germ layer starting from the foregut, and ending with the Hirschsprung disease (HSCR), a congenital anomaly of the ganglion cells of the hindgut. Some of the more commonly seen anomalies, such as pancreas divisum (PD), are dealt in detail wherever required.

Small and Large Intestine

Anatomy and Embryogenesis

At 4 weeks of gestation, the alimentary tract is divided into three parts: foregut, midgut, and hindgut. The duodenum originates from the terminal portion of the foregut and cephalic part of the midgut. With rotation of the stomach, the duodenum becomes C-shaped and rotates to the right. The midgut gives rise to the duodenum distal to the ampulla, to the entire small bowel, and to the cecum, appendix, ascending colon, and the proximal two-thirds of the transverse colon. The distal third of the transverse colon, the descending colon and sigmoid, the rectum, and the upper part of the anal canal

originate from the hindgut. The anal canal's proximal portion is formed from the hindgut endoderm whereas the distal portion arises from the ectoderm of the cloacal membrane.

The colon has a rich blood supply, with a specific vascular arcade formed by union of branches of superior mesenteric, inferior mesenteric, and internal iliac arteries. Despite its presence, the colon vasculature has two weak points: the splenic flexure and the rectosigmoid junction which are supplied by the narrow terminal branches of superior mesenteric artery (SMA) and inferior mesenteric artery (IMA), respectively. These two watershed areas are most vulnerable to ischemia during systemic hypotension.

Aberrations in midgut development may result in a variety of anatomic anomalies (Table 1.1), and these are broadly classified as:

- Rotation and fixation
- Duplications

Practical Gastroenterology and Hepatology: Small and Large Intestine and Pancreas, 1st edition. Edited by Nicholas J. Talley, Sunanda V. Kane and Michael B. Wallace. © 2010 Blackwell Publishing Ltd.

Table 1.1 Congenital anomalies of upper gastrointestinal tract.

Anomaly	Incidence	Symptoms and Signs	Treatment
Esophageal stenosis	1 : 25 000 to 50 000	Emesis dysphagia	Dilation, myotomy, or resection with anastomosis
Esophageal duplication	1 : 8000	Respiratory symptoms, vomiting, neck mass	Resection
Gastric, antral, or pyloric atresia	3 : 100 000, when combined with webs	Non-bilious emesis	Gastroduodenostomy, gastrojejunostomy
Pyloric or antral membrane	As above	Failure to thrive, emesis	Incision or excision, pyloroplasty
Microgastria	Rare	Emesis, malnutrition	Continuous-drip feedings or jejunal reservoir pouch
Pyloric stenosis	US, 3 : 1000 (range, 1–8 : 1000 in various regions); male/female, 4 : 1	Non-bilious emesis	Pyloromyotomy
Gastric duplication	Rare male/female, 1 : 2	Abdominal mass, emesis, hematemesis	Excision or partial gastrectomy
Gastric volvulus	Rare	Emesis, feeding refusal	Reduction of volvulus, anterior gastropexy
Duodenal atresia or stenosis	1 : 20 000	Bilious emesis, upper abdominal distension	Duodenojejunostomy or gastrojejunostomy
Annular pancreas	1 : 10 000	Bilious emesis, failure to thrive	Duodenojejunostomy
Duodenal duplication	Rare	Pain, gastrointestinal bleeding	Excision
Malrotation and midgut volvulus	Rare	Abdominal distension, bilious emesis	Reduction, division of bands, possibly resection

• Atresias and stenoses: these occur most frequently and are either due to failure of recanalization or a vascular accident. Atresias have a reported incidence rate of 1 in 300 to 1 in 1500 live births, and are more common than stenoses. Atresias are more common in black infants, low birth-weight infants, and twins. Clinically, the presentation is that of a proximal intestinal obstruction with bilious vomiting on the first day of life. Treatment is surgical correction.

The other major congenital anomalies of the intestine and abdominal cavity are related to abnormalities with development of abdominal wall, the vitelline duct, and innervation of the gastrointestinal tract.

Abdominal Wall Congenital Anomalies

The congenital anomalies of the abdominal wall are:
• Gastrochisis: caused by an intact umbilical cord with evisceration of the bowel, but no covering membranes, through a defect in the abdominal wall [1]. Gastrochisis is commonly associated with intestinal atresia and cryptorchism.
• Omphalocele: characterized by herniation of the bowel, liver, and other organs into the intact umbilical cord; unlike gastrochisis, these tissues are covered by a membrane formed from fusion of the amnion and peritoneum.

Diagnosis
An abdominal wall defect may be diagnosed during routine prenatal ultrasonography. Both gastroschisis and omphalocele are associated with elevation of maternal serum α-fetoprotein.

Management
Recommended management for both these conditions is operative reduction of the contents back in to the abdominal cavity. The size of the omphalocele deter-

mines whether a primary repair or delayed primary closure is selected as the surgical approach.

Vitelline Duct Congenital Anomalies

Persistence of the duct communication between the intestine and the yolk sac beyond the embryonic stage may result in several anomalies of the omphalomesenteric or vitelline duct.

The most common congenital abnormality of the gastrointestinal tract is omphalomesenteric duct, or Meckel diverticulum, which results from the failure of the vitelline duct to obliterate during the fifth week of fetal development [2].

Clinical presentation

Meckel diverticulum may remain completely asymptomatic or it may mimic such disorders as Crohn disease, appendicitis, and peptic ulcer disease. Bleeding is the most common complication of Meckel diverticulum, related to acid-induced ulceration of adjacent small intestine from the presence of ectopic gastric mucosa. Obstruction, intussusception, diverticulitis, and perforation may also occur, especially in adults, due to the active ectopic pancreatic tissue or gastric mucosa.

Diagnosis

The most useful method of detection of a Meckel diverticulum is technetium-99m pertechnetate scanning. Technetium uptake depends on the presence of heterotopic gastric tissue. The test has 85% sensitivity and 95% specificity. The sensitivity of the scan can be increased minimally with use of cimetidine [3]. Other tests useful in diagnosis are superior mesenteric artery angiography, laparoscopy, and double balloon enteroscopy.

Management

Meckel diverticulectomy either by laparoscopy or open laparotomy approach is the procedure of choice for symptomatic diverticulum.

Less Common Vitelline Duct Abnormalities

Other, less common congenital abnormalities of vitelline duct include:
• Omphalomes-enteric or vitelline cyst: central cystic dilatation in which the duct is closed at both ends but patent in its center

• Umbilical-intestinal fistula: a patent duct throughout its length
• Omphalomesenteric band: complete obliteration of the duct, resulting in a fibrous cord or ligament extending from the ileum to the umbilicus.

Enteric Nervous System Anomalies

The most common enteric nervous system congenital anomaly is Hirschsprung (HSCR) disease; other associated anomalies include intestinal neuronal dysplasia (IND) and chronic intestinal pseudo-obstruction.

HSCR is characterized by the absence of ganglion cells in the submucosal (Meissner) and myenteric (Auerbach) plexuses along a variable length of the hindgut. It is classified as short-segment HSCR (80% of cases), when the aganglionic segment does not extend beyond the upper sigmoid, and long-segment HSCR when aganglionosis extends proximal to the sigmoid. Twelve percent of children with Hirschsprung disease have chromosomal abnormalities, 2 to 8% of which are trisomy 21 (Down syndrome) [4].

Clinical Presentation

In most cases, HSCR presents at birth as non-passage of meconium, abdominal distension, feeding difficulties, and/or bilious emesis. Some patients are diagnosed later in infancy or in adulthood with severe constipation, chronic abdominal distension, vomiting, and failure to thrive.

Diagnosis

The diagnosis in a symptomatic individual may be made by one or a combination of the following tests: barium enema, rectal biopsy, and anal manometry.

Management

Definitive treatment of Hirschsprung disease is surgical, and the specific method of surgery is operator dependent.

Pancreas

Anatomy and Embryogenesis

The pancreas first appears during the fourth week of gestation as ventral and dorsal outpouchings from the endodermal lining of the duodenum. The normal adult

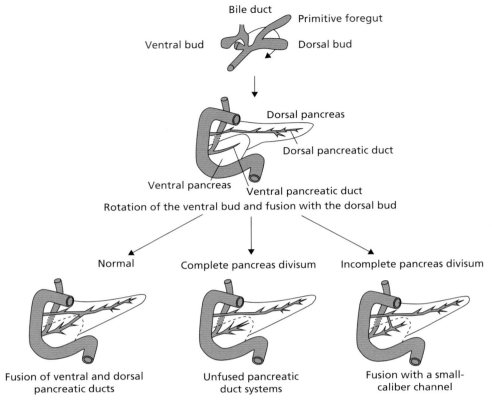

Figure 1.1 Schematic illustration of embryology of normal pancreas and pancreas divisum. (Reproduced with kind permission from Springer & Business Media. Kamisawa T. Clinical significance of the minor duodenal papilla and accessory pancreatic duct. *Journal of Gastroenterology* 2004; 39: 606.)

pancreas results from the fusion of these dorsal and ventral pancreatic buds during the second month of fetal development. The tail, body, and part of the head of the pancreas are formed by the dorsal component; the remainder of the head and the uncinate process derive from the ventral pancreas.

The dorsal duct arises directly from the duodenal wall, and the ventral duct arises from the common bile duct. On fusion of the ventral and dorsal components of the pancreas, the ventral duct anastomoses with the dorsal one, forming the main pancreatic duct of Wirsung (Figure 1.1). The proximal end of the dorsal duct becomes the accessory duct of Santorini in the adult [5]. The pancreatic acini appear in the third month of gestation as derivatives of the side ducts and termini of these primitive ducts.

Pancreas Divisum (PD)

PD occurs when the dorsal and ventral ducts fail to fuse; the dorsal duct drains the majority of the pancreas via the minor papilla, while the short ventral duct drains the inferior portion of the head via the major papilla (Figure 1.1). Pancreas divisum has been observed in 5 to 10% of autopsy series and in about 2 to 7% of patients undergoing endoscopic retrograde cholangiopancreatography (ERCP) [6]. Most patients with pancreas divisum are asymptomatic, and the diagnosis is made incidentally. However, some patients develop abdominal pain, recurrent acute pancreatitis, or chronic pancreatitis. The causal relationship between divisum and pancreatitis is still a matter of debate. PD is usually diagnosed by ERCP although endoscopic ultrasonography and magnetic resonance cholangiopancreatography (MRCP) may be useful for diagnosis [7]. Therapeutic intervention (either endoscopic sphincterotomy with placement of stents through the accessory papilla or surgical sphincteroplasty of the accessory papilla) may benefit some patients with PD and recurrent, acute pancreatitis associated with accessory papilla stenosis [8].

Ectopic Pancreas

Ectopic pancreas is pancreatic tissue found outside the usual anatomic confines of the pancreas. Although it may occur throughout the gastrointestinal tract it is most commonly found in the stomach and small intestine. Usually an incidental finding, it may rarely become clinically evident when complicated by inflammation, bleeding, obstruction, or malignant transformation [9].

Pancreatic Agenesis

Agenesis of the pancreas is very rare and may be associated with other congenital disease states. In addition, isolated agenesis of the dorsal or, less commonly, the ventral pancreas can occur as silent anomalies [10].

Congenital Cysts

Congenital cysts of the pancreas are rare and are distinguished from pseudocysts by the presence of an epithelial lining. True congenital cysts occur as a result of developmental anomalies related to the sequestration of primitive pancreatic ducts. They are generally asymptomatic, although abdominal distension, vomiting, jaundice, or pancreatitis can be observed requiring surgical removal.

Anomalous Pancreaticobiliary Ductal Union (APBDU)

APBDU is a congenital malformation of the confluence of the pancreatic and bile ducts. A classification has been developed for APBDU: if the pancreatic duct appears to join the common bile duct, this is classified as a P–B type. If the common bile duct joins the main pancreatic duct, this is a B–P type. A long common channel is denoted Y type. The frequency of APBDU varies from 1.5 to 3 2%. APBDU is associated with pancreatitis (with long >21 mm and wide >5 mm common channel), choledochal cysts, and neoplastic abnormalities like cholangiocarcinoma and pancreatic cancer in adults [11].

Take-home points

Small and large intestine:
- The colon vasculature has two weak points; the splenic flexure and the rectosigmoid junction which are supplied by the narrow terminal branches of SMA and IMA, respectively. These two watershed areas are most vulnerable to ischemia during systemic hypotension.

- The two common congenital anomalies of the abdominal wall presenting at birth are gastrochisis and omphalocele.

- The most common congenital abnormality of the gastrointestinal tract is omphalomesenteric duct, or Meckel diverticulum, which results from the failure of the vitelline duct to obliterate during fetal development.

- The most common enteric nervous system congenital anomaly is Hirschsprung (HSCR) disease, which is characterized by the absence of ganglion cells in the submucosal (Meissner) and myenteric (Auerbach) plexuses along a variable length of the hindgut.

Pancreas:
- Pancreas divisum occurs when the dorsal and ventral ducts fail to fuse; the dorsal duct drains the majority of the pancreas via the minor papilla, while the short ventral duct drains the inferior portion of the head via the major papilla.

References

1 Weber T, Au-Fliegner M, Downard C, Fishman S. Abdominal wall defects. *Curr Opin Pediatr* 2002; **14**: 491–7.

2 Turgeon D, Barnett J. Meckel's diverticulum. *Am J Gastroenterol* 1990; **85**: 777–81.

3 Petrokubi R, Baum S, Rohrer G. Cimetidine administration resulting in improved pertechnetate imaging of Meckel's diverticulum. *Clin Nucl Med* 1978; **3**: 385–8.

4 Skinner M. Hirschsprung's disease. *Curr Probl Surg* 1996; **33**: 389–460.

5 Kleitsch W. Anatomy of the pancreas; a study with special reference to the duct system. *AMA Arch Surg* 1955; **71**: 795–802.

6 Delhaye M, Engelholm L, Cremer M. Pancrease divisum: congenital anatomic variant or anomaly? Contribution of endoscopic retrograde dorsal pancreatography. *Gastroenterology* 1985; **89**: 951–8.

7 Bret P, Reinhold C, Taourel P, *et al.* Pancreas divisum: evaluation with MR cholangiopancreatography. *Radiology* 1996; **199**: 99–103.

8 Lans J, Geenen J, Johanson J, Hogan W. Endoscopic therapy in patients with pancreas divisum and acute pancreatitis: a

prospective, randomized, controlled clinical trial. *Gastroin-test Endosc* 1992; **38**: 430–4.

9 Eisenberger C, Gocht A, Knoefel W, *et al.* Heterotopic pancreas—clinical presentation and pathology with review of the literature. *Hepatogastroenterology* 2004; **51**: 854–8.

10 Fukuoka K, Ajiki T, Yamamoto M, *et al.* Complete agenesis of the dorsal pancreas. *J Hepatobiliary Pancreat Surg* 1999; **6**: 94–7.

11 Wang H, Wu M, Lin C, *et al.* Pancreaticobiliary diseases associated with anomalous pancreaticobiliary ductal union. *Gastrointest Endosc* 1998; **48**: 184–9.

CHAPTER 2
Physiology of Weight Regulation

Louis Chaptini, Christopher Deitch, and Steven Peikin

Division of Gastroenterology and Liver Diseases, Cooper University Hospital, Robert Wood Johnson Medical School, University of Medicine and Dentistry of New Jersey, Camden, NJ, USA

Summary

The interest in the physiology of weight regulation has increased in recent years due to the major deleterious effects of the obesity epidemic on public health. A complex neuroendocrine network involving peripheral organs and the central nervous system is responsible for maintaining a balance between energy intake and expenditure. Major change in weight can result from an imbalance in this network. Gut and adipose tissue are the main peripheral organs involved in weight regulation. Hormones are secreted from these peripheral organs in response to nutrient intake and weight fluctuation. They are subsequently integrated by the central nervous system. Unraveling these peripheral and central signals and their complex interaction at multiple levels has an essential role in understanding the physiology of weight regulation.

Introduction

The physiology of weight regulation has gained tremendous interest in recent decades because of the major deleterious effects of overweight and obesity on public health. More than 300 000 deaths per year are attributed to obesity [1] and poor diet and inactivity may soon overtake tobacco as a leading cause of death in the USA [2]. Complex brain–gut interaction constitutes the basis of weight regulation and involves intricate mechanisms, some of which are not fully elucidated thus far and are focus of extensive ongoing research. This chapter reviews the current understanding of the mechanisms of weight regulation with emphasis on the role of the gastrointestinal system.

Concept of Energy Homeostasis

Fat is the primary form of energy storage in the human body. According to the first law of thermodynamics, the amount of stored energy is equal to the difference between energy intake and energy expenditure. Under normal conditions, homeostatic mechanisms maintain the difference between energy intake and energy expenditure close to zero. A very small imbalance in those mechanisms over a long period of time can result in large cumulative effects, leading to a major change in weight. In order to keep a perfect balance between energy intake and expenditure, homeostatic mechanisms rely on neural signals that emanate from adipose tissue, endocrine, neurological, and gastrointestinal systems and are integrated by the central nervous system (CNS) [3,4]. The CNS subsequently sends signals to multiple organs in the periphery in order to control energy intake and expenditure and maintain energy homeostasis over long periods of time (Figure 2.1).

Role of the Central Nervous System

During recent decades, extensive research has focused on the role of the CNS in the regulation of food intake and the pathogenesis of obesity. Eating in humans is thought to follow a dual model: "reflexive" eating that represents automatic impulses to overeat in anticipation for a coming food shortage and "reflective eating" that incorporates a cognitive dimension involving social

Practical Gastroenterology and Hepatology: Small and Large Intestine and Pancreas, 1st edition. Edited by Nicholas J. Talley, Sunanda V. Kane and Michael B. Wallace. © 2010 Blackwell Publishing Ltd.

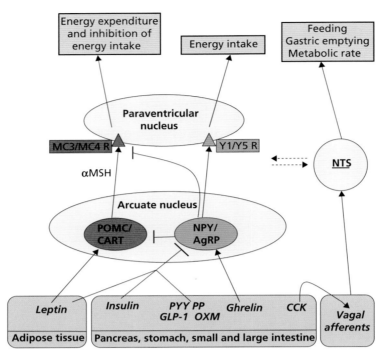

Figure 2.1 Pathways of regulation of food intake. Representation of the potential action of gut peptides on the hypothalamus. Primary neurons in the arcuate nucleus contain multiple peptide neuromodulators. Appetite-inhibiting neurons (red) contain pro-opiomelanocortin (POMC) peptides such as α melanocyte-stimulating hormone (αMSH), which acts on melanocortin receptors (MC3 and MC4) and cocaine- and amphetamine-stimulated transcript peptide (CART), whose receptor is unknown. Appetite-stimulating neurons in the arcuate nucleus (blue) contain neuropeptide Y (NPY), which acts on Y receptors (Y1 and Y5), and agouti-related peptide (AgRP), which is an antagonist of MC3/4 receptor activity. Integration of peripheral signals within the brain involves interplay between the hypothalamus and hindbrain structures including the nucleus of the tractus solitarius (NTS), which receives vagal afferent inputs. Inputs from the cortex, amygdala, and brainstem nuclei are integrated as well, with resultant effects on meal size and frequency, gut handling of ingested food, and energy expenditure. →, direct stimulatory; ⊣, direct inhibitory; PYY, peptide tyrosine tyrosine; PP, pancreatic polypeptide; GLP-1, glucagon-like peptide-1; OXM: oxyntomodulin; CCK: cholecystokinin. (Adapted from Badman and Flier [4]).

expectations of body shape and long-term health goals [5]. Reflexive eating is represented by the brainstem and the arcuate nucleus. Two populations of neurons are responsible for the regulation of food intake in the arcuate nucleus, one expressing neuropeptide Y (NPY) and agouti-related peptide (AgRP), which when activated leads to an orexigenic response and reduced energy expenditure, and the other containing pro-opiomelanocortin (POMC) and cocaine and amphetamine-regulated transcript (CART), where increased activity results in an increase in energy expenditure and a decrease in food intake [6]. NPY is one of the hormones that constitute

the pancreatic polypeptide family, which includes two other hormones, pancreatic polypeptide (PP) and peptide YY (PYY). NPY is present in large quantities in the hypothalamus and is one of the most potent orexigenic factors [7]. Among NPY receptors, the Y5 receptors have been implicated as important mediators of the feeding effect and the Y5 receptors antagonists have been involved in recent weight loss studies [8]. The brain cortex seems to play a role in the regulation of food intake and represents the "reflective eating" [5]. The right prefrontal cortex (PFC) has been specifically involved in the cognitive inhibition of food intake.

Role of Adipose Tissue

Insulin and leptin are adiposity signals that play an important role in the physiology of weight regulation.

Insulin receptors are widely present in the CNS. Insulin levels have been shown to correlate with body adiposity. Increase in food intake and adiposity can result from hypothalamic defects in insulin signaling [9].

Circulating levels of leptin, an adipocyte-derived hormone, reflect the adipose tissue mass as well as recent nutritional status. The action of leptin in the CNS results in decrease in food intake and increase in energy expenditure through the inhibition of NPY/AgRP neurons and activation of POMC neurons [10]. Most obese humans have elevated serum leptin levels, which suggests leptin resistance may be important in human obesity. Manipulating leptin resistance may provide an interesting target for obesity treatment.

Adiponectin and resistin are two other peptides produced by adipocytes. Low levels of the former are associated with insulin resistance, dyslipidemia, and atherosclerosis, whereas the latter has proinflammatory effects and has also been implicated in insulin resistance [11,12].

Role of the Gastrointestinal Tract

The gastrointestinal tract elicits neural and endocrine signals that play a major role in food intake regulation. The interaction of gastrointestinal hormones with the brain constitutes the gut–brain axis which has been extensively studied in the past decade.

Role of the Stomach in Food Intake Regulation

Gastric distension
Gastric distension has been shown in multiple studies to serve as a signal for satiety. Instillation of a volume load in the stomach leads to distension of gastric wall, which in turn induces satiety regardless of the nature of the load: in rats, studies have shown that equivalent volumes of saline or different nutrient solutions produce equivalent reduction in food intake [13,14].

Ghrelin
Ghrelin is a peptide predominantly produced by the stomach and its secretion is increased by fasting and in response to weight loss and decreased by food intake. Ghrelin is the only known circulating appetite stimulant. It stimulates appetite by acting on arcuate nucleus NPY/AgRP neurons and may also inhibit POMC neurons [15]. There is also evidence that the vagus nerve is required to mediate the orexigenic effect of ghrelin. Ghrelin plays a role in meal initiation which is demonstrated by a premeal surge in plasma ghrelin levels in humans and animals. In addition to its role in short-term regulation of food intake (meal initiator), ghrelin appears to participate in long-term energy homeostasis, which is suggested by its fluctuation in response to body weight variations [16].

Role of the Pancreas and Small Intestine in Food Intake Regulation

Cholecystokinin (CCK)
CCK is the prototypical satiety hormone, produced by cells in the duodenum and jejunum. It is produced in response to the presence of nutrients within the gut lumen, specifically fat and protein. The satiating effect of CCK is mediated through paracrine interaction with sensory fibers of the vagus nerve. It inhibits food intake by reducing meal size and duration [17]. CCK has a short half-life which makes it a very short-term modulator of appetite.

Peptide Tyrosine Tyrosine (PYY) and Pancreatic Polypeptide (PP)
PYY and PP are members of the pancreatic polypeptide family which also includes NPY discussed earlier. PYY is secreted by enteroendocrine L-cells, mainly in the distal portion of the gastrointestinal tract. It is released following meals (acting as meal terminator) and suppressed by fasting, exactly opposite to the pattern of secretion seen with ghrelin [17]. PP is secreted in response to a meal, in proportion to the caloric load, and has been shown to reduce appetite and food intake [18]. It is produced mainly in the endocrine pancreas, but also in the exocrine pancreas, colon, and rectum.

Glucagon-like peptide-1 (GLP-1) and Oxyntomodulin
GLP-1 and oxyntomodulin derive from the posttranslational processing of proglucagon, which is expressed in the gut, pancreas, and brain. GLP-1 is secreted by enteroendocrine L-cells in the distal small bowel in response to direct nutrient stimulation in the

distal small intestine as well as indirect neurohumoral stimulation in proximal regions of the small intestine. The actions of GLP-1 include inhibition of gastric emptying, stimulation of insulin release, inhibition of glucagon release and inhibition of appetite [19]. Oxyntomodulin is secreted in the distal small intestine as well. It binds but has lower affinity to the GLP-1 receptor. It has been shown to decrease energy intake and, moreover, increase energy expenditure [20].

Conclusion

The physiology of weight regulation involves intricate interaction between the brain and the gut. Tremendous progress in the understanding of the different components of the gut brain axis has been achieved and extensive research is underway to create agents targeting these different components to accomplish significant and lasting weight reduction.

Take-home points

- Understanding the physiology of weight regulation is fundamental in the fight against the obesity epidemic.
- Maintaining a stable weight involves complex homeostatic mechanisms responsible for a perfect balance between energy expenditure and energy intake.
- Signals originating from peripheral organs, such as adipose tissue and gastrointestinal system, and integrated by the central nervous system constitute the homeostatic mechanisms responsible for weight regulation.
- Gut hormones are produced in response to nutrient intake and weight fluctuation.
- Targeting complex peripheral and central signals involved in weight regulation is the mainstay in the development of weight reduction therapeutic agents.

References

1 Fontaine KR, Redden DT, Wang C, *et al.* Years of life lost due to obesity. *JAMA* 2003; **289**: 187–93.

2 Allison DB, Fontaine KR, Manson JE, *et al.* Annual deaths attributable to obesity in the United States. *JAMA* 1999; **282**: 1530–8.

3 Strader AD, Woods SC. Gastrointestinal hormones and food intake. *Gastroenterology* 2005; **128**: 175–91.

4 Badman MK, Flier JS. The gut and energy balance: visceral allies in the obesity wars. *Science* 2005; **307**: 1909–14.

5 Alonso-Alonso M, Pascual-Leone A. The right brain hypothesis for obesity. *JAMA* 2007; **297**: 1819–22.

6 Morton GJ, Cummings DE, Baskin DG, *et al.* Central nervous system control of food intake and body weight. *Nature* 2006; **443**: 289–95.

7 Arora S, Anubhuti. Role of neuropeptides in appetite regulation and obesity—a review. *Neuropeptides* 2006; **40**: 375–401.

8 Aronne LJ, Thornton-Jones ZD. New targets for obesity pharmacotherapy. *Clin Pharmacol Ther* 2007; **81**: 748–52.

9 Niswender KD, Schwartz MW. Insulin and leptin revisited: adiposity signals with overlapping physiological and intracellular signaling capabilities. *Front Neuroendocrinol* 2003; **24**: 1–10.

10 Badman MK. Flier JS. The adipocyte as an active participant in energy balance and metabolism. *Gastroenterology* 2007; **132**: 2103–15.

11 Qi Y, Takahashi N, Hileman SM, *et al.* Adiponectin acts in the brain to decrease body weight. *Nat Med* 2004; **10**: 524–9.

12 Fantuzzi G. Adipose tissue, adipokines, and inflammation. *J Allergy Clin Immunol* 2005; **115**: 911–9.

13 Phillips RJ, Powley TL. Gastric volume rather than nutrient content inhibits food intake. *Am J Physiol* 1996; **271**: R766–9.

14 Powley TL, Phillips RJ. Gastric satiation is volumetric, intestinal satiation is nutritive. *Physiol Behav* 2004; **82**: 69–74.

15 Cowley MA, Smith RG, Diano S, *et al.* The distribution and mechanism of action of ghrelin in the CNS demonstrates a novel hypothalamic circuit regulating energy homeostasis. *Neuron* 2003; **37**: 649–61.

16 Soriano-Guillen L, Barrios V, Campos-Barros A, Argente J. Ghrelin levels in obesity and anorexia nervosa: effect of weight reduction or recuperation. *J Pediatr* 2004; **144**: 36–42.

17 Wren AM, Bloom SR. Gut hormones and appetite control. *Gastroenterology* 2007; **132**: 2116–30.

18 Batterham RL, Le Roux CW, Cohen MA, *et al.* Pancreatic polypeptide reduces appetite and food intake in humans. *J Clin Endocrinol Metab* 2003; **88**: 3989–92.

19 Baggio LL, Drucker DJ. Biology of incretins: GLP-1 and GIP. *Gastroenterology* 2007; **132**: 2131–57.

20 Wynne K, Park AJ, Small CJ, Meeran K, *et al.* Oxyntomodulin increases energy expenditure in addition to decreasing energy intake in overweight and obese humans: a randomised controlled trial. *Int J Obes* 2006; **30**: 1729–36.

CHAPTER 3
Small Intestinal Hormones and Neurotransmitters

Nithin Karanth[1] and James C. Reynolds[2]
[1] Department of Gastroenterology, Drexel University College of Medicine, Philadelphia, PA, USA
[2] Department of Medicine, Drexel University College of Medicine, Philadelphia, PA, USA

Summary

Gastrointestinal hormones provide critically important regulation of normal digestive physiological processes, become altered in several common disease states, result in rare but classic syndromes when secreted in high concentrations by neuroendocrine tumors, and are used in a variety of therapeutic applications. Digestion is regulated by complex interactions between the endocrine system, intrinsic neural systems, and the autonomic nervous system. The importance of hormones in the regulation of normal physiological processes is evident from the diversity of their influences, their sheer numbers, and their complexity. In addition to being localized in the pancreas, hormone-secreting neuroendocrine cells are interspersed throughout the mucosal surfaces of the luminal digestive tract. Thus, the gut endocrine system is the largest endocrine organ system of the body, has a major influence on normal physiology of digestion, and is altered in several disease states. In this chapter, we describe the key peptide hormones, their physiological and pathophysiological roles, and their clinical applications.

Introduction

Gastrointestinal hormones provide critically important regulation of normal digestive physiological processes, become altered in several common disease states, result in rare but classic syndromes when secreted in high concentrations by neuroendocrine tumors, and are used in a variety of therapeutic applications [1,2]. Digestion is regulated by complex interactions between the endocrine system, intrinsic neural systems, and the autonomic nervous system. The importance of hormones in the regulation of normal physiological processes is evident from the diversity of their influence, their sheer numbers, and their complexity. A generation ago, the normal physiological process of the gut was thought to be regulated by the triad of gastrin, secretin, and cholecystokinin

(CCK). Since then, more than 100 active transmitters have been identified [1,2]. Thirty peptide hormones divided into eight families (Table 3.1) regulate the motility, secretion, and blood flow of the gut. Rather than being localized to the pancreas and upper digestive tract, hormone-secreting neuroendocrine cells are interspersed throughout the mucosal surfaces of the luminal digestive tract. Although many of these cells release peptide transmitters into the bloodstream by a classic hormonal mechanism, many others release transmitters into the local milieu to exert a paracrine effect. A third mechanism is the feedback effect of the released hormone on the cell itself, an autocrine effect.

A number of disorders are caused by disturbances in endocrine functions. The most common is peptic ulcer disease, which may result from hypergastrinemia from a variety of mechanisms. Obesity may be caused by irregularities of several hormones including leptin and CCK. Other disorders that may be due to abnormal hormone or neuropeptide secretion include irritable bowel syndrome, gall stones, various diarrheal disorders, achalasia,

Table 3.1 Neuropeptide families.

Family	Hormones
Secretin	Secretin, glucagon, glucagon-like peptides, VIP, peptide histidine isoleucine, growth hormone-releasing hormone, pituitary adenyl cyclase-activating peptide
Insulin	Insulin, insulin-like growth factors I and II, relaxin
Epidermal growth factor	Epidermal growth factor, transforming growth factor-α, amphiregulin
Gastrin	Gastrin, CCK, cerulean, cionin
Pancreatic polypeptide-fold	Pancreatic polypeptide, peptide YY, neuropeptide Y
Tachykinin	Substance P, neurokinins
Somatostatin	Somatostatin, corticostatin
Ghrelin	Ghrelin, motilin

CCK, cholecystokinin; VIP, vasoactive intestinal peptide.

and Hirschsprung disease (Table 3.2). The expression of neuropeptides and hormones by neoplastic cells has recently been shown to exert paracrine and autocrine effects on malignant tumor growth.

Medications often alter hormone levels and commonly lead to patient symptoms and medical complications. Patients who receive total parenteral nutrition intravenously do not experience the normal cyclical increases of CCK, which contributes to stasis of gall-bladder content and to the risk for both calculous and acalculous cholecystitis. Potent suppression of acid secretion by proton pump inhibitors results in a rebound increase in serum gastrin levels. When proton pump inhibitors are used for several weeks, the increase in the concentration of gastrin can lead to increases in parietal cell mass and the potential for acid secretion. When these medications are discontinued abruptly, the patient has a rebound increase in acid secretion that can exacerbate symptoms and perpetuate the need for acid suppression [3].

Gastrointestinal hormones are used in a variety of therapeutic strategies. Somatostatin and its analogues constitute first-line therapy for life-threatening bleeding from esophageal varices. Somatostatin is also used to reduce the quantity of hormone released from neuroendocrine tumors, to reduce chronic diarrhea in patients with advanced HIV infections, and to close pancreatic

and enteric fistulae. It was hoped that agonists and antagonists to motilin and CCK receptors could provide important therapeutic agents to treat motility disorders. Although efforts to develop these agents thus far have been disappointing, erythromycin acting on motilin receptors has become a standard means of emptying the stomach of its contents before emergency endoscopy is performed.

Peptide hormones are valuable as diagnostic tools. For example, serum measurements of circulating hormones are helpful to diagnose and monitor neuroendocrine tumors such as gastrin in Zollinger–Ellison syndrome (ZES), vasoactive intestinal peptide (VIP) in Verner–Morrison syndrome, and somatostatin in somatostatinoma (Table 3.2). The paradoxical effect of secretin on gastrin levels in ZES is another important diagnostic use of peptide hormones. Receptors for somatostatin, particularly subtypes 2 and 5, are present in a variety of neurohormone-secreting tumors of the digestive system and elsewhere. Radiolabeled somatostatin analogues also provide a sensitive diagnostic tool for locating neuroendocrine tumors with octreotide scans.

Characteristics of Gastrointestinal Hormones

Gastrointestinal hormone-secreting cells are located in the islets of Langerhans of the pancreas and in the enterochromaffin cells of the gastrointestinal mucosa, interspersed among epithelial cells. They release their peptide transmitters by endocrine, paracrine, and autocrine secretion. Secretion from enterochromaffin cells is regulated by input from local enteric neurons and from afferent receptors located on specialized apical microvilli that reach between epithelial cells to sample luminal contents. They can secrete multiple bioactive substances from the same cell, which may occur through the secretion of different translational products of the same gene by alternative splicing of the primary transcript, translation of hormones with the same active sequence but distinct lengths, or by synthesis of distinct structures. In fact, the endocrine system contains 100 distinct chemical messengers [4]. All gastrointestinal hormones are single-chain polypeptides synthesized from single-copy genes. Once synthesized, peptides are released into the blood or adjacent interstitial spaces by exocytosis. Peptides

Table 3.2 Clinical importance of peptide hormones.

Hormone	Disease state	Clinical application
Gastrin	(↑) Zollinger–Ellison syndrome Severe peptic ulcer disease Diarrhea	Reduce secretion via use of proton pump inhibitors
Cholecystokinin	(↓) Seen in bulimia, celiac disease, delayed gastric emptying	Evaluate gall-bladder contractility Sphincter of Oddi manometry
Vasoactive intestinal polypeptide	(↑) Verner–Morrison syndrome Voluminous diarrhea Hypokalemia Flushing (↓) Hirschsprung disease Achalasia	
Secretin		Secretin stimulation test to diagnose gastrinomas (paradoxical rise in gastrin levels with administration of secretin) Aid in cannulation of minor duct during endoscopic retrograde cholangiopancreatography

Somatostatin	(↑) Somatostatinoma
	Diabetes
	Malabsorptive diarrhea
	Gall-stone disease
		Octreotide (analog) used to treat:
		  Secretory diarrheas
		  Gastrointestinal/ variceal bleeding
		Used to image neuroendocrine tumors
		Can treat certain neuroendocrine tumors

Motilin		Macrolide antibiotics stimulate motilin receptors (↑) Gastric emptying (diabetic gastroparesis, increased visibility in emergent endoscopy for upper gastrointestinal bleed
Pancreatic polypeptide Peptide YY	(↑) PYY is seen in surgical resections that result in increased transit of food products to ileum/ colon	In animal studies: (↑) PP led to reduced food intake (↓) PYY led to insulin resistance and obesity

PP, pancreatic polypeptide; PYY, peptide YY.

released into the circulation can influence a wide variety of cell functions throughout the digestive tract and may influence multiple cellular roles simultaneously (i.e., motility, secretion, and absorption). The widespread, multifunctional capacity of gastrointestinal hormones is exemplified by CCK. CCK enhances contraction of the pyloric sphincter to delay gastric emptying while increasing gall-bladder contraction and emptying of the gall-bladder bile duct. It also influences secretion of digestive enzymes by the acinar cells of the pancreas and other upper digestive luminal organs.

Secretin was the first hormone to be described. Bayliss and Starling isolated this bioactive substance from mucosal scrapings of the duodenum in 1902 [5]. In 1905, Starling proposed the word hormone to describe this function [6]. In that same year, Edkins described a second hormone, gastrin, a bioactive substance of the antrum [7]. CCK soon followed. The development by McGuigan and others of radioimmunoassay for gastrin, and later its various subtypes, led to a much better understanding of the importance of this hormone's normal and abnormal physiological processes and led others to use this important tool to discover the location and physiological functions of other hormones and neuropeptides [8].

As more neuropeptides were discovered, they were placed in eight families on the basis of their peptide sequence homologies rather than by location or function (Table 3.1). The logic of this approach is apparent from the fact that a single peptide transmitter may be found in neurons and endocrine cells as well as have an autocrine function. In fact, endocrine and neuropeptides are also found throughout other organs of the body including the brain. Hormones that have no structural analogs are orphan peptides. The orphan peptides include gastrin-releasing peptide, neurotensin, galanin, and pancreastatin. It is important to note that Table 3.1 does not include many other clinically important peptides that are primarily neurotransmitters such as calcitonin gene-related peptide and enkephalins. Perhaps the most fascinating fact about this expanding array of newly discovered neurohormonal transmitters is that several functions of the gastrointestinal tract have been described for which the responsible transmitter has yet to be identified.

Peptide hormones interact with three broad classes of receptors. The most common class includes single transmembrane receptors with intrinsic ligand-triggered enzyme activity. Other classes have multiple transmembrane-crossing sequences that are either associated with ligand-gated channels or G proteins.

Neuroendocrine Tumors

Gastrointestinal hormone-secreting tumors can result in severe ulcerations, diarrheal syndromes, and other progressive symptom complexes (Table 3.2). These tumors are relatively rare, representing only 2% of all gastrointestinal tumors and fewer than half of all endocrine tumors. The incidence of such tumors is 1 to 2 per 100 000 persons per year. Neuroendocrine tumors may originate from the foregut (stomach, duodenum, pancreas, lung, and thymus), midgut (jejunum, ileum, appendix, and ascending colon), or hindgut (transverse, descending, and sigmoid colon and rectum). The carcinoid tumor is the most common neuroendocrine tumor. Twenty percent occur in the ileum. The most common agent secreted by carcinoids is serotonin. Whereas pancreatic neuroendocrine tumors most commonly arise from islet cells of the pancreas, others are found within the "gastrinoma triangle," composed of the neck of the pancreas, the duodenum, and the confluence of the cystic and common bile ducts. Carcinoid tumors are derived from the neuroendocrine tissues of the more distal digestive tract, most commonly in the ileum and rectum. The most common symptom-producing tumors are those secreting insulin, gastrin, glucagon, and VIP. The majority of neuroendocrine tumors may grow silently despite

the secretion of a variety of peptide hormones. The syndromes associated with a predominance of specific hormones are described in more detail in each of the sections below.

Neuroendocrine tumors are often slow growing and relatively benign, but approximately 40% show malignant behavior, including metastasis to distant organs and local invasiveness [9]. A critical step in the management of patients with these tumors is to determine whether the tumor occurs in isolation or as a manifestation of multiple endocrine neoplasia type 1. Patients with this condition may have tumors of the pituitary, parathyroid gland, and pancreas. Recognizing patients with this syndrome is important, not only because of the potential risk for other family members who may be affected but also because such patients have multifocal neuroendocrine tumors of the gastrointestinal tract that are rarely benefited by surgical intervention. In some patients, the tumors grow so slowly that the optimal management is cautious observation. Patients with more aggressive tumors may require surgery, chemoembolization, and chemotherapy [9]. In carefully selected patients, surgery provides long-term remission and hope for cure in up to 80% of cases. When metastases extend to the liver, surgical debulking procedures can lead to 5-year survival rates exceeding 60%. When tumor growth continues despite chemotherapy, long-acting somatostatin analogs can provide a valuable long-term palliative benefit.

Although a detailed description of all endocrine peptides is beyond the scope of this article, a review of the most clinically important ones follows. The role of leptin and other hormones in the development of obesity is discussed elsewhere.

Endocrine Peptides

Gastrin

Gastrin is a clinically important peptide hormone that affects both normal and abnormal gastric acid secretion and contributes to an understanding of autocrine mechanisms of peptide transmitters. Gastrin is secreted by G cells in the gastric antrum in response to luminal, hormonal, and neural regulation. Sham feeding is a potent stimulus of gastrin release. Gastric distension in response to a meal and to outlet obstruction increases gastrin release. Gastrin-releasing peptide, the human analog of bombesin, is a potent stimulant. Luminal stimuli include alkaline solutions, calcium, and amino acids, particularly aromatic amino acids such as tryptophan and phenylalanine. In contrast, carbohydrates and fat, the digestion of which is not influenced by acid or pepsin, have little effect on gastrin secretion. G-cell secretion is inhibited by the presence of luminal acid, secretin, and, most importantly, somatostatin. Autonomic system inputs from the parasympathetic nervous system have complex influences on gastrin secretion. Gastrin is not involved in the intestinal phase of acid secretion.

Gastrin is secreted in multiple bioactive forms that vary by the length of the peptide but all share the same pentapeptide active site. The major biologically active peptides are chains of 17 and 34 amino acids. The longer chain has a half-life that is much longer (30 min) than that of the shorter chain (7 min). The clinically important effects of gastrin on normal physiological processes are mediated by its stimulation of acid secretion by parietal cells through the G protein-coupled receptor (the type B CCK receptor). Gastrin also increases parietal cell secretion of intrinsic factor through a mechanism that is not linked to proton pump activity. The effects of gastrin on parietal cell secretion of acid are greatly enhanced in the presence of acetylcholine or histamine. CCKB receptors are also found on gastric mucosal cells and smooth muscle cells of the digestive tract. In addition to these effects on secretion and motility, gastrin can increase gastric mucosa cell proliferation. Patients treated with proton pump inhibitors have increased gastrin levels that are associated with both hypertrophy and increased proliferation of parietal cells. Acid rebound greater than pretreatment levels can occur when these medications are discontinued [3]. The autocrine and endocrine effects of gastrin on neoplastic cells of other organs remain a key target for investigation. Current data indicate, however, that the incidence or prognosis of colon cancer is not influenced by the mild hypergastrinemia seen in response to acid suppression by proton pump inhibitors.

Hypergastrinemia from non-beta cell tumor of the pancreas leads to severe peptic ulcer disease and diarrhea, known as Zollinger–Ellison syndrome (ZES). It is important to note, however, that most patients with ZES present with a solitary ulcer. Diarrhea is present in half of the patients because of the increased volume of fluid secretion, precipitation of bile salts, deactivation of pancreatic enzymes, and mucosal flattening due to acid injury that can be misdiagnosed as sprue. Whereas all of the adverse manifestations of the hypergastrinemia are due to acid hypersecretion, ZES patients often also secrete a variety of other neuropeptides. Approximately half of gastrin-secreting tumors arise in the gastrinoma triangle. Patients who have undergone partial gastrectomy may have hypergastrinemia-induced acid hypersecretion due to retained antral tissue that is not exposed to intraluminal acid. Other conditions associated with increased acid secretion and hypergastrinemia include short gut syndrome, antral G-cell hyperplasia, gastric outlet obstruction, and hypercalcemia. More commonly, elevated gastrin levels are due to hypochlorhydria. Common causes of reduced acid secretion include proton pump inhibition, atrophic gastritis, and pernicious anemia.

Cholecystokinin

The isolation of a peptide extract from the canine duodenum that had potent contractile effects on the gall bladder led to the description of CCK in 1928 [10]. Although it is produced from a single gene, circulating CCK is found in several molecular forms as a result of post-translational processing. The principal form is composed of 58 amino acids that have a carboxyl terminus sequence identical to that of gastrin. CCK derives its biologic activity from this region; it is not surprising that CCK has weak gastrin-like activity and is a member of the gastrin family [4,11].

The cells that release CCK, known as I cells, are located predominantly in the proximal small bowel, with decreasing numbers in the distal jejunum and ileum. The apical surfaces of I cells are exposed to intestinal contents, which allows detection of ingested fats and proteins, the primary stimulants for secretion of CCK. The release of CCK results in gall-bladder contraction and relaxation of the sphincter of Oddi, enabling delivery of bile into the intestine. Furthermore, gastric emptying is delayed and pancreatic secretion is stimulated (via CCK-mediated release of acetylcholine by the vagus nerve), putting in order the events needed for normal digestion to occur [4,11,12]. It is hypothesized that intestinal releasing factors control the secretion of CCK and that degradation of these factors by pancreatic enzymes completes the negative feedback loop [13]. In addition, CCK has been implicated in induction of satiety via gastric receptors that relay the effect into afferent vagal fibers. This signal then reaches the hypothalamus via the vagus nerve [4].

Two CCK receptors have been identified, CCKA and CCKB, both of which are G protein-coupled receptors. These receptors are found in the pancreas, gall bladder, stomach, lower esophageal sphincter, ileum, colon, and peripheral nerves. The CCKB receptor, which is identical to the gastrin receptor, is the predominant form found in the pancreas. Given the increased affinity of this receptor for gastrin, CCK probably stimulates pancreatic secretion by its influence on acetylcholine release by the vagus nerve [4,11].

CCK is used clinically primarily for diagnostic testing. It has been used with nuclear imaging to evaluate gallbladder contractility and during sphincter of Oddi manometry. Low levels of CCK have been reported in patients with bulimia nervosa, celiac disease, and delayed gastric emptying, whereas no disease is known to be caused by an excess of CCK. The well-described exaggeration of the gastrocolic reflex leading to increased colonic contractions after fat ingestion in patients with irritable bowel syndrome was hypothesized to be a valuable target for pharmaceutical intervention. Unfortunately, the CCK antagonists that were developed have not yet been shown to be clinically useful.

Vasoactive Intestinal Polypeptide

VIP is a neurohormone that is released from nerve terminals and a paracrine molecule that acts locally on cells bearing its receptor. VIP is mainly localized in neurons and is expressed in both the enteric and central nervous systems. The peptide is a precursor molecule that is cleaved to the final active peptide, which is composed of 28 amino acids. Peptide histidine isoleucine is an alternative peptide derived from VIP that also stimulates intestinal fluid secretion. The VIP receptors, which are G protein coupled, are plentiful on the smooth muscle sphincters of the lower esophagus, ampulla of Vater, and rectum; on pancreatic acinar and duct cells; and on enteric mucosal cells. Binding of VIP to its receptor leads to the activation of G protein and subsequent increase in cAMP, initiating the signaling cascade responsible for the physiological actions of the cell [14].

VIP serves multiple functions in the gastrointestinal tract. It acts principally to stimulate gut secretion and absorption and to promote fluid and bicarbonate secretion from bile duct cholangiocytes. VIP is a potent inducer of smooth muscle relaxation throughout the digestive tract. It is often co-localized in cells containing nitric oxide, particularly in sphincters such as the lower esophageal sphincter, the sphincter of Oddi, the ileocolonic sphincter, and the anal sphincters. VIP causes relaxation by inducing smooth muscle cell membrane hyperpolarization. Another characteristic of this peptide is its vasodilatory properties [14,15].

Patients with VIP tumors (VIPoma) present with voluminous diarrhea and flushing. This condition has several names: pancreatic cholera, watery diarrhea–hypokalemia–achlorhydria (WHDA syndrome), and Verner–Morrison syndrome [16]. On the other hand, a dearth of neurons secreting VIP has also been associated with multiple disease processes. Scarcity of VIP ganglion cells in the myenteric plexus of the colon is seen in patients with Hirschsprung disease [17]; a reduced number in the distal esophagus is noted in those with achalasia [18]. Both conditions share the inability to effectively relax the smooth muscle of the affected region.

Secretin

Discovered in 1902 by Bayliss and Starling [5], secretin has the distinction of being the first hormone discovered, thereby igniting the field of endocrinology. Nearly 50 years after its landmark discovery, the 27-amino-acid-sequence was identified. Secretin is the founding member of the "secretin/ glucagon/ VIP" family of gastrointestinal hormones. It is encoded by a gene expressed in specialized enteroendocrine cells of the small intestine known as S cells. The apical surfaces of S cells are exposed to luminal contents, where they are triggered by a low pH (<4.5) to release secretin from their basolateral membrane into the circulation [19,20].

The receptors for this hormone are densely populated on pancreatic duct and acinar cells, allowing for secretin-stimulated enzyme secretion. In addition, receptors are also found in the vagus nerve, allowing secretin to enhance postprandial pancreatic secretion. Secretin receptors are G protein coupled, whereby the binding of secretin activates the G protein leading to elevation of cellular cAMP levels. This second messenger then triggers a signaling cascade that activates the physiological responses of the cells [20].

Stimulation of pancreatic fluid and bicarbonate secretion by secretin leads to the neutralization of acidic chyme in the small intestine. Furthermore, secretin inhibits gastric acid release and gastric motility. In combination, these physiological actions raise the duodenal pH, which serves as negative feedback to halt further secretin release. An intestinal secretin-releasing factor is responsible for the regulation of secretin. In this model, release of secretin occurs until sufficient quantities of pancreatic enzymes are present to degrade the secretin-releasing factor, stopping the additional release of hormone [21].

The most notable clinical application of the hormone is diagnosis of gastrinomas by the secretin stimulation test. Under normal conditions, secretin inhibits gastrin release. Conversely, in gastrinomas, administration of secretin leads to a paradoxical rise in gastrin levels [22]. Another practical use is administration of secretin during endoscopic retrograde cholangiopancreatography to aid in ductal cannulation of the minor duct; the increase in pancreatic secretions causes a temporary dilation of the pancreatic ducts.

Somatostatin

Originally discovered as an inhibitor of growth hormone release, somatostatin exists in two molecular forms resulting from differing post-translational processing of the same preprohormone. Somatostatin is prevalent throughout the body and is especially plentiful in the central and enteric nervous systems and in the gastrointestinal tract and pancreas. In the nervous system, somatostatin is released by nerves functioning as neurotransmitters. In the gastrointestinal tract and pancreas, it is produced by D cells that either release the peptide into the circulation or direct secretion onto a neighboring cell. The somatostatin receptor is an inhibitory G protein-coupled receptor that, when activated, results in reduced cAMP levels leading to the appropriate cell response [23,24].

Somatostatin is produced by endocrine, enteroendocrine, and neural cells and has an exceptionally short half-life—less than 3 min. Gastrointestinal D cells are stimulated to produce somatostatin by meal ingestion and gastric acid secretion. Furthermore, the autonomic nervous system stimulates somatostatin production by the cholinergic effect and inhibits its production with catecholamines. The overall physiological effect of somatostatin is inhibitory. It reduces gut motility and gallbladder contraction, decreases blood flow, and retards endocrine and exocrine secretion of most other gastrointestinal hormones [23,24].

In its natural state, somatostatin would have little clinical utility given its short half-life. However, the development of octreotide, a somatostatin analogue with a half-life of more than 90 min, has yielded a number of practical applications. Newer, slow-release formulations of octreotide have been developed that require only one dose per month. This advancement is likely to improve patient compliance and further increase clinical utility of the peptide [25]. Octreotide has been used in the treatment of secretory diarrheas (VIPomas, carcinoid) and gastrointestinal bleeding (especially variceal hemorrhage). Furthermore, a meta-analysis suggested that octreotide might reduce morbidities following pancreatic surgery [26]. The fact that a majority of neuroendocrine tumors express somatostatin receptors on their cell surfaces provides the basis for using octreotide in the imaging of these lesions. Given that neuroendocrine tumors are often small and difficult to identify using standard radiological techniques (i.e., CT, US, MRI), the use of radiolabeled octreotide has proved to be a valuable tool in localizing these tumors. Furthermore, activation of somatostatin receptors in several of these tumors can result in induction of cell cycle arrest as well as inhibition of tumor angiogenesis, making octreotide a useful therapeutic option [27].

The physiological consequences of excess somatostatin are illustrated by the clinical presentation of a rare tumor, a somatostatinoma. As a result of the inhibition of insulin secretion, pancreatic exocrine secretion, and gall-bladder contraction, patients typically exhibit diabetes, malabsorptive diarrhea, and gall-stone disease [19]. These tumors most commonly develop in the pancreas, duodenum, or ampulla of Vater, either in isolation or as part of the multiple endocrine neoplasia type 1 syndrome (50% of cases) [23].

A complex relationship exists between somatostatin secretion and *Helicobacter pylori* infection. Acute inflammation induced by *H. pylori* infection reduces somatostatin secretion, leading to increased gastrin release, hyperchlorhydria, and risk of peptic ulcers. The effect of chronic *H. pylori* infection is more complex and varies by site and severity of infection [23,24].

Motilin

Motilin is the peptide released by enterochromaffin cells in the duodenum and proximal intestine that is the primary stimulant of phase III of the migrating motor complex, often known as the "intestinal housekeeper".

This forceful contraction begins at the lower esophageal sphincter and progresses down the upper digestive tract to the lower or terminal ileum, sweeping undigested solids and other postdigestive waste into the colon. Antibodies to motilin disrupt the regularity of this important interorgan physiological event, whereas intravenous administration of motilin can initiate (but perhaps not continuously propagate) the intestinal housekeeper. Acid in the duodenum antagonizes this effect of motilin.

Macrolide antibiotics and their analogs stimulate motilin receptors. Erythromycin has a potent effect on gastric emptying, even in diabetic patients with severe enteroneuropathy. This observation led to extensive efforts to develop macrolide analogs that had much greater affinity for motilin receptors than did erythromycin. Regrettably, the development of these agents by several pharmaceutical companies never reached phase III testing. Nevertheless, clinicians have continued to find erythromycin valuable in treating severe diabetic gastroparesis and to promote gastric emptying in patients who require emergency endoscopy to treat upper gastrointestinal bleeding.

Pancreatic Polypeptide/ Peptide YY/ Neuropeptide Y

PP, the founding member of the pancreatic polypeptide family, was originally isolated in 1968 during the preparation of insulin [28]. Two other major members of this family include PYY and NPY. Each of these peptides is composed of 36 amino acids and, despite sharing significant structural similarities, they have varying biological functions and are found in different locations throughout the gastrointestinal tract and nervous system. PP is produced by PP cells, which are distinct, specialized pancreatic islet cells. PYY is created from enteroendocrine cells of the gastrointestinal tract, most densely populating the ileum (in the form of L cells) and colon (in H cells). NPY is found principally in the sympathetic neurons where it functions as a neurotransmitter. PP and PYY function in both a paracrine and endocrine fashion, whereas NPY is a true neurotransmitter. An assortment of receptor subtypes exists for this family, all of which are called Y receptors. These peptides bind to the typical G protein-coupled receptors, which causes inhibition of adenylyl cyclase [29,30].

PP hinders exocrine secretion of the pancreas and decreases gall-bladder contraction and gut motility. Its

release is triggered by vagal-cholinergic stimulation following a meal. The main catalyst for PYY release by cells in the ileum is incompletely digested nutrients, especially fats, although the levels of PYY increase only sluggishly in the postprandial state. PYY impedes vagally stimulated gastric acid secretion and, most notably, delays gastric emptying and intestinal motility. These properties allow this hormone to delay further transit of food into the intestine, an action known as the "ileal break." NPY, one the most abundant peptides in the central nervous system, is the strongest known stimulant of food intake [30].

Patients with increased transit of food products to the ileum and colon resulting from surgically altered anatomy have elevated levels of PYY. The potential clinical applications for this peptide family have focused largely on the regulation of food intake. In animal studies, overexpression of PP led to reduced food intake and body weight, whereas absence of PYY resulted in insulin resistance and obesity [31,32]. PYY may be diminished in functional dyspepsia [33].

> ### Take-home points
>
> - More than 30 peptide hormones divided into eight families (Table 3.1) regulate the motility, secretion, and blood flow of the gut.
>
> - Gut hormones can mediate their influence through more than 100 active forms in a classical endocrine fashion after being released into the bloodstream or via more localized paracrine or autocrine mechanisms.
>
> - Gut hormone irregularities are associated with a variety of clinical syndromes, regulate food intake and digestion, and are found in abnormal circulating levels in common disorders such as dyspepsia and obesity and in rare neuroendocrine tumor syndromes.
>
> - Physicians need to understand the clinical importance and effects of gastrin to properly manage patients with acid peptic disorders and to be able to recognize at its early stages patients affected by Zollinger–Ellison syndrome.
>
> - Hypergastrinemia is most commonly due to achlorhydria, but acid-secreting tumors or other causes of aberrant gastrin secretion must be identified to avoid potentially life-threatening acid peptic disorders and their complications.
>
> - Somatostatin analogues, secretin, and cholecystokinin (CCK) are used in a variety of diagnostic algorithms that can provide invaluable data in difficult-to-diagnose disorders.

- Low levels of CCK have been reported in patients with bulimia nervosa, celiac disease, and gastroparesis, but measuring CCK levels is not clinically useful at present.
- Although many peptide hormones are being investigated for potential uses, somatostatin is the only hormone used commonly in both therapeutic and diagnostic gastroenterology.

References

1 Rehfeld JF. A centenary of gastrointestinal endocrinology. *Horm Metab Res* 2004; **36**: 735–41.

2 Ahlman H, Nilsson O. The gut as the largest endocrine organ in the body. *Ann Oncol* 2001; **12** (Suppl. 2): S63–S68.

3 Reimer C, Sondergaard B, Hilsted L, Bytzer P. Proton-pump inhibitor therapy induces acid-related symptoms in healthy volunteers after withdrawal of therapy. *Gastroenterology* 2009; **137**: 80–7.

4 Rehfeld J. Clinical endocrinology and metabolism. Cholecystokinin. *Best Pract Res Clin Endocrinol Metabol* 2004; **18**: 569–86.

5 Bayliss WM, Starling EH. The mechanism of pancreatic secretion. *J Physiol (London)* 1902; **28**: 325–53.

6 Starling EH. Croonian Lecture: On the chemical correlation of the functions of the body I. *Lancet* 1905; **2**: 339–41.

7 Edkins JS. The chemical mechanism of gastric secretion. *J Physiol (London)* 1906; **34**: 133–44.

8 McGuigan JE, Trudeau WL. Immunochemical measurement of elevated levels of gastrin in the serum of patients with pancreatic tumors of the Zollinger-Ellison variety. *N Engl J Med* 1968; **278**: 1308–13.

9 Delaunoit T, Neczyporenko F, Rubin J, *et al.* Medical management of pancreatic neuroendocrine tumors. *Am J Gastroenterol* 2008; **103**: 475–83.

10 Ivy AC, Oldberg E. A hormone mechanism for gall-bladder contraction and evacuation. *Am J Physiol* 1928; **86**: 599–613.

11 Liddle RA. Cholecystokinin. In: Walsh JH, Dockray GJ, eds. *Gut Peptides: Biochemistry and Physiology*. New York: Raven Press, 1994: 175.

12 Owyang C, Logsdon CD. New insights into neurohormonal regulation of pancreatic secretion. *Gastroenterology* 2004; **127**: 957–69.

13 Liddle RA. Regulation of cholecystokinin secretion by intraluminal releasing factors. *Am J Physiol* 1995; **269**: G319–G327.

14 Dockray GJ. Vasoactive intestinal polypeptide and related peptides. In: Walsh JH, Dockray GJ, eds. *Gut Peptides: Biochemistry and Physiology*. New York: Raven Press, 1994: 447.

15 Gozes I, Furman S. Clinical endocrinology and metabolism. Potential clinical applications of vasoactive intestinal peptide: a selected update. *Best Pract Res Clin Endocrinol Metab* 2004; **18**: 623–40.

16 Masel SL, Brennan BA, Turner JH, *et al.* Pancreatic vasoactive intestinal polypeptide-oma as a cause of secretory diarrhoea. *J Gastroenterol Hepatol* 2000; **15**: 457–60.

17 Larsson LT, Sundler F. Is the reduction of VIP the clue to the pathophysiology of Hirchsprung's disease? *Z Kinderchir* 1990; **45**: 164–6.

18 Aggestrup S, Uddman R, Sundler F, *et al.* Lack of vasoactive intestinal polypeptide nerves in esophageal achalasia. *Gastroenterology* 1983; **84**: 924–7.

19 Delvalle J, Yamada T. The gut as an endocrine organ. *Annu Rev Med* 1990; **41**: 447–55.

20 Leiter AB, Chey WY, Kopin AS. Secretin. In: Walsh JH, Dockray GJ, eds. *Gut Peptides: Biochemistry and Physiology*. New York: Raven Press, 1994: 144.

21 Li P, Lee KY, Chang TM, Chey WY. Mechanism of acid-induced release of secretin in rats. Presence of a secretin-releasing peptide. *J Clin Invest* 1990; **86**: 1474–9.

22 Brady CE 3rd. Secretin provocation test in the diagnosis of Zollinger-Ellison syndrome. *Am J Gastroenterol* 1991; **86**: 129–34.

23 Low MJ. Clinical endocrinology and metabolism. The somatostatin neuroendocrine system: physiology and clinical relevance in gastrointestinal and pancreatic disorders. *Best Pract Res Clin Endocrinol Metabol* 2004; **18**: 607–22.

24 Schubert ML. Gastric secretion. *Curr Opin Gastroenterol* 2005; **21**: 636–43.

25 Lamberts SW, van der Lely AJ, de Herder WW, Hofland LJ. Octreotide. *N Eng J Med* 1996; **334**: 246–54.

26 Connor S, Alexakis N, Garden OJ, *et al.* Meta-analysis of the value of somatostatin and its analogues in reducing complications associated with pancreatic surgery. *Br J Surg* 2005; **92**: 1059–67.

27 Florio T. Molecular mechanisms of the antiproliferative activity of somatostatin receptors (SSTRs) in neuroendocrine tumors. *Front Biosci* 2008; **13**: 822–40.

28 Kimmel JR, Pollock HG, Hazelwood RL. Isolation and characterization of chicken insulin. *Endocrinology* 1968; **83**: 1323–30.

29 Adrian TE, Ferri GL, Bacarese-Hamilton AJ, *et al.* Human distribution and release of a putative new gut hormone, peptide YY. *Gastroenterology* 1985; **89**: 1070–7.

30 Strader AD, Woods SC. Gastrointestinal hormones and food intake. *Gastroenterology* 2005; **128**: 175–91.

31 Batterhan RL, Cohen MA, Ellis SM, *et al.* Inhibition of food intake in obese subjects by peptide YY3-36. *N Engl J Med* 2003; **349**: 941–8.

32 Hazelwood RL. The pancreatic polypeptide (PP-fold) family: gastrointestinal, vascular, and feeding behavioral implications. *Proc Soc Exp Biol Med* 1993; **202**: 44–63.

33 Pilichiewicz AN, Feltrin KL, Horowitz M, *et al.* Functional dyspepsia is associated with a greater symptomatic response to fat but not carbohydrate, increased fasting and postprandial CCK, and diminished PYY. *Am J Gastronenterol* 2008; **103**: 2613–23.

CHAPTER 4

Mucosal Immunology of the Intestine

Steven J. Esses[1] and Lloyd Mayer[2]

[1] Division of Gastroenterology, Mount Sinai School of Medicine, New York, NY, USA
[2] Divisions of Clinical Immunology and Gastroenterology, Mount Sinai Medical Center, New York, NY, USA

Summary

In the intestine, the mucosal immune system is separated from a significant bacterial and dietary antigen load by an epithelial cell layer. The immunologic tone is one of tolerance towards non-pathogenic bacteria and food antigens. However, the system maintains the capacity to exclude and eliminate pathogenic microbes. This tolerance exists as a result of multiple innate and adaptive responses, but the presence of adequate regulatory cells, which are common in mucosal sites, is probably the most important factor. Defects in mucosal tolerance underlie the development of inflammatory intestinal diseases such as inflammatory bowel disease (IBD), celiac disease, and food allergy.

Introduction

In the intestine, the mucosal immune system is separated from a significant bacterial and dietary antigen load by an epithelial cell layer. The immunologic tone is one of tolerance towards non-pathogenic bacteria and food antigens. However, the system maintains the capacity to exclude and eliminate pathogenic microbes.

The mucosal barrier, intestinal epithelial cell layer, innate and adaptive immune systems, and luminal bacteria flora all contribute to maintaining the balance of suppression and microbial defense.

Mucosal and Epithelial Barrier

Barriers to entry for pathogenic bacteria or toxins include pancreatic and gastric proteases, bile acids, and extremes of pH in the intestine such as the harsh acidic environment of the stomach and the alkaline pH in the upper small bowel.

Practical Gastroenterology and Hepatology: Small and Large Intestine and Pancreas, 1st edition. Edited by Nicholas J. Talley, Sunanda V. Kane and Michael B. Wallace. © 2010 Blackwell Publishing Ltd.

Another key barrier is the goblet cell-produced mucus layer, which lines the surface epithelium from the nasal cavity to the rectum. MUC2 is the main mucin glycoprotein secreted by goblet cells, while MUC3A and B are two predominant, membrane-bound isoforms [1]. Bacteria, particles, and viruses are trapped in this layer of mucus and are expelled by the peristaltic contractions of the gut.

Another family of secreted goblet cell proteins, called trefoil factors, promotes restoration of the barrier in response to injury. Trefoil factors bind mucin to form the hydrophobic mucus barrier [2]. In absence of these factors, the host is susceptible to uncontrolled inflammation.

The main component of the barrier is the epithelial cell. Tight junctions between epithelial cells prevent passage of macromolecules that might elicit antigenic responses. Defects in the tight junction barrier may be involved in the aberrant immune responses seen in inflammatory bowel disease (IBD) and food allergy [3]. Agents that affect the epithelial barrier, such as non-steroidal anti-inflammatory drugs, antibiotics, and microbial infections, are common triggers of IBD. Certain pathogenic bacteria mediate their damage through tight junction and barrier disruption. For example, enteropathogenic *E. coli* dephosphorylates and dissociates occludin from the epithelial tight junctions [4]. In addition, intestinal epithelial cells are immunologically active. They process and present antigen and secrete cytokines and chemokines that initiate protective immune responses [5].

Innate Immune System

The innate immune response is the body's first line of defense against invading microbes. Its objective is to localize and eradicate threats quickly.

Paneth cells are unique intestinal epithelial cells that participate in innate immunity and inhibit excessive microbial growth by secreting α-defensins, which are cationic antimicrobial peptides. The importance of Paneth cells was emphasized by reports that defensins confer protection from *Salmonella typhi* infection [6].

Other components of the innate system include membrane-bound Toll-like receptors (TLR) and the CARD15/NOD2 intracellular pattern recognition receptor. TLR4 and TLR5 recognize lipopolysaccharides and flagellin respectively, while the intracellular sensor CARD15/NOD2 recognizes peptidoglycan, MDP. These receptors are expressed on epithelial cells and other innate immune cells, and their trigger leads to a proinflammatory response. CARD15/NOD2 mutations were the first identified genetic susceptibility locus in Crohn disease [7]. The CARD15/NOD2 mutation may affect the innate system's ability to localize and eradicate bacteria that gain entry to the host. The resulting persistence of a microbial stimulus may lead to an adaptive immune response towards an otherwise harmless stimulus. Interestingly, patients with genetic defects in innate immunity, such as chronic granulomatous disease or Herman–Pudlak syndrome, can have an IBD-like disease [8].

Antigen Uptake and Induction of a Mucosal Immune Response

Peyer patches and mesenteric lymph nodes are the main inductive sites of the mucosal immune system. Peyer patches are aggregates of lymphoid tissue composed of a large B-cell follicle, an interfollicular T cell zone, and interspersed dendritic cells and macrophages.

Antigen uptake in the gut occurs through a number of different mechanisms. Dendritic cells underneath the epithelium of the distal small bowel insert dendrites between intestinal epithelial cells to sample luminal content [9]. Specialized epithelial cells known as microfold (M) cells overlie Peyer patches and mediate the uptake of luminal antigen (particulate) and microorganisms, as well as their transfer to subepithelial dendritic cells and B cells for further processing [10]. Finally, intestinal epithelial cells ingest soluble antigen by fluid-phase endocytosis. This is a slow and stable process, the kinetics of which is dependent on solubility, not size.

Naïve lymphocytes home to Peyer patches, and are exposed to antigen. They then traffic to mesenteric lymph nodes where there is further antigen exposure, expansion, and maturation. These newly activated T cells leave the mesenteric lymph nodes and enter into the circulation through the thoracic duct, where they subsequently home back to all mucosal effector sites (lamina propria) under the guidance of tissue-specific integrins on the high endothelial venules (HEV). This last step is mediated by the interaction between the $\alpha_4\beta_7$ integrin, expressed on mucosally derived lymphocytes, and mucosal addressin cell adhesion molecule MadCAM-1, which is expressed on HEVs in the lamina propria [11]. Activation of mucosal lymphocytes at any site along the intestine can generate protective responses at all mucosal sites.

Adaptive Immune System

The adaptive immune system is characterized by specificity and memory that is largely mediated by T and B cells. T cells produce cytokines, thereby orchestrating an organized and directed immune response that eradicates infections and gives rise to memory cells (Figure 4.1).

Exposed to a vast array of microbial and food antigens, the mucosal immune system mounts a constant "controlled" immune response, as evidenced by the presence of activated CD4+ helper T cells [12]. This suppression is characterized by hyporesponsive lymphocytes and antigen-presenting cells (APCs) [13] and is mediated by a variety of regulatory cells that produce immunosuppressive cytokines such as transforming growth factor-β (TGF-β) and interleukin-10 (IL-10).

CD4+ T helper 1 (Th1) cells are characterized by the production of interferon-γ (IFN-γ), tumor necrosis factor-α (TNF-α), and IL-2. APC-derived IL-12 drives their differentiation. The cytokines produce enhanced intracellular killing (IFN-γ, TNF-α), inflammatory cell

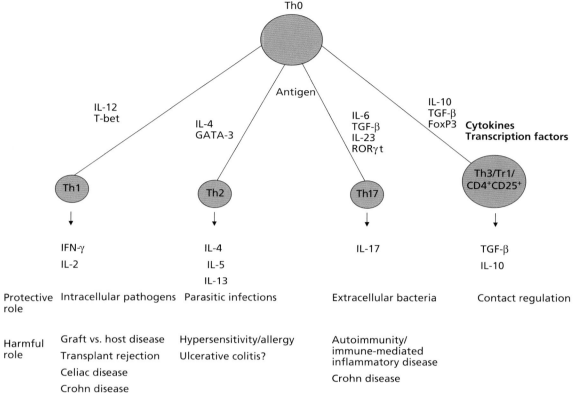

Figure 4.1 CD4+ helper T cells differentiate along different pathways and assume various protective or harmful roles. IFN, interferon; IL, interleukin; TGF, transforming growth factor.

recruitment (TNF-α), and promote tissue destruction. The Th1 response leads to the formation of granulomas, whose chief role is to wall off infectious agents. Tissues from patients with graft-versus-host disease, transplant rejection, and celiac disease also display Th1 profiles of cytokines.

Crohn disease was initially thought to be the result of aberrant Th1 responses because of increased mucosal levels of IFN-γ, IL-2, and IL-12, as well as the presence of mucosal granulomas in patients. However, evidence has steadily accumulated to support a prominent role for a second T helper subset, Th17. IL-17 and IL-22 are increased in inflamed Crohn mucosa [14], while a recently discovered mutation in the IL-23 receptor protects hosts from developing Crohn disease [15]. The recent paradigm shift in CD pathogenesis from a Th1 to a Th17 response is underscored by the lack of efficacy of an anti-IFN-γ mAb in the treatment of Crohn patients.

Th2 cells produce cytokines IL-4, IL-5, and IL-13 and are involved in hypersensitivity reactions, food allergy, helminthic infections, and ulcerative colitis (UC). UC was thought to be a Th2-mediated disease because of increased mucosal levels of IL-5, and more recently of IL-13 [16]. However, patients with UC exhibit decreased production of mucosal IL-4. Natural killer T cells may be responsible for the aberrant production of IL-13, which targets epithelial cells of the mucosal barrier to become dysfunctional. This may explain why UC is a superficial epithelial injury disorder [17].

Humoral Response and Secretory IgA

The mucosal immune system is characterized by secretory IgA, which is produced more than any other antibody in the body and is transported by intestinal epithelial cells. It is protected from luminal proteases by an epithelial-derived glycoprotein known as secretory component that envelopes the Fc portion of sIgA and protects potential proteolytic cleavage sites. Secretory IgA functions mainly to inhibit the adhesion of viruses and bacteria to the epithelium by agglutinating the bacteria and other antigens, trapping them in the mucus layer and facilitating their removal from the host [18].

Secretory IgA derived from breast milk provides newborns with passive immunity against pathogens. It may also aid tolerance by preventing exposure of the immune system to commensal bacteria and food antigen, a process is known as immune exclusion. In IgA deficiency, there is a greater incidence of serum antibody to food antigen. However, it is unknown whether this plays a role in food allergy since the majority of patients with food-allergy are not IgA deficient.

IgE is not a dominant antibody of the gastrointestinal tract. In food allergy, however, IgE is present in the gastrointestinal tract and facilitates antigen uptake and trans-epithelial transfer to mucosal mast cells [19].

Tolerance and Regulatory T Cells

Tolerance to non-pathogenic bacteria and food antigens is mediated by regulatory cells, and is perhaps the most critical immune pathway in the intestine.

Oral tolerance is defined as a lack of systemic immune response to orally introduced antigen. Tolerance is dependent on a number of factors, including the dose of the antigen. High-dose antigen leads to anergy or deletion of responsive T cells [20], while low-dose antigen activates regulatory T cells that secrete IL-10 and TGF-β [21].

The regulatory T cells in the gut include Tr1, Th3, and CD4$^+$CD25$^+$ T cells. CD4$^+$ Tr1 T cells secrete IL-10, which suppresses the response to flora [22]. Interestingly, IL-10 deficient mice develop a Crohn-like inflammatory disease [23]. CD4$^+$ Th3 cells produce TGF-β, which promotes IgA production and inhibits T- and B-cell activation. CD4$^+$CD25$^+$ Treg cells are located systemically and are dependent on the transcription factor FoxP3. FoxP3 deficiency leads to a multiorgan autoimmune disease know as IPEX syndrome, with little in the way of gastrointestinal tract disease [24]. Populations of CD8$^+$ regula-

tory T cells have been described in the gut as well, and have been shown to be deficient in IBD patients [25].

Tolerance to food and/or bacteria is broken in disease states including IBD and celiac disease. Antibodies against microbial products such as anti-*Saccharomyces cerevisiae* (ASCA) [26] and the anti-flagellin antibody Cbir1 [27] have been found in the serum of IBD patients. Furthermore, defective oral tolerance has been demonstrated in both IBD patients and healthy relatives [28].

Celiac disease is characterized by an immune response to gluten that involves aberrant IL-15 production by intestinal epithelial cells and IFN-γ by T cells. This results in flattening of the villi of the upper small intestine, crypt hyperplasia, and intraepithelial lymphocytosis [29].

Commensal Flora

The intestinal flora plays a major role in both immune system development and defense. These bacteria aid in digestion, promote epithelial cell growth, and produce required vitamins. They also play a major role in shaping the immune system. Previous studies show that germ-free animals are relatively immunodeficient, and [30] colonization of these animals with normal flora establishes both the mucosal and systemic immune system.

The commensal flora occupies all available ecological niches of the intestine, preventing outgrowth of pathogenic bacteria such as *Clostridium difficile*. When the flora is altered, outgrowth may occur, leading to disease processes such as pseudomembranous colitis.

Take-home points

- In the intestine, the mucosal immune system is separated from a vast bacterial and dietary antigen load by an epithelial cells layer.

- The immunologic tone in the intestine is one of suppression, with tolerance and controlled physiologic inflammation being examples of this suppressed state.

- Tolerance exists as a result of multiple innate and adaptive responses, but the presence of adequate regulatory cells is probably the most important factor.

- Defects in mucosal tolerance, as well as underlying deficits in the innate and adaptive immune response, leads to the unchecked inflammation that results in intestinal diseases such as IBD, celiac disease, and food allergy.

References

1 Kyo K, Muto T, Nagawa H, *et al.* Associations of distinct variants of the intestinal mucin gene MUC3A with ulcerative colitis and Crohn's disease. *J Hum Genet* 2001; **46**: 5.

2 Sands BE, Podolsky DK. The trefoil peptide family. *Annu Rev Physiol* 1996; **58**: 253–73.

3 de Boissieu D, Matarazzo P, Rocchiccioli F, Dupont C. Multiple food allergy: a possible diagnosis in breastfed infants. *Acta Paediatr* 1999; **86**: 1042–6.

4 Simonovic I, Rosenberg J, Koutsouris A, *et al.* Enteropathogenic *Escherichia coli* dephosphorylates and dissociates occludin from intestinal epithelial tight junctions. *Cell Microbiol* 2000; **2**: 305.

5 Kagnoff MF, Eckmann L. Epithelial cells as sensors for microbial infection. *J Clin Invest* 1997; **100**: 6.

6 Salzman NH, Ghosh D, Huttner KM, *et al.* Protection against enteric salmonellosis in transgenic mice expressing a human intestinal defensin. *Nature* 2003; **422**: 522–6.

7 Hugot JP, Chamaillard M, Zouali H, *et al.* Association of NOD2 leucine-rich repeat variants with susceptibility to Crohn's disease. *Nature* 2001; **411**: 599–603.

8 Korzenik JR. Is Crohn's disease due to defective immunity? *Gut* 2007; **56**: 2–5.

9 Rescigno M, Urbano M, Valzasina B, *et al.* Dendritic cells express tight junction proteins and penetrate gut epithelial monolayers to sample bacteria. *Nat Immunol* 2001; **2**: 361.

10 Miller H, Zhang J, Kuolee R, *et al.* Intestinal M cells: the fallible sentinels? *World J Gastroenterology* 2007; **13**: 1477–86.

11 De Keyser F, Elewaut D, De Wever N, *et al.* The gut associated addressins: Lymphocyte homing in the gut. *Baillieres Clin Rheumatol* 1996; **10**: 25.

12 MacDonald TT, Pender SL. Lamina propria T cells. *Chem Immunol* 1998; **71**: 103–17.

13 Smythies LE, Sellers M, Clements RH, *et al.* Human intestinal macrophages display profound inflammatory anergy despite avid phagocytic and bacteriocidal activity. *J Clin Invest* 2005; **115**: 66.

14 Fujino S, Andoh A, Bamba S, *et al.* Increased expression of interleukin 17 in inflammatory bowel disease. *Gut* 2003; **52**: 65–70.

15 Duerr RH, Taylor KD, Brant SR, *et al.* A genome-wide association study identifies IL23R as an inflammatory bowel disease gene. *Science* 2006; **314**: 1461–3.

16 Heller F, Florian P, Bojarski C, *et al.* Interleukin-13 is the key effector Th2 cytokine in ulcerative colitis that affects epithelial tight junctions, apoptosis, and cell restitution. *Gastroenterology* 2005; **129**: 550–64.

17 Fuss IJ, Heller F, Boirivant M, *et al.* Nonclassical CD1d-restricted NK T cells that produce IL-13 characterize an atypical Th2 response in ulcerative colitis. *J Clin Invest* 2004; **113**: 1490–7.

18 Cunningham-Rundles C. Physiology of IgA and IgA deficiency. *J Clin Immunol* 2001; **21**: 303–9.

19 Berin MC, Kiliaan AJ, Yang PC, *et al.* Rapid transepithelial antigen transport in rat jejunum: impact of sensitization and the hypersensitivity reaction. *Gastroenterology* 1997; **113**: 856–64.

20 Benson JM. T cell activation and receptor down-modulation precede deletion induced by mucosally administered antigen. *J Clin Invest* 2000; **106**: 1031.

21 Neurath MF, Fuss I, Kelsall BL, *et al.* Experimental granulomatous colitis in mice is abrogated by induction of TGF-beta-mediated oral tolerance. *J Exp Med* 1996; **183**: 2605.

22 Groux H, O'Garra A, Bigler M, *et al.* A CD4[+] T-cell subset inhibits antigen-specific T-cell responses and prevents colitis. *Nature* 1997; **389**: 737–42.

23 Kühn R, Löhler J, Rennick D, *et al.* Interleukin-10-deficient mice develop chronic enterocolitis. *Cell* 1993; **75**: 263–74.

24 Bennett CL, Christie J, Ramsdell F, *et al.* The immune dysregulation, polyendocrinopathy, enteropathy, X-linked syndrome (IPEX) is caused by mutations of FOXP3. *Nat Genet* 2001; **1**: 20–1.

25 Allez M, Brimnes J, Dotan I, Mayer L. Expansion of CD8[+] T cells with regulatory function after interaction with intestinal epithelial cells. *Gastroenterology* 2002; **123**: 1516–26.

26 Landers CJ, Cohavy O, Misra R, *et al.* Selected loss of tolerance evidenced by Crohn's disease-associated immune responses to auto- and microbial antigens *Gastroenterology* 2002; **123**: 689–99.

27 Lodes MJ, Cong Y, Elson CO, *et al.* Bacterial flagellin is a dominant antigen in Crohn disease. *J Clin Invest* 2004; **113**: 1296–306.

28 Kraus TA, Toy L, Chan L, *et al.* Failure to induce oral tolerance to a soluble protein in patients with inflammatory bowel disease. *Gastroenterology* 2004; **126**: 1771–8.

29 Kagnoff MF. Celiac disease: pathogenesis of a model immunogenetic disease. *J Clin Invest* 2007; **117**: 41–9.

30 Bealmear PM, Mirand EA, Holtermann OA. Miscellaneous immune defects in gnotobiotic and SPF mice. *Prog Clin Biol Res* 1983; **132C**: 423–32.

CHAPTER 5

Motor and Sensory Function

Eamonn M.M. Quigley

Department of Medicine, Alimentary Pharmabiotic Centre, University College Cork, Cork, Ireland

Summary

Studies of small intestinal and colonic motor activity in man have been limited by the relative inaccessibility of both organs and by issues related to the presence of stool in the colon. Nevertheless, considerable knowledge has been learned, from animal and human tissues, of the basic morphology and physiology of the small intestine and colon, and the primary patterns of motor activity in both organs have been described in normal man. The role of the gut as a sensory organ is increasingly recognized and the various neural elements involved in conveying sensory information to the central nervous system, as well as the areas in the brain activated by such input, have been identified. From these studies the importance of the intrinsic electrophysiological properties of gut smooth muscle cells, the primacy of interstitial cells of Cajal as pacemakers, and the ability of the enteric nervous system to generate and coordinate much of the motor activity of the gut regions have emerged as essential factors in gut motility and sensation.

Introduction

Through its role in digestion, absorption, secretion and excretion, the gastrointestinal tract and its associated organs play a central role in homeostasis. The various physiological functions of the gastrointestinal tract subserve these roles. Thus, in the small intestine, motility propels food, chyme, and stool along the gut, promotes mixing of chyme with intestinal enzymes to promote digestion, and increases contact time between luminal contents and the mucosa, promoting absorption [1]. In the colon, meanwhile, motility also supports the important roles of this organ in absorption, storage, and defecation. Thus tone is an important feature of motor activity in the colon, permitting changes in volume to accommodate stool; the colon is also capable of periodically generating high-amplitude phasic contractions that traverse the organ and propel stool into the rectum and coordinated activity in the rectum, sphincters, pelvic

floor. and abdominal musculature and diaphragm effect defecation [2].

The gut is also a sensory organ. While the roles of sensation in maintaining continence, generating defecation, and differentiating stool from gas are obvious examples of the importance of sensory input, much has been learned of late of other sensory activity in the small intestine and colon.

Gut Muscle and Nerve

The past several years have witnessed dramatic advances in our understanding of the physiology and morphology of the gastrointestinal motor apparatus. The ultrastructure and basic biochemistry of both gastrointestinal smooth muscle and nerve cells have been examined in detail and the complex properties of the enteric nervous system and its interactions with the autonomic and central nervous systems revealed [3–5]. Gut motor function is regulated by an elaborate neurohumoral system. Levels of control include: gut muscle, through its intrinsic properties and the close connections (nexi) that exist between individual smooth muscle cells, interstitial cells

Practical Gastroenterology and Hepatology: Small and Large Intestine and Pancreas, 1st edition. Edited by Nicholas J. Talley, Sunanda V. Kane and Michael B. Wallace. © 2010 Blackwell Publishing Ltd.

of Cajal (ICCs), acting as pacemakers in the small intestine and colon, the enteric nervous system, the extrinsic (autonomic) nervous input to the gut, and the central nervous system (CNS).

Throughout the small intestine, gut muscle is arranged in two circumferential layers, an outer longitudinal and an inner circular layer; in the cecum and colon the longitudinal layer is condensed into three bands, the taenia coli, which are arrayed equidistant from each other along the length of the large intestine as far as the rectum, where they are replaced by a complete longitudinal layer. In the anorectum, smooth muscle fibers of the internal anal sphincter function work in concert with striated muscle of the external anal sphincter and pelvic floor musculature to control continence and participate in the act of defecation.

Intracellular recordings from gut muscle in the small intestine have revealed its distinctive properties. These cells generate an omnipresent slow wave; a depolarization of the resting membrane potential which does not reach the critical level for firing of the action potential. While, in general, slow waves do not generate contractions, they do determine the frequency of contractions, given that action potentials (or spikes), which do cause contractions, occur on the summit of slow waves. In this manner, the frequency of phasic contractions, in a given part of the gut, is "phase-locked" to its slow wave frequency. Colonic smooth muscle electrophysiology is more complex [6] and includes differences between the electrical activity of the longitudinal and circular muscles and the observation that, unlike the small intestine, slow wave activity in colonic circular muscle is more variable in frequency and amplitude, averaging between two and four cycles per minute, is not omnipresent, and is sensitive to stretch and markedly altered by excitatory and inhibitory substances, *in vitro* properties that mirror the sensitivity of the colon to such factors as stress and meal ingestion in life. Recordings from human and canine colon have also identified a more rapid, oscillatory activity, which seems to originate along the outer border of the circular and longitudinal muscle layer [6]. Again in contrast to the small intestine, tone, a state of more sustained contraction, is an important function in the colon and is also critical to the function of sphincters.

Areas of close contact (nexi) between smooth muscle cells facilitate the transmission of electrical events between smooth muscle cells, allowing smooth muscle to function as a syncitium. Action potentials may result from neurogenic or neurochemical stimuli; the response of the smooth muscle cell to an incoming stimulus may also be influenced by modulatory events at the neuromuscular junction.

For decades it was assumed that slow waves originated in smooth muscle cells and ICCs, first described more than a century ago and found at various locations in the gut wall, including within the myenteric plexus, at the myenteric border between the circular and longitudinal smooth muscle cell layers (ICC-MY), and at the interface between the circular muscle and the submucosa (ICC-SM), were regarded as no more than a curiosity. How things have changed. We now know that, as summarized by Sanders *et al.* [7]: firstly, ICCs are pacemakers and actively propagate electrical slow waves in gastrointestinal muscles; secondly, ICCs mediate both inhibitory and excitatory motor neurotransmission; thirdly, ICCs serve as non-neural stretch receptors in gut muscle, affecting both smooth muscle excitability and slow wave frequency; and, finally, that ICCs form intimate associations with the intramuscular terminals of vagal afferents and, thereby, may have a role in afferent signaling. While their morphology varies according to location and may, in some instances, bear some resemblance to smooth muscle cells, it is now evident that these cells are neither neurons nor smooth muscle cells and are more likely to be derived from fibroblasts [8]. The recognition of the distinctive morphological, electrophysiological and biochemical properties of ICCs has led to the conclusion that the slow wave mechanism is an exclusive feature of the interstitial cells and that the active propagation of slow waves occurs through the interstitial cell network; slow waves are then electrotonically conducted into and depolarize smooth muscle cells [7,8]. There are important differences in the organization of electrical pacemaker activity between the small and large intestine. In the small bowel, electrical slow waves are generated by ICC-MYs; slow waves in the colon, in contrast to the small intestine, originate in ICC-SMs and actively propagate along the submucosal surface into the circular muscle [9]. Those ICCs which lie in close proximity to enteric nerves are those that play a role in the modulation of neurotransmission. It should be no surprise that absence of, or abnormalities in, ICCs have been demonstrated in a variety of clinical disorders of intestinal motility, including constipation [8].

The most important level of control of gut function resides within the gut itself, in the neurons and plexi of the enteric nervous system (ENS). It is now abundantly evident that the ENS is capable of generating and modulating many functions within the gastrointestinal tract without input from the autonomic or central nervous systems. Through variations in morphology, in the interconnections between neurons and plexi, as well as through the presence of a wide variety of neurotransmitters and neuromodultors, the ENS is capable of exhibiting striking plasticity in generating responses to stimuli, whether their origin is in the lumen, in the gut wall, or external to the gut. This plasticity is illustrated by the regulation and modulation of transmission of an electrical signal within the ENS. Such transmission may be influenced at either the presynaptic or postsynaptic level. For example, inhibitory or excitatory postsynaptic potentials may either "down-regulate" or "upregulate"/prime the postsynaptic neuron and thereby either diminish or accentuate, respectively, the likelihood of an action potential traveling down the presynaptic neuron and generating a response in the postsynaptic neuron. By virtue of variations in the longitudinal, circumferential, or cross-sectional extent of neuronal interactions the ENS can generate highly varied, complex, and, where appropriate, extensive responses to local stimuli. Such responses can involve one or other or both muscle layers in concert with, or in isolation from, the mucosa, as appropriate.

Support for the concept of the ENS as a "mini-brain" comes from the recognition that the neurally-isolated gut can generate and propagate such sophisticated motor events as the peristaltic reflex and the migrating motor complex. Indeed, it has become increasingly clear that input to the gut from the traditional branches of the autonomic nervous system influences gut function, not through direct synapses with the effector organs, gut muscle, and mucosa, but through the modulation of enteric neurons.

The characteristic structural feature of the enteric nervous system is the ganglionated plexus. There are two major ganglionated plexi within the wall of the hollow viscera of the gut, the submucosal (Meissner) plexus and the myenteric (Auerbach) plexus. The submucosal plexus is located in the submucosa and the more prominent myenteric plexus is found in the plane between the longitudinal and circular layers of the muscularis propria.

The submucosal and myenteric plexi consist of numerous ganglia—localized collections of nerve cell bodies, extensively interconnected by nerve bundles or strands. This gives the plexi the appearance of a flat meshwork with nodes (ganglia) at junctions in the mesh. The myenteric plexus is architecturally more than a network of ganglia and interconnecting nerve bundles; it also has a secondary structure that consists of nerve bundles that do not connect ganglia and a tertiary structure consisting of fine nerve fibers that ramify over the smooth muscle within the plane of the myenteric plexus. The plexi are continuous around the circumference of the gut wall and along the length of the gastrointestinal tract. The vast majority of neural elements in the ganglionated plexi are intrinsic in origin. Nerve bundles do run between the myenteric and submucosal plexi, thereby providing communication between them. The ganglia also contain glial cells. The neurons and the glial cells of enteric ganglia are tightly packed together so that only a basal lamina is present between them. Not even connective tissue elements or blood vessels penetrate the ganglion. Ganglia are partially enclosed by interstitial cells and connective tissue elements found between the muscle layers or in the submucosa.

The lack of a continuous connective tissue sheath means that neuronal cell bodies, dendrites, and glial cells, covered only by a basal lamina, are exposed to the extracellular milieu. Therefore, neurohumoral agents in the interstitial fluid have ready access to cells of the ganglia. Small blood vessels, in close proximity to ganglia of the myenteric plexus, create periganglionic networks in some species.

The organization of the plexus differs in the distal colon where bundles, referred to as shunt fascicles, which convey myelinated (parasympathetic and sympathetic efferents) and unmyelinated fibers (arising from the intrinsic nerves of the plexus) from the hypogastric plexi lie on the ganglia of the myenteric plexus.

Gut Sensation

Unlike the skin, specialized sensory receptors are not a feature of the intestinal mucosa; here, free nerve endings act as polymodal receptors responding to touch, acid, and other chemical stimuli [10]. Sensory information is conveyed from receptors in one of three types of primary afferent neuron:

1 Intrinsic primary afferent neurons (IPANs) whose cell bodies lie in the submucous or myenteric plexus

2 Vagal afferents whose cell bodies lie in the nodose ganglion and input primarily to the nucleus of the tractus solitarius

3 Splanchnic or spinal primary afferents whose cell bodies lie in the dorsal horn of the spinal cord and who synapse with second order neurons that ascend in the spinothalamic and spinoreticular tracts and the dorsal columns.

IPANs provide the sensory arm of intrinsic enteric reflexes while vagal and splanchnic afferents facilitate vagovagal and spinal reflexes and also the transmission of visceral sensory input to the higher centers. IPANs are present in both myenteric and submucosal ganglia and respond to luminal chemical stimuli, mechanical deformation of the mucosa, and muscle stretch and tension. IPANs may also be activated by serotonin, released locally, in a paracrine fashion, by enterochromaffin cells. Visceral sensory axons are almost exclusively thin myelinated Aδ or unmyelinated C fibers. Spinal afferents include a population of capsaicin-sensitive unmyelinated C fibers which contain neuropeptides such as calcitonin gene-related peptide (CGRP), VIP, somatostatin, and dynorphin and the tachykinins substance P and neurokinin A and are the primary route for the transmission of a variety of nocicepitve stimuli from the gut. These fibers respond to a variety of inflammatory mediators; stimuli which also awaken silent nociceptor fibers. Vagal afferent axons ramify extensively in the enteric plexi and infiltrate muscle sheets where they course with ICCs. Vagal afferents include mucosal chemosensitive and mechanosensitive neurons as well as neurons conveying input from tension receptors in the muscle layers. Mucosal receptors on vagal afferents are primarily activated by "physiological" mechanical and chemical stimuli; their proximity to enteroendocrine and mast cells suggests that they may also be activated by serotonin (e.g., in the induction of nausea and vomiting) and other neuropeptides. While vagal afferents are viewed as predominantly involved in the transmission of non-noxious stimuli, they should not be viewed as irrelevant to nociception. Indeed, vagal fibers may not only transmit nociceptive input but may also play an important role in the modulation of nociceptive information traversing other pathways

through the activation of antinociceptive descending spinal pathways.

The Autonomic Nervous System

Most of the constituent nerve fibers of the vagus nerve are afferent neurons; that is, neurons carrying sensory information away from the gut and toward more central nervous structures.

Vagal efferent fibers, that is neurons carrying information from the CNS to the gastrointestinal tract, arise from cell bodies in the dorsal motor nucleus of the vagus and the nucleus ambiguous. Those originating in the dorsal motor nucleus are preganglionic parasympathetic fibers that project to the smooth muscle esophagus, stomach, the small intestine, and the proximal half of the colon. Tracer studies indicate that these efferent fibers terminate in the myenteric ganglia, but that most of the neuronal elements in the ganglia are not contacted by the vagal efferent fibers. The density of the vagal efferent innervation decreases steadily from the stomach to the ileocecal junction.

The mesenteric nerves arise in the prevertebral (celiac, superior mesenteric, and inferior mesenteric) ganglia and travel through the mesentery to the stomach and intestine. Most of the axons in the mesenteric nerves are efferent adrenergic fibers arising from cell bodies in the prevertebral ganglia. These are the postganglionic sympathetic fibers that make up the adrenergic neural supply to the gut. Neurons of the prevertebral ganglia receive synaptic inputs from the preganglionic sympathetic fibers which, in turn, arise from cell bodies in the inferomediolateral columns from levels T4 to L4 of the spinal cord. They also receive inputs from afferent neurons located in the wall of the gut.

The pelvic plexus is a ganglionated plexus that is located on either side of the rectum. Nerves from this plexus project to the aboral part of the gastrointestinal tract and to the urogenital organs.

The autonomic nerves act not only as the conduit for information between the gut and the CNS but also function as the afferent and efferent arcs of so-called "long" reflexes in the gut, such as the gastrocolonic and intestinointestinal reflexes. In this manner, the autonomic nerves permit the rapid transmission of information between distant parts of the gut and, thereby, to the generation of rapid responses in one organ to a stimulus in another. Were these signals to be transmitted through gut muscle and the enteric nervous system, the response would be much delayed or non-existent.

The "Big" Brain and Gut Function

Anther area of well-documented interaction between the CNS and the gut relates to the effects of stress on gut function. A variety of stressors have been clearly and consistently demonstrated to profoundly affect gut motor and absorptive function through both neural and hormonal mechanisms. The hypothalamic–pituitary–adrenal (HPA) axis plays a key role in the latter [11]. The development of relatively non-invasive and accurate techniques for dynamic cerebral imaging has permitted an exploration of the afferent side of the inter-action—the responses of the brain to gut events [12]. Let us now turn to a discussion of the motor patterns generated by gut muscle and nerve and their regulatory systems in man.

Small Intestinal Motor Activity

The definition of normality in any area of gastrointestinal motility continues to pose a formidable clinical challenge. First and foremost, testing small intestinal motility is invasive and studies in normal volunteers have therefore been limited. Indeed, as more are performed the extent of the range of normal variation is increasingly appreciated.

The first detailed observations of small intestinal motor patterns were those performed by Walter Cannon in the unanesthetized cat almost a century ago [13]. From prolonged, meticulous observations on the movement of a radiopaque marker through the gut and based on his drawings, Cannon described the basic patterns of the movement of intestinal contents. Later, recordings from intraluminal balloons and non-perfused catheters identified individual contractions at a limited number of sites in the proximal small intestine. More recent, technical advances have permitted recordings from multiple sites over prolonged periods of time and along the entire length of the intestine. Currently, recordings of small intestinal motor activity, in man, are performed using

either low compliance perfusion or solid-state systems. The former involves the peroral or pernasal placement of a multilumen catheter assembly into the intestine, each lumen being attached to a pneumohydraulic, low-compliance perfusion apparatus, a system that, though usually performed with the subject recumbent and stationary, can be modified to ambulatory recordings [14]. One major advantage of the perfused system is that multiple catheters and, therefore, recording sites at variable intervals are possible. Solid-state systems involve the intraluminal placement of a catheter assembly containing miniaturized strain gauges. These are, in turn, connected either to a stationary recorder or, more commonly, to an ambulatory recording system, similar to ambulatory pH recorders, which the patient wears around their waist. While initially limited to a maximum of six to eight sensors, recent progress in the development of solid-state systems for esophageal manometry has seen the incorporation of 36 solid state sensors in a single assembly [15]. By combining the output from circumferentially sensitive sensors spaced at just 1-cm intervals, with sophisticated algorithms to display the expanded manometric dataset as pressure topography plots rather than overlapping line tracings, the age of high-resolution manometry had arrived [16].

Regardless of the system used, the basic motor patterns recorded are similar, being organized, in the fasted state, into recurring cycles of the migrating motor complex (MMC), and featuring a fed response to meal administration (Figure 5.1). Each MMC cycle comprises three phases, which occur in sequence and continue to recur as long as the individual remains fasted. Each cycle begins with a period of quiescence (phase 1), is followed by a period of apparently irregular contractions which increase in frequency and amplitude (phase 2), and culminates in a burst of uninterrupted phasic activity (phase 3) which slowly migrates along the intestine from the proximal duodenum. Simultaneous with the onset of phase 3 activity in the duodenum, related activity occurs in the stomach, gall bladder, and biliary tree. In man, in contrast to some animal species, phase 3 tends to peter out in the terminal ileum. Following the administration of a meal of adequate caloric composition, two things happen; the MMC is interrupted and is replaced by the fed pattern, a period of irregular but intense contractions which last from 2 to 6 h, depending on meal size and content (Figure 5.2).

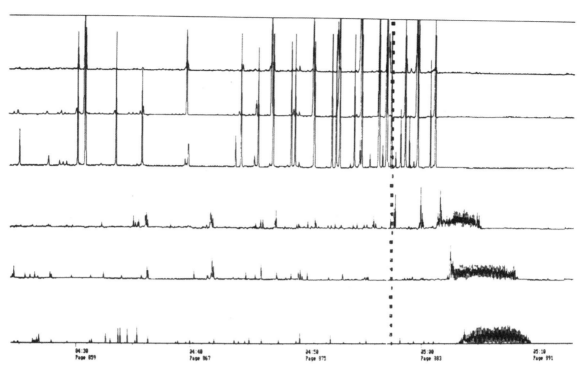

Figure 5.1 Fasting motor activity from the human antrum (top three tracings) small intestine (lower three tracings). Note irregular activity (phase 2) recorded from all sites, culminating in a burst of rhythmic activity (phase 3) which slowly traverses the segment and is followed by quiescence (phase 1) of the next cycle.

What is the normal range of variation of these patterns? Twenty-four hour recordings in a fully ambulatory state of normal individuals going about their usual activities have revealed the extreme variability in the frequency of the migrating motor complex [17]; the number recorded in a given individual varying, from as few as one, to as many as eight. These 24-h studies also emphasize the significance of diurnal variations in normal small bowel motility. Other factors also contribute to variability. For example, recordings performed along the length of the small intestine have revealed the extent of regional variations. In man, the ileocolonic junctional region demonstrates quite different patterns; here the migrating motor complex peters out and is replaced by irregular activity, grouped or clustered contractions, and occasional high-amplitude, prolonged, propagated contractions [18]. Clustered activity is also prominent in the proximal duodenum where motor activity is closely synchronized with that of the distal antrum. Gender may also be relevant; variations in such motor parameters as

gastric emptying have been demonstrated in relation to the phase of the menstrual cycle, as well as during pregnancy. Finally, both acute and chronic stress have been shown to be capable of causing significant disruption to motor patterns in the stomach and small intestine. Certain stresses can, indeed, completely interrupt the postprandial response and lead to its replacement by phase type 3 activity. Given the invasive nature of small intestinal manometry, one cannot discount the possible, and variable, effects of stress on recorded motor activity.

Colonic Motility

Because of its relative inaccessibility and the difficulties posed by the presence of solid or semisolid fecal material, our understanding of colonic motility lags far behind that of the small intestine [19]. Initially studies of colonic motor function focused on phasic contractile activity.

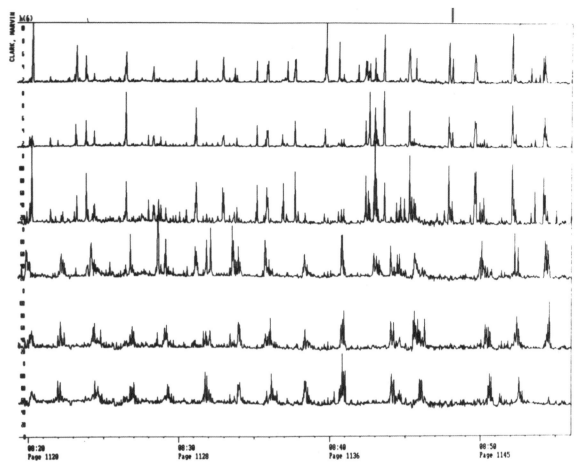

Figure 5.2 The fed motor pattern; same recording sites as Figure 5.1. The migrating motor complex has been abolished and is replaced by intense, irregular activity at all sites.

Because of the challenges posed by the prolonged recordings that are necessary to describe normal phasic motor patterns in this organ, there is surprisingly little information on colonic motility in man, in health or in disease. While consensus is lacking in this area, it seems reasonable to summarize the current status of our knowledge of colonic motor patterns by stating that colonic motility, in man, presents alternating periods of activity and quiescence (Figure 5.3). Some recognizable patterns have been described in the active periods: individual phasic contractions, propagating contractions, propagating bursts or clusters of contractions and, most recognizable of all, high amplitude propagating contractions (HAPCs). The latter are more prevalent in children than in adults,

are associated with the mass movement of fecal material over segments of the colon and may be accompanied by the passage of flatus or the urge to defecate. HAPCs typically propagate from the cecum or ascending colon to the sigmoid colon at a velocity of 1 cm/min. They may be induced by the administration of laxatives such as cascara and bisacodyl. Given the distinctive nature of this motor phenomenon and the fact that it can be induced, as described, it has served as a marker of the integrity of colonic motor function in diseases states. While there is a surprising degree of between-study variability in this area, most studies have indicated that colonic motility is affected by food intake (the so-called gastrocolonic reflex, whose intensity is influenced considerably by the

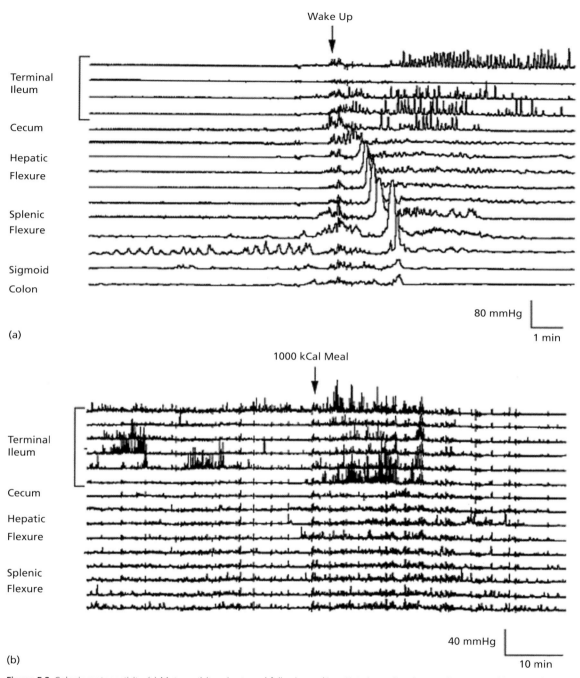

Figure 5.3 Colonic motor activity. (a) Motor activity prior to and following waking. Note immediate increase in motor activity on waking which includes a high-amplitude propagating contraction (HAPC) in the more distal sites. (b) Fed motor response. Note immediate increase in motor activity. (Reproduced from Bampton PA *et al*. [20], by permission from Macmillan Publishers Ltd.)

location of the recording sensor, being more intense in the sigmoid colon), diurnal variation, exercise, and stress. It is certainly clear that, in comparison to the small intestine, the colon is more susceptible to the influences of the autonomic and central nervous systems, a fitting arrangement given our necessity to regulate the time and place of voluntary defecation.

The most complete assessment of normal human colonic motility has been provided by Bampton and colleagues [20]. They advanced a 16-channel perfused side-hole catheter assembly through the nares in an antegrade fashion into the colon in 14 healthy volunteers. They identified a number of patterns of propagated activity, antegrade and retrograde, high amplitude and low amplitude. High-amplitude contractions, corresponding to HAPCs, propagated more slowly but over greater lengths of the colon, were more prominent after a meal, and were more likely to result in an urge to defecate. All propagated activity diminished at night and during sleep, only to increase dramatically on waking. A pattern of non-propagated clusters of phasic contractions, which had been recognized by others in the rectum and had therefore been referred to as the rectal motor complex, were observed by Bampton and colleagues to also occur in the right colon [20].

The advent of such techniques as the barostat has permitted the examination of patterns of tonic activity in the colon and has revealed the importance of fluctuations in tone in colonic homeostasis. In the colon, tone is low during sleep, rises on waking, and increases further following meal ingestion or the instillation of short-chain fatty acids. Again, between-study variations, related in part to technical and protocol issues, limit our ability to draw firm conclusions in this area.

Motor Activity of the Anorectum

When colonic contents reach the rectum, a sensation of rectal fullness is generated by rectal afferents, probably arising from activation of stretch receptors in the mesentery or pelvic floor muscles. In response to this, a "sampling" reflex, also known as the rectoanal inhibitory or rectosphincteric reflex, is generated and leads to internal anal sphincter relaxation and external sphincter contractions. At this stage, the individual can decide to postpone or, if it is considered socially acceptable, proceed with defecation. To facilitate the process, the puborectalis muscle and external anal sphincter relax, thereby straightening the rectoanal angle and opening the anal canal. The propulsive force for defecation is then generated by contractions of the diaphragm and the muscles of the abdominal wall which now propel the rectal contents through the open sphincter. The internal anal sphincter is a continuation of the smooth muscle of the rectum and is under sympathetic control. It provides approximately 80% of normal resting anal tone. The external anal sphincter and pelvic floor muscles are striated muscles, innervated, respectively, by sacral roots 3 and 4 and the pudendal nerve. The anorectum represents, therefore, the other site of convergence of the somatic and autonomic nervous systems and is susceptible to disorders of both striated and smooth muscle, as well as to diseases of the central, peripheral, and autonomic nervous systems.

Small Intestinal, Colonic, and Anorectal Sensation

In contrast to our understanding of the aforementioned role of sensation in the anorectum, our knowledge of sensory activity in the remainder of the colon and small intestine is far from complete. Visceral afferent input is conveyed to the central nervous system by rapidly conducting myelinated Aδ fibers, and slower, non-myelinated C fibers. These nerve fibers reach the central nervous system via either the vagus nerve (which consists of 60% afferent fibers at the level of the diaphragm) or spinal afferents. Spinal afferents have their cell bodies in the dorsal root ganglia, and constitute the first in a chain of three neurons conveying gut afferent input to conscious perception. The second-order neuron is the dorsal horn neuron in the spinal cord which sends information along the lateral spinothalamic or spinoreticular tracts. In addition, there is a mid-line dorsal column nociceptive pathway conveying pain sensation from abdominal and pelvic viscera to brainstem centers. The third-order neurons project from the latter to cortical or subcortical centers that convey the specific sensation (somewhat localized to the gut area), and the associated symptoms such as affective responses, appetite changes, or autonomic features. It is thought that pain results when sensory fibers are inflamed or stimulated more intensely. Sensations have a diffuse nature, unless the parietal peritoneum is stimulated with resultant stimulation of somatic afferents. The dorsal horn neuron to which visceral fibers project also receives input from somatic nerves.

Most stimuli in the gut are, however, not consciously perceived. What leads to such stimuli from the small intestine and colon being not only being perceived but becoming noxious is a topic of much interest to those who study painful functional disorders, such as irritable bowel syndrome (IBS). Studies of colonic sensation have focused, in particular, on the role of visceral hypersensitivity and/or hyperalgesia in IBS. Here, the barostat has proven to be valuable tool in generating reproducible and clinically relevant levels of distension in the rectum and colon. Distension studies have revealed the poorly localized nature of colonic discomfort and pain; stimuli in the rectum, for example, giving rise, in some subjects, to symptoms localized to various parts of the abdomen. Advanced and dynamic brain imaging techniques have also permitted the mapping of those areas of the CNS that respond to stimuli applied to various parts of the gut and have been widely applied to the study of brain responses to rectal and colonic distension.

Take-home points

- Gut smooth muscle, the interstitial cells of Cajal, and the enteric nervous system work in unison to generate, propagate, and modulate most motor events in the small intestine and colon.

- Extrinsic neural influences exert a greater impact on the colon than the small intestine.

- Sensation is an important but poorly understood phenomenon in the normal colon and small intestine.

- During fasting, motor activity in the small intestine is organized into recurring cycles of the migrating motor complex; on meal ingestion this is abolished and replaced by the fed motor response.

- Motor activity in the colon is more complex and less readily characterized but features diurnal variation, a meal response, and powerful contractions that can traverse much of the colon and induce an urge to defecate.

References

1 Quigley EMM. Gastric and small intestinal motility in health and disease. *Gastroenterol Clin N Am* 1996; **25**: 113–46.

2 Quigley EMM. Colonic motility and colonic motor function. In: Pemberton JH, Swash M, Henry MM, eds. *The Pelvic Floor, its Function and Disorders.* Philadelphia: WB Saunders, 2002: 84–93.

3 Furness JB, Costa M. *The Enteric Nervous System.* Edinburgh: Churchill Livingstone, 1986.

4 Goyal RK, Hirano I. Mechanisms of disease: the enteric nervous system. *New Engl J Med* 1996; **334**: 1106–15.

5 Furness JB. The enteric nervous system: normal functions and enteric neuropathies. *Neurogastroenterol Motil* 2008; **20** (Suppl. 1): 32–8.

6 Rae MG, Fleming N, McGregor DB, *et al.* Control of motility patterns in the human colonic circular muscle layer by pacemaker activity. *J Physiol* 1998; **510**: 309–20.

7 Sanders KM, Koh SD, Ward SM. Interstitial cells of Cajal as pacemakers in the gastrointestinal tract. *Annu Rev Physiol* 2006; **68**: 307–43.

8 Streutker CJ, Huizinga JD, Driman DK, Riddell RH. Interstitial cells of Cajal in health and disease. Part I: normal ICC structure and function with associated motility disorders. *Histopathology* 2007; **50**: 176–89.

9 Lee HT, Hennig GW, Park KJ, *et al.* Heterogeneities in ICC Ca2+ activity within canine large intestine. *Gastroenterology* 2009; **136**: 2226–36.

10 Kellow JE, Azpiroz F, Delvaux M, *et al.* Applied principles of neurogastroenterology: physiology/ motility sensation. *Gastroenterology* 2006; **130**: 1412–20.

11 Taché Y, Bonaz B. Corticotropin-releasing factor receptors and stress-related alterations of gut motor function. *J Clin Invest* 2007; **117**: 33–40.

12 Sharma A, Lelic D, Brock C, *et al.* New technologies to investigate the brain-gut axis. *World J Gastroenterol* 2009; **15**: 182–91.

13 Quigley EMM. Intestinal manometry in man: an historical and clinical perspective. *Dig Dis Sci* 1994; **12**: 199–209.

14 Samsom M, Smout AJPM, Hebbard G, *et al.* A novel portable perfused manometric system for recording of small intestinal motility. *Neurogastroenterol Motil* 1998; **10**: 149–56.

15 Pandolfino JE, Kahrilas PJ. New technologies in the gastrointestinal clinic and research: impedance and high-resolution manometry. *World J Gastroenterol* 2009; **15**: 131–8.

16 Kahrilas PJ, Ghosh SK, Pandolfino JE. Challenging the limits of esophageal manometry. *Gastroenterology* 2008; **134**: 16–8.

17 Wilson P, Perdikis G, Hinder RA, *et al.* Prolonged ambulatory antroduodenal manometry in humans. *Am J Gastroenterol* 1994; **89**: 1489–95.

18 Quigley EMM, Borody TJ, Phillips SF, *et al.* Motility of the terminal ileum and ileocaecal sphincter in healthy man. *Gastroenterology* 1984; **87**: 857–66.

19 Camilleri M, Ford MJ. Colonic sensorimotor physiology in health and its alteration in constipation and diarrheal disorders. *Aliment Pharmacol Ther* 1998; **12**: 287–302.

20 Bampton PA, Dinning PG, Kennedy ML, *et al.* Prolonged multi-point recording of colonic manometry in the unprepared human colon: providing insight into potentially relevant pressure wave parameters. *Am J Gastroenterol* 2001; **96**: 1838–48.

CHAPTER 6
Neoplasia

John M. Carethers

Department of Internal Medicine, University of Michigan, Ann Arbor, MI, USA

Summary

Neoplasia, the abnormal proliferation of cells, causes a macroscopic tumor that is often benign initially, but can progress to malignancy due to successive waves of clonality caused by genomic instability. The genetic damage to cause the genomic instability comes from environmental and genetic stresses that ultimately damage a stem cell's DNA, allowing that stem cell to evade normal mechanisms that typically regulate its growth and proliferation. Neoplasms occur anywhere in the gastrointestinal tract, and each organ that is affected has different gender distributions as well as a differing prognosis. Benign neoplasms are often found incidentally or at screening, while malignant neoplasms typically present symptomatically. Multiple neoplasms in one person as well as family history may identify individuals at high risk and who can be targeted for surveillance. Gastrointestinal neoplasms are removed surgically or at endoscopy, but malignant ones may need additional chemoradiation treatment.

Case

A 43-year-old male with a family history of colorectal cancer presented with iron-deficiency anemia. Colonoscopy revealed a circumferential sigmoid adenocarcinoma (stage II) and was surgically resected. Follow-up colonoscopy 2 years later revealed a large (stage II) transverse adenocarcinoma. Genetic testing revealed a germline *hMLH1* gene mutation identifying Lynch syndrome, and the patient was recommended to have a subtotal colectomy, but refused and had a segmental resection, then was lost to follow up. Five years later, he returned for routine care, offered a colonoscopy that revealed a circumferential (stage IV) cecal adenocarcinoma, and the remainder of his colon was resected. He was treated with chemotherapy, but the patient succumbed to metastatic colonic adenocarcinoma a year later.

Definition and Epidemiology

Neoplasia refers to the abnormal proliferation of cells. At the macroscopic level, neoplasia results in a neoplasm, or

Practical Gastroenterology and Hepatology: Small and Large Intestine and Pancreas, 1st edition. Edited by Nicholas J. Talley, Sunanda V. Kane and Michael B. Wallace. © 2010 Blackwell Publishing Ltd.

tumor. Neoplasms within the gastrointestinal tract generally start out as benign lesions that, if discovered and treated, have no untoward effect on patient survival. Often, neoplasms may indolently grow and transform into malignant tumors, which then can threaten survival [1].

The gastrointestinal tract, including the hollow organs of the gut, pancreas, liver, and biliary tree, is the site of more cancers and the source of more cancer mortality than any other organ system in the body. As shown in Table 6.1, cancer incidence from the gastrointestinal tract for 2009 in the US is over 275 000 cases [2]. However, this number greatly underestimates the incidence for all gastrointestinal neoplasms because those that are benign or remain indolent are not included, and probably would increase the neoplasm incidence at least fivefold or more. Table 6.1 also shows that there are differences in the male-to-female incidence, as well as the gastrointestinal cancers that are relatively more deadly, such as esophageal, pancreas, and liver cancers. These differences may be related to a multitude of factors but include: (i) gender and hormone differences, (ii) differing levels of exposure to environmental carcinogens, (iii) the late presentation and discovery of certain neoplasms clinically, (iv) genetic

Table 6.1 Incidence and mortality of gastrointestinal cancers in the US (2009).

Cancer	Incidence	Male incidence	Female incidence	Deaths	Annual deaths/incidence (%)
Esophagus	16 470	12 940	3530	14 530	88
Stomach	21 130	12 820	8310	10 620	50
Small intestine	6230	3240	2990	1110	18
Pancreas	42 470	21 050	21 420	35 240	83
Liver and intrahepatic duct	22 620	16 410	6210	18 160	80
Gall bladder and biliary ducts	9760	4320	5440	3370	35
Colon and rectum	146 970	75 590	71 380	49 920	34
Anus and anorectum	5290	2100	3190	710	13
Other digestive organs	4780	1550	3230	2170	45
Total	**275 720**	**150 020**	**125 700**	**135 830**	**49**

Adapted from Jemal A, Siegel R, Ward E, Hao Y, Xu J, Thun MJ. Cancer statistics, 2009. *CA Cancer J Clin* 2009; **59**: 225–49.

factors, and (v) the response to therapy for specific cancers [1].

Clinical Features

Benign neoplasms often are asymptomatic, and are typically discovered incidentally or during screening or surveillance. The best recognized benign lesion in the gastrointestinal tract is the colonic adenoma due to the screening of all persons over the age of 50 years, with only a few percent of adenomas progressing to cancer. Size and histology of adenomas can predict future risk for colon cancer, and these features are used in algorithms for surveillance [1]. Other gastrointestinal organs may have begun as benign neoplasms prior to malignancy and include: pancreatic intraepithelial neoplasia, adenomas of the stomach, small intestine, and colon, and benign neuroendocrine tumors.

Malignant neoplasms can be discovered incidentally, but are more often brought to medical attention due to patient symptoms. Esophageal cancers often present with solid-food dysphagia; pancreatic, liver, and gastric cancers may present with abdominal pain and weight loss; colon and small intestinal cancers may present with weight loss, bowel obstruction, and iron-deficiency anemia. Anal cancers may present with rectal pain and bleeding.

In some cases that are important to recognize, a familial component to gastrointestinal tract and other cancers may exist [3]. Clues such as young age of presen-tation, a strong family history for cancers, multiple neoplasms in an individual, and some clinical features in a patient may determine if the patient should be evaluated for genetic counseling and genetic testing. Identifying these high-risk individuals will make them targets for regular surveillance strategies which will extend their life span.

Pathophysiology

The abnormal cellular growth that defines neoplasia is born out of alterations to normal cellular proteins which change the normal cellular responses and checkpoints in cells. The alterations may occur via environmental factors (e.g., toxin exposure such as tobacco or alcohol for pancreatic, liver, and esophageal squamous cell cancer; acidic bile exposure for esophageal adenocarcinoma; ingested fats and microbiome changes for colorectal cancer; certain viral etiologies for liver and anal cancers; and *Helicobacter pylori* for gastric cancer) as well as inherited genetic factors that affect key growth regulatory genes in affected patients, predisposing them to neoplastic growth [3–5].

The paradigm of environmental or inherited genetic damage to a stem cell (termed genomic instability) [1,6,7] followed by subsequent clonal expansion with continued genetic alteration during accelerated cellular proliferation, which transforms normal cells to an initially benign but rapidly growing lesion to a malignant tumor capable of metastasizing to distant organs, holds for most gastrointestinal neoplasms [1]. Stem cell proteins can ultimately be altered by a number of DNA damage mechanisms, including: mutation, loss of heterozygosity or chromosome breakage, rearrangement, amplification, methylation, acetylation and deacetylation, inactivation of DNA repair mechanisms, telomerase damage, as well as non-DNA mechanisms such as microRNA expression [1,6–8]. Damaged cells have deregulated growth pathways, subvert normal cell cycle checkpoints, and avoid programmed cell death mechanisms. The best studied of these is the adenoma-to-carcinoma sequence in the colon, due to the accessibility of the colon with colonoscopy. Specific genetic changes have been detected and can be predicted during each wave of clonal expansion which matches the histology of the growing adenoma and its transformation into cancer [1,5–7,9,10]. As depicted in Figure 6.1, sporadic colon adenomas may take three to five decades of life to form, with another one to two decades to become malignant, and may be a consequence of environmental exposure in the colon plus some genetic factors. In familial adenomatous polyposis (FAP), the development of adenomas is greatly accelerated due to an inherited germline mutation in the *APC* gene, but the malignant transformation rate is the same as in the sporadic condition. With Lynch syndrome, adenomas form at the same rate as sporadic ones, but malignant transformation is accelerated due to loss of function of the DNA mismatch repair system [1,3].

Diagnosis

Because of the internal nature of the organs that make of the gastrointestinal tract, diagnosis of neoplasms involves the use of radiologic imaging studies (e.g., computed tomography, magnetic resonance imaging, ultrasound, contrast X-ray), direct endoscopic viewing (e.g., esophagogastroduodenoscopy, colonoscopy, wireless capsule video endoscopy, double balloon enteroscopy), or

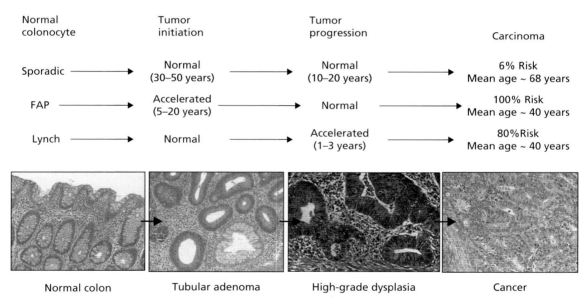

Figure 6.1 Depiction of colorectal tumor progression in sporadic and high-risk genetic syndromes. The general paradigm is that a tumor is initiated from a normal colonocyte stem cell that has sustained genetic damage over time due to the local environment and any germline genetic mutation that has been inherited. The damaged DNA provides a growth advantage that drives tumor progression as successive clonal outgrowths are generated, ultimately forming carcinoma. In familial adenomatous polyposis, tumor initiation is accelerated with the inheritance of a germline *APC* mutation, and in Lynch syndrome, tumor progression is accelerated due to the hypermutable phenotype that occurs with loss of DNA mismatch repair. Photomicrographs depict, in order, normal colon, tubular adenoma, high-grade dysplasia, and cancer.

Table 6.2 Examples of oncofetal antigen markers in the gastrointestinal tract.

Marker	Epitope	Primary tumor with serum elevation	Other tumors with serum elevation
CEA	Multiple glycosylation sites on an immunoglobin-like protein	Colorectum	Stomach, pancreas, biliary tract, liver
CA 19-9	Sialylated Lewis A	Pancreas	Stomach, biliary tract, liver, colorectum
CAM 17.1	Sialyl I blood group antigen	Pancreas	Biliary tract
CA 50	Sialylated Lewis A	Pancreas	Stomach, biliary tract, liver, colorectum
CA 242	Mucin-like antigen	Colorectum	Pancreas
CA 72-4	Mucin-like glycoprotein (sialosyl-2-6-6-alpha-N-acetylgalactosaminyl)	Pancreas, ovary	Colorectum
CA 125	Mucin-like molecule	Ovary	Colorectum
α-Fetoprotein	Multiple isoforms of an albuminoid molecule	Liver	Biliary tract, stomach

CEA, carcinoembryonic antigen; CA, cancer antigen; CAM, cancer antigen immunoglobin M antibody.

combined radiologic and endoscopic modalities (e.g., endoscopic ultrasound, endoscopic retrograde cholangiopancreatography). Many of these modalities allow tissue sampling for pathological diagnosis.

Many gastrointestinal neoplasms secrete oncofetal antigens, usually in the malignant stage (Table 6.2). These serum biomarkers are useful for confirming a diagnosis of a cancer, or can be used in surveillance for recurrence. Oncofetal antigens have not been useful as the sole primary diagnostic modality for gastrointestinal tumors.

Treatment

Most gastrointestinal neoplasms are removed at surgery or at endoscopy. Patients are cured of their neoplasm if a benign lesion is completely removed. Malignant neoplasms often will require surgery for attempted cure, and depending on the staging of the tumor, may require pre- and/or postsurgical chemoradiation [11,12]. Chemoprevention may be effective in some patients that belong to high-risk groups, such as FAP [13]. Advances in the understanding of the molecular pathogenesis of some tumors have led to the development of targeted drugs that may dramatically shrink a tumor, such as imatinib for use in gastrointestinal stromal tumors [14].

Take-home points

- Abnormal cell growth, or neoplasia, can occur anywhere in the GI tract from the mouth to the anus.
- Neoplasia can commence as a benign but altered growth process or mass, and can progress to a malignant process, eventually affecting survival.
- Neoplasms reflect altered cellular processes that change the balance of cell proliferation and cell death in favor of proliferation.
- Genetic predisposition and environmental factors affect an individual's neoplastic risk, and surveillance programs for high-risk individuals may improve detection and survival.
- Some gastrointestinal neoplasms secrete oncofetal antigens, which can be used as markers for the presence or recurrence of a neoplasm.

Acknowledgments

Supported by the United States Public Health Service (DK067287), the UCSD Digestive Diseases Research Development Center (DK080506), the SDSU/UCSD Comprehensive Cancer Center Partnership (CA132379 and CA13238), and the VA Research Service (Merit Review Award).

References

1 Grady WM, Carethers JM. Genomic and epigenetic instability in colorectal cancer pathogenesis. *Gastroenterology* 2008; **135**: 1079–99.

2 Jemal A, Siegel R, Ward E, *et al.* Cancer statistics, 2009. *CA Cancer J Clin* 2009; **59**: 225–49.

3 Boland CR, Koi M, Chang DK, Carethers JM. The biochemical basis of microsatellite instability and abnormal immunohistochemistry and clinical behavior in Lynch syndrome: from bench to bedside. *Familial Cancer* 2008; **7**: 41–52.

4 Anderson AR, Weaver AM, Cummings PT, Quaranta V. Tumor morphology and phenotypic evolution driven by selective pressure from the microenvironment. *Cell* 2006; **127**: 905–15.

5 Kinzler KW, Vogelstein B. Cancer-susceptibility genes. Gatekeepers and caretakers. *Nature* 1997; **386**: 761, 3.

6 Vogelstein B, Fearon ER, Hamilton SR, *et al.* Genetic alterations during colorectal-tumor development. *N Engl J Med* 1988; **319**: 525–32.

7 Issa JP. CpG island methylator phenotype in cancer. *Nat Rev Cancer* 2004; **4**: 988–93.

8 Kim DH, Rossi JJ. Strategies for silencing human disease using RNA interference. *Nat Rev Genet* 2007; **8**: 173–84.

9 Markowitz S, Wang J, Myeroff L, *et al.* Inactivation of the type II TGF-beta receptor in colon cancer cells with microsatellite instability. *Science* 1995; **268**: 1336–8.

10 Jung B, Doctolero RT, Tajima A, *et al.* Loss of activin receptor type 2 protein expression in microsatellite unstable colon cancers. *Gastroenterology* 2004; **126**: 654–9.

11 Carethers JM. Systemic treatment of advanced colorectal cancer—tailoring therapy to the tumor. *Ther Adv Gastroenterol* 2008; **1**: 33–42.

12 Potti A, Dressman HK, Bild A, *et al.* Genomic signatures to guide the use of chemotherapeutics. *Nat Med* 2006; **12**: 1294–300.

13 Steinbach G, Lynch PM, Phillips RK, *et al.* The effect of celecoxib, a cyclooxygenase-2 inhibitor, in familial adenomatous polyposis. *N Engl J Med* 2000; **342**: 1946–52.

14 Heinrich MC, Blanke CD, Druker BJ, Corless CL. Inhibition of KIT tyrosine kinase activity: a novel molecular approach to the treatment of KIT-positive malignancies. *J Clin Oncol* 2002; **20**: 1692–703.

PART 2

Colonoscopy, Endoscopic Retrograde Cholangiopancreato-graphy, and Endoscopic Ultrasound

CHAPTER 7
Technique of Colonoscopy

Anna M. Buchner[1] and Michael B. Wallace[2]

[1] Department of Gastroenterology, University of Pennsylvania, Philadelphia, PA, USA
[2] Division of Gastroenterology and Hepatology, Mayo Clinic, Jacksonville, FL, USA

Summary

Colonoscopy has been essential in the evaluation of colorectal symptoms and screening of colorectal cancer. Colonoscopy remains the gold standard for detecting and removal of colon polyps in hope of preventing colorectal cancer. This chapter will review the basic techniques of successful colonoscopy exam including colonoscopy intubation and extubation. It will also discuss the adjunctive imaging techniques such as chromoendoscopy and magnification endoscopy developed to help in detection of neoplastic lesions during the colonoscopy exam.

Introduction

Colonoscopy is widely accepted as the gold standard procedure for the detection and prevention of colorectal cancer and evaluation of colorectal symptoms. Colonoscopies with polypectomies are estimated to prevent 76 to 90% of incident colorectal cancers [1]. However colonoscopy remains still as an imperfect tool for neoplasia detection, with missing rates ranging from 17 to 48% [2,3]. It carries also the risk of complications with bleeding and perforation [4]. Thus, the successful colonoscopy has the goals of maximizing detection of adenomas and cancers during colonoscopy and avoidance of procedure-related complications.

Basic Techniques

Colonoscopy Intubation

The success rates of cecal intubation ranges from 90 to 95% [5,6]. Colonoscopy involves passage of the colonoscope through colons of variable length, mobility, and fixation. This procedure is reported to be more difficult

Practical Gastroenterology and Hepatology: Small and Large Intestine and Pancreas, 1st edition. Edited by Nicholas J. Talley, Sunanda V. Kane and Michael B. Wallace. © 2010 Blackwell Publishing Ltd.

in slender female patients with acute rectosigmoid angle and prior pelvic surgeries [7].

Anus and Rectum

The colonoscopic exam starts from the inspection of the perianal area and digital rectal exam. This allows identification of skin lesions, anal fissure, hemorrhoids, or prolapsed abnormalities. The colonoscope's tip is slowly introduced in the direction indicated by digital palpation up to 5 cm, followed by advancement to the rectosigmoid junction.

To complete an examination of the rectum (at the end of extubation) retroflexion is required. This involves a selection of the widest part of rectal vault, applying full upward with lateral angulation, followed by pushing inward. In some instances, where there is scarring or severe inflammation, the exam should be performed only in the prograde view.

Sigmoid Colon

The sigmoid colon is located intraperitoneally. Advancing the colonoscope through the sigmoid colon toward the descending colon can be challenging in slender patients as the sigmoid colon is pushed into the left upper abdomen which narrows the junction with the descending colon. In such cases, changing the position of the patient from left lateral to supine position or, particularly in slender patients, to right lateral will move the sigmoid colon to the middle and right abdomen. With the techniques of inward push followed by withdrawal, as well as minimizing air insufflations, the endoscope can reach the sigmoid-descending junction. Once the sigmoid-descending junction is reached it is important to straighten the colonoscope by pulling back, clockwise rotation, and deflating techniques. Once the colonoscope is straightened in the descending colon, it can usually be advanced without forming loops and discomfort to the patient. This technique named "right turn shortening techniques" has become a basic technique of straight scope insertion [8].

Other techniques such as "jiggling" of the colonoscope and application of water infusion may facilitate the passage of the colonoscope. Once an angulated sigmoid colon has been passed, again straightening the colonoscope is important.

Looping of the colonoscope in the sigmoid colon represents a challenge. In order to prevent creation of loops, the use of external abdominal pressure can be helpful in fixing sigmoid colon. After reaching the rectosigmoid junction, external pressure could be placed in the lower left abdomen to splint the sigmoid colon and to prevent looping. Prior to re-attempts at advancing, the colonoscopy should be fully shortened as evidenced by one-to-one back and forth movement of the tip during push and

pull of the shaft. If pressure applied in this position does not allow advancement, changing the pressure location or changing the patient's position to supine position followed by application of mid-abdominal pressure may help. This can be further enhanced by additional external pressure applied on the patient's left lateral side, thus preventing movement of the sigmoid colon to this direction.

Recognizing the formation of spiral loops in the sigmoid colon is also very important. These include an alpha loop, intermediate N-loops and the shortest spiral loops formed with pulling and twisting maneuvers.

• **Alpha loop**: Formation of an alpha loop occurs when the sigmoid loop is long (assessed by amount of the scope inserted) and has an alpha configuration (counterclockwise spiral) allowing advancement of the tip to the descending colon without reaching any point of angulation. In the presence of an alpha loop, an endoscopist does not pull the scope back but advances its tip to the splenic flexure at the about 90 cm of insertion. This maneuver is followed by pulling back and clockwise twisting which straightens the colonoscope at the splenic flexure. Figure 7.1 illustrates the concept of alpha loop technique.

• **Spiral loop**: Passing through the sigmoid colon can lead to creation of spiral loops, called N-loops, created by stretching of the sigmoid loop from its normal, vari-

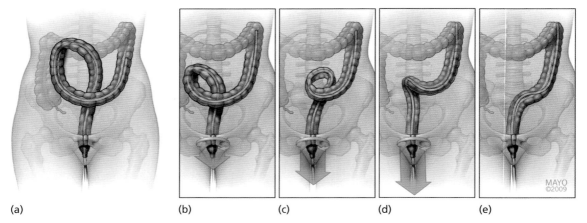

| (a) | (b) | (c) | (d) | (e) |

Figure 7.1 The alpha loop technique. (a–b) Formation of the loop with the alpha configuration (counterclockwise spiral) within the long sigmoid with the scope advancement until splenic flexure. (c–e) Pulling back and clockwise twisting of the colonoscope lead to straightening of the colonoscope at the splenic flexure and the loop reduction.

able tortuous features into a clockwise spiral. Anticlockwise twist exaggerates looping whereas clockwise twisting combined with withdrawal will straighten the loop.

Warm water infusion serve is an adjunct to the usual air insufflations and improves the cecal intubation rate and speed through severe mechanisms [9–12]. Water infusion likely works by a combination of lubrication and straightening of the sigmoid under the weight of the water-filled lumen. It may lead to local distension and decrease spasm, facilitating the advance of the colonoscope. Furthermore, water infused into the sigmoid colon flows to the left colon thus opening passage through the loops and bends.

Redundant or excessively long colons represent another challenge. Straightening of the endoscope, maximal reductions of all loops, and external pressure application are all critically important steps. The use of additional accessories such as a variable stiffness of colonoscope, overtube, or a stiffing guidewire are alternatives, though there is only limited clinical evidence supporting these techniques [6,13].

Descending Colon and Splenic Flexure
The descending colon is fixed on the posterior abdominal wall. Looping can prevent further advancement of the colonoscope beyond the sigmoid-descending junction, thus the application of alpha loop techniques as well as external pressure techniques described above can advance the colonoscope to the descending colon. The proximal descending colon ends with the splenic flexure with a variable position and angulation. The splenic flexure is described either as a high flexure beneath the diaphragm with the angle greater than 90° degree between descending and transverse colon. The colonoscopy can usually be passed around this angulation by a combination of tip deflection and slow withdrawal in order to stay as close to the "inside" of the curvature as possible. Once passed, as with nearly all acute angulations, suctioning to shorten the colon length, and withdrawing the colonoscope will reduce the loop formation, and when combined with external pressure will prevent new loops from forming.

Transverse Colon and Hepatic Flexure
The position of transverse colon can vary from complete horizontal to "drooping" position because of its intraperitoneal location and fixation of both splenic and

hepatic flexures on either end of the transverse. The application of upward external pressure in the midabdomen over the transverse colon and changing positions from left lateral to supine can lift a drooping colon and facilitate passage (Figure 7.2). The techniques for passage around the hepatic flexure resemble those for the splenic flexure; tip angulation, taking the "inside" curve, and suctioning/withdrawal once the tip has passed around to the lumen on the other side. If these difficulties are present, changing positions from left lateral to supine or right lateral is strongly encouraged. Then, the scope should be further advanced to the beginning of ascending colon and then pulling back techniques should be applied. Applying further external pressure to the right flank over the hepatic flexure can be very helpful in passing this angulation.

Ascending Colon, Cecum, and Terminal Ileum
Pushing with application of external hand pressure over the cecum or in some cases changing position to supine or right lateral can be helpful in reaching the cecum. Additionally, deflation can play a role in shortening and flattening of the ascending colon. Frequent looping of the colonoscope is common in the last 5–10 cm of the colon; usually due to bowing of the transverse colon downwards. This can be prevented by upward external pressure on the mid abdomen to counter the transverse bow. Once the cecum is identified, careful inspection of the base and the medial wall of the cecum proximal to the ileocecal valve is recommended. The intubation of the ileocecal (IC) valve is an important part of the colonoscope exam. If the valve is easily notable, then advancement of the scope to the terminal ileum should be achieved without difficulties (Video 1). However, if the opening of the valve is not identified, then suctioning air out of the cecum can visualize the valve, otherwise in some cases retroflexion at the base of the cecum may be required to visualize the IC valve.

Colonoscopy Extubation—Withdrawal Technique and Basic Principles
Withdrawal of the endoscope is technically a simpler part of the examination. However, careful inspection of colonic folds, proximal sides of flexures, and valves is a key step to maximize adenoma detection [14]. The most important of the withdrawal techniques remains back and forth inspection behind folds, at the proximal sites

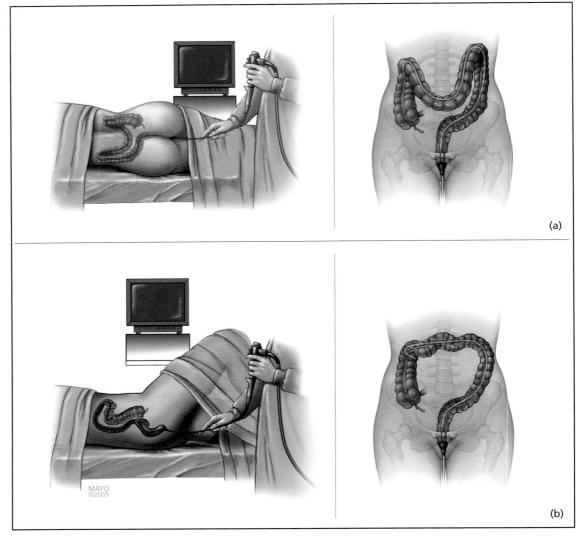

Figure 7.2 (a) The drooping transverse colon in the patient being in the left lateral position. (b) Changing position of the patient from left lateral to supine can lift the drooping colon and facilitate the colonoscope passage.

to flexures and valves with an adequate time of inspection (Video 2). Barclay *et al.* [15] demonstrated that endoscopists who spend more than 6 min on withdrawal inspecting the colonic mucosa had 10-fold higher adenoma detection rates. Careful attention to subtle areas of erythema (or pallor relative to surrounding erythema), rough/ villiform surface, and puckering of folds can help detect flat and depressed lesions. Quality of bowel preparation and rational use of sedatives are strongest predictors of successful colonoscopy with cecal intubation [15]. Use of irrigation pumps or hand-held water syringes to wash mucous and stool from the surface can improve visualization, even when the preparation is not ideal (Video 3). Sufficient air insufflation is often necessary to flatten colonic folds and this applies to all parts of the colon, from cecum to rectum.

Colonoscopy Imaging Technologies

In spite of efforts to improve colonoscopy techniques, small, flat, and depressed neoplastic lesions remain often undetected during regular, standard, white-light endoscopy [16]. New technologic advances combine optical physics and biomedical engineering to improve imaging of colonic mucosa and detection of adenomas by increasing the contrast between abnormal and normal tissue and a field of view. It should be emphasized though that the careful, slow, and deliberate inspection for flat lesions remains the most important "technology" available. These methods include dye-based or digital-based chromoendoscopy, such as narrow-band imaging (NBI), Fujinon Intelligent Contrast Enhancement imaging (FICE; Fujinon, Ft Wayne, NJ, USA), and iScan (Pentax, Montvale, NJ, USA) [17–19] (Video 4).

The key role of chromoendoscopy is the identification of flat lesions with the determination of surface staining mucosal and vessels pattern, with the irregular microvascular and mucosal patterns serving as a predictor of neoplasia [17,20]. The use of dye-based chromoendoscopy techniques improved the detection rates of flat adenomas [21] and small adenomas in some studies [22,23]. However, other studies did not reveal an overall difference in the adenoma detection using chromoendoscopy techniques [17,24,25].

Technologies exposing the whole mucosal surface, such as wide-angle colonoscopies, could be of essential importance. However, Pellise et al. [26] demonstrated that the use of colonoscopes with a field of view of 170° (30% more than conventional models) does not lead to an improvement in adenoma detection.

Conclusions

The improvement of detection of cancer lesions can be achieved with better education of colonoscopy techniques, as opposed to application of new technology alone. However, it is certain that all these colonoscopy techniques and technologies discussed above, when combined together, will lead to better outcome in colorectal cancer prevention. Careful inspection of folds during withdrawal and basic colonoscopic techniques remain of paramount importance independently of advances in endoscopic technologies.

Take-home points

- Successful colonoscopy exam relies on mastering the basic techniques of cecal intubation and extubation.
- Basic insertion techniques include avoidance of looping, passing angulations by shortening the scope, applying external pressure, and changing positions of patients.
- Water immersion during intubation was recently shown to have potential of assisting colonoscopy intubation by improving lubrication between the colonoscope and mucosa, relieving colon spasm, and straightening of the left colon.
- Improving basic withdrawal techniques, including time spent on inspection of colonic mucosa, achieving adequate visualization of all folds, proximal flexures and valves, remains the key for the successful extubation of a colonoscopy exam.
- Traditional chromendoscopy, though considered in general practice as impractical, is effective for detection of small adenoma, dysplasia in chronic irritable bowel disease, and characterization of flat lesions. Digital chromoendoscopy may be also very useful in detection and characterization of colorectal lesions, including flat, small lesions.

References

1 Winawer SJ, Zauber AG, Ho MN, et al. Prevention of colorectal cancer by colonoscopic polypectomy. The National Polyp Study Workgroup. N Engl J Med 1993; 329: 1977–81.

2 Gross SA, Buchner AM, Cangemi J, et al. A prospective randomized back-to-back trial comparing narrow band imaging to conventional colonoscopy for adenoma detection. Gastroenterology 2008; 134 (4 Suppl.): 69.

3 Rex DK. Colonoscopic miss rates of adenomas determined by back-to-back colonoscopies. Gastroenetrology 1997; 112: 24–8.

4 Rabeneck L, Paszat LF, Hilsden RJ, et al. Bleeding and perforation after outpatient colonoscopy and their risk factors in usual clinical practice. Gastroenterology 2008; 2008: 1899–906.

5 Rex DK, Petrini JL, Baron TH, et al. Quality indicators for colonoscopy. Am J Gastroenterol 2006; 101: 873–85.

6 Rex DK. Achieving cecal intubation in the very difficult colon. Gastrointest Endosc 2008; 67: 938–44.

7 Rex DK, Goodwine BW. Method of colonoscopy in 42 consecutive patients presenting after prior incomplete colonoscopy. Am J Gastroenterol 2002; 97: 1148–51.

8 Waye JD. Colonoscopy. CA Cancer J Clin 1992; 42: 350–65.

9 Baumann UA. Water intubation of the sigmoid colon: water instillation speeds up left-sided colonoscopy. *Endoscopy* 1999; **31**: 314–7.

10 Church JM. Warm water irrigation for dealing with spasm during colonoscopy: simple, inexpensive, and effective. *Gastrointest Endosc* 2002; **56**: 672–4.

11 Brocchi E, Pezzilli R, Tomassetti P, *et al.* Warm water or oil-assisted colonoscopy: toward simpler examinations? *Am J Gastroenterol* 2008; **103**: 581–7.

12 Leung FW. Water-related techniques for performance of colonoscopy. *Dig Dis Sci* 2008; **53**: 2847–50.

13 Subramania S, Rex DK. Variable stiffness colonoscopes: do they offer a better examination? *Curr Opin Gastroenterol* 2003; **19**: 492–6.

14 Rex DK. Colonoscopic withdrawal technique is associated with adenoma miss rates. *Gastrointestinal Endosc* 2000; **51**: 33–6.

15 Barclay RJ, Vicaril JJ, Doughty AS, *et al.* Colonoscopic withdrawal times and adenoma detection during screening colonoscopy. *N Engl J Med* 2006; **355**: 2533–41.

16 Rex DK. Maximizing detection of adenomas and cancers during colonoscopy. *Am J Gastroenterol* 2006; **101**: 2866–77.

17 Curvers WL, Singh R, Song LM, *et al.* Endoscopic tri-modal imaging for detection of early neoplasia in Barrett's oesophagus: a multi-centre feasibility study using high-resolution endoscopy, autofluorescence imaging and narrow band imaging incorporated in one endoscopy system. *Gut* 2008; **57**: 167–72.

18 Pohl J, Nguyen-Tat M, Pech O, *et al.* Computed virtual chromoendoscopy for classification of small colorectal lesions: a prospective comparative study. *Am J Gastroenterol* 2008; **103**: 562–9.

19 Hoffman A, Basting N, Goetz M. High definition colonoscopy (HD) with I-scan function allows to recognize and characterize flat and neoplastic changes as precisely as chromoendoscopy. *Endoscopy* 2009; **41**: 107–12.

20 Yoshida T, Inoue H, Usui S, *et al.* Narrow-band imaging system with magnifying endoscopy for superficial esophageal lesions. *Gastrointest Endosc* 2004; **59**: 288–95.

21 Soetikno RM, Kaltenbach T, Rouse RV, *et al.* Prevalence of nonpolypoid (flat and depressed) colorectal neoplasms in asymptomatic and symptomatic adults. *JAMA* 2008; **299**: 1027–35.

22 Le Rhun M, Coron E, Parlier D, *et al.* High resolution colonoscopy with chromoendoscopy versus standard colonoscopy for the detection of colonic neoplasia: a randomized study. *Clin Gastroenterol Hepatol* 2006; **4**: 349–54.

23 Hurlstone DP, Cross SS, Slater R, *et al.* Detecting diminutive colorectal lesions at colonoscopy: a randomized controlled trial of pancolonic versus targeted chromoscopy. *Gut* 2004; **53**: 376–80.

24 Wo JM, Ray MB, Mayfield-Stokes S, *et al.* Comparison of methylene blue-directed biopsies and conventional biopsies in the detection of intestinal metaplasia and dysplasia in Barrett's esophagus: a preliminary study. *Gastrointest Endosc* 2001; **54**: 294–301.

25 Dave U, Shousha S, Westaby D. Methylene blue staining: is it really useful in Barrett's esophagus? *Gastrointest Endosc* 2001; **53**: 333–5.

26 Pellise M, Fernandez-Esparrach G, Cardenas A, *et al.* Impact of wide-angle, high definition endoscopy in the diagnosis of colorectal neoplasia: a randomized controlled trial. *Gastroenterology* 2008; **135**: 1062–8.

CHAPTER 8

Advanced Colonoscopy, Polypectomy, and Colonoscopic Imaging

Douglas K. Rex

Indiana University Hospital, Indianapolis, IN, USA

Summary

Technically difficult colonoscope insertions can generally be categorized as either a very difficult sigmoid or a redundant colon. These categories guide instrument selection and the technical approach to achieving cecal intubation. Endoscopic submucosal dissection is the newest approach to endoscopic resection of colorectal polyps, but is rarely used in the United States, where piecemeal polypectomy is still preferred. The Third Eye Retroscope produced a 12% gain in adenoma detection in an initial uncontrolled study. Wide-angle colonoscopy and cap-fitted colonoscopy have been studied more, and have generally not been useful in increasing adenoma detection. Likewise, although chromoendoscopy produces small gains in small adenoma detection, the more practical electronic forms of highlighting polyps (e.g., narrow-band imaging) have not successfully increased adenoma detection. A variety of imaging methods, including confocal laser microscopy, endocytoscopy, narrow-band imaging, Fujinon Intelligent Chromo Endoscopy, and the Pentax I-Scan, allow real-time differentiation of polyp histology, at least for adenomatous versus hyperplastic histology.

Insertion Techniques in Difficult Colons

Technically challenging colons that defy cecal intubation can be grouped into two categories: one is the redundant colon and the other is the narrowed or angulated sigmoid colon [1]. When faced with a difficult sigmoid, the approach is narrower colonoscopes, first a pediatric colonoscope, and if that fails a thin upper endoscope. An upper endoscope will pass almost all benign left colon strictures. Aggressive loop reduction and abdominal pressure, sometimes applied with four hands, will advance an upper endoscope to the cecum in about two-thirds of cases [1]. If that fails, passage can be attempted with a double

Practical Gastroenterology and Hepatology: Small and Large Intestine and Pancreas, 1st edition. Edited by Nicholas J. Talley, Sunanda V. Kane and Michael B. Wallace. © 2010 Blackwell Publishing Ltd.

balloon enteroscope or with the technique of guidewire exchange. The latter technique is performed by advancing a long, stiff guidewire with a soft tip into the transverse colon (or the furthest extent to which the upper endoscope can be passed), followed by withdrawal of the upper endoscope. The stiff end of the guidewire is then passed backwards through a pediatric colonoscope by protecting it in the sheath of a polypectomy snare that has been passed forward through the colonoscope. The pediatric colonoscope is then advanced over the guidewire. The wire itself straightens the angulation in the sigmoid sufficiently to allow the pediatric colonoscope to be passed.

In the very redundant colon, an initial attempt with a standard colonoscope and excellent standard technique is often successful. Special tools may be needed, such as the push enteroscope, double balloon enteroscope, or a standard colonoscope with overtube. A simple 60-cm overtube is available from Olympus (Center Valley, PA) but the USGI Shapelock (San Clemente, CA) device is a safe and highly effective alternative. The device is back loaded onto the colonoscope.

Water immersion (filling the left colon with water and colonoscope passage without air insufflation) can also be used to pass redundant colons and difficult sigmoids [2–5], though additional study is needed. Water immersion in the left colon causes the left colon to sink into the left lower quadrant when the patient is in the left lateral decubitus position, thereby straightening the sigmoid. Warm water can also relieve spasm and water or corn seed oil may improve the hydrophilic forces between the colonoscope and the mucosa.

Advanced Techniques for Polyp Resection

The newest method of advanced polypectomy is endoscopic submucosal dissection (ESD) [6]. The technique was developed for resection of early gastric cancers in Japan but has been used (primarily by Japanese physicians) to resect large, broad colorectal polyps. A long-acting solution such as hyaluronidate is injected into the submucosa. A needle knife is then used to make an incision into the submucosa around the circumference of the lesion. A special knife such as the "insulated tip (IT) knife," or the "hook knife," is then used to dissect through the submucosa under the polyp. The advantages include an extremely high rate of cure on the initial resection compared to piecemeal polypectomy (98% versus a maximum of 85% for piecemeal polypectomy). Additionally, the quality of the pathologic specimens is superior to piecemeal polypectomy. The downsides include a long learning curve, longer procedural times, and an approximate 5% risk of perforation, though most perforations have been closed with endoscopic clips [6].

In the United States, most large sessile polyps are still removed endoscopically using piecemeal snare resection after submucosal injection. Aggressive application of argon plasma coagulation to flat polyp remaining after snare resection, as well as to the perimeter of the polypectomy site, can reduce the risk of local recurrence [7]. Patients should undergo an initial follow-up examination 3 to 6 months after the initial resection. If the base of the polypectomy site is clear at 3 to 6 months, a second follow-up examination a year later is warranted to look for so-called "late recurrences."

Inclusion of epinephrine in submucosal injection fluid has been shown in randomized controlled trials to prevent immediate bleeding, but there is no effect on delayed bleeding [8–11]. For large pedunculated polyps with sufficient stalk length, placement of detachable snares has been shown to prevent postpolypectomy bleeding [11,12].

Endoscopic resection of large sessile polyps has one-fifth the cost of surgical resection [13]. All pedunculated colorectal polyps are endoscopically resectable, as are nearly all sessile polyps less than 2 cm in size, and a substantial fraction of those greater than 2 cm in size are also endoscopically resectable.

The use of a cap for endoscopic mucosal resection has been less important in the colon than in the esophagus or stomach. However, the cap can facilitate resection of extremely flat lesions that cannot be otherwise snared. Barb snares and spiral snares can also sometimes enable the resection of extremely flat lesions.

Endoscopic Imaging in the Colon

Detection of Neoplasia
Colonoscopy misses neoplastic lesions when the bowel preparation is inadequate, when lesions are hidden on the proximal sides of folds, and when flat lesions are present on the television screen but not recognized by colonoscopists. Technical aids to detection have focused on exposing more colorectal mucosa or highlighting flat lesions.

Exposing Hidden Mucosa
Wide-angle colonoscopy refers to the use of lenses with wider than standard 140° angle of view in most commercial colonoscopes. In Olympus 180 series colonoscopes, the angle of view is 170° as a standard feature. The benefits of wide-angle colonoscopy appear to be operator dependent but individual examiners have achieved improved adenoma detection and greater efficiency of examination [14]. Efficiency is provided because there is less work and time expended in exposing the proximal sides of folds and flexures during withdrawal.

Cap-fitted colonoscopy refers to the use of a clear plastic hood on the tip of the colonoscope to flatten haustral folds. Eight randomized controlled trials have been performed and several have shown small increases in polyp detection, but only one tandem study showed an increase in adenoma detection [15]. Further, in the positive trial the detection rate of adenomas in the control arm was considerably lower than in prior tandem studies. Therefore, no substantial benefit for adenoma detection has been shown with cap-fitted colonoscopy.

The Third Eye Retroscope (Avantis Medical Systems, Sunnyvale, CA) is a disposable device that is inserted down the instrument channel of the colonoscope. After exiting the channel, it is advanced 3 to 4 cm, where it automatically retroflexes. The device has a lens on the tip with a CMOS (complementary-symmetry metal-oxide semiconductor) video chip and 135° angle of view. The colonoscopist watches both the forward view from the colonoscope and the retroflexed view through the Third Eye Retroscope. In an initial study, there was an apparent 12% gain in adenomas provided by use of the Third Eye Retroscope [16]. The device is FDA approved but there are practical obstacles to its use, including its cost, the need to remove it for each polyp that is detected, difficulty keeping the lens clear in a poorly prepared colon, and currently a relatively poor-quality image.

Highlighting Flat and Depressed Lesions

The best studied technique for this purpose is chromoendoscopy or dye spraying. Chromoendoscopy has two uses. One is to evaluate already detected lesions by examination of the pit pattern in combination with high-magnification endoscopy. The other use is pancolonic spraying to highlight and detect flat lesions. Several randomized controlled trials have been performed for the latter indication [17]. Generally, chromoendoscopy has been associated with higher detection rates of adenomas, although the detected adenomas are typically small, tubular adenomas with low-grade dysplasia. The technique requires time for application and is generally not considered practical for routine use. Pancolonic dye spraying has greater value in chronic ulcerative colitis, where randomized controlled trials have shown that it allows targeted biopsying of dysplasia. Detection of dysplasia in ulcerative colitis is improved with chromoendoscopy, even though fewer (but targeted) biopsies are taken.

Narrow-band imaging (NBI) has been evaluated as an aid to detection of adenomas in several tandem studies and randomized controlled trials. NBI could potentially improve adenoma detection because the color contrast between adenomas in blue light (adenomas appear brown in blue light) compared to normal mucosa is greater in blue than in white light; however, adenomas seen in blue light are invariably still visible when viewed in white light. In a European multicenter study, adenoma detection was initially higher in blue light than white light, but by the end of the study detection rates were equal with blue light and white light [18]. This suggests that high-level adenoma detectors do not achieve improved adenoma detection using NBI [19] but NBI may have a useful learning effect in low-level adenoma detectors [18].

Fujinon (Wayne, NJ) makes a postimage processing color enhancement system (FICE: Fujinon Intelligent CE) that has been tested in randomized controlled trials and found to not improve adenoma detection [20]. In a single randomized controlled trial, high definition resulted in the highest level of adenoma detection ever reported, but this was true with either white light or FICE. High definition has not been directly tested for its impact on adenoma detection.

Determination of Histology in Real Time

A variety of endoscopic imaging techniques have been developed to allow determination of histology of colon polyps in real time. Real time histology could be used to determine the appropriateness of endoscopic versus surgical resection in the case of early cancers, or to decide whether or not to remove a non-neoplastic polyp, or to remove polyps and discard them (rather than send them to pathology) and then determine postpolypectomy surveillance intervals based on the endoscopic evaluation.

The most sophisticated system for real-time histology is the Pentax (Montvale, NJ) endoscopic confocal laser endomicroscopy (eCLE) system which allows actual histologic images of endoscopically visualized tissue. eCLE is capable of determining adenomatous versus hyperplastic histology, the degree of dysplasia, and the presence of cancer [21]. However, the endoscopes are expensive and the learning curve is substantial, and therefore the use of confocal is at this time confined to research centers. A probe-based confocal laser endomicroscopy (pCLE) system is now available (Mauna Kea Technologies, Paris, France) and early studies suggest pCLE is capable of accurate classification of hyperplastic and adenomatous polyps without removal [22]. CLE systems, although still under investigation, offer the potential to definitively diagnose polyp histology *in vivo* and thus avoid removal of small hyperplastic polyps, and to resect and discard small tubular adenomatous polyps. The Olympus endocytoscopy system also provides information regarding neoplastic versus non-neoplastic histology and the degree of dysplasia [23].

Narrow-band imaging, when combined with high-magnification endoscopy, can differentiate adenomatous from hyperplastic histology, identify the presence of cancer, and in recent studies determine the degree of dysplasia in adenomatous polyps. The evaluation is based on the appearance of microcapillaries in the polyp surface as well as the appearance of pits. Olympus endoscopes in the United States do not typically have high magnification, and both narrow-band imaging and high magnification are needed for consistent high accuracy [24]. The Fujinon FICE system allows accurate differentiation of adenomatous from hyperplastic histology [20]. Pentax also offers a postprocessing system called I-Scan and at the time of writing little evidence is available regarding its effectiveness in differentiating adenomatous from hyperplastic histology [25].

- No method of improving detection of flat lesions during colonoscopy has proven to be both effective and practical, including chromoendoscopy, narrow-band imaging, the Fuji Intelligent Chromo Endoscopy system, and high-definition colonoscopy.
- Several methods allow accurate determination of polyp histology in real time. Confocal laser endomicroscopy provides "virtual histology" of these lesions. The Olympus endocystoscopy system and the Olympus narrow-band imaging with high-magnification systems can both provide detailed histologic information. The Fujinon FICE system, Olympus NBI without magnification, and Pentax I-Scan are all reasonably effective at differentiation of adenomas from hyperplastic histology.

Take-home points

- Technically difficult colonoscopies can be categorized as difficult sigmoids or redundant colons. Narrower instruments should be used for angulated sigmoids. Redundancy can be overcome in most cases by meticulous standard technique, longer colonoscopes, overtubes, double balloon enteroscopy, and perhaps water immersion.
- Endoscopic submucosal dissection is seldom used in the United States at the time of writing. Advantages include higher initial cure rates and better pathologic specimens. Disadvantages include longer procedure times and higher perforation rates.
- Piecemeal resection of large sessile polyps is followed by substantial failure rates. Careful follow-up is needed.
- Detachable snares can be used to prevent bleeding from pedunculated polyps.
- Submucosal injection of epinephrine reduces immediate bleeding from polypectomy.
- No method of increasing exposure of hidden mucosa during colonoscopy (wide-angle colonoscopy, cap-fitted colonoscopy, Third Eye Retroscope) has yet been proven to be both effective and practical.

References

1 Rex DK. Achieving cecal intubation in the very difficult colon. *Gastrointest Endosc* 2008; **67**: 938–44.

2 Church JM. Warm water irrigation for dealing with spasm during colonoscopy: simple, inexpensive, and effective. *Gastroint Endosc* 2002; **56**: 672–4.

3 Brocchi E, Pezzilli R, Tomassetti P, *et al.* Warm water or oil-assisted colonoscopy: toward simpler examinations? *Am J Gastroenterol* 2008; **103**: 581–7.

4 Baumann UA. Water intubation of the sigmoid colon: water instillation speeds up left-sided colonoscopy. *Endoscopy* 1999; **31**: 314–7.

5 Hamamoto N, Nakanishi Y, Morimoto N, *et al.* A new water instillation method for colonoscopy without sedation as performed by endoscopists-in-training. *Gastrointest Endosc* 2002; **56**: 825–8.

6 Fujishiro M, Yahagi N, Kakushima N, *et al.* Outcomes of endoscopic submucosal dissection for colorectal epithelial neoplasms in 200 consecutive cases. *Clin Gastroenterol Hepatol* 2007; **5**: 678–83.

7 Brooker JC, Saunders BP, Shah SG, *et al.* Treatment with argon plasma coagulation reduces recurrence after piecemeal resection of large sessile colonic polyps: a randomized trial and recommendations. *Gastrointest Endosc* 2002; **55**: 371–5.

8 Shioji K, Suzuki Y, Kobayashi M, *et al.* Prophylactic clip application does not decrease delayed bleeding after colonoscopic polypectomy. *Gastrointest Endosc* 2003; **57**: 691–4.

9 Paspatis GA, Paraskeva K, Theodoropoulou A, *et al.* A prospective, randomized comparison of adrenaline injection in combination with detachable snare versus adrenaline injection alone in the prevention of postpolypectomy bleeding in large colonic polyps. *Am J Gastroenterol* 2006; **101**: 2805–9.

10 Hsieh YH, Lin HJ, Tseng GY, *et al.* Is submucosal epinephrine injection necessary before polypectomy? A prospective, comparative study. *Hepatogastroenterology* 2001; **48**: 1379–82.

11 Di Giorgio P, De Luca L, Calcagno G, *et al.* Detachable snare versus epinephrine injection in the prevention of postpolypectomy bleeding: a randomized and controlled study. *Endoscopy* 2004; **36**: 860–3.

12 Iishi H, Tatsuta M, Narahara H, *et al.* Endoscopic resection of large pedunculated colorectal polyps using a detachable snare. *Gastrointest Endosc* 1996; **44**: 594–7.

13 Onken JE, Friedman JY, Subramanian S, *et al.* Treatment patterns and costs associated with sessile colorectal polyps. *Am J Gastroenterol* 2002; **97**: 2896–901.

14 Fatima H, Rex DK, Rothstein R, *et al.* Cecal insertion and withdrawal times with wide-angle versus standard colonoscopes: a randomized controlled trial. *Clin Gastroenterol Hepatol* 2008; **6**: 109–14.

15 Horiuchi A, Nakayama Y. Usefulness of a transparent retractable extension device on colorectal adenoma detection. *Gastrointest Endosc* 2008; **67**: AB89.

16 Waye JD, Heigh RI, Fleischer DE, *et al.* A prospective efficacy evaluation of the third eye retroscope auxiliary endoscopy system. *Gastrointest Endosc* 2008; **67**: AB101–2.

17 Rex DK. Maximizing detection of adenomas and cancers during colonoscopy. *Am J Gastroenterol* 2006; **101**: 2866–77.

18 Adler A, Pohl H, Papanikolaou IS, *et al.* A prospective randomised study on narrow-band imaging versus conventional colonoscopy for adenoma detection: does narrow-band imaging induce a learning effect? *Gut* 2008; **57**: 59–64.

19 Rex DK, Helbig CC. High yields of small and flat adenomas with high-definition colonoscopes using either white light or narrow band imaging. *Gastroenterology* 2007; **133**: 42–7.

20 Pohl J, Nguyen-Tat M, Pech O, *et al.* Computed virtual chromoendoscopy for classification of small colorectal lesions: a prospective comparative study. *Am J Gastroenterol* 2008; **103**: 562–9.

21 Kiesslich R, Goetz M, Rafoud K, *et al.* Staging of colorectal neoplasia with confocal laser endomicroscopy using two contrast agents simultaneously. *Gastrointest Endosc* 2008; **67**: AB123.

22 Buchner AM, Murli K, Wolfsen HC, Wallace MB. High resolution confocal endomicroscopy probe system for in vivo diagnosis of colorectal neoplasia [abstract]. *Gastroenterology* 2008; **135**: 295.

23 Wakamura K, Kudo SE, Kashida H, *et al.* Endocytoscopy in the colorectum. *Gastrointest Endosc* 2008; **67**: AB131.

24 Parra-Blanco A, Matsuda T, Fujii T, *et al.* Diagnostic advantage of optical vs electronic magnification for the diagnosis of colonic polyps. *Gastrointest Endosc* 2008; **67**: AB126.

25 Hoffman A, Kagel C, Goetz M, *et al.* High definition colonoscopy (HD+) with I-Scan function allows to recognize and characterize flat neoplastic changes as precisely as chromoendoscopy. *Gastrointest Endosc* 2008; **67**: AB125.

CHAPTER 9

Complications of Colonoscopy

Ana Ignjatovic and Brian Saunders

Wolfson Unit for Endoscopy, St Mark's Hospital, Harrow, UK

Summary

Colonoscopy is widely accepted as the investigation of choice for patients with colonic symptoms, and for screening those at increased or average risk for colorectal cancer. Most colonoscopy procedures are straightforward with a very low risk of complications and procedure-related mortality is very rare (0.007–0.07%). However, given the high volume of colonoscopy and the increasingly therapeutic nature of procedures, colonoscopists and patients must be aware of procedural risk. Bleeding and perforation of the colon are the commonest complications following therapeutic colonoscopy. Recognition of complications and their prompt and effective management is an essential part of ensuring quality at colonoscopy and in maintaining wide acceptability of the procedure.

Introduction

Colonoscopy is widely accepted as the investigation of choice for patients with colonic symptoms, and for screening those at increased or average risk for colorectal cancer. It is probably the commonest gastrointestinal procedure performed in the Western World and more than 7 million screening colonoscopies are performed annually in the USA alone [1]. Most colonoscopy procedures are straightforward with a very low risk of complications and procedure-related mortality is very rare (0.007–0.07%) [2,3]. However, given the high volume of colonoscopy and the increasingly therapeutic nature of procedures colonoscopists and patients must be aware of procedural risk. Recognition of complications and their prompt and effective management is an essential part of ensuring quality at colonoscopy [4] and in maintaining wide acceptability of the procedure. This chapter describes the common complications that can occur at colonoscopy, which can be broadly divided into those

relating to the period immediately before colonoscopy, to the insertion of the instrument to cecum, and to withdrawal of colonoscope, including therapeutic interventions.

Precolonoscopy

Bowel Preparation

Good bowel preparation is a prerequisite for a good quality colonoscopy—poor preparation has been identified as a factor predictive of technically difficult colonoscopy and increases the chance of missing clinically significant lesions [5].

There is little evidence that one form of bowel preparation is better than any other [6] but general measures to ensure patient safety such as clear written instructions with a telephone patient help line, admission to the hospital and intravenous hydration for frail or elderly patients, and administration of supervised enemas prior to the procedure if the preparation has failed, all help ensure a successful procedure. The most common, serious, bowel preparation-related complication is electrolyte disturbances. These have been described with all types of preparation but particularly with lower-volume

Practical Gastroenterology and Hepatology: Small and Large Intestine and Pancreas, 1st edition. Edited by Nicholas J. Talley, Sunanda V. Kane and Michael B. Wallace. © 2010 Blackwell Publishing Ltd.

phosphate-based preparations, which should be avoided in patients with severe renal impairment (see Chapter 7).

Sedation

Sedation practice for colonoscopy varies worldwide with some colonoscopists using little or no sedation whilst most use conscious or deep sedation with a combination of opiate and benzodiazepine or propofol. Apart from hypersensitivity reactions to sedation, endoscopists need to be aware of the potential cardiovascular and respiratory complications, predominantly respiratory depression and consequent hypoxia (0.3–5.6%) [7], and hemodynamic instability [8,9]. This is of particular importance in patients with pre-existing cardiovascular or respiratory problems. All patients should be fully assessed prior to the administration of sedation and given supplemental oxygen with pulse oximetry monitoring as routine. Deeper sedation necessitates a practitioner skilled in airway management to be present. Reversal agents for sedation (naloxone and flumazenil) and a fully equipped resuscitation trolley should be available in the Endoscopy Unit at all times (see Chapter 7).

Intubation

Traumatic Bowel Perforation

Traumatic bowel perforation is uncommon with modern flexible instruments but its early recognition and treatment are associated with improved patient outcomes

[10]. Most traumatic perforations occur when force is applied to a fixed bowel segment and therefore are often in the setting of pre-existing pathology such as diverticular disease, cancer, inflammatory bowel disease, or post-surgical pericolic adhesions. Excessive force should never be applied during colonoscopy, whether inserting or withdrawing the colonoscope, and in technically difficult cases alternatives to colonoscopy such as computed tomography colonography (CTC) should always be considered. Traumatic perforation can occur from the scope tip (most commonly at the rectosigmoid or sigmoid/descending junction [10]) or from the shaft when excessive force is used to push through a loop (typically a linear split on the antimesenteric border of the midsigmoid is seen), or from barotrauma when excessive gas is inflated. The later cause may occur if there is an enclosed space such as when the colonoscope tip becomes impacted in a diverticulum or if gas is introduced above a colonic stricture where the perforation usually occurs in the cecum.

Diagnostic colonoscopy perforation rates reported in recent literature range from 0 to 0.3% (Table 9.1). Most published studies are from tertiary centers and this may lead to an underestimation of the true incidence of perforation. Reassuringly, in a meta-analysis of 27 studies, Wexner *et al.* [11] observed that the rate of traumatic perforation had reduced greatly since 1990 (0.34% in 1970s and 0.16% in 1990s).

Early recognition and identification of perforation is critical. Small, linear tears can occasionally be approximated with endoscopic clips and a conservative manage-

Table 9.1 Complications of colonoscopy: perforation rate.

Study	Number of colonoscopies	Perforation rate, n (%)		
		Overall	Diagnostic	Therapeutic
Waye 1993 [33]	2097	2 (0.10%)	0%	2/777 (0.3%)
Eckardt *et al.* 1999 [34]	2500	2 (0.08%)	1/2071 (0.05%)	1/429 (0.23%)
Sieg *et al.* 2001 [2]	82416	4 (0.005%)	NA	9/14249 (0.06%)
Anderson *et al.* 2000 [35]	10486	20 (0.19%)	12†	8†
Wexner *et al.* 2001 [7]	13580	10 (0.07%)	2/8473 (0.02%)	8/5107 (0.15%)
Dafnis *et al.* 2001 [36]	6066	8 (0.1%)	5/4677 (0.1%)	3/1389 (0.2%)
Nelson *et al.* 2002 [15]	3196	0 (0%)	0/1524 (0%)	0/1672 (0%)
Bowles *et al.* 2004 [3]	9223	12 (0.13%)	8/7382 (0.11%)	4/1841 (0.22%)
Rathgaber, Wick 2006 [37]	12210	2 (0.016%)	2/7136 (0.03%)	0/5074 (0%)
Paspatis *et al.* 2008 [14]	9648	4 (0.04%)	3/7617 (0.04%)	1/2031 (0.05%)

†No data given for the number of diagnostic and therapeutic procedures.

ment strategy adopted in the form of close observation with intravenous fluids and antibiotics. Most traumatic perforations, however, do require early surgical intervention before the advent of peritoneal contamination. In a review of 258 248 colonoscopies, Iqbal *et al.* identified 165 iatrogenic perforations (0.07%) that were managed surgically. Patients presenting within 24 h were more likely to have minimal peritoneal contamination and have a primary repair or resection with anastomosis than patients presenting later [10].

Splenic Trauma

Splenic trauma, with hemodynamic compromise, although a serious complication, is thought to be rare, with less than 60 cases reported worldwide since the 1970s but the frequent delay in presentation may mean that the incidence is under-reported [12,13]. Likely mechanisms for injury include forceful pushing when passing the splenic flexure and aggressive withdrawal maneuvers, pulling back on the splenocolic ligament or pre-existing adhesions between the spleen and the colon. Splenic trauma is probably more likely in patients with enlarged or diseased spleens. Abdominal pain without free gas and hemodynamic compromise with a drop in hemoglobin should alert the clinician to the possibility of splenic injury postcolonoscopy. CT of the abdomen is the most sensitive and specific test to assess splenic laceration and rupture. Most patients with significant splenic injury will require splenectomy, although percutaneous transarterial embolization may be attempted in hemodynamically stable patients.

Cardiopulmonary Complications

Vasovagal events are relatively common during colonoscopy (0.08–5.4%) [14,15] and occur as a result of visceral pain due to mesenteric stretch or over distension. Aspiration of air and temporary scope withdrawal reduce visceral stimulation and the anticholinergic effect of antispasmodics such as hyoscine may also be protective. Minor cardiac arrhythmias are common during colonoscopy but appear to have little consequence and routine ECG monitoring appears to be unnecessary. Of more concern are the occasional reports of major cardiovascular events in the pericolonoscopy time period, particularly of acute myocardial infarction—0.06% in one study [16]. It is unclear whether this is a true association. Possible mechanisms include stimulation of sympathetic nervous system and electrolyte disturbance as a result of bowel preparation.

Infection

Transmission of infection through colonoscopes is rare—cases of *Salmonella*, *Klebsiella*, and *Enterobacter* as well as hepatitis B and C have been described although, to date, not HIV. Transmission of hepatitis C is of particular concern but can usually be linked to inadequate decontamination of scopes and accessories [17,18]. Theoretical risk of transmission of prion proteins (identified as causative agents of Creutzfeldt–Jakob disease(CJD)) exists as they are not destroyed by current sterilization procedure and any endoscope used in a patient at risk of CJD must be quarantined [19,20]. Risk of bacterial endocarditis following diagnostic and therapeutic colonoscopy is thought to be low and deemed not to warrant prophylactic antibiotics in most patients (for full details see ASGE guidelines [21]). Colonoscopists are frequently exposed to bodily fluids and protective clothing should be worn in order to minimize the theoretical risk of transmission of infection from patients.

Extubation

Missed Lesion

Lesions could be missed as a result of incomplete colonoscopy, poor bowel preparation, inadequate use of patient position change to open the dependent loops of bowel especially at splenic and hepatic flexures, and too rapid extubation. Numerous tandem colonoscopy studies have revealed that even expert colonoscopists can miss up to 25% of small polyps and 2–6% of significant lesions [22,23]. Moving the patient to left lateral position to examine the right colon, supine to examine the transverse, and right lateral to examine the left colon increases adenoma detection rate [24]. Barclay *et al.* [25] found that colonoscopists who had at least 6 min extubation time detected significantly more polyps that those who had shorter withdrawal time. Use of antispasmodics and adequate insufflation with use of targeted dye spray also probably aid detection in routine colonoscopy.

Biopsy and Polypectomy

Bleeding is the commonest serious colonoscopic complication. Generally, simple cold biopsy with standard

Table 9.2 Complications of colonoscopy: bleeding rate.

Study	Number of colonoscopies	Bleeding, n (%)		
		Overall	Diagnostic (with cold biopsy)	Therapeutic
Eckardt *et al.* 1999 [34]	2500	6 (0.24)	0/2071 (0)	6/429 (1.40)
Sieg *et al.* 2001 [2]	82416	1 (0.001)	NA	37/14249 (0.36)§
Wexner *et al.* 2001 [7]	13580	10 (0.07)	0/8473 (0.00)	10/5107 (0.19)
Dafnis *et al.* 2001 [36]	6066	12 (0.20)	0/4677 (0)	12/1389 (0.86)
Nelson *et al.* 2002 [15]†	3196	7 (0.22)	0/1524 (0)	7/1672 (0.42)
Bowles *et al.* 2004 [3]†	9223	6 (0.07%)	3/7382 (0.04)	3/1841
Rathgaber, Wick 2006 [37]†	12210	25 (0.20)	0/7136 (0.00)	23/5074 (0.46)*
Levin *et al.* 2006 [16]	16318	53 (0.32)	0/5235 (0)‡	53/11083 (0.48)
Paspatis *et al.* 2008 [14]	9648	83 (0.8)	2/7617 (0.03)	81/2031 (3.99)

*Postpolypectomy.
†Data for patients requiring hospitalization only.
‡Diagnostic without biopsies.
§Bleeding rate per polypectomy performed.

pinch biopsy forceps is safe, even in patients on anticoagulation, with rates of 0–0.04% reported (Table 9.2). As expected rates of bleeding after polypectomy are higher (0–4% in studies performed in the last decade). Patients undergoing polypectomy or dilatation should have anticoagulation withdrawn prior to colonoscopy to reduce the risk of bleeding. ASGE recommends that aspirin does not need to be stopped prior to polypectomy [26]. Patients on clopidogrel are particularly at risk and ideally this drug should be stopped for 10 days prior to therapeutic intervention bearing in mind the risk of in-stent thrombosis in patients with recent insertion of drug-eluting coronary stents.

Bleeding after therapy can be immediate or delayed for up to 3 weeks after colonoscopy. In a multivariate analysis, Kim *et al.* found that old age, cardiovascular and chronic renal disease, anticoagulant use, polyp size greater than 1 cm, pedunculated or laterally spreading tumors, use of cutting rather than blended or coagulation current, and poor bowel preparation were all risk factors for immediate postpolypectomy bleeding [27].

Delayed bleeding presents with hemotochesia, decrease in hemoglobin, and subsequent hemodynamic instability. Risk factors associated with delayed bleeding include increasing polyp size and resumption of anticoagulation following polypectomy [28]. The majority of patients stop bleeding spontaneously with conservative management, which includes correction of any clotting abnor-mality and blood transfusion. Repeat colonoscopy may be necessary to identify the bleeding point and apply therapy. Clips, endoloops, adrenaline injection, and thermal modalities have all been used successfully either as single modalities or in combination. If endoscopic therapy fails, angiography and segmental embolization may be attempted prior to segmental colonic resection.

Perforation following polypectomy can be immediate, recognized at colonoscopy, or delayed [29,30], with rates ranging from 0 to 0.3%. If a small perforation is recognized at colonoscopy, an attempt to close it using endoscopic clips can be made. The patient should be admitted to hospital for close observation and intravenous antibiotics as well as surgical review [31]. Larger perforations usually need a surgical repair. Delayed perforations can occur several days after polypectomy and patients should be warned to seek medical help if they develop abdominal pain or fever in that time period. Anecdotally, delayed perforations may occur more often when pure coagulating rather than cutting or blended current is used [29].

Postpolypectomy syndrome refers to a transmural burn postpolypectomy causing serosal irritation, but without free perforation. This occurs following 0.5–1% of polypectomies [32]. Patients present with fever, localized peritonitis, and leukocytosis, without free gas in the abdomen. Management includes intravenous fluids, antibiotics, and close clinical observation.

Conclusion

Colonoscopy is generally a safe procedure but with recognized minor and occasionally serious complications. Careful patient assessment prior to the procedure helps to identify and reduce the risk of complications whilst early recognition and treatment leads to improved patient outcomes.

Take-home points

- Patient assessment prior to the procedure can identify those at higher risk of colonoscopy complications and alternative, less invasive investigations such as CTC should be considered.
- Most major complications at colonoscopy relate to therapy, the most common being bleeding and perforation.
- Patients need to be made aware of the possible symptoms of postcolonoscopy complications (bleeding, severe pain, fever, vomiting) and have immediate access to appropriate emergency medical care.
- Early recognition of complications leads to improved patient's outcome.

References

1 Seeff LC, Manninen DL, Dong FB, *et al.* Is there endoscopic capacity to provide colorectal cancer screening to the unscreened population in the United States? *Gastroenterology* 2004; **127**: 1661–9.

2 Sieg A, Hachmoeller-Eisenbach U, Eisenbach T. Prospective evaluation of complications in outpatient GI endoscopy: a survey among German gastroenterologists. *Gastrointest Endosc* 2001; **53**: 620–7.

3 Bowles C, Leicester R, Romaya C, *et al.* A prospective study of colonoscopy practice in the UK today: are we adequately prepared for national colorectal cancer screening tomorrow? *Gut* 2004; **53**: 277–83.

4 Rex DK, Petrini JL, Baron TH, *et al.* Quality indicators for colonoscopy. *Am J Gastroenterol* 2006; **101**: 873–85.

5 Froehlich F, Wietlisbach V, Gonvers JJ, *et al.* Impact of colonic cleansing on quality and diagnostic yield of colonoscopy: the European Panel of Appropriateness of Gastrointestinal Endoscopy European multicenter study. *Gastrointest Endosc* 2005; **61**: 378–84.

6 Belsey J, Epstein O, Heresbach D. Systematic review: oral bowel preparation for colonoscopy. *Aliment Pharmacol Ther* 2007; **25**: 373–84.

7 Wexner S, Garbus J, Singh J. A prospective analysis of 13580 colonoscopies—Re-evaluation of credentialing guidelines. *Surg Endoc* 2001; **15**: 251–61.

8 Holm C, Christensen M, Rasmussen V, *et al.* Hypoxaemia and myocardial ischaemia during colonoscopy. *Scand J Gastroenterol* 1998; **33**: 769–72.

9 Ristikankare M, Julkunen R, Laitinen T, *et al.* Effect of conscious sedation on cardiac autonomic regulation during colonoscopy. *Scand J Gastroenterol* 2000; **35**: 990–6.

10 Iqbal CW, Cullinane DC, Schiller HJ, *et al.* Surgical management and outcomes of 165 colonoscopic perforations from a single institution. *Arch Surg* 2008; **143**: 701–6; discussion 6–7.

11 Wexner SD, Garbus JE, Singh JJ. A prospective analysis of 13,580 colonoscopies. Reevaluation of credentialing guidelines. *Surg Endosc* 2001; **15**: 251–61.

12 Petersen CR, Adamsen S, Gocht-Jensen P, *et al.* Splenic injury after colonoscopy. *Endoscopy* 2008; **40**: 76–9.

13 Shah P, Raman S, Hraray P. Splenic rupture following colonoscopy: Rare in the UK? *Surgeon* 2005; **3**: 293–5.

14 Paspatis GA, Vardas E, Theodoropoulou A, *et al.* Complications of colonoscopy in a large public county hospital in Greece A 10-year study. *Dig Liv Dis* 2008; **40**: 951–7.

15 Nelson D, McQuaid K, Bond J, *et al.* Procedural success and complications of large-scale screening colonoscopy. *Gastrointest Endosc* 2002; **55**: 307–14.

16 Levin T, Zhao W, Connell C, *et al.* Complications of colonoscopy in an intergrated health care delivery system. *Ann Intern Med* 2006; **145**: 880–6.

17 Bronowicki JP, Venard V, Botte C, *et al.* Patient-to-patient transmission of hepatitis C virus during colonoscopy. *N Engl J Med* 1997; **337**: 237–40.

18 DiMarino AJ, Bond WW. Flexible gastrointestinal endoscopic reprocessing. *Gastrointest Endosc* 1996; **43**: 522–4.

19 Bramble MG, Ironside JW. Creutzfeldt–Jakob disease: implications for gastroenterology. *Gut* 2002; **50**: 888–90.

20 Axon AT, Beilenhoff U, Bramble MG, *et al.* Variant Creutzfeldt–Jakob disease (vCJD) and gastrointestinal endoscopy. *Endoscopy* 2001; **33**: 1070–80.

21 ASGE. Guidelines for antibiotic prophylaxis for GI endoscopy. *Gastrointest Endosc* 2008; **67**: 791–8.

22 Rex DK, Cutler CS, Lemmel GT, *et al.* Colonoscopic miss rates of adenomas determined by back-to-back colonoscopies. *Gastroenterology* 1997; **112**: 24–8.

23 Rex D. Colonoscopic withdrawal technique is associated with adenoma miss rates. *Gastrointest Endosc* 2000; **51**: 33–6.

24 East JE, Suzuki N, Arebi N, *et al.* Position changes improve visibility during colonoscope withdrawal: a randomized, blinded, crossover trial. *Gastrointest Endosc* 2007; **65**: 263–9.

25 Barclay RL, Vicari JJ, Doughty AS, *et al.* Colonoscopic withdrawal times and adenoma detection during screening colonoscopy. *N Engl J Med* 2006; **355**: 2533–41.

26 Zuckerman MJ, Hirota WK, Adler DG, *et al.* ASGE guideline: the management of low-molecular-weight heparin and nonaspirin antiplatelet agents for endoscopic procedures. *Gastrointest Endosc* 2005; **61**: 189–94.

27 Kim HS, Kim TI, Kim WH, *et al.* Risk factors for immediate postpolypectomy bleeding of the colon: a multicenter study. *Am J Gastroenterol* 2006; **101**: 1333–41.

28 Sawhney MS, Salfiti N, Nelson DB, *et al.* Risk factors for severe delayed postpolypectomy bleeding. *Endoscopy* 2008; **40**: 115–9.

29 Fatima H, Rex DK. Minimizing endoscopic complications: colonoscopic polypectomy. *Gastrointest Endosc Clin N Am* 2007; **17**: 145–56, viii.

30 Repici A, Tricerri R. Endoscopic polypectomy: techniques, complications and follow-up. *Tech Coloproctol* 2004; **8** (Suppl. 2): s283–90.

31 Magdeburg R, Collet P, Post S, Kaehler G. Endoclipping of iatrogenic colonic perforation to avoid surgery. *Surg Endosc* 2008; **22**: 1500–4.

32 Waye JD, Lewis BS, Yessayan S. Colonoscopy: a prospective report of complications. *J Clin Gastroenterol* 1992; **15**: 347–51.

33 Waye JD. Management of complications of colonoscopic polypectomy. *Gastrenterologist* 1993; **1**: 158–64.

34 Eckardt V, Kanzler G, Scmitt T, *et al.* Complications and adverse effects of colonoscopy with selective sedation. *Gastrointest Endosc* 1999; **49**: 560–5.

35 Anderson ML, Pasha TM, Leighton JA. Endoscopic perforation of the colon: lessons from a 10-year study. *Am J Gastroenterol* 2000; **95**: 3418–22.

36 Dafnis G, Ekbom A, Pahlman L, Blomqvist P. Complications of diagnostic and therapeutic colonoscopy within a defined population in Sweden. *Gastrointest Endosc* 2001; **54**: 302–9.

37 Rathgaber S, Wick T. Colonoscopy completion and complication rates in a community gastroenterology practice. *Gastrointest Endosc* 2006; **64**: 556–62.

CHAPTER 10

Pancreatography (Including Pancreatic Sphincterotomy and Difficult Cannulation)

Nalini M. Guda[1] and Martin L. Freeman[2]

[1] University of Wisconsin School of Medicine and Public Health and St Luke's Medical Center, Milwaukee, WI, USA

[2] Division of Gastroenterology, Hepatology and Nutrition, University of Minnesota, Minneapolis, MN, USA

Summary

Endoscopic retrograde cholangiopancreatography (ERCP) is now mostly indicated for biliary and pancreatic therapeutic interventions. Diagnostic pancreatography has been largely replaced by other non/less invasive techniques including magnetic resonance cholangiopancreatography (MRCP) and endoscopic ultrasound. ERCP complications are best reduced by performing the procedures only when indications are appropriate. ERCP is still a dominant technique for relief of biliary and pancreatic obstruction, whether benign or malignant. Temporary pancreatic duct stenting has shown to reduce the incidence of post-ERCP pancreatitis in high-risk patients. Inadvertent or intentional pancreatic duct cannulation can facilitate biliary cannulation and allow placement of a pancreatic stent to reduce risk. Pancreatoscopy is now feasible, but its utility and safety are not well established. Understanding the risks and benefits of diagnostic and interventional aspects is essential, as well as proper training for the level of procedure performed.

Case

A 36-year-old female executive at a bank is admitted to the hospital with sudden-onset abdominal pain in the epigastric area radiating to the back, nausea, and vomiting. In the emergency department she was noted to have a serum lipase of 2000 U/L (normal 300 U/L). Her serum liver chemistries and triglycerides were normal. She has had three similar episodes in the past 4 years. She does not drink any alcohol, smoke cigarettes, or take any medications. After the last episode 1 year ago, she underwent cholecystectomy for suspected gall-bladder sludge.

During the current admission, a CT scan of the abdomen showed peripancreatic fat stranding suggestive of inflammation, without evidence of necrosis or fluid collections. The common bile duct and pancreatic ducts were not dilated. She recovered uneventfully after 4 days of hospitalization with intravenous hydration and parenteral pain control. She subsequently underwent an endoscopic ultrasound which did not show any parenchymal or ductal features of chronic pancreatitis, but there was a suspicion for possible pancreas divisum. A secretin-stimulated MRCP confirmed pancreas divisum with presence of a prominent dorsal pancreatic duct crossing the bile duct and absence of communication with a small ventral duct. She subsequently underwent an endoscopic retrograde cholangiography with minor papilla papillotomy and temporary small-caliber dorsal pancreatic duct stent placement.

Anatomical/Embryological Considerations

Normal Anatomy. Embryologically, the pancreas is formed by fusion of the dorsal and ventral segments. The tail, body, and portion of the head of the pancreas are formed by the dorsal segment and the uncinate process and the remaining portions of the head are formed by

---

Practical Gastroenterology and Hepatology: Small and Large Intestine and Pancreas, 1st edition. Edited by Nicholas J. Talley, Sunanda V. Kane and Michael B. Wallace. © 2010 Blackwell Publishing Ltd.

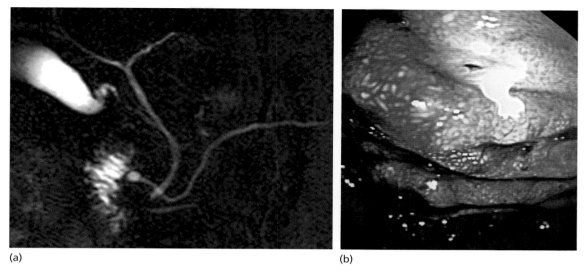

(a)   (b)

Figure 10.1 (a) Secretin MRCP showing pancreas divisum with Santorinicele. (b) Minor papilla orifice in patient with recurrent acute pancreatitis, revealed after administration of intravenous secretin and topical spray of methylene blue.

the ventral segment. The main duct of the pancreas (duct of Wirsung) starts in the tail and reaches the ampulla of Vater by traversing caudally and posteriorly in the head. The pancreatic duct may have a separate opening in the ampulla of Vater or may join the common bile duct to have a short common segment (1–12 mm). The accessory pancreatic duct (Santorini) drains a portion of the head and is developed from the duodenal wall. It usually communicates with the main pancreatic duct and is patent in about 70% of individuals. It drains into the minor papilla which is cephalad and anterior to the main pancreatic duct. The main pancreatic duct typically has a diameter of 2–4 mm in the head, 2–3 mm in the body, and 1–3 mm in the tail, increasing with age.

Pancreas Divisum. This is a congenital anomaly in which there is a failure of fusion of dorsal and ventral ducts, and is reported in 5–10% at autopsy series and as many as 25% of patients with recurrent acute pancreatitis. Failure to cannulate/opacify the pancreatic duct when intended should raise a suspicion of pancreas divisum; minor papilla cannulation is technically challenging and carries a high risk of post-ERCP pancreatitis. As MRCP (especially secretin enhanced) and endoscopic ultrasound have been shown to be effective in diagnosing this condition, ERCP to establish a diagnosis is mostly unnecessary

[1,2] (Figure 10.1). The role of pancreas divisum in acute recurrent pancreatitis and treatment responses to minor papillotomy are not clear. Response to papillotomy when performed for alleviation of chronic pain, whether or not it is associated with acute recurrent pancreatitis, is limited [3].

Annular Pancreas. This is a rare condition in which the second part of the duodenum is surrounded by a ring of pancreatic tissue continuous with the head of the pancreas. It is detected in 1 out of 12 000 to 15 000 newborns, when it typically presents with gastric outlet obstruction, but may remain asymptomatic, or present with duodenal obstruction, and/or recurrent acute or chronic pancreatitis later in life.

Pancreatic Duct Cannulation and Sphincterotomy

Pancreatic duct can be cannulated via the major papilla using a standard or tapered tip catheter, a sphincterotome, or a guidewire [4]. The pancreatic duct is generally medial and pedal (to the right and below) the bile duct orifice as visualized through a duodenoscope. Once the duct is cannulated, care should be taken not to overfill

Table 10.1 Indications for pancreatic sphincterotomy.

Pancreatic sphincterotomy (major papilla)
  Pancreatic duct strictures (usually with dilation + stenting)
  Pancreatic duct leaks (usually with transpancreatic stent or
    nasopancreatic drain)
  Palliation of malignant obstruction with stenting
  Treatment of chronic pancreatitis (stone removal/stricture dilation
    and or stenting)
  Sphincter of Oddi dysfunction
  Pancreatic duct evaluation/sampling (pancreatoscopy, intraductal
    ultrasound)
Pancreatic sphincterotomy (minor papilla)
  In those with pancreas divisum:
    Relief of obstruction in those with acute recurrent pancreatitis,
    chronic pancreatitis or chronic pain with obstruction of
    dorsal duct flow (same as in major papilla pancreatic
    sphincterotomy)
  In those without pancreas divisum:
    Same as in major papilla pancreatic sphincterotomy when best
    access to the duct is through minor papilla

Adapted from Freeman ML, Guda NM. Endoscopic biliary and pancreatic sphincterotomy. *Curr Treat Options Gastroenterol* 2005; **8**: 127–13.

the pancreatic duct with contrast. Post-ERCP pancreatitis is thought to be increased with the degree of duct opacification and the complexity of endoscopic intervention [5–8]. Acinarization (parenchymal blush from local or diffuse high pressure injection) of the pancreas has been shown to increase the risk of pancreatitis in univariate but not multivariate analyses, suggesting that other factors are more important.

Pancreatic duct sphincterotomy is generally performed for treatment of acute and chronic pancreatitis, pancreatic duct strictures, removal of pancreatic stones, or treatment of sphincter of Oddi dysfunction (Table 10.1). Pancreatic sphincterotomy should be done in centers performing advanced endoscopic interventions and by endoscopists with advanced training. It can be done with or without biliary sphincterotomy. Concomitant biliary sphincterotomy is usually recommended for treatment of papillary stenosis or sphincter of Oddi dysfunction.

Pancreatic sphincterotomy of the major papilla is done either by using a standard traction-type sphincterotome or by using a needle knife over a stent or guidewire. For either technique, deep cannulation of the duct and passage of a guidewire at least a few cm into the duct is

a prerequisite. For pull-type sphincterotomy, a sphincterotome is advanced with just a short segment of the wire in contact with the tissue, the sphincter is divided usually in the direction of the biliary sphincterotomy (between 11 and 1 o'clock position). Sphincterotomy should be done in 1 to 2-mm increments. Pure cutting current or a cut-effect on automated delivery systems is generally preferred to minimize thermal injury to the pancreas and duct, although specific data are not available. Pancreatic stent placement is required in almost all patients, although patients with severe chronic pancreatitis and large ducts may be the exception [9]. Needle knife sphincterotomy over a stent or guidewire is an alternate option [10–12].

A recent, randomized controlled trial show significantly reduced rates of pancreatitis for needle knife pancreatic sphincterotomy performed over a pancreatic stent compared with pull-type sphincterotomy [11]. Precut/access papillotomy of the pancreatic duct is seldom done except when the orifice is obstructed by a protruding stone, as the anatomy is so variable and unpredictable, or occasionally for minor papilla access, usually after secretin administration (Video 5).

Pancreatic Duct Guidewire or Sphincterotomy as an Aid to Biliary Cannulation. During ERCP performed for biliary access, sometimes the pancreatic duct is inadvertently cannulated, injected, or instrumented. In this situation placement of a pancreatic duct guidewire can facilitate biliary cannulation [7,8,13–16]. This serves several functions including opening of a stenotic papillary orifice, straightening the angle of the papilla so that biliary cannulation can be readily achieved, and facilitating placement of a pancreatic stent (Figure 10.2). Placement of a guidewire into the pancreatic duct does carry some risk. The reported risk of pancreatitis in those where a stent was not placed after passage of a wire is high, perhaps due to trauma to the main pancreatic duct or sidebranch perforation [14]. Certain anatomical variations of the pancreatic duct such as ansa configuration (a 360° turn of the pancreatic duct in the head of the pancreas) may render pancreatic wire and stent placement difficult. Failure to place a stent in high-risk individuals where pancreatic duct stenting was intended increases the risk of post-ERCP pancreatitis; in these instances a short stent can be placed in virtually all cases, even if the wire can be advanced into the pancreatic duct for a short distance, by

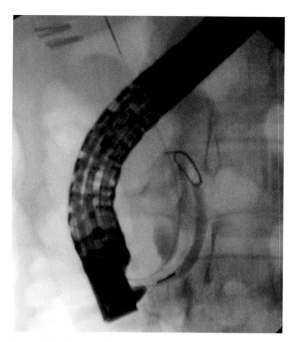

Figure 10.2 Fluoroscopic image during endoscopic retrograde cholangiopancreatography showing a 0.018 inch guidewire knuckled in the pancreatic duct with bile duct cannulated beside the pancreatic wire.

using an 0.018-inch platinum-tipped wire with a knuckle on the end to stabilize the wire [14].

Placement of a stent or cannula into the pancreatic duct have both been described to facilitate cannulation of the bile duct [8]. Any of these techniques might obviate the need for other riskier techniques such as needle knife precut sphincterotomy.

Transpancreatic septotomy for biliary access has also been described. In this technique once pancreatic duct is accessed, the pancreatic sphincter is cut using a traction papillotome. The initial results reported by a single operator were promising with an overall complication rate of less than 2% [17]. Subsequent results from a large case series have shown a high risk of complications (10% compared to their background rate of <1%) [18]. Another randomized study has shown a lower complication rate with this technique compared to precut sphincterotomy, but results were difficult to interpret because of inconsistent use of pancreatic stents [19]. Because the long-term complications of pancreatic sphincterotomy are unclear, this technique should be used with caution,

and in most cases placement of a temporary pancreatic stent is recommended.

Pancreas Divisum and Minor Papilla Interventions

Minor papillotomy with temporary stent placement may be indicated for treatment of acute relapsing pancreatitis in the setting of pancreas divisum, or severe chronic pancreatitis with dorsal dominant drainage or pancreas divisum. Data supporting efficacy in this context are ample but not universally accepted [20]. Relief of chronic pain in context of pancreas divisum is inconsistent at best. Minor papilla cannulation, stent placement, and papillotomy can be technically challenging, requiring small-caliber guidewires and cannulas, and specialized approaches including administration of secretin, and chromoendoscopy to aid in localizing and accessing minor papilla [21] (Video 5).

Pancreatography, Endoscopic, and Other Methods for Chronic Pancreatitis

Since chronic pancreatitis involves the gland as well as the duct, pancreatography alone is often inadequate to make a diagnosis. Earlier classifications including the most widely used Cambridge criteria were based on pancreatogam obtained at ERCP demonstrating abnormalities of the main pancreatic duct and sidebranches [22]. Less-invasive techniques have replaced this method. Computed tomography (CT) of the pancreas is sensitive mostly in detecting calcifications or dilated main pancreatic duct, which occur only in advanced disease. Endoscopic ultrasound can identify ductal dilation, calcifications, cysts, and prominent side branches, which along with the parenchymal changes can be used to make the diagnosis. Endoscopic ultrasound is thought to be quite sensitive for diagnosis of chronic pancreatitis, depending on the number and type of criteria used [23]. MRCP has a very high specificity in evaluation of chronic pancreatitis though the sensitivity is relatively low [24]. MRCP and magnetic resonance imaging (MRI) can identify changes in the duct, including obstruction from calcifications, strictures, and cysts that are not in

Table 10.2 Utility of various techniques in evaluating pancreatic diseases.

Condition	ERCP	MRCP	EUS	CT
Pancreas divisum	✓	✓	✓	?
Sphincter of Oddi dysfunction	✓	?	X	X
Chronic pancreatitis	✓	✓	✓	✓
Duct disruption/disconnection (pseudocyst/trauma/fistula)	✓*	✓**	✓	✓

*If cyst is not in communication with the main pancreatic duct or if the cyst contents are viscous ERCP is not helpful. Also ERCP does not show the upstream duct in case of duct disruption and MRCP might be beneficial.
**MRCP useful to delineate the up and down stream ducts and show the disruption and fluid collection.
ERCP, endoscopic retrograde cholangiopancreatography; MRCP, magnetic resonance cholangiopancreatography; EUS, endoscopic ultrasound; CT, computed tomography.

communication with the main pancreatic duct. T1 and T2-weighted images give substantial additional information about parenchymal changes. Administration of secretin improves not only imaging of the duct during MRCP but may provide functional information about the degree of obstruction and may allow assessment of exocrine function [24].

Utility of various tests in evaluating pancreatic disease are listed (Table 10.2). Sensitivity and specificity data are limited since most studies are small and ERCP has been the gold/reference standard for chronic pancreatitis, pancreas divisum. Newer imaging modalities are being increasingly used and are at least comparable or better. Due to the risk of complications, ERCP with pancreatography should be performed primarily when the intention is for treatment.

Pancreatoscopy

Direct per oral pancreatoscopy is now feasible during ERCP in order to evaluate the pancreatic duct. A newly developed, single operator, direct access cholangiopancreatoscope has made it easier compared to the conventional "mother–daughter" duodenoscope, although the current large diameter (10 F) limits its use to markedly dilated pancreatic ducts [25]. The fiberoptic guidewire

can also be passed through a standard 5 French ERCP cannula if limited visualization of the distal pancreatic duct is the only goal. Digital video, small-caliber pancreatoscopes will facilitate this procedure. Any utility of pancreatoscopy for tissue acquisition remains to be investigated. Direct pancreatoscopic lithotripsy and stone extraction from the main pancreatic duct to relieve obstruction appears to be feasible, although it has not been compared to extracorporeal shock wave lithotripsy, which has been widely used and shown to be both effective and safe [26].

Take-home points

- Diagnostic ERCP and pancreatography should generally be avoided, and can largely be supplanted by endoscopic ultrasound and/or MRCP.
- After inadvertent pancreatography during ERCP for bile duct access, placing a guidewire in the pancreatic duct can aid biliary cannulation and facilitate pancreatic stent placement to reduce risk of post-ERCP pancreatitis.
- Pancreatic duct stents have been shown to reduce post ERCP pancreatitis in high-risk patients.
- Pancreatic sphincterotomy can be done as traction sphincterotomy or as needle knife sphincterotomy over a pancreatic duct stent.
- Pancreatoscopy is now possible although data regarding benefits, limitations, and complications are limited.

References

1 Lai R, Freeman ML, Cass OW, Mallery S. Accurate diagnosis of pancreas divisum by linear-array endoscopic ultrasonography. *Endoscopy* 2004; **36**: 705–9.
2 Vitellas KM, Keogan MT, Spritzer CE, Nelson RC. MR holangiopancreatography of bile and pancreatic duct abnormalities with emphasis on the single-shot fast spin-echo technique. *Radiographics* 2000; **20**: 939–57.
3 Gerke H, Byrne MF, Stiffler HL, *et al.* Outcome of endoscopic minor papillotomy in patients with symptomatic pancreas divisum. *JOP* 2004; **5**: 122–31.
4 Freeman ML, Guda NM. Endoscopic biliary and pancreatic sphincterotomy. *Curr Treat Options Gastroenterol* 2005; **8**: 127–34.
5 Buscaglia JM, Simons BW, Prosser BJ, *et al.* Severity of post-ERCP pancreatitis directly proportional to the invasiveness of endoscopic intervention: a pilot study in a canine model. *Endoscopy* 2008; **40**: 506–12.

6 Cheon YK, Cho KB, Watkins JL, *et al.* Frequency and severity of post-ERCP pancreatitis correlated with extent of pancreatic ductal opacification. *Gastrointest Endosc* 2007; **65**: 385–93.

7 Freeman ML, Guda NM. Prevention of post-ERCP pancreatitis: a comprehensive review. *Gastrointest Endosc* 2004; **59**: 845–64.

8 Freeman ML, Guda NM. ERCP cannulation: a review of reported techniques. *Gastrointest Endosc* 2005; **61**: 112–25.

9 Freeman ML. Pancreatic stents for prevention of post-endoscopic retrograde cholangiopancreatography pancreatitis. *Clin Gastroenterol Hepatol* 2007; **5**: 1354–65.

10 Attwell A, Borak G, Hawes R, *et al.* Endoscopic pancreatic sphincterotomy for pancreas divisum by using a needle-knife or standard pull-type technique: safety and reintervention rates. *Gastrointest Endosc* 2006; **64**: 705–11.

11 Maple JT, Keswani RN, Edmunowicz SA, *et al.* Wire-assisted access sphincterotomy of the minor papilla. *Gastrointest Endosc* 2009; **69**: 57–64.

12 Varadarajulu S, Wilcox CM. Randomized trial comparing needle-knife and pull-sphincterotome techniques for pancreatic sphincterotomy in high-risk patients. *Gastrointest Endosc* 2006; **64**: 716–22.

13 Ito K, Fujita N, Noda Y, *et al.* Pancreatic guidewire placement for achieving selective biliary cannulation during endoscopic retrograde cholangio-pancreatography. *World J Gastroenterol* 2008; **14**: 5595–600.

14 Freeman ML, Overby C, Qi D. Pancreatic stent insertion: consequences of failure and results of a modified technique to maximize success. *Gastrointest Endosc* 2004; **59**: 8–14.

15 Wang P, Li ZS, Liu F, *et al.* Risk factors for ERCP-related complications: a prospective multicenter study. *Am J Gastroenterol* 2009; **104**: 31–40.

16 Freeman ML, DiSario JA, Nelson DB, *et al.* Risk factors for post-ERCP pancreatitis: a prospective, multicenter study. *Gastrointest Endosc* 2001; **54**: 425–34.

17 Goff JS. Long-term experience with the transpancreatic sphincter pre-cut approach to biliary sphincterotomy. *Gastrointest Endosc* 1999; **50**: 642–5.

18 Akashi R, Kiyozumi T, Jinnouchi K, *et al.* Pancreatic sphincter precutting to gain selective access to the common bile duct: a series of 172 patients. *Endoscopy* 2004; **36**: 405–10.

19 Catalano MF, Linder JD, Geenen JE. Endoscopic transpancreatic papillary septotomy for inaccessible obstructed bile ducts: Comparison with standard pre-cut papillotomy. *Gastrointest Endosc* 2004; **60**: 557–61.

20 Romagnuolo J, Guda N, Freeman M, Durkalski V. Preferred designs, outcomes, and analysis strategies for treatment trials in idiopathic recurrent acute pancreatitis. *Gastrointest Endosc* 2008; **68**: 966–74.

21 Park SH, de Bellis M, McHenry L, *et al.* Use of methylene blue to identify the minor papilla or its orifice in patients with pancreas divisum. *Gastrointest Endosc* 2003; **57**: 358–63.

22 Sai JK, Suyama M, Kubokawa Y, Watanabe S. Diagnosis of mild chronic pancreatitis (Cambridge classification): comparative study using secretin injection-magnetic resonance cholangiopancreatography and endoscopic retrograde pancreatography. *World J Gastroenterol* 2008; **14**: 1218–21.

23 Catalano MF, Sahai A, MD, Levy M, *et al.* EUS-based criteria for the diagnosis of chronic pancreatitis: the Rosemont classification *Gastrointest Endosc* 2009; **69**: 1251–61.

24 Kinney TP, Freeman ML. Pancreatic imaging: current state of the art. *Gastroenterology* 2009; **136**: 776–9.

25 Judah JR, Draganov PV. Intraductal biliary and pancreatic endoscopy: an expanding scope of possibility. *World J Gastroenterol* 2008; **14**: 3129–36.

26 Guda NM, Partington S, Freeman ML. Extracorporeal shock wave lithotripsy in the management of chronic calcific pancreatitis: a meta-analysis. *JOP* 2005; **6**: 6–12.

CHAPTER 11
Endoscopic Ultrasound

David J. Owens and Thomas J. Savides
Division of Gastroenterology, University of California, San Diego, CA, USA

Summary

Endoscopic ultrasound (EUS) has become critically important for evaluating a variety of pancreatic, small bowel, and colorectal diseases. In the absence of distant metastatic disease, locoregional EUS staging of pancreatic, ampullary, and rectal cancer impacts cancer management. EUS is excellent in the evaluation of benign pancreatic lesions such as pancreatic cysts, chronic pancreatitis, and autoimmune pancreatitis. EUS fine needle aspiration (FNA) is especially accurate for obtaining diagnostic cytologic material for pancreatic lesions. Anal EUS is one of the best modalities for evaluating prior obstetrical trauma as a cause of fecal incontinence. Interventional EUS techniques are becoming increasingly used for therapies, such as pancreatic pseudocyst drainage, injection therapy to assist pancreatic cancer treatment, and even transcolonic drainage of perirectal fluid collections.

Case

A 65-year-old woman has a 1-month history of diarrhea with floating oil droplets. Her referring gastroenterologist found she had a normal colonoscopy and also a normal esophagogastroduodenoscopy (EGD) with duodenal biopsies. Since the initial evaluation, over the past 2 weeks she developed dark urine and unintentionally lost 6.8 kg (15 pounds). Pancreatic EUS reveals a 3-cm mass in the pancreatic head causing upstream dilation of both the bile duct and pancreatic and with abutment of the superior mesenteric vein. EUS-guided transduodenal fine needle aspiration (FNA) reveals pancreatic adenocarcinoma. Along with referral to a pancreatic surgeon, she is started on oral pancreatic enzymes before meals, which resolves her diarrhea and fecal incontinence.

Introduction

Endoscopic ultrasound (EUS) incorporates an ultrasound transducer on the tip of an endoscope. EUS can be performed with a radial echoendoscope, which provide images perpendicular to the axis of the scope and corresponds to the axial computed tomography (CT) or magnetic resonance imaging (MRI) slices in the rectum, esophagus, and stomach, or with a linear array EUS scope, which provides an image parallel to the shaft of the endoscope and allows real-time visualization of needle aspiration or therapeutic maneuvers. This chapter will focus on pancreatic, small bowel, and colorectal EUS.

Pancreatic EUS

Pancreatic Cancer

EUS can detect pancreatic masses in patients with abnormal CT scans or unexplained biliary obstruction (Figure 11.1). When a solid pancreatic mass is identified, EUS FNA has a sensitivity and specificity of 85% and 95%, respectively, for diagnosing malignancy [1]. When solid pancreatic masses undergo EUS FNA, a large multicenter study found the overall cancer diagnosis yield to be 72%, with variation among endosonographers possibly related to the underlying rates of chronic pancreatitis in the population, as well as technical, cytopathology, and operator issues [2].

Once pancreatic cancer is diagnosed or highly suspected, the next important step is determining resectability. CT or MRI scan should first be obtained to

Practical Gastroenterology and Hepatology: Small and Large Intestine and Pancreas, 1st edition. Edited by Nicholas J. Talley, Sunanda V. Kane and Michael B. Wallace. © 2010 Blackwell Publishing Ltd.

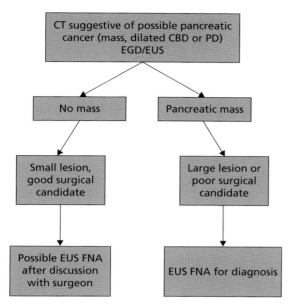

Figure 11.1 Algorithm for endoscopic ultrasound-guided approach to suspected pancreatic mass. CT, computed tomography; CBD, common bile duct; PD, pancreatic duct; EGD, esophagogastroduodenoscopy; EUS, endoscopic ultrasound; FNA, fine needle aspiration.

exclude distant metastases. Although traditionally invasion of the superior mesenteric artery, superior mesenteric vein, or portal vein have been considered unresectable for cure, more recently some expert pancreatic surgeons may attempt resection with vascular reconstruction in selected patients [3]. EUS accuracy for determining resectability of pancreatic cancers ranges from 62 to 93%, and recent studies comparing EUS to CT and MRI have not yielded a clearly superior test for determining respectability [4].

Interventional EUS can play a role in the palliation of unresectable pancreatic cancer patients. EUS fine needle injection can implant metal radiopaque fiducials to assist stereotactic radiation therapy, as well as inject experimental chemotherapy directly into the lesion for localized treatment [5,6] (Video 6 and 7).

Pancreatic Cysts

Pancreatic cysts are an increasingly common problem, because they are frequently found as incidental lesions. Approximately 3% of abdominal CT scans will incidentally detect small pancreatic cysts less than 3 cm [7]. Serial

CT scan studies usually show no change in these lesions over a several-year period, suggesting the natural history of small incidentally found cysts is benign. The challenge is trying to determine which cysts are actually cancer or could turn into cancer.

Pancreatic cystic lesions are described in detail in Chapter 58, but can be separated into three categories: those that are benign (simple cysts, pseudocysts, branch-type intraductal papillary mucinous neoplasm (IPMN)), those that are cancer (adenocarcinoma or endocrine tumor), and those that have malignant potential (cystadenoma, main duct IPMN). The natural history of lesions with malignant potential is unknown, and it is quite likely that for many patients the risk of developing a life-threatening cancer is less than the risk of surgical cyst resection.

EUS is extremely useful in the initial evaluation of pancreatic cysts to determine if there is an associated mass which likely would represent cancer. EUS FNA can aspirate cysts to obtain fluid for CEA, amylase, and cytology, which can help distinguish between mucinous and non-mucinous lesions (Video 8 and 9). However, the actual utility of pancreatic cyst aspiration is uncertain as the results are often confusing to interpret and cannot indicate which patient will go on to develop cancer. Pancreatic cyst aspiration is associated with rare risks of bleeding, pancreatitis, and cyst infection. If a pancreatic cyst is aspirated, a common practice to reduce complications is to completely aspirate the cyst and provide the patient with intravenous and/or oral antibiotics for 3–7 days. Benign-appearing cysts can generally be observed with serial imaging studies.

Large and/or symptomatic pancreatic pseudocysts can be safely and effectively drained with EUS-guided transgastric stent placement to form a cystgastrostomy [8].

Chronic Pancreatitis

The use of EUS in the evaluation of chronic pancreatitis is debated, and true accuracy estimates are hampered by lack of an available gold standard. EUS findings suggestive of chronic pancreatitis include stones/calcifications, echogenic foci, echogenic stranding, hyperechoic main pancreatic duct, dilated pancreatic duct, irregular pancreatic duct, visible pancreatic size branches, lobular echotexture, and cysts. Agreement among expert endosonographers is moderate for diagnosing "early" chronic pancreatitis [9] except in the presence of obvious pancreatic stones/calcifications, which can generally be diagnosed with other less-invasive imaging studies. Due to its high sensitivity, the main role of EUS is likely to exclude chronic pancreatitis in patients with chronic, pancreatic-type, epigastric pain.

Autoimmune Pancreatitis

Autoimmune pancreatitis is an infrequent, but increasingly recognized, cause of biliary obstruction which is important to consider because patients are treated with steroids rather than surgery. Most patients are male over age 55. The most commonly described CT finding is a diffusely swollen, sausage-shaped pancreas with a narrowed pancreatic duct, but the CT can also find pancreatic masses and isolated biliary strictures. EUS is very helpful in identifying possible autoimmune pancreatitis, because the pancreas will appear diffusely hypoechoic and enlarged. EUS FNA with core biopsy, as well as serum IgG subtype 4 levels, support the diagnosis of autoimmune pancreatitis [10,11].

Pancreatic Endocrine Tumors

Pancreatic endocrine tumors are classified as either functional or non-functional depending upon their production of symptomatic hormones (i.e., insulin, gastrin, glucagon, vasoactive intestinal peptide, and somatostatin). The majority of pancreatic endocrine tumors do not cause endocrine symptoms, but are found either due to pain or on an incidental imaging study. EUS is extremely useful for detecting small symptomatic hormone-producing pancreatic endocrine tumors, such as insulinomas or gastrinomas, with confirmation by EUS FNA cytology.

Small Bowel EUS

Ampullary Adenomas and Cancers

EUS can accurately assess ampullary adenomas or superficial ampullary adenocarcinomas which are being considered for possible endoscopic resection. If EUS shows extension into the bile duct, pancreatic duct, or peripancreatic lymph nodes, then invasive cancer should be suspected and surgical resection considered rather than endoscopic ampullectomy.

Duodenal Polyps and Cancers

EUS can evaluate mucosal/submucosal lesions of the duodenum prior to endoscopic resection. These lesions can include carcinoid tumors, cysts, adenomas, paraganglionomas, and others. EUS has a more limited role for evaluation of duodenal adenocarcinoma, as this is usually treated surgically.

Colorectal EUS

Colon Cancer

There is no role for EUS in staging colon cancer. This is because colon cancer can easily and safely be resected with wide margins, which allows complete removal and locoregional staging in one step.

Rectal Cancer

In contrast to colon cancer, rectal cancer surgery is limited by the ability to get sufficient radial and proximal/distal resection margins due to limitations from the pelvic bones and the anus. Because of risks of local recurrence after rectal cancer resection, preoperative chemoradiation is generally recommended for locally advanced rectal cancers. EUS is ideally suited for evaluating rectal cancer (Figure 11.2), because if it finds tumor extending into the perirectal fat (T3) or with adjacent lymph nodes (N1), then preoperative chemoradiation is given (Video 10). If the tumor is found to be limited to the mucosa/submucosal layer (T1), then it is amenable to transanal resection or endoscopic mucosal resection. The overall accuracy of EUS for the T and N-staging of rectal cancers is approximately 85% and 75%, respectively [12]. EUS has much diminished staging accuracy after radiation therapy.

Anal Cancer

EUS has limited utility in anorectal cancer evaluation because staging of this is based on length of tumor and more distant lymph node metastases (iliac and femoral nodes), rather than local extension.

Fecal Incontinence

Fecal incontinence is usually due to prior obstetrical trauma, which can either result in trauma to the anal sphincters and/or pudendal nerve damage. Fecal incontinence becomes more common in women greater than 60 years of age, which is felt due to age-related weakening of already damaged anal sphincters and nerves. Postobstetrical damage to the anal sphincters is seen after 40%

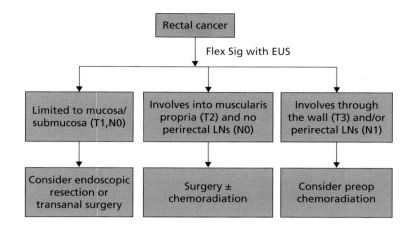

Figure 11.2 Algorithm for endoscopic ultrasound-guided management of rectal cancer. Flex Sig, flexible sigmoidoscopy; LN, lymph node; EUS, endoscopic ultrasound.

of vaginal deliveries based on EUS studies [13]. Patients with a significant defect of the anal sphincters on EUS may be considered for overlapping surgical sphincteroplasty.

Anal Fistulae

EUS can also detect such perianal findings as fistula, abscesses, and fissures in patients with perirectal pain or a history of Crohn disease. These exams are challenging given the complexity of these fistulae, and might better be done with endoanal coil MRI or complete examination under anesthesia by an experienced colorectal surgeon.

Complications of EUS

Complications associated with EUS are similar to standard EGD, except that the rigid long tip of the echoendoscope can lead to a higher rate of esophageal or duodenal perforation. The risks of pancreatic EUS FNA are approximately 1%, and include bleeding, infection, perforation, and pancreatitis [14].

Take-home points

- EUS can detect small pancreatic masses which may not be visualized well with CT or MRI.
- EUS is complimentary to CT and MRI for staging of pancreatic cancer.

- EUS FNA has a high accuracy rate for obtaining tissue diagnosis of pancreatic cancer.
- Pancreatic cysts can be evaluated by EUS to help stratify risk of malignancy.
- EUS is a sensitive method to exclude chronic pancreatitis in patients with epigastric pain.
- Therapeutic interventional endoscopic ultrasound is a growing field that includes pseudocyst drainage, celiac plexus block, and fine needle injection to aid in targeted chemotherapy and radiation.
- EUS is accurate for staging rectal cancer but plays no significant role in staging colon cancer.
- Anal EUS can detect postobstetrical anal sphincter damage which may contribute to fecal incontinence.

References

1 Eloubeidi MA, Chen VK, Eltoum IA, *et al.* Endoscopic ultrasound-guided fine needle aspiration biopsy of patients with suspected pancreatic cancer: diagnostic accuracy and acute and 30-day complications. *Am J Gastroenterol* 2003; **98:** 2663–8.

2 Gress F, Savides T, Cummings O, *et al.* Radial scanning and linear array endosonography for staging pancreatic cancer: a prospective randomized comparison. *Gastrointest Endosc* 1997; **45:** 138–42.

3 Al-Haddad M, Martin JK, Nguyen J, *et al.* Vascular resection and reconstruction for pancreatic malignancy: a single center survival study. *J Gastrointest Surg* 2007; **11:** 1168–74.

4 Dewitt J, Devereaux B, Chriswell M, *et al.* Comparison of endoscopic ultrasonography and multidetector computed tomography for detecting and staging pancreatic cancer. *Ann Intern Med* 2004; **141**: 753–63.

5 Chang KJ, Lee JG, Holcombe RF, *et al.* Endoscopic ultrasound delivery of an antitumor agent to treat a case of pancreatic cancer. *Nat Clin Pract Gastroenterol Hepatol* 2008; **5**: 107–11.

6 Pishvaian AC, Collins B, Gagnon G, *et al.* EUS-guided fiducial placement for CyberKnife radiotherapy of mediastinal and abdominal malignancies. *Gastrointest Endosc* 2006; **64**: 412–7.

7 Laffan TA, Horton KM, Klein AP, *et al.* Prevalence of unsuspected pancreatic cysts on MDCT. *AJR Am J Roentgenol* 2008; **191**: 802–7.

8 Varadarajulu S, Tamhane A, Blakely J. Graded dilation technique for EUS-guided drainage of peripancreatic fluid collections: an assessment of outcomes and complications and technical proficiency (with video). *Gastrointest Endosc* 2008; **68**: 656–66.

9 Wallace MB, Hawes RH, Durkalski V, *et al.* The reliability of EUS for the diagnosis of chronic pancreatitis: interobserver agreement among experienced endosonographers. *Gastrointest Endosc* 2001; **53**: 294–9.

10 Farrell JJ, Garber J, Sahani D, Brugge WR. EUS findings in patients with autoimmune pancreatitis. *Gastrointest Endosc* 2004; **60**: 927–36.

11 Levy MJ, Reddy RP, Wiersema MJ, *et al.* EUS-guided trucut biopsy in establishing autoimmune pancreatitis as the cause of obstructive jaundice. *Gastrointest Endosc* 2005; **61**: 467–72.

12 Savides TJ, Master SS. EUS in rectal cancer. *Gastrointest Endosc* 2002; **56** (4 Suppl.): S12–S18.

13 Sultan AH, Kamm MA, Hudson CN, *et al.* Anal-sphincter disruption during vaginal delivery. *N Engl J Med* 1993; **329**: 1905–11.

14 Al Haddad M, Wallace MB, Woodward TA, *et al.* The safety of fine-needle aspiration guided by endoscopic ultrasound: a prospective study. *Endoscopy* 2008; **40**: 204–8.

PART 3

Other Investigations of the Intestine and Pancreas

CHAPTER 12
Capsule Endoscopy

Blair S. Lewis

Henry D. Janowitz Division of Gastroenterology, Mount Sinai School of Medicine, New York, NY, USA

Summary

Capsule endoscopy is the test of choice when dealing with obscure gastrointestinal bleeding once colonoscopy and esophagogastroduodenoscopy (EGD) have proved negative. Yields of capsule endoscopy average 70% and are improved when the test is performed close to the bleeding episode. In addition, capsule endoscopy guides subsequent therapy with double balloon enteroscopy by using the percentage of the small bowel transit time to guide either per oral or transrectal double balloon approaches. A normal capsule study indicates a low risk of further bleeding.

Case

A 72-year-old man with a history of atrial fibrillation maintained on warfarin presents with progressive weakness and fatigue. In his doctor's office, he is seen to be pale and a stat blood count reveals a hemoglobin of 8 g. He is referred to the local emergency room where he is transfused with 2 units of packed cells. Further laboratory studies reveal an international normalized ratio (INR) of 2.5. His warfarin is held and both colonoscopy and esophagogastroduodenoscopy (EGD) are performed the next day. These exams are normal. He is discharged home back on warfarin with a hemogoblin of 10 g. Capsule endoscopy is performed 2 weeks later in his gastroenterologist's office. This reveals a single large angioectasia in the small bowel (Figure 12.1).

Review of the capsule study showed that the vascular lesion was located at 1 h 39 min into the study. The gastric transit time was 1 h 4 min and the small bowel transit time was 5 h 58 min. As outlined above, the lesion was calculated to be 99 min minus 64 past the pylorus or 35 min. The lesion was thus calculated to be 35/294 or approximately 12% of the capsule small bowel transit time. Per oral double balloon enteroscopy (DBE) was arranged. It was elected to perform this exam on an ambulatory basis and the patient's warfarin

was not discontinued for the exam. At DBE the lesion was reached and endoscopy cauterization using a plasma argon coagulator was applied. The patient has been free of bleeding for more than 1 year.

Introduction

Capsule endoscopy of the small bowel was first cleared for marketing in the USA by the Food and Drug Administration (FDA) in August 2001. In addition to the small bowel capsule, a capsule for viewing the esophagus has also been granted FDA clearance. The third development in the field of capsule endoscopy is a capsule for evaluation of the colon. A colon capsule has been developed and tested internationally but is not an FDA approved device at present. The endoscopic capsule was initially developed by Dr Gavriel Idan in 1981 as a means to evaluate the entire small intestine. Two capsule systems are currently available for small bowel imaging (Given Imaging, Israel, and Olympus, Japan). The capsule system from Given Imaging measures 11×26 mm and contains six light emitting diodes (LEDs), a lens, a color camera chip, two silver oxide batteries, a radiofrequency transmitter, and an antenna [1]. The capsule obtains two images per second and transmits the data via

Practical Gastroenterology and Hepatology: Small and Large Intestine and Pancreas, 1st edition. Edited by Nicholas J. Talley, Sunanda V. Kane and Michael B. Wallace. © 2010 Blackwell Publishing Ltd.

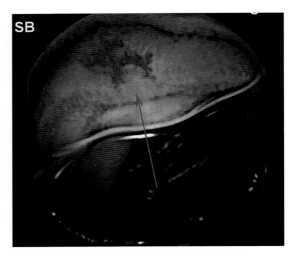

Figure 12.1 Vascular lesion in the small bowel (arrow).

radiofrequency to a recording device. Once the acquisition time is reached, the recording device is downloaded to a computer workstation whose software provides the images to the computer screen. The capsule is disposable and does not need to be retrieved by the patient as it is passed naturally. The Olympus capsule system is similar.

Contraindications

Contraindications to capsule endoscopy include swallowing disorders, pacemakers, and small bowel obstruction. The capsule can be placed in the small bowel endoscopically in cases where patients are unable to swallow the it. Pacemakers are contraindicated for regulatory reasons. Clinical research has shown that there is no interference between the capsule and the implanted device, including implanted defibrillators [2]. Small bowel obstruction is contraindicated due to the risk of capsule retention. Capsule retention has been reported in a small percentage of capsule exams but only upstream of areas of pathology [3]. A dissolving capsule has been designed to test small bowel passage prior to video capsule endoscopy to in patients who are felt to be at increased risk for retention [4].

Clinical Experience

Small bowel capsule endoscopy is the state-of-the-art method of small bowel evaluation, due to the length of the small bowel examined, quality of the examination, and non-invasive nature of the test. This has been supported by the most recent ICCE International Conference of Capsule Endoscopy (ICCE) consensus statement [5], the American Society for Gastrointestinal Endoscopy (ASGE) technical assessment [6], and the American Gastroenterological Association (AGA) medical position statement [7]. Worldwide experience suggests that capsule endoscopy should be the third test in the evaluation of patients with gastrointestinal bleeding, once EGD and colonoscopy have been found to be negative. A pooled data analysis of company-sponsored trials has shown capsule endoscopy to have a significantly increased pathology detection capability as compared to push enteroscopy, small bowel series, and colonoscopy with ileal intubation for suspected disease of the small intestine [8]. Capsule endoscopy identified a potential cause of bleeding in approximately 70% of the exams in the pooled data analysis of 530 exams. This was double the yield of other methods. Approximately 90% of 1349 pathologies were not identified by any method other than capsule endoscopy. Capsule endoscopy is considered to be the superior method in the diagnosis of bleeding from the small intestine. A meta-analysis of both published trials and abstracts also attests to this increased yield [9]. A total of 14 studies comparing capsule endoscopy to push enteroscopy were reviewed with a combined yield of 63% and 28%, respectively. A meta-analysis by Marmo *et al.* also attests to this increased yield of capsule endoscopy [10].

Long term follow-up studies have allowed calculation of sensitivity and specificity for capsule endoscopy by obtaining a final diagnosis during the follow-up period. Pennazio *et al.* reported 1-year follow-up of 100 patients with obscure bleeding [11]. Sensitivity, specificity, and positive and negative predictive values of capsule endoscopy were 88.9%, 95%, 97%, and 82.6%, respectively, in the 56 patients in whom a definite confirmed diagnosis was obtained. Delvaux *et al.* reported 1-year follow-up experience in 44 patients [12]. The positive predictive value of capsule endoscopy was 94% in those with findings at capsule endoscopy and the negative predictive value was 100% in patients with normal capsule exam findings.

The findings at capsule endoscopy are reliable, as confirmed by a prospective study comparing capsule endoscopy to intraoperative endoscopy in 47 patients [13]. The overall yield for capsule endoscopy was 74% and for both procedures was 77%. Bleeding sites were identified by both techniques in 36, by capsule endoscopy only in two, and by intraoperative enteroscopy only in one. Both exams were negative in 11. The calculated sensitivity for capsule endoscopy was 95%, specificity 75%, and positive and negative predictive values of 95% and 86%.

Patient Selection

Investigators have looked at patient selection for capsule endoscopy to determine if this influences the yield of the exam. Bresci *et al.* reported a greater yield for capsule endoscopy of 91% versus 34% if capsule endoscopy were performed within 2 weeks of a bleeding episode [14]. May *et al.* also reported that patient selection for capsule endoscopy affected yields [15]. Patients who had been enrolled in a study of capsule endoscopy where inclusion criteria included a drop of hemoglobin below 10 g, anemia or bleeding persisting more than 6 months, and the occurrence of more than one bleeding episode were more likely to have a source of bleeding identified. The yield of capsule endoscopy in these patients was higher than in this selected group than in those tested as part of routine clinical practice: 66% versus 45%. Despite this, capsule endoscopy has shown a significant yield in patients with unexplained iron deficiency anemia [16].

Therapeutic Impact

The therapeutic impact of capsule endoscopy has been measured. Kraus *et al.* reported that in 33% of cases, capsule exam findings guided additional diagnostic and therapeutic steps [17]. Ben Soussan *et al.* reported that in 37% of exams, new steps in management were undertaken, including endoscopic management in 10, surgery in two, and medical therapy in one [18]. Mylonaki *et al.* reported that capsule endoscopy led to an alteration of therapy in 66% of patients with positive findings [19]. Pennazio *et al.* reported that in 20 of 23 patients in whom capsule endoscopy was performed for ongoing overt bleeding, directed treatments led to resolution of bleeding in 87% [11]. Overall, follow-up data of 91 patients during a mean follow-up period of 18 months showed that subsequent management dictated by capsule

endoscopy led to the resolution of the bleeding in 59 (65%).

Capsule identification of a bleeding site in the small bowel aids in the performance of subsequent successful enteroscopy. In one of the initial reports of capsule endoscopy, Lewis and Swain detailed a yield of capsule endoscopy of 55% in 21 patients with obscure gastrointestinal bleeding [20]. Twenty-two push enteroscopies had been performed in nine of the patients prior to enrollment in the trial and all of these exams had been negative. Following capsule endoscopy, four of these patients were found to have lesions within reach of push enteroscopy and repeat examination led to the identification of the bleeding site and the application of cautery. Having the capsule show a lesion in a particular area drives the endoscopist at subsequent enteroscopy to reidentify the lesion. Thus, primary enteroscopy without prior capsule endoscopy is generally avoided.

Localization of Bleeding Site

An area of ongoing investigation has been the localization of a bleeding site seen on capsule endoscopy to determine if the finding is within reach of push enteroscopy or DBE using an oral or transrectal approach. Initial attempts to use capsule passage time from the pylorus to the lesion proved inaccurate since total small bowel passage times vary, attesting to varied peristalsis between individuals. Appleyard has advocated using percentage of passage times to determine where a finding is located (personal communication). The capsule passage time from the pylorus to the lesion is divided by the total small bowel passage time (Figure 12.2). He has suggested that passage percentages less than 10% are within reach of a push enteroscope. Lesions within 70% can be reached using an oral approach, while those longer than 70% can only be reached by transrectal passage. This has also been confirmed by Gay *et al.* who performed 47 DBE exams in 42 patients [21]. They used a cut-off of 75% to decide between oral and transrectal approaches for DBE. They concluded that capsule endoscopy is a useful "filter" for DBE and can help choose the route of the DBE exam.

A negative capsule exam is predictive of a low likelihood of recurrent blood loss. Lai *et al.* reported a negative predictive value of capsule endoscopy of 94% in a study of 49 patients with obscure bleeding in whom the median follow-up period was 19 months [22]. Thus, the risk of

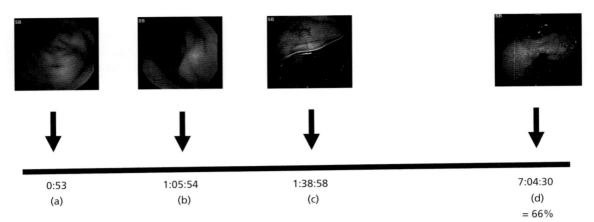

0:53	1:05:54	1:38:58	7:04:30
(a)	(b)	(c)	(d)
			= 66%

Figure 12.2 Calculation of the location of a bleeding site in the small bowel. (a) First gastric image; (b) first duodenal image; (c) the vascular lesion (arrow); and (d) the first cecal image. Gastric time = b − a; small bowel transit time = d − b; time to the lesion = [c − b/d − b].

recurrent bleeding rate in a normal exam is approximately 6%.

Take-home points

- Capsule endoscopy should be performed as closely to the bleeding episode as possible.

- If a bleeding site is identified, the percentage should be calculated of the small bowel transit time to the lesion from the pylorus. If less than 70%, a per oral DBE should be requested; and if greater than 70%, a transrectal DBE.

- If a capsule study is normal, there is a very low likelihood of further bleeding.

References

1 Meron G. The development of the swallowable video capsule (M2A). *Gastrointest Endosc* 2000; **6**: 817–9.

2 Bandorski D, Irnich W, Bruck M, Beyer N, Kramer W, Jakobs R. Capsule endoscopy and cardiac pacemakers: investigation for possible interference. *Endoscopy* 2008; **40**: 36–9.

3 Cave D, Legnani P, deFranchis R, Lewis B. ICCE consensus for capsule retention. *Endoscopy* 2005; **37**: 1065–7.

4 Herrerias J, Leighton J, Costamagna G, *et al.* Agile patency system eliminates risk of capsule retention in patients with known intestinal strictures who undergo capsule endoscopy. *Gastrointest Endosc* 2008; **67**: 902–9.

5 Mergener K, Ponchon T, Gralnek I, *et al.* Literature review and recommendations for clinical application of small-bowel capsule endoscopy, based on a panel discussion by international experts. *Endoscopy* 2007; **39**: 895–909.

6 Mishkin DS, Chuttani R, Croffie J, *et al*; Technology Assessment Committee, American Society for Gastrointestinal Endoscopy. ASGE Technology Status Evaluation Report: wireless capsule endoscopy. *Gastrointest Endosc* 2006; **63**: 539–45.

7 Raju GS, Gerson L, Das A, Lewis B; American Gastroenterological Association. American Gastroenterological Association (AGA) Institute medical position statement on obscure gastrointestinal bleeding. *Gastroenterology* 2007; **133**: 1694–6.

8 Lewis B, Eisen G, Friedman S. A pooled analysis to evaluate results of capsule endoscopy trials. *Endoscopy* 2005; **37**: 960–5.

9 Triester SL, Leighton JA, Leontiadis GI, *et al.* A meta-analysis of the yield of capsule endoscopy compared to other diagnostic modalities in patients with obscure gastrointestinal bleeding. *Am J Gastroenterol* 2005; **100**: 2407–18.

10 Marmo R, Rotondano G, Piscopo R, Bianco MA, Cipolletta L. Meta-analysis: capsule enteroscopy vs. conventional modalities in diagnosis of small bowel diseases. *Aliment Pharmacol Ther* 2005; **22**: 595–604.

11 Pennazio M, Santucci R, Rondonotti E, *et al.* Outcome of patients with obscure gastrointestinal bleeding after capsule endoscopy: report of 100 consecutive cases. *Gastroenterology* 2004; **126**: 643–53.

12 Delvaux M, Fassler I, Gay G. Clinical usefulness of the endoscopic video capsule as the initial intestinal investigation in patients with obscure digestive bleeding: validation of a diagnostic strategy based on the patient outcome after 12 months. *Endoscopy* 2004; **36**: 1067–73.

13 Hartmann D, Schmidt H, Bolz G, *et al.* A prospective two-center study comparing wireless capsule endoscopy with intraoperative enteroscopy in patients with obscure GI bleeding. *Gastrointest Endosc* 2005; **61**: 826–32.

14 Bresci G, Parisi G, Bertoni M, Tumino E, Capria A. The role of video capsule endoscopy for evaluating obscure gastrointestinal bleeding: usefulness of early use. *J Gastroenterol* 2005; **40**: 256–9.

15 May A, Wardak A, Nachbar L, Remke S, Ell C. Influence of patient selection on the outcome of capsule endoscopy in patients with chronic gastrointestinal bleeding. *J Clin Gastroenterol* 2005; **39**: 684–8.

16 Apostolopoulos P, Liatsos C, Gralnek IM, *et al.* The role of wireless capsule endoscopy in investigating unexplained iron deficiency anemia after negative endoscopic evaluation of the upper and lower gastrointestinal tract. *Endoscopy* 2006; **38**: 1127–32.

17 Kraus K, Hollerbach S, Pox C, Willert J, Schulmann K, Schmiegel W. [Diagnostic utility of capsule endoscopy in occult gastrointestinal bleeding]. *Dtsch Med Wochenschr* 2004; **129**: 1369–74.

18 Ben Soussan E, Antonietti M, Herve S, *et al.* Diagnostic yield and therapeutic implications of capsule endoscopy in obscure gastrointestinal bleeding. *Gastroenterol Clin Biol* 2004; **28**: 1068–73.

19 Mylonaki M, Fritscher-Ravens A, Swain P. Wireless capsule endoscopy: a comparison with push enteroscopy in patients with gastroscopy and colonoscopy negative gastrointestinal bleeding. *Gut* 2003; **52**: 1122–6.

20 Lewis B, Swain S. Capsule endoscopy in the evaluation of patients with suspected small intestinal bleeding: results of a pilot study. *Gastrointest Endosc* 2002; **56**: 349–53.

21 Gay G, Delvaux M, Fassler I. Outcome of capsule endoscopy in determining indication and route for push-and-pull enteroscopy. *Endoscopy* 2006; **38**: 49–58.

22 Lai L, Wong G, Lau J, Sung J, Leung W. Long-term follow-up of patients with obscure gastrointestinal bleeding after negative capsule endoscopy. *Am J Gastroenterol* 2006; **101**: 1224–8.

CHAPTER 13

Enteroscopy

G. Anton Decker and Jonathan A. Leighton

Division of Gastroenterology, Mayo Clinic, Scottsdale, AZ, USA

Summary

New methods of enteroscopy enable potential visualization of the entire small bowel, and allow for biopsies and therapeutic intervention in areas previously out of reach of push enteroscopy or ileocolonoscopy. The technique for advancement, using the double balloon enteroscopy (DBE) method, uses a push-and-pull method, with inflation and deflation of two balloons and telescoping of the intestine onto an overtube. DBE can be done in an antegrade and/or retrograde fashion with visualization of the entire small bowel reported in up to 86% of cases, usually by a combination of antegrade and retrograde approaches.

Equipment and Review of Technology

Modern enteroscopy includes several currently available technologies; double balloon enteroscopy (DBE) (Fujinon Inc, Saitama, Japan), single balloon enteroscopy (Olympus, Japan) and rotational enteroscopy using a spiral overtube (Spirus Medical, Stoughton, MA, USA). The equipment and techniques differ but the principles are the same: plicating or foreshortening the small bowel so that the depth of insertion exceeds the endoscope length. Because DBE has been available for a longer period of time and has led to more published data, this chapter will focus only on DBE; however, the principles are common to all methods.

The DBE system consists of three components: a high-resolution videoendoscope with an inflatable balloon at the tip, an overtube with an inflatable balloon at the tip, and a balloon pump controller. Both a diagnostic and therapeutic endoscope and overtube are available. The

Practical Gastroenterology and Hepatology: Small and Large Intestine and Pancreas, 1st edition. Edited by Nicholas J. Talley, Sunanda V. Kane and Michael B. Wallace. © 2010 Blackwell Publishing Ltd.

main difference between the two is the larger diameter on the therapeutic scope and overtube. The specifications of the endoscopes are given in Table 13.1 and of the overtubes in Table 13.2. The balloon pump controller has a remote switch as well as foot pedals to inflate and deflate the balloons. The maximum flow rate of the pump is 170 mL/10 s and it inflates the balloons to a pressure of 5.6 ± 2 kPa.

How to Perform Double Balloon Enteroscopy (Video 11)

Endoscopy Technique

The technique of DBE was first described by Yamamoto *et al.* in 2001 [1]. A technician loads the balloon onto the overtube which is then back-loaded onto the endoscope. The second balloon is then loaded onto the tip of the endoscope. Both balloons are connected to the balloon pump controller via flexible plastic tubing. The procedure can be done in an antegrade or a retrograde fashion and is dependent on an assistant holding the overtube. Single-operator DBE has been reported but is not widely practiced. Fluoroscopy can be used to monitor advancement and minimize loop formation but is not essential.

Table 13.1 Endoscope specifications.

	EN-450P5/20	EN-450T5
Distal diameter (mm)	8.5	9.4
Field of view (degrees)	120	140
Working length (cm)	200	200
Total length (cm)	230	230
Forceps channel diameter (mm)	2.2	2.8

Table 13.2 Overtube specifications.

	TS-12140	TS-13140
Outer diameter (mm)	12.2	13.2
Inner diameter (mm)	10	10.8
Distal end diameter (mm)	8.7	9.8
Outer diameter with the balloon (mm)	40	40
Working length (cm)	135	135
Total length (cm)	145	145

Antegrade Double Balloon Enteroscopy
With both balloons deflated, the endoscope and the overtube are advanced to the duodenum. Inflation of the balloons in the area of the ampulla should be avoided because the trauma or duodenal hypertension may cause pancreatitis. The balloon on the overtube is inflated and holds the overtube in a stationary position while the endoscope is advanced to its maximal extent (Figure 13.1a). The balloon at the end of the endoscope is then inflated while the balloon on the overtube is deflated (Figure 13.1b). The overtube is advanced to the distal end of the endoscope when the overtube balloon is inflated. At this point the balloons approximate each other (Figure 13.1c). The endoscopist then gently withdraws the overtube and the endoscope together, allowing the intestine to be pleated over the overtube (Figure 13.1d). This is the most important step in the process and is what prevents looping of the endoscope. The balloon at the tip of the endoscope is then deflated, followed by advancement of the endoscope, and then the sequence is repeated until the desired depth of insertion is reached or the scope cannot be advanced any further. It is advised to inject an india ink tattoo at the most distal extent reached, allowing its identification should a retrograde procedure be necessary. Withdrawing the scope follows a similar sequence, but in reverse. The overtube is withdrawn and

anchored by inflating the balloon. The endoscope balloon is then deflated and the endoscope withdrawn until the tip reaches the tip of the overtube. After inflating the balloon on the endoscope, the overtube balloon is deflated and the sequence is repeated.

Retrograde Double Balloon Enteroscopy
The principles are exactly the same as for the antegrade procedure, once the small bowel is intubated. It is critical that all loops are reduced in the colon if subsequent advancement in the small bowel is to be successful. It can be challenging to get both endoscope and overtube across the ileocecal valve, but abdominal pressure, patient rotation, and subtle adjustments in endoscope and overtube positions are helpful.

Sedation and Anesthesia
DBE can be a lengthy procedure and patients find the distension of the small bowel uncomfortable. Moderate sedation can be used, similar to esophagogastroduodenoscopy (EGD) and colonoscopy [2]. Particularly with antegrade procedures, monitored anesthesia care (MAC) or general anesthesia with intubation and ventilation may be required. Glucagon may also be utilized to slow the peristalsis of the small intestine.

Bowel Preparation
Antegrade DBE does not require any specific bowel preparation but patients are asked to fast for 8 h prior to the procedure. Retrograde DBE requires a standard bowel cleansing regimen as is used for colonoscopy.

Diagnostic and Therapeutic Methods

Virtually all diagnostic and therapeutic modalities that can be performed with a standard esophagogastroduodenoscope or colonoscope can also be performed during DBE. The limited outcomes data on DBE are addressed below.

Indications
The most common indication is obscure gastrointestinal bleeding (69%). The other, less common, indications include abnormal radiology exams, polyposis syndromes, Crohn disease, and/or abdominal pain.

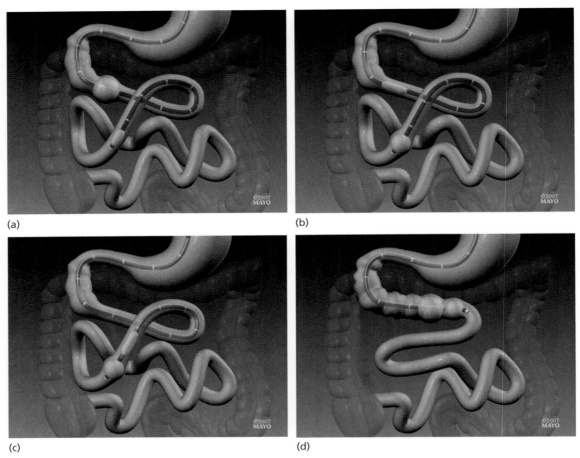

(a)

(b)

(c)

(d)

Figure 13.1 Double balloon enteroscopy. (a) Step 1: The overtube is fixed by the inflated balloon and the enteroscope with the deflated balloon is advanced. (b) Step 2: The balloon on the enteroscope is inflated and the balloon on the overtube is deflated. (c) Step 3: The enteroscope is fixed by the inflated balloon and the overtube is advanced to the level of the enteroscope balloon. (d) Step 4: The balloons on the enteroscope and the overtube are inflated before both tubes are pulled back, thereby plicating the small bowel over the overtube (Used with permission of the Mayo Foundation for Medical Education and Research.)

Depth of Insertion

The pliable nature of the small bowel makes it difficult to judge endoscopic advancement. The only true gauge of insertion depth is when total enteroscopy is achieved; by reaching the ileocecal valve during an antegrade procedure or reaching the tattoo during a DBE performed from the opposite direction to the first DBE. When this is not achieved, the advancement with each push–pull cycle needs to be estimated and totaled at the end of the procedure. The average depth of insertion by the antegrade approach ranges from 220 cm [3] to 360 cm [4].

The average depth of insertion into the small bowel from a retrograde approach ranges from 120 cm [3] to 180 cm [4].

Total Enteroscopy

Total enteroscopy from an antegrade approach is technically possible, but variably achieved [5]. The true rate of total enteroscopy is difficult to come by as most endoscopists do not set out to achieve this; in other words, once the lesion(s) has been found, then scope advancement is usually halted. Yamamoto *et al.* did report total enteroscopy by combining antegrade and retrograde approaches in 84% of patients when this was the *a priori* goal [5]. Zhong *et al.* have also reported high total enteroscopy rates of 56% [6]. The USA, Australia, and Europe have reported lower rates of total enteroscopy, ranging from 0% in a small series from Australia [7] to 45% in Germany [8]. In a large study from the Mayo Clinic, total enteroscopy rates were related to the endoscopist's experience with 8% being achieved in the first 50 cases but greater than 63% after 150 cases [9].

Diagnostic Yield

The diagnostic yield is broadly defined as the rate of finding the cause for the patient's symptoms or finding the lesion identified on pre-DBE small bowel imaging. There are geographic differences in diagnostic yield reported in larger series, ranging from 42% in a US multicenter study [4] to 65.3% in a Chinese study [6] and 80% in a European study [8].

The diagnostic yield in cases of obscure gastrointestinal bleeding ranges from 51% [4] to 81% [6]. The most common cause for gastrointestinal bleeding in Western countries is arteriovenous malformations [4,10], whereas Eastern countries report more ulcerations [5,11]. The higher rate of ulceration in Eastern countries may be because capsule endoscopy is not widely available or approved for clinical use.

With the ability to take biopsies, DBE is potentially useful in the diagnosis of Crohn disease and to monitor mucosal healing [12]. Because there is no single gold standard diagnostic test for Crohn disease of the small bowel, DBE is complimentary to other imaging modalities, such a capsule endoscopy, computed tomography enterography (CTE), and magnetic resonance enterography (MRE). Retrograde DBE also allows inflammatory changes to be reached that might be beyond the capability of ileocolonoscopy [13].

Comparison to Other Imaging Modalities of the Small Bowel

The depth on insertion and the yield of antegrade DBE is significantly greater than with push enteroscopy [14]. A meta-analysis of 11 studies by Pasha *et al.* also found

that DBE had a comparable diagnostic yield to capsule endoscopy; however, when full-length articles of prospective studies only were analyzed, then capsule endoscopy had a 19% higher diagnostic yield compared to DBE [15]. This is not surprising as capsule endoscopy is able to visualize the entire small bowel in the majority of cases whereas DBE is not. Because of this and also because of the non-invasive nature of capsule endoscopy, the authors recommend capsule endoscopy to precede DBE. Capsule endoscopy also helps direct the route of DBE. Gay *et al.* showed that if the lesion was seen after 75% of the capsule transit time, then an anal route DBE had a positive predictive value of 94.7% and a negative predictive value of 96.7% [16]. There is a lack of data comparing DBE to radiologic studies, in particular CTE, MRE, and barium small bowel follow-through, but these tests are best thought of as complimentary rather than exclusive of DBE.

DBE is new technology and therefore the data on its ability to affect long term clinical outcome are lacking. Zhong *et al.* reported outcomes 6 months after DBE. Of 247 patients with positive findings on DBE that led to specific endoscopic or medical treatment, relevant symptoms disappeared or were controlled in 76.9% [6]. The results were best when DBE led to specific treatments such as endoscopic therapy, surgery, or medical treatment as opposed to symptomatic treatment.

Therapeutic Role

DBE has an advantage over other small bowel diagnostic tools as it allows for biopsies and therapeutic interventions. In a large series, May *et al.* reported that endoscopic therapy was used in 41.5% of DBE cases, including argon plasma coagulation (APC), polypectomy, foreign body extraction, dilation and injection therapy [8]. Ell *et al.* reported the use of endoscopic therapy in 62% of DBE procedures, mostly involving APC.

DBE allows for the endoscopic balloon dilation of small bowel strictures in Crohn disease, either native or anastomotic. Morini *et al.* reported successful endoscopic dilation in 34 of 43 patients with ileal or ileocolonic anastomotic strictures [17]. In doing so, surgery was avoided in about half the patients during a mean follow-up period of 7 years. Repeated dilations are often required. Others have reported success with endoscopic dilations in Crohn disease but with rare reports of perforation [18,19].

DBE can be used in patients with altered anatomy, such as gaining access to the excluded stomach or biliopancreatic limb after Roux-en-Y gastric bypass [20]. In these cases, DBE can also be used to facilitate endoscopic retrograde cholangiopancreatography (ERCP) or retrograde percutaneous endoscopic gastrostomy (PEG) placement [21].

Complications

In a multicenter survey, Mensink *et al.* reported 40 complications in 2362 DBE procedures (1.7%) [22]. The complication rate was higher in therapeutic DBE (4.3%) than in diagnostic DBE (0.8%). Typical complications include bleeding and perforation but also self-limiting abdominal pain in up to 20% of patients [10]. May *et al.* reported severe complications in 3.4% of therapeutic DBEs, including bleeding or perforation in 10.8% of patients undergoing polypectomy [2]. In a multicenter US study, Gerson *et al.* reported major complications in 0.9% of 2254 DBE examinations. Perforation was more likely to occur in patients with altered surgical anatomy, such as ileoanal anastomosis [23]. Pancreatitis is a relatively unique complication, first reported by Honda *et al.* [24]. The rate of clinically significant pancreatitis has been reported to be in the range of 0.2–1% [10,23]. Post-DBE asymptomatic hyperamylasemia appears to be common. In a study by Honda *et al.*, hyperamylasemia was found in six of 13 cases after DBE, although only one patient had clinical pancreatitis [25]. The pathogenesis of acute pancreatitis from DBE has not been determined, but it might involve direct trauma to the pancreas or duodenal hypertension as a result of balloon insufflation. The current authors do not recommend routine measurement of pancreatic enzymes in patients with post-DBE abdominal pain. However, in the patient with severe or persistent abdominal pain, pancreatitis must be considered.

Take-home points

- Double balloon enteroscopy (DBE) is one of several new technologies for performing enteroscopy

---

- DBE allows for potential visualization of the entire small bowel.
- DBE also allows for biopsies and therapeutic interventions.
- DBE can be done in an antegrade (per os) or retrograde fashion (per rectum).
- The DBE system consists of a high-resolution videoendoscope with an inflatable balloon at the tip, an overtube with an inflatable balloon at the tip, and a balloon pump controller.
- Push–pull cycles allow the small bowel to be pleated over the overtube.
- Total enteroscopy is rarely achieved by antegrade DBE alone and usually requires combined antegrade and retrograde procedures.
- Complications are higher in patients with altered anatomy and after polypectomy.
- Pancreatitis occurs in 0.3–1% but asymptomatic hyperamylasemia is common.

References

1 Yamamoto H, Sekine Y, Sato Y, *et al.* Total enteroscopy with a nonsurgical steerable double-balloon method. *Gastrointest Endosc* 2001; **53**: 216–20.

2 May A, Nachbar L, Pohl J, Ell C. Endoscopic interventions in the small bowel using double balloon enteroscopy: feasibility and limitations [see comment]. *Am J Gastroenterol* 2007; **102**: 527–35.

3 Ell C, May A, Nachbar L, *et al.* Push-and-pull enteroscopy in the small bowel using the double-balloon technique: results of a prospective European multicenter study. *Endoscopy* 2005; **37**: 613–6.

4 Mehdizadeh S, Ross A, Gerson L, *et al.* What is the learning curve associated with double-balloon enteroscopy? Technical details and early experience in 6 U.S. tertiary care centers. *Gastrointest Endosc* 2006; **64**: 740–50.

5 Yamamoto H, Kita H, Sunada K, *et al.* Clinical outcomes of double-balloon endoscopy for the diagnosis and treatment of small-intestinal diseases. *Clin Gastroenterol Hepatol* 2004; **2**: 1010–6.

6 Zhong J, Ma T, Zhang C, *et al.* A retrospective study of the application on double-balloon enteroscopy in 378 patients with suspected small-bowel diseases. *Endoscopy* 2007; **39**: 208–15.

7 Kaffes AJ, Koo JH, Meredith C. Double-balloon enteroscopy in the diagnosis and the management of small-bowel diseases: an initial experience in 40 patients. *Gastrointest Endosc* 2006; **63**: 81–6.

8 May A, Nachbar L, Ell C. Double-balloon enteroscopy (push-and-pull enteroscopy) of the small bowel: feasibility and diagnostic and therapeutic yield in patients with suspected small bowel disease. *Gastrointest Endosc* 2005; **62**: 62–70.

9 Gross S, Stark M. Initial experience with double-baloon enteroscopy at a U. S. center. *Gastrointest Endosc* 2008; **67**: 890–7.

10 Heine GD, Hadithi M, Groenen MJ, Kuipers EJ, Jacobs MA, Mulder CJ. Double-balloon enteroscopy: indications, diagnostic yield, and complications in a series of 275 patients with suspected small-bowel disease. *Endoscopy* 2006; **38**: 42–8.

11 Ohmiya N, Yano T, Yamamoto H, *et al.* Diagnosis and treatment of obscure GI bleeding at double balloon endoscopy. *Gastrointest Endosc* 2007; **66** (3 Suppl): S72–7.

12 Decker GA, Pasha SF, Leighton JA. Utility of double balloon enteroscopy for the diagnosis and management of Crohn's disease. *Tech Gastrointest Endosc* 2008; **10**: 83.

13 Oshitani N, Yukawa T, Yamagami H, *et al.* Evaluation of deep small bowel involvement by double-balloon enteroscopy in Crohn's disease. *Am J Gastroenterol* 2006; **101**: 1484–9.

14 Matsumoto T, Moriyama T, Esaki M, Nakamura S, Iida M. Performance of antegrade double-balloon enteroscopy: comparison with push enteroscopy. *Gastrointest Endosc* 2005; **62**: 392–8.

15 Pasha SF, Leighton JA, Das A, *et al.* Double-balloon enteroscopy and capsule endoscopy have comparable diagnostic yield in small-bowel disease: A meta-analysis. *Clin Gastroenterol Hepatol* 2008; **6**: 671–6.

16 Gay G, Delvaux M, Fassler I. Outcome of capsule endoscopy in determining indication and route for push-and-pull enteroscopy. *Endoscopy* 2006; **38**: 49–58.

17 Morini S, Hassan C, Lorenzetti R, *et al.* Long-term outcome of endoscopic pneumatic dilatation in Crohn's disease. *Dig Liver Dis* 2003; **35**: 893–7.

18 Ferlitsch A, Reinisch W, Püspök A, *et al.* Safety and efficacy of endoscopic balloon dilation for treatment of Crohn's disease strictures. *Endoscopy* 2006; **38**: 483–7.

19 Nomura E, Takagi S, Kikuchi T, *et al.* Efficacy and safety of endoscopic balloon dilation for Crohn's strictures. *Dis Colon Rectum* 2006; **49** (10 Suppl): S59–67.

20 Kuga R, Safatle-Ribeiro AV, Faintuch J, *et al.* Endoscopic findings in the excluded stomach after Roux-en-Y gastric bypass surgery. *Arch Surg* 2007; **142**: 942–6.

21 Ross AS, Semrad C, Alverdy J, Waxman I, Dye C. Use of double-balloon enteroscopy to perform PEG in the excluded stomach after Roux-en-Y gastric bypass. *Gastrointest Endosc* 2006; **64**: 797–800.

22 Mensink PB, Haringsma J, Kucharzik T, *et al.* Complications of double balloon enteroscopy: a multicenter survey. *Endoscopy* 2007; **39**: 613–5.

23 Gerson LB, Tokar J, Chiorean M, *et al.* Complications associated with double balloon enteroscopy at nine US centers. *Clin Gastroenterol Hepatol* 2009; **7**: 1177–82.

24 Honda K, Mizutani T, Nakamura K, *et al.* Acute pancreatitis associated with peroral double-balloon enteroscopy: a case report. *World J Gastroenterol* 2006; **12**: 1802–4.

25 Honda K, Itaba S, Mizutani T, *et al.* An increase in the serum amylase level in patients after peroral double-balloon enteroscopy: an association with the development of pancreatitis. *Endoscopy* 2006; **38**: 1040–3.

CHAPTER 14

Other Investigations of the Intestine and Pancreas: Diagnostic Imaging

Saravanan Krishnamoorthy[1], Bobby Kalb[2], Sonali Sakaria[3], Shanthi V. Sitaraman[3], and Diego R. Martin[4]

[1] Department of Diagnostic Radiology, Yale University, New Haven, CT, USA
[2] Department of Radiology, Emory University School of Medicine, Atlanta, GA, USA
[3] Division of Digestive Diseases, Emory University School of Medicine, Atlanta, GA, USA
[4] Department of Radiology, Emory University School of Medicine, Atlanta, GA, USA

Summary

A variety of inflammatory and neoplastic diseases of the gastrointestinal tract can be accurately evaluated with cross sectional imaging studies. While computed tomography (CT) has played a pivotal role in depicting these diseases, recent advances in magnetic resonance imaging (MRI), such as faster T2 and T1-weighted sequences and superior fat suppression techniques, have allowed for detailed visualization of the bowel and pancreas. The lack of radiation exposure is especially pertinent due to concerns regarding cancer induction risks, particularly in children and young adults. In this chapter we will highlight the imaging modality of choice for various diseases of the bowel and pancreas and discuss MR applications and findings in more detail. Small bowel follow through and small bowel enteroclysis will be mentioned briefly as their use has become increasingly uncommon and largely replaced with newer small bowel imaging techniques including capsule endoscopy, double balloon enteroscopy, and MRI.

Intestine

Recent advances in magnetic resonance imaging (MRI) have enabled differentiation of the tubular configuration of bowel from abnormal collections or inflammatory processes. MRI is able to identify processes in the bowel wall and distinguish submucosal inflammation from fibrosis. Current common applications of MRI in non-neoplastic diseases include: (i) differentiating the type and severity of inflammatory bowel disease (IBD) [1–7]; (ii) diagnosing inflammatory processes such as appendicitis, diverticulitis; and (iii) identifying enteric abscesses and fistulae [8].

Practical Gastroenterology and Hepatology: Small and Large Intestine and Pancreas, 1st edition. Edited by Nicholas J. Talley, Sunanda V. Kane and Michael B. Wallace. © 2010 Blackwell Publishing Ltd.

Inflammatory Bowel Disease (IBD)

Radiologic evaluation via computed tomography (CT) and MRI has served to assess complications of IBD such as abscesses, fistulae, and stricture formation. Other radiologic techniques, such as small bowel follow through and enteroclysis, are now largely replaced by capsule endoscopy and MRI. Here we discuss the utility of MRI as an adjunct to endoscopy in the diagnosis, assessment of disease severity, and response to treatment in patients with IBD.

Crohn Disease

Changes of luminal Crohn disease are well delineated on MRI (Figure 14.1). Assessment of submucosal disease on MRI serves as a complement to mucosal assessment using video capsule endoscopy or conventional endoscopy. Severe disease is characterized by wall thickness more than 1 cm, length of involvement more than 15 cm,

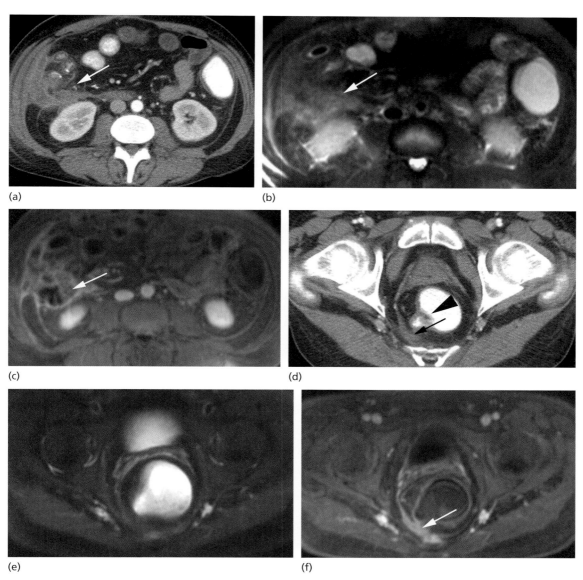

Figure 14.1 A 40-year-old male with known Crohn disease presented with severe right abdominal pain and perirectal drainage. Axial images from a CT with intravenous and oral contrast (a) demonstrated a heterogeneous collection with surrounding fat stranding and possible wall thickening (arrow). On MRI, T2 fat-saturated (b) and T1 fat-saturated delayed postgadolinium contrast-enhanced (c) images confirmed that this abscess was acute given the extensive edema and avid enhancement (arrows). Two distinct fistulous tracts were identified on MRI from the terminal ileum to the abscess (not shown). In the pelvis, there was a fistula from the rectum that filled with rectal contrast on the CT (d, arrowhead). The adjacent fat stranding (d, arrow) is an abnormal finding that may be related to any combination of fluid, inflammatory, or fibrotic mass. T2 fat-saturated MRI image (e) shows negligible signal, an indicator corresponding to no active inflammation or infection and no fluid. Postgadolinium T1-weighted image (f) shows that the soft tissue is enhancing. This combination of features indicates chronic fibrotic reactive tissue.

and mural enhancement. T2-weighted single-shot spin-echo and gadolinium-enhanced T1-weighted fat-suppressed spoiled gradient echo (SGE) images demonstrate characteristic findings: transmural involvement, skip lesions, and mesenteric inflammatory changes. Edema on T2 fat-suppressed images is associated with acute disease activity [1,4,5]. Enhancement of the bowel wall equal to or greater than renal cortex is an indicator of inflammatory changes [9]. In patients with longstanding disease, marked enhancement of the mucosa with substantially thickened wall and minimal enhancement of the outer layer is suggestive of acute-on-chronic involvement, and may have a role in the evaluation of acute exacerbations of Crohn disease.

Ulcerative Colitis

Compared to colonoscopy, the current gold standard for diagnosing ulcerative colitis, MRI examination may be better suited for patients in active disease state due to the risk of perforation with endoscopy in flare states. The MRI appearance of ulcerative colitis reflects the underlying physiology: (i) rectal involvement progressing in a retrograde fashion and (ii) submucosal sparing. The latter is especially well seen on MRI images showing marked mucosal enhancement and negligible submucosal enhancement. MRI cannot, however, distinguish other forms of colitis such as cytomegalovirus (CMV) or *C. difficile* which can co-exist with IBD.

Fistula

Fistulae (Figure 14.1 d,e) may be sequelae of infection, inflammation, neoplasia, radiation therapy, and ischemia. Fistulae on CT may appear as tracts containing orally or rectally administered contrast. However, MRI is more sensitive and very effective for evaluating colonic fistulae [8,10–12] as well as perianal fistulae. Fluid-filled tracts are high in signal intensity on T2-weighted MRI sequences, whereas gas-filled tracts show a signal void. Fat suppression and intravenous gadolinium delineates the enhancing tracts [8,10]. The multiplanar capability of MRI is useful for surgical planning in perianal fistulae because the relationship of fistulae to the levator ani muscle is well shown on a combination of transverse, coronal, and sagittal plane images. Fluoroscopic fistulograms are an alternative modality widely used for evaluation of enterocutaneous and colocutaneous fistulae.

Radiation Enteritis/Colitis

Early complications of radiation treatment occurring within hours to days include ulceration, necrosis, bleeding, perforation, and abscess formation. Chronic radiation enteritis develops months to years after exposure, resulting from vascular damage. The subsequent parenchymal atrophy and progressive fibrosis can cause strictures, fistulae, bowel fixation, and angulation that are apparent on imaging. The small bowel is the most sensitive portion of the gastrointestinal tract to radiation therapy while the rectum is the most susceptible. The routine use of gadolinium-enhanced T1-weighted fat-suppressed imaging is effective for evaluating postradiation changes due to the high sensitivity of this technique for inflammatory changes. High-resolution T2-weighted images further demonstrate the findings of submucosal edema in acute radiation proctocolitis. MRI has excellent sensitivity but limited specificity [13] in diagnosing radiation injury. Therefore, detailed clinical history is vital for proper imaging interpretation.

Ischemia

Initial diagnostic tests in patients with suspected ischemic colitis include an abdominal plainfilm which may show the classic "thumbprinting sign." Further clinical investigation including changes to the bowel wall (Figure 14.2), the arterial supply through the celiac axis, superior mesenteric artery, and inferior mesenteric artery, as well as the venous drainage via the superior mesenteric vein and portal system, can be evaluated with more advanced modalities including CT with intravenous contrast or magnetic resonance angiography (MRA)/MRI, the latter the preferred modality due to precision of findings and lack of contrast or radiation exposure. Mucosal ischemia on CT may present as bowel wall thickening, pneumatosis, or portal venous air.

Diverticulitis

Cross-sectional imaging via CT or MRI is equivalent or superior to barium enema in the diagnosis of diverticulitis [14,15]. CT findings depict wall thickening and adjacent fat stranding in the location of the inflamed diverticulum, as well as possible abscess formation. Bowel wall thickening and diverticular abscesses are well demonstrated with gadolinium-enhanced fat-suppressed T1-weighted SGE images and T2-weighted images (Figure 14.3) [16]. Sinus tracts and fistulae can also be identified

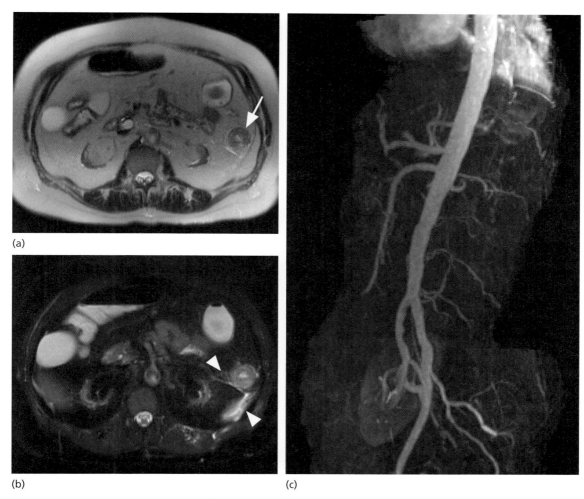

(a)

(b)

(c)

Figure 14.2 A 57-year-old female with non-specific abdominal pain and history of prior renal transplant. Axial T2-weighted image (a) demonstrates wall thickening of the descending colon (arrow). There are extensive acute inflammatory changes surrounding the thickened descending colon, findings that are more conspicuous on corresponding T2-weighted images with fat-saturation (b, arrowheads). Three-dimensional MR angiography with maximum intensity projection (c) demonstrates diffuse luminal irregularity of the arterial structures, in keeping with moderate diffuse atherosclerotic disease. Subsequent biopsy of the inflamed descending colon demonstrated changes of ischemic colitis.

with this technique (Figure 14.3). On unenhanced, non-fat suppressed T1-weighted SGE images, inflammatory changes appear as low-signal intensity curvilinear strands within the high signal intensity of the pericolonic fat.

Appendicitis

CT imaging with intravenous and oral contrast is currently the test of choice to diagnose appendicitis in adults. This modality has now largely replaced ultra-sound. Appendiceal diameter larger than 6 mm, wall thickening, surrounding fat stranding, and periappendiceal abscess formation are features suspicious for acute appendicitis. MRI can also be used to diagnose appendicitis when available (Figure 14.4).

Abscess

CT imaging and ultrasound are the mainstays of diagnosis of abdominal abscesses and have the added advantage

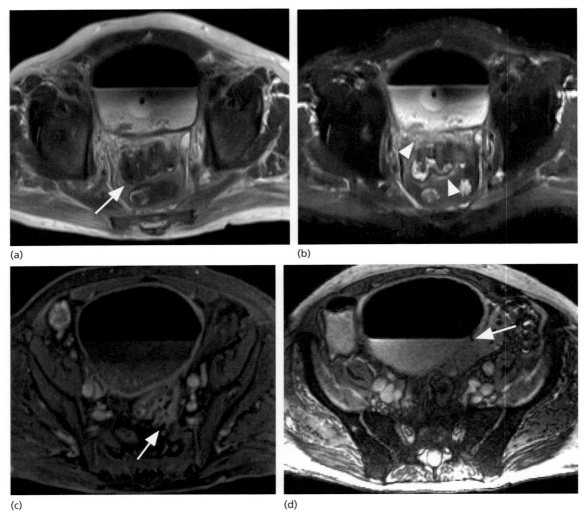

(a)

(b)

(c)

(d)

Figure 14.3 A 79-year-old male with complaints of pelvic pain and air in urine. Axial T2-weighted image (a) demonstrates thickening of the sigmoid colon (arrow) with associated diverticula, while corresponding fat-saturated T2-weighted image (b) depicts associated surrounding acute inflammatory changes (arrowheads), findings in keeping with acute diverticulitis. Three-dimensional contrast-enhanced T1-weighted image (c) shows extraluminal inflammatory tissue (arrow) that is in keeping with focal perforation. Steady-state free precession image (d) demonstrates a small focus of gas (arrow) extending through the bladder wall, communicating with the adjacent, inflamed sigmoid colon, in keeping with a colovesical fistula that developed as a sequela of acute diverticulitis.

Figure 14.4 CT and MR abdominal and pelvic images in a 29-year-old male with an acute flare of chronic, intermittent, non-specific abdominal pain and borderline leukocytosis over a period of several months. Axial (a) and coronally reconstructed (b) CT images with intravenous and oral contrast show apparent bowel wall thickening and enhancement of the cecum and adjacent bowel loops (arrows). The terminal ileum could not be distinguished from these adjacent loops. This appearance can be seen with acute and chronic processes, including acute appendicitis and inflammatory bowel disease. Axial T2 (c) and T2 with fat-saturation MR images (d) demonstrate edema in the thickened wall of the appendix and in the surrounding fat (arrows). Note that fat suppression allows distinction from high-signal edematous fluid and the surrounding fat, which would otherwise have high signal and obscure this finding (compare c and d) thereby diagnosing acute inflammation. Gadolinium-enhanced axial (e) and coronal (f) T1-weighted images with fat suppression show diffuse enhancement of the appendix and abnormal wall thickening (white arrow). The combination of enhancement and edema makes the diagnosis of acute appendicitis straightforward on MRI. The patient underwent appendectomy and pathological evaluation confirmed this diagnosis.

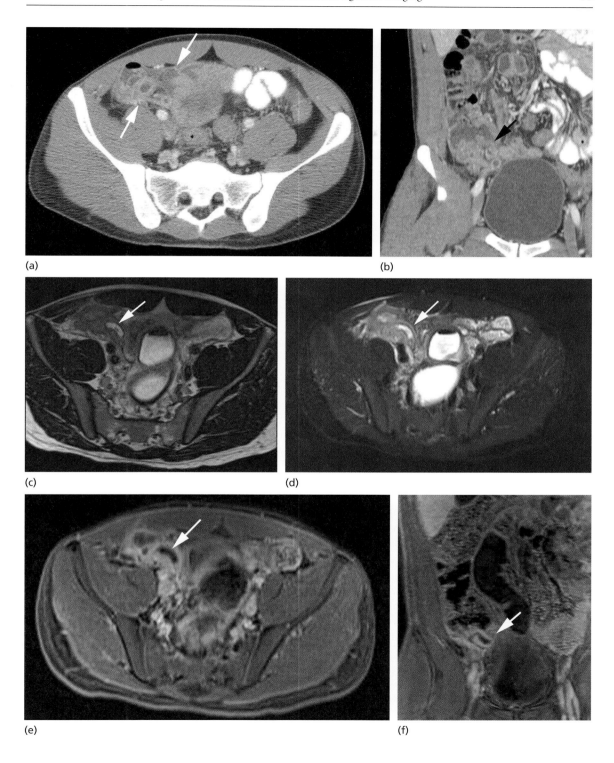

(a)

(b)

(c)

(d)

(e)

(f)

of ease of percutaneous drainage capabilities. CT with intravenous and oral contrast will identify an extraluminal, loculated fluid collection. On ultrasound, abscesses demonstrate a complex, hypoechoic fluid collection, often with internal debris and an irregular wall. MRI has also diagnostic accuracy in evaluating suspected acute intraperitoneal abscess [17]. Abscesses are visualized as well-defined fluid collections with peripheral rim enhancement on gadolinium-enhanced T1-weighted fat-suppressed images. In patients with a contraindication to iodinated intravenous contrast, MRI should be considered for the evaluation of abscess.

Pancreas

Non-invasive imaging of the pancreas and pancreatic duct is a critical component of the diagnosis and severity assessment of acute and chronic pancreatic disease. The goal of any comprehensive method of pancreatic imaging should be to accurately and safely assess the pancreatic parenchyma, the ductal system, the vasculature, and the surrounding soft tissues in a single examination, and also to exclude other causes of abdominal pain that may mimic the symptoms of pancreatic disease.

Types of Imaging

There are several methodologies available for imaging the pancreas and the pancreatic duct, including both invasive and non-invasive techniques. Non-invasive techniques include ultrasound, CT, and MRI. Ultrasound is relatively less expensive and uses non-ionizing radiation, but the diagnosis of pancreatic disease is markedly limited when employing a transabdominal approach due to poor penetration of sound waves into the retroperitoneum and also secondary to overlying bowel gas. Endoscopic ultrasound provides relatively improved parenchymal evaluation compared to the transabdominal approach, but is more invasive and requires specific technical skills to perform accurately. CT is another modality frequently used to image the pancreas, often in an emergency setting, and has the ability to diagnose moderate and severe cases of acute pancreatitis, in addition to vascular involvement when iodinated contrast is administered. Although CT produces images with good spatial resolution, it generally lacks soft tissue contrast, which is the

most important feature required in an imaging methodology to provide specificity in diagnosis. Other concerns with the use of CT include the exposure to ionizing radiation in patients that may require repeated exams to follow disease progression, in addition to iodinated contrast-induced nephropathy (CIN) [18]. Given these factors, when available, MRI is the imaging modality of choice in the evaluation of pancreatic disease. The soft tissue detail of MRI allows clear delineation of pancreatic tissues, and multiple imaging sequences act as different "stains" (similar to pathology) that are able to interrogate different aspects of normal tissue and also disease states. Excellent sensitivity to fluid and edema allow for the diagnosis of very mild cases of pancreatitis that may be missed on other imaging examinations. MRI can be performed with rapid imaging sequences that can be used even in very sick, free-breathing patients. MRI is non-invasive, uses non-ionizing radiation and does not hold the same risks of contrast-induced nephropathy as for CT. Nephrogenic systemic fibrosis (NSF) is a cutaneous disease resembling scleroderma that has recently been associated with the administration of specific gadolinium-based MR contrast agents (>95% of cases attributed to gadodiamide) in the setting of severe (primarily Stage V, glomerular filtration rate (GFR) less than 15 mL/min) renal disease. However, the use of more stable gadolinium agents at lower doses reduces this risk to a significantly lower level. Endoscopic retrograde cholangiopancreatography (ERCP) and endoscopic ultrasound (EUS) are additional diagnostic methods for imaging the pancreatic ductal system and are discussed elsewhere.

Acute Pancreatitis

Very mild cases of pancreatitis may show a morphologically normal pancreas, but with a small amount of retroperitoneal fluid that may extend along the psoas musculature. MRI is quite sensitive for even very small amounts of edema with the use of fat-saturated, fluid-sensitive T2-weighted sequences, and can identify early cases of pancreatitis that would be undetectable by other imaging modalities, including CT (Figure 14.5). Studies have found MRI to be superior to CT in the evaluation of acute pancreatitis, specifically in the ability to characterize biliary stone disease and pancreatic fluid collections [19,20]. More severe cases of acute pancreatitis are

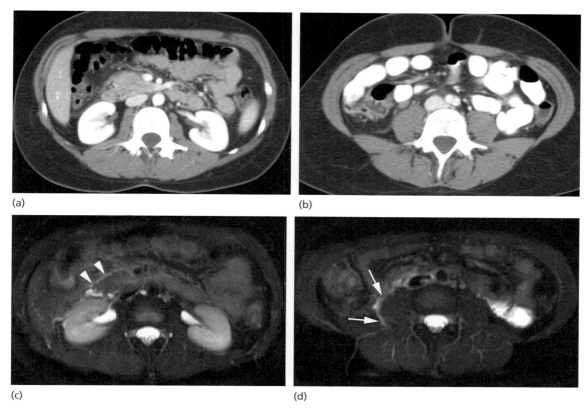

Figure 14.5 Subtle, early pancreatitis on CT and MRI. The patient presented with diffuse, non-specific abdominal pain, and axial CT images at the level of the pancreatic head (a) and retroperitoneum (b) show no evidence of inflammation to suggest pancreatitis. Subsequent MRI clearly demonstrates edema and fluid surrounding the pancreatic head (c, arrowheads) and right psoas muscle (d, arrows), in keeping with mild, acute pancreatitis. Superior soft tissue contrast makes MRI a more sensitive exam for detection of mild pancreatitis.

associated with complications which include pseudocyst formation, abscess, and pancreatic necrosis. Evaluation of parenchymal enhancement is possible with both MRI and CT. However evaluation of peripancreatic fluid collections and pseudocyst formation is best performed with MRI, which allows improved depiction of the internal cyst content compared with other imaging modalities. Assessment of the internal cyst content is important for evaluating the possibility of superinfection, which will prompt more aggressive therapeutic interventions, including percutaneous drainage (Figure 14.6).

MRI is also useful for grading and prognosis of more advanced cases of acute pancreatitis. Severe inflammation is associated with hemorrhage and fat necrosis, findings that demonstrate increased T1 signal in the peripancreatic tissues. CT is relatively insensitive for peripancreatic hemorrhage compared with MRI (Figure 14.7). Severe, elevated peripancreatic T1 signal has been associated with progressively poor outcomes in patients with acute pancreatitis. In addition to imaging the soft tissues, MRI can also evaluate the vascular structures of the abdomen in a non-invasive fashion. Vascular thrombosis (Figure 14.8) or aneurysm formation are common complications of acute pancreatitis that are relatively simple diagnostic entities with standard imaging protocols.

Chronic Pancreatitis

Although ERCP and pancreatic function testing have traditionally been considered gold standards for evaluation

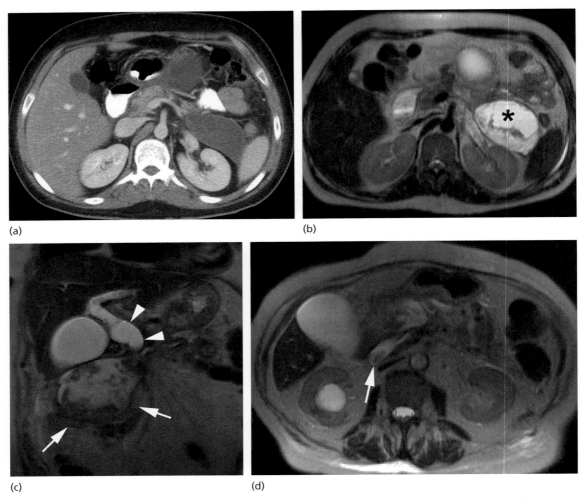

(a)　　　　(b)

(c)　　　　(d)

Figure 14.6 Infected pseudocyst. Axial CT (a) shows a retroperitoneal fluid collection in the setting of acute pancreatitis. However, MRI is better able to demonstrate the complexity of the internal fluid content with standard T2-weighted images (b), showing sepatations and internal debris (*) that are invisible on CT. Coronal T2-weighted image (c) demonstrates another pseudocyst with extensive complex internal debris (arrows). This image provides additional anatomic depiction of the dilated biliary tree (arrowheads), resulting from an obstructing common duct stone which is best shown on axial T2-weighted images (d, arrow).

of chronic pancreatitis, both have major limitations of risk (of pancreatitis) and reproducibility. EUS has emerged as a safe, highly sensitive method but is less specific and is very dependent on the expertise of the endoscopist. All methods assess chronic pancreatitis primarily by assessing morphologic changes in the main pancreatic duct, side branch dilation, and the presence of parenchymal calcifications. MRI allows for earlier detec-

tion of chronic pancreatitis since it can detect early parenchymal changes such as fibrosis that decrease the intrinsic T1 signal of the pancreas. In addition, the fibrotic tissue uptake of gadolinium contrast is characteristically delayed, which causes a chronically diseased pancreas to enhance most avidly in the later, interstitial phase of enhancement (Figure 14.9). These changes on a cellular level produce imaging findings on MRI that

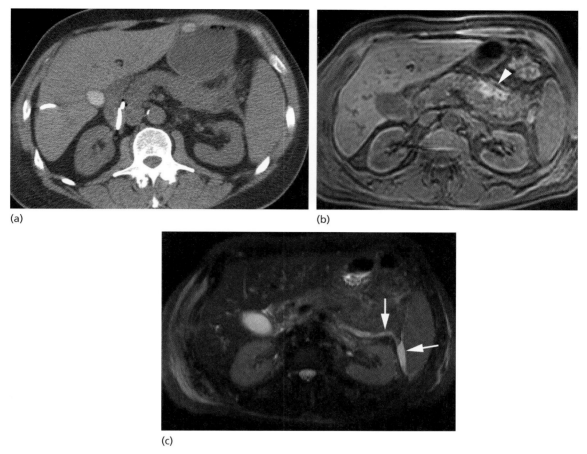

(a)

(b)

(c)

Figure 14.7 Hemorrhagic pancreatitis. Non-contrast axial CT (a) demonstrates inflammatory changes of acute pancreatitis surrounding the pancreatic tail. However, CT fails to demonstrate areas of hemorrhagic fat necrosis which manifest as regions of increased T1 signal on precontrast T1-weighted images (b, arrowhead), a finding with significant prognostic implications for patient outcome. The associated inflammation and edema manifest as increased signal on fat-saturated T2-weighted images (c, arrows) within and surrounding the pancreas.

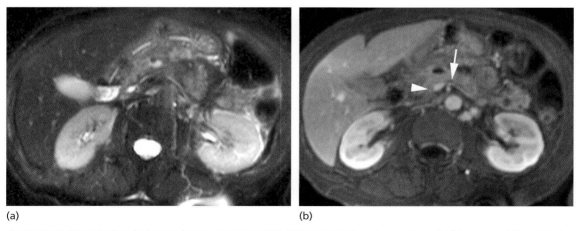

(a)

(b)

Figure 14.8 Splenic vein thrombosis secondary to acute pancreatitis. Peripancreatic edema is present on axial fat-suppressed T2-weighted images (a), while postcontrast T1-weighted images (b) show a narrowed portal venous confluence (arrowhead) and thrombosis of the splenic vein (arrow).

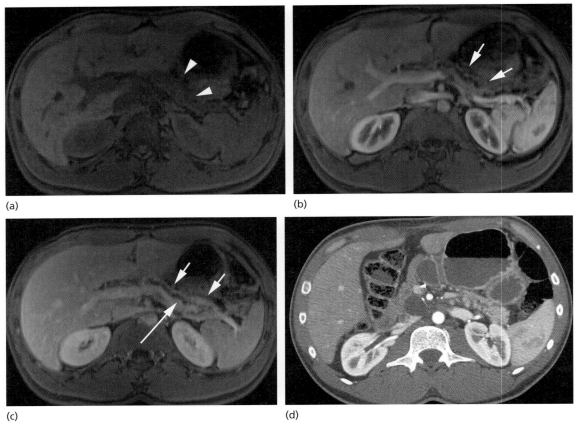

(a)   (b)

(c)   (d)

Figure 14.9 Chronic pancreatitis. Axial precontrast T1-weighted image (a, arrowheads) shows loss of the normal increased pancreatic T1 signal. Arterial (b) and later interstitial phase (c) postcontrast images show progressive uptake of contrast within the pancreatic parenchyma (short arrows), in keeping with chronically diseased and fibrotic tissue. In addition, a dilated, irregular pancreatic duct (c, long arrow) is identified even without the use of conventional MRCP sequences. Axial contrast-enhanced CT (d) in the same patient cannot show the same parenchymal fibrotic changes identified on MRI, due to a relative lack of soft tissue contrast. The irregular ductal dilation is also less apparent with CT.

provide earlier detection of disease compared to evaluating just the morphologic changes of the pancreatic duct in isolation via ERCP.

In addition to parenchymal assessment, evaluation of the pancreatic duct remains an important aspect of the imaging evaluation of chronic pancreatitis. The Cambridge classification is used to classify ductal changes of chronic pancreatitis on ERCP or EUS [21]. Using heavily T2-weighted sequences, MRI provides imaging of the ductal system that is comparable to ERCP, however without the attendant risks or complications, and can evaluate both the main pancreatic duct and dila-

tion of side branches (Figure 14.10). Evaluation of the pancreatic duct may be further enhanced with the administration of secretin prior to MR imaging, which some groups have found to improve the sensitivity of MRI for ductal abnormalities [22]. However, the secretin magnetic resonance cholangiopancreatography (MRCP) study adds complexity to the scan procedure and has never been evaluated in systematic trials to compare against combined, newer, fast-imaging T2-weighted and T1-weighted pre- and postcontrast techniques, used in a comprehensive examination with overall short scan times. Other advantages of MRI

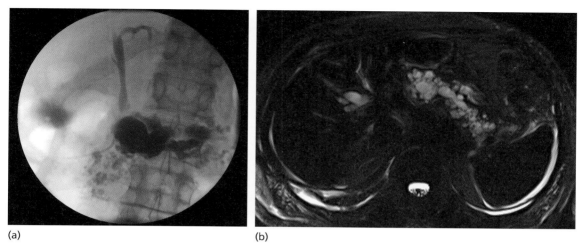

(a)   (b)

Figure 14.10 Chronic pancreatitis with dilated side branches. ERCP (a) in a patient with advanced chronic pancreatitis demonstrates marked irregular dilation of the pancreatic ducts after injection of contrast. Axial MRCP (b) in another patient with severe, advanced chronic pancreatitis also clearly demonstrates an irregular, dilated main pancreatic duct in addition to extensive side-branch dilation. MRI is non-invasive and not limited by high-grade duct obstruction that may preclude passage of contrast material, and provides an excellent road map for subsequent endoscopic interventions.

include the provision of soft tissue detail that is not obtained with ERCP.

Pancreas Divisum

MRI can depict both the main pancreatic duct and the presence of an accessory duct draining into the minor ampulla, which is clearly identified on both conventional MRCP and axial T2-weighted images [23] (Figure 14.11).

Conclusions

CT and MRI have become integral tools for gastrointestinal imaging. CT scans are generally favored in acute infectious conditions such as appendicitis and diverticulitis and have the advantage of widespread availability and lower cost. MRI continues to evolve into a highly sophisticated method of both structural and functional imaging of soft tissue and luminal organs and has become

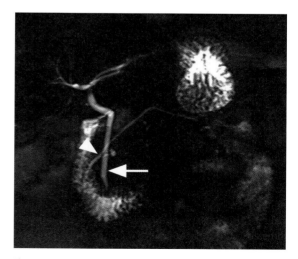

Figure 14.11 Coronal MRCP slab image demonstrates a prominent accessory duct (arrowhead) that drains the majority of the pancreatic parenchyma through the minor ampulla. Note the distal common bile duct (arrow) extends caudally to drain into the ampulla of Vater.

the method of choice for pancreatic and liver imaging. Both methods have associated risks which can usually be managed with appropriate patient selection and risk reduction measures.

Take-home points

- While CT has played a pivotal role in diagnosing small bowel, large bowel, and pancreatic disease, recent advances in MRI have allowed more detailed visualization of the bowel and pancreas.

- MRI can be used as an adjunct to video capsule endoscopy and traditional endoscopy in the diagnosis and assessment of patients with inflammatory bowel disease.

- Fistulae may be diagnosed using CT imaging, MRI, or fluoroscopic fistulograms.

- The use of gadolinium-enhanced T1-weighted fat-suppressed imaging on MRI has high sensitivity but limited specificity in diagnosing postradiation changes seen in radiation enteritis or colitis.

- The initial diagnostic test in patients with suspected ischemic colitis includes an abdominal plain film which may show the classic "thumb printing sign" followed by further visualization of the vasculature with contrast CT or MRA/MRI.

- Cross-sectional imaging via CT scan is generally first-line diagnostic test in the diagnosis of diverticulitis.

- CT imaging with intravenous and oral contrast is test of choice to diagnose appendicitis in adults.

- When available, MRI is the imaging modality of choice in acute pancreatitis. Specifically, it can detect early cases of pancreatitis that may be missed by other modalities and is useful in the grading and prognosis of acute pancreatitis.

- While ERCP and EUS are sensitive methods for evaluating chronic pancreatitis, MRI provides an alternative, non-invasive modality to evaluate the pancreatic duct and its side branches.

References

1 Shoenut JP, Semelka RC, Silverman R, *et al*. Magnetic resonance imaging in inflammatory bowel disease. *J Clin Gastroenterol* 1993; **17**: 73–8.

2 Semelka RC, Shoenut JP, Silverman R, *et al*. Bowel disease: prospective comparison of CT and 1.5 T pre- and postcontrast MR imaging with T1-weighted fat-suppressed and breath-hold FLASH sequences. *J Magn Reson Imaging* 1991; **11**: 625–32.

3 Shoenut JP, Semelka RC, Magro CM, *et al*. Comparison of magnetic resonance imaging and endoscopy in distinguishing the type and severity of inflammatory bowel diseases. *J Clin Gastroenterol* 1994; **19**: 31–5.

4 Kettritz U, Isaacs K, Warshauer DM, Semelka RC. Crohn's disease: Pilot study comparing MRI of the abdomen with clinical evaluation. *J Clin Gastroenterol* 1995; **21**: 249–53.

5 Shoenut JP, Semelka RC, Silverman R, *et al*. Magnetic resonance imaging evaluation of the local extent of colorectal mass lesions. *J Clin Gastroenterol* 1993; **17**: 248–53.

6 Martin DR, Lauenstein T, Sitaraman SV. Utility of magnetic resonance imaging in small bowel Crohn's disease. *Gastroenterology* 2007; **133**: 385–90.

7 Udayasankar U, Martin DR, Rutherford R, *et al*. The role of spectral presaturation attenuated inversion-recovery fat-suppressed T2-weighted MR imaging in active inflammatory bowel disease. *J Magn Reson Imaging* 2008; **28**: 1133–40.

8 Outwater E, Schiebler ML. Pelvic fistulas: findings on MR images. *AJR Am J Roentgenol* 1993; **160**: 327–30.

9 Marcos HB, Semelka RC. Evaluation of Crohn's disease using half-fourier RARE and gadolinium-enhanced SGE sequences initial results. *Mag Reson Imaging* 2000; **18**: 263–8.

10 Semelka RC, Hricak H, Kim B. Pelvic fistulas: appearances on MR images. *Abdom Imaging* 1997; **22**: 91–5.

11 Cho KC, Morehouse HT, Alterman DD, Thornhill BA. Sigmoid diverticulitis: Diagnostic role of CT—comparison with barium enema studies. *Radiology* 1990; **170**: 111–15.

12 Chung JJ, Semelka RC, Martin DR, Marcos HB. Colon diseases: MR evaluation using combined T2-weighted single-shot echo train spin-echo and gadolinium-enhanced spoiled gradient-echo sequences. *J Magn Reson Imaging* 2000; **12**: 297–305.

13 Eisenberg RL. Solitary filling defects in the jejunum and ileum. In: Eisenberg RL, ed. *Gastrointestinal Radiology*. Philadelphia: Lippincott, 1983: 492–504.

14 Bartolo D, Goepel JR, Parsons MA. Rectal malignant lymphoma in chronic ulcerative colitis. *Gut* 1982; **23**: 164–8.

15 Dragosics B, Bauer P, Radaasziewicz T. Primary gastrointestinal non-Hodgkin's lymphomas. *Cancer* 1985; **55**: 1060–73.

16 Jetmore AB, Ray JE, Gathright BJ, McMullen KM. Rectal carcinoids: the most frequent carcinoid tumor. *Dis Colon Rectum* 1992; **35**: 717–25.

17 Acheson ED. The distribution of ulcerative colitis and regional enteritis in United States veterans with particular reference to the Jewish religion. *Gut* 1960; **1**: 291–3.

18 Wong GT, Irwin MG. Contrast-induced nephropathy. *Br J Anaesth* 2007; **99**: 474–83.

19 Stimac D, Miletic D, Radic M, *et al*. The role of nonenhanced magnetic resonance imaging in the early assessment

of acute pancreatitis. *Am J Gastroenterol* 2007; **102**: 997–1004.

20 Ward J, Chalmers AG, Guthrie AJ, *et al.* T2-weighted and dynamic enhanced MRI in acute pancreatitis: comparison with contrast enhanced CT. *Clin Radiol* 1997; **52**: 109–14.

21 Balci NC, Alkaade S, Magas L, *et al.* Suspected chronic pancreatitis with normal MRCP: findings on MRI in correlation with secretin MRCP. *J Magn Reson Imaging* 2008; **27**: 125–31.

22 Yu J, Turner MA, Fulcher AS, Halvorsen RA. Congenital anomalies and normal variants of the pancreaticobiliary tract and the pancreas in adults: part 2, Pancreatic duct and pancreas. *AJR Am J Roentgenol* 2006; **187**: 1544–53.

23 Bret PM, Reinhold C, Taourel P, *et al.* Pancreas divisum: evaluation with MR cholangiopacreatography. *Radiology* 1996; **199**: 99–103.

CHAPTER 15
Motility Testing of the Intestine

Eamonn M.M. Quigley

Department of Medicine, Alimentary Pharmabiotic Centre, University College Cork, Cork, Ireland

Summary

Motor disorders of the small intestine, colon, and anorectum are common and present significant diagnostic and therapeutic challenges for the clinician. A plethora of tests have been developed and advocated to aid in diagnosis and guide the management of these disorders. Few have been subjected to rigorous, objective assessment in terms of their true impact on patient outcome. Some, and especially the more complex and invasive methodologies such as small intestinal or colonic manometry, are available only at a few, highly specialized centers. In terms of clinical utility, a normal small intestinal manometry may prove of critical value, in the appropriate context, in directing patient management; studies of colon transit, which are relatively easy to perform and widely available, can define slow-transit constipation; and anorectal manometry and an endoanal study of sphincter morphology provide valuable information in the context of fecal incontinence. On the other hand, a variety of techniques are available for the assessment of anorectal and pelvic floor function; the clinician should select tests based on both evidence of their impact and available local expertise.

Introduction

Tests of small intestinal, colonic, and anorectal motility seek to provide an anatomical and/or physiological basis for a patient's symptoms and to guide management and, especially, decisions regarding the appropriateness of surgical intervention and, in the case of the anorectum, biofeedback therapy. Given its relative inaccessibility and the rarity of motor disorders of the small intestine, studies of its motor function are not widely available and data on their validation and influence on clinical outcome are scanty. In contrast, colonic transit and anorectal and pelvic floor function are quite readily amenable to study and a relative plethora of instruments and protocols are available. While many of these tests, with the possible exception of the radiopaque marker study of colon transit and anorectal manometry, have failed to gain universal acceptance as definitive in the evaluation of the

patient with either constipation or incontinence, the clinician can gain a good appreciation of the nature of the underlying deficit(s) and assist management by employing a logical and complementary range of tests.

Equipment, Review of Technology, and Indications

Small Intestine

Clinical indications for motility testing of the small intestine are relatively infrequent and, for this reason, as well as the relative inaccessibility of the organ, experience in the relevant techniques has been concentrated in a few specialized tertiary referral centers [1,2]. The principal indications for studies of small bowel motility are, firstly, to determine if abnormalities of enteric neuromuscular function are responsible for unexplained gastrointestinal symptoms, when structural abnormalities have been excluded and known causes of dysmotility are not present, and, secondly, to evaluate the degree of enteric dysfunction so as to optimize clinical management.

Practical Gastroenterology and Hepatology: Small and Large Intestine and Pancreas, 1st edition. Edited by Nicholas J. Talley, Sunanda V. Kane and Michael B. Wallace. © 2010 Blackwell Publishing Ltd.

The range of options for the assessment of small bowel motor function is limited to studies of transit and direct manometry.

Transit Studies

While some general inferences with regard to the status of small intestinal transit (i.e., rapid or delayed) can be garnered from radiological studies, this approach cannot provide an accurate assessment of transit. On the other hand, orocecal transit can be estimated with some degree of reproducibility by means of the lactulose breath hydrogen test. The equipment involved is identical to that required for other breath hydrogen tests [3].

More formal measures of transit can be obtained using radionuclide approaches and, with some of the more sophisticated techniques, separate assessments of gastric emptying, small bowel transit, and colon transit can be derived [4–9]. Most recently, the transit of a capsule capable of monitoring intraluminal pH and temperature and recording intraluminal pressure has been advocated for the assessment of small bowel transit, the abrupt pH changes that occur on leaving the stomach and reaching the cecum providing an opportunity to estimate small bowel transit [10].

Manometry

The manometric study of the small intestine presents formidable challenges which include the need to place the manometric assembly in the small intestine, the tremendous intrinsic variability of patterns of small intestinal motility in normal individuals, and the relative paucity of validated diagnostic criteria for disorders such as enteric myopathy or neuropathy. Small intestinal manometry is not widely practiced and it is this author's impression that enthusiasm for this approach has waned considerably in recent decades. Recordings may be obtained using either continuously perfused catheter assemblies or catheters incorporating multiple solid-state sensors. The only difference between the equipment required for the performance of small intestinal and esophageal manometry relates to the overall length of the assembly and the total number (which varies considerably from center to center, though a minimum of three is recommended) and relative positioning of pressure sensors, be they perfused side-holes or solid state, on the assembly. While ambulatory systems have been developed based on both of these approaches, perfusion manometry is usually performed in a stationary setting while solid-state systems are most commonly employed for ambulatory studies [1]. To date, high-resolution manometry has not been applied to the assessment of small intestinal motor function in the clinical setting.

Colon

Constipation is a common symptom and severe idiopathic constipation a not infrequent source of much suffering and social debility. Two basic forms of chronic idiopathic constipation have been defined: slow-transit constipation (or colonic inertia) and outlet-type constipation (incorporating such terms as dyssynergic defecation, pelvic floor dysfunction, difficult defecation, and anismus). The primary goal of colonic function testing is to identify the patient whose principal abnormality resides in the colon itself and who, therefore, will be amenable to approaches that stimulate colonic motility or, in very rare and extreme cases, who may be considered for colectomy.

Transit Studies

The popularity of colon transit as a clinical measurement owes much to the validation of a simple test of transit: the radiopaque marker study. The only "equipment" that is required is a capsule containing a defined number of radiopaque markers (usually 20–24) and access to a radiology department for the performance of a plain abdominal X-ray(s) at a timed interval(s) following marker ingestion. This approach has been shown to provide not only an accurate and reproducible assessment of overall colonic transit, but has also been shown to facilitate separation of colonic inertia from normal transit (but probably cannot identify "outlet" problems.)

More accurate and dynamic assessments of colon transit, including the determination of transit within various segments of the colon, can be obtained from radioisotopic approaches though these methodologies have been largely confined to a few centers and to clinical research protocols [4–8].

Manometry

Colonic manometry presents formidable challenges foremost among these being that of positioning the catheter assembly in the first place and ensuring that it retains its position throughout the period of study. Furthermore, patterns of colonic motility are poorly defined and subject to tremendous variation between normal individuals, not to mind in disease states. While the absence of the most recognizable pressure wave pattern, the high amplitude power contraction (HAPC), during a recording period of accurate duration, as well as following exposure to adequate stimulation, has been proposed as being of diagnostic value among children, there is at present no consensus with regard to the utility of colonic manometry in clinical practice in the adult patient [1].

Anorectum and Pelvic Floor

In the constipated patient, defects in the defecatory process are especially challenging to define and manage and, as the affected individual may require a somewhat different therapeutic approach to that of the patient with slow-transit constipation or colonic inertia, considerable effort has been expended in developing reliable and clinically useful tests for the assessment of anorectal and pelvic floor function. Symptoms alone have not proven to be especially useful in differentiating between the two main categories of constipation. Furthermore, the identification of abnormalities in anorectal or pelvic floor function is regarded as a contraindication to colectomy in the patient who, on the basis of symptoms or other tests, appears to have colonic inertia.

These same anatomical structures also contribute to the maintenance of fecal continence and a somewhat similar array of tests may also be applied to the evaluation of their function in the patient with fecal incontinence.

In contrast to the relative paucity of tests available for the assessment of small intestinal or colonic motility, a relative plethora of approaches has been applied to the study of anorectal and pelvic floor function. Most experts would advocate the application of a number of tests, each assessing somewhat different parameters, to the assessment of the patient with constipation or incontinence.

Anatomy

Though not strictly speaking a "motility" test, approaches that evaluate the integrity of the various structures that comprise the pelvic floor and anal sphincters are of considerable value in the evaluation of the patient with fecal incontinence [11]. Both endoanal ultrasound and endoanal magnetic resonance imaging (MRI) are widely employed to define anatomical (usually obstetric or postsurgical) defects in the internal and external anal sphincters, with ultrasound being the preferred modality for the

former and MRI for the latter [12]. Static images of the anorectal angle can be obtained during defecography (whether performed using fluoroscopy or MRI), a procedure employed to describe the movements of the pelvic floor musculature in relation to the anorectum during various maneuvers, which is described below.

Transit Studies

Transit of feces (or, more usually, a simulated stool) is typically assessed by means of defecography using standard contrast imaging, scintigraphy, or MRI. The first two involve radiation exposure and the use of a customized "throne" on which the patient sits and performs various maneuvers following the insertion of a material to simulate the consistency of feces into the rectum. In this manner, the behavior of the pelvic floor musculature can be recorded as the patient attempts to retain or expel stool. Magnetic resonance imaging offers many advantages over barium defecography but for a truly physiological test, requires a dedicated "open" system, a facility that is available at only a few highly specialized centers [12].

The balloon expulsion test has been developed and validated by some centers as a simple method to assess defecatory function. A balloon is placed in the rectum and inflated with 50 cc of air; the ability of the subject to expel the balloon either unaided or with the addition of external weights is assessed [13].

Manometry

Anorectal manometry has been used for decades to assess the integrity of the internal and external sphincters and is a well-established technique for the identification of Hirschsprung disease and the definition of poor sphincter tone in patients with incontinence [14]. In the latter context, the clinician can go on to employ manometry as the basis for biofeedback approaches to improving sphincter function.

A variety of manometric assemblies have been employed: multiple balloon, perfused catheter, solid-state, and high-resolution. The most widely used assembly incorporates an inflatable balloon at its tip (used to test sensation and elicit the rectoanal inhibitory reflex) and a radially arranged array of closely spaced sensors (either perfused side holes or miniaturized solid-state sensors) which records pressure transients in the sphincters.

Electromyography

Electromyographic approaches have been employed to study both the integrity and responsiveness of the anal sphincters (typically using an intraluminal electrode assembly incorporated in a manometric assembly) and the innervation of the external sphincter and the pelvic floor musculature (using concentric needle, fine needle, or single fiber techniques). While the former is quite commonly employed in some centers as an aid to biofeedback, the latter approaches are employed in some centers to define neurogenic incontinence [15,16]. Approaches involving relatively large-bore needles have been criticized on the basis of procedure-related artifact. Formerly, pudendal nerve terminal motor latency (measured by a customized device which incorporated both stimulating and recording electrodes fixed 3 cm apart on a rubber finger stall and mounted on the index finger which was then inserted into rectum) was advocated as a valuable technique for identifying injury or neuropathy of the pudendal nerve [17] but has fallen out of favor because of poor reproducibility in some hands.

Barostat

While rectal sensation, compliance, and capacity can be estimated using the inflatable balloon mounted on a typical manometric assembly, these parameters can be most accurately and objectively measured using a barostat system [18]. As has been the case elsewhere in the gastrointestinal tract, barostat balloon systems, with electronic control of inflation and deflation, have been widely employed in research studies of the colon and anorectum but their clinical application has been limited. Nevertheless, whether assessed by a simple balloon or by the barostat, abnormalities of rectal sensation, both hypo- and hypersensation, have been well documented and considered of pathophysiological importance among patients with both constipation and incontinence.

Techniques

Only the more accessible and more commonly used techniques will be described.

Small Bowel Transit

The techniques most commonly utilized are the lactulose breath hydrogen test and one of the several scintigraphic approaches.

This lactulose breath hydrogen test is based on the fact that carbohydrate fermentation by the gut flora is the only source of H_2 production in the body [3]. H_2 produced in this manner diffuses into the systemic circulation and is excreted via the lung in the expired air; about one-fifth of the gas produced is exhaled. Generally, the generation of a detectable peak in H_2 in expired air following lactulose ingestion requires high concentrations of intestinal bacteria. For this reason, the test has been widely used to measure the orocecal transit time (OCTT), the arrival of the lactulose in the caecum, where it comes into contact with its abundant flora, leading to the generation of a detectable peak.

To perform the study 10 mL of lactulose in 250 mL of water is taken by mouth and breath samples for hydrogen analysis obtained at 15-min intervals for at least 90 min.

The most widely used scintigraphic technique simply involves an extension of a traditional ^{99m}Tc-labeled meal gastric emptying study to assess ileal arrival or colonic filling. A region of interest is developed in the area of the terminal ileum/cecum and arrival of the radiolabeled meal in this location defined.

Small Bowel Manometry

Two basic protocols for recording small intestinal motility have been described; a shorter stationary study and a more prolonged (typically 24 h duration) ambulatory study. Both require intubation through either the mouth or, more commonly, the nasopharynx with advancement of the catheter (sometimes facilitated by the presence of an inflatable balloon at the tip) under fluoroscopic guidance until a satisfactory location is encountered. For the detection of motility patterns and their propagation, at least three sites are recommended as a minimum standard, with one site at, or preferably just beyond the ligament of Treitz. For a stationary study, recordings are first performed in the fasted state for 6 h and then for at least a further 2 h following ingestion of a meal of adequate caloric load to induce a fed motor response [19].

Colon Transit

In the most widely used test of colon transit, the radioopaque marker (ROM) study, one of two basic protocols is employed. In the original protocol described by Metcalf and colleagues, a capsule containing 20 radiopaque markers was ingested on days 1, 2, and 3 and X-rays of the abdomen obtained on days 4 and 7 [20]. More recently that protocol has been simplified to involve the ingestion of 24 markers on day 1 only, followed by a single X-ray on day 4. In the other protocol, described by Martelli and colleagues, 20 markers are ingested on day 1 and a single X-ray performed on day 5 [21].

Scintigraphic studies of colon transit involve the ingestion of a methacrylate-coated delayed-release gelatin capsule which dissolves in the alkaline milieu of the terminal ileum [22]. Scans are taken at intervals and regions of interest defined in various segments of the large bowel; in this way the movement of the colonic contents can be tracked over time.

The so-called Smart Pill® technology (SmartPill Corp., Buffalo, NY, USA) involves the use of a $26 \times 13\,mm$ capsule which houses sensors for pH, temperature, and pressure and transmits sensed data at 434 MHz [10]. A battery-operated data receiver worn on a belt clip or on a lanyard around the neck collects and stores the test data. The data receiver may be removed but must be maintained within 1.5 m (5 feet) of the patient. A truly ambulatory study can be performed in the patient's usual environment. After completion of the test, the data receiver is connected to a PC using a special docking station employing a standard USB-type 2.0 interface and data analysis performed.

For defecography, material (which varies depending on whether a barium-based or MRI methodology is used) is inserted into the rectum and the patient seated on a customized commode; using either fluoroscopy or an "open" magnet, dynamic images are obtained with the patient at rest, while they contract the pelvic floor (or "lift") and while they attempt to expel the rectal contents ("strain"). As well as observing the dynamics of the process, static images can be obtained during these various maneuvers to permit definition of changes in the anorectal angle. During the MRI study, images of adjacent organs and tissues may also be obtained [12].

The balloon expulsion test involves the inflation of a 50-mL balloon in the rectum which the patient is then asked to expel while squatting; if the balloon cannot be expelled spontaneously weights are added to a lead attached to the balloon in an incremental manner and the degree of assistance required (in g of added weights) calculated [13].

Anorectal Manometry

In the most commonly employed approach [14] a perfused catheter assembly, incorporating multiple radially-arrayed (to allow for sphincter asymmetry), closely spaced side holes (typically 0.5 to 1 cm apart) and with an inflatable balloon at its tip, is placed in the rectum and anal canal so the sensors straddle the sphincter which has been identified by a series of slow pull-through maneuvers. In this location, basal and maximal squeeze pressures are recorded and the rectoanal inhibitory response (RAIR, also referred to as the sampling reflex or recto-sphincteric reflex, Figure 15.1) to balloon inflation defined. Rectal sensation may also be assessed through balloon inflation. Multiple modifications of this basic system and protocol are in use and include the use of solid-state sensors, high-resolution manometry, or the incorporation of electromyography (EMG) electrodes as well as variations on the technique for identifying the sphincter. For most situations, the essential elements of the procedure are the definition of the basal and squeeze pressure (apparently the most discriminating parameter in the assessment of fecal incontinence) and the elicitation of the RAIR.

Interpretation

Lactulose breath hydrogen test of orocecal transit. Using the lactulose breath hydrogen test, the OCTT is defined as the time interval between the administration of lactulose and the detection of a sustained (i.e., two consecutive values) rise of H_2 by at least 20 ppm above the basal level. The normal range varies considerably between studies; the average being around 75–100 min.

Scintigraphy. Scintigraphic studies have defined either the arrival of the meal in the region of interest or the rate of filling of the cecum; from the former, an average value for small bowel transit of approximately 80 min has been described among healthy adult males and females [22]; from the latter, rates of cecal filling in excess of 70% at 6 h have been documented among control subjects [23].

Small intestinal manometry. The primary objective of a small intestinal manometry study is to demonstrate normal interdigestive motility and a normal fed response [1,2,19]. Interdigestive motility is usually defined by

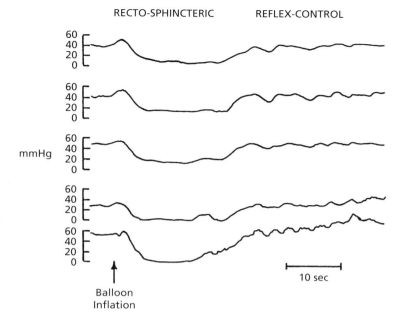

RECTO-SPHINCTERIC   REFLEX-CONTROL

mmHg

Balloon
Inflation

10 sec

Figure 15.1 An example of a normal recto-anal inhibitory (recto-sphincteric) reflex. Five closely spaced and radially arrayed perfused side holes straddle the anal sphincter. Note normal response to balloon inflation in the rectum: a brief contraction (generated by the external sphincter) followed by a prolonged relaxation (of the internal sphincter).

identifying its most recognizable feature, phase III, or the activity front as it migrates along the intestine. There is tremendous intrinsic variability in the frequency of phase III complexes; in some normal individuals they may be as rare as one per day. For this reason and as phase III complexes are typically most prominent overnight, some prefer 24-h ambulatory studies over the shorter duration stationary approach. On ingesting an adequate meal, interdigestive activity should be abolished and replaced by intensive but irregular activity—the fed response. Various authors have championed other parameters and motor patterns but none have achieved consensus.

Radiopaque markers. The ROM study calculates colon transit based on the number of radiopaque markers retained. Using the original Metcalf technique, a mathematical formula is used to calculate colon transit with a colon transit time in excess of 68h being regarded as abnormal [20]. Using the single film technique of Martelli and colleagues, the retention of more than 20% of the ingested markers at day 5 is considered to indicate abnormal transit [21]. The distribution of markers, whether dispersed throughout the colon or aggregated in the pelvis, may serve as an indicator of the basic type of constipation present. Scintigraphic studies of

colonic transit can track the movement of the labeled material through the colon and a geometric center of the material at certain timed intervals (typically 24 and 48h) calculated.

Smart Pill®. The read-out from a Smart Pill® study can be interpreted on the basis of shifts in intraluminal pH, a sudden rise in pH of 2 or more units indicating egress of the capsule from the stomach while a subsequent rise of 1 or more pH units is taken as indicating arrival in the cecum; its expulsion, as recorded by the patient or as indicated by a sudden drop in temperature recorded, is taken to indicate its exit from the large bowel [10]. From these various detection points gastric residence time, small bowel transit, and colon transit can be calculated and results, in the case of colon transit, similar to those obtained with the radiopaque technique, obtained [10].

Anorectal manometry. While a number of parameters may be derived from an anorectal manometry study, the basal sphincter pressure, the squeeze response, and the elicitation of the rectoanal inhibitory response have been the most useful in clinical practice [14]. As with many other test results in this area, results vary considerably in relation to both technical and technique factors. Bearing these variations in mind, the normal ranges for resting and squeeze pressures are from 40 to 80 mmHg and from 80 to 160 mmHg (i.e., squeeze pressure is approximately double that of resting pressure), respectively. It is assumed that resting pressure is largely a reflection of internal anal sphincter tone whereas the squeeze response is generated by the external sphincter. A normal RAIR should feature relaxation of the internal sphincter and contraction of the external sphincter; the elicitation of this reflex indicates the integrity of the enteric nervous system thus explaining the loss of this reflex in aganglionic conditions such as Hirschsprung disease.

Role and Therapeutic Implications

Small Intestine

Clinical studies of small intestinal motor function are typically considered in one of two circumstances [1,2,19]:
1 In a patient with chronic or recurrent gastrointestinal symptoms which could be attributable to an underlying motility disorder and where prior testing raised the possibility of motor dysfunction (e.g., delayed gastric emptying, slow transit of barium through the small bowel). In most such circumstances, a functional disorder is the

most likely explanation but a motor disorder needs to be definitively ruled out. In this context, scintigraphy may provide supportive evidence either way but a normal manometry provides the best evidence against the presence of a primary or secondary motor disorder. A normal study is of critical value in this situation as it prevents the patient from commencing on an inexorable path that may lead from enteral feeding, through opiate use to total parenteral nutrition, and, even, surgical interventions.
2 Small bowel manometry studies have also been advocated in the patient with intractable slow-transit constipation who is being considered for surgery and, especially, where upper gastrointestinal-type symptoms suggest the presence of a more diffuse motor abnormality. There is some limited evidence to indicate that a normal small bowel study is a predictor of a good surgical outcome.

Colon and Anorectum

The principal indications for motor and sensory testing of the colon, anorectum, and pelvic floor are in the investigation of constipation and incontinence [1,2,14,24,25]. While investigations in the patient with constipation are reserved for the patient with chronic non-responsive symptoms, the threshold for investigation in the incontinent patient is, typically, lower given the distress associ-

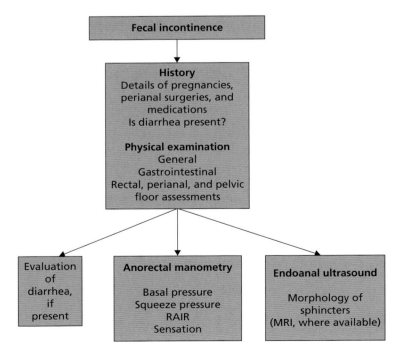

Figure 15.2 An approach to the evaluation of fecal incontinence.

ated with this symptom and the paucity of simple medical remedies.

The goals of testing in constipation are, firstly, to differentiate slow-transit constipation from defecatory dysfunction, and, secondly, in the patient with defecatory dysfunction, to define as best as possible the anatomical and functional defects that may be responsible for the patient's symptoms and that may be amenable to specific therapy. In the case of incontinence, the goals of testing are more straightforward and are to define the presence of anatomical defects and/or neurogenic incontinence. In the patient with defecatory dysfunction, as well as in the patient with incontinence, a defect identified on physiological testing may form the basis for biofeedback therapy. There are very few prospective studies which have critically assessed the impact of a given test or, indeed, compared the relative merits of two or more similar tests, in terms of their impact on a therapeutic intervention or strategy, be it pharmacologic, surgical, or biofeedback. Motility laboratories have varying experience with various tests and each tends to have its own preferences in terms of an assessment algorithm.

Figures 15.2 and 15.3 seek to represent a reasonable consensus in regard to the application of the aforemen-

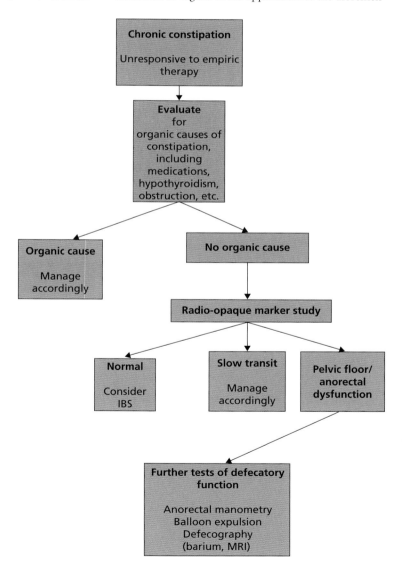

Figure 15.3 An approach to the assessment of chronic constipation. IBS, irritable bowel syndrome.

tioned motility tests to the investigation of constipation and incontinence.

Complications

While motility tests tend to fall short when it comes to hard and fast data on sensitivity, specificity, and evidence-based clinical impact, they are, in general, remarkably safe.

Radiological and scintigraphic studies will, of course, involve radiation exposure as will small intestinal manometry, if fluoroscopy is used to guide the assembly into place. The investigator should be aware of the radiation exposure doses related to each of these studies and, in the case of small intestinal manometry, in particular, should strive to minimize fluoroscopy time.

Small bowel manometry necessitates intubation and may be attended by any of the associated risks; prolonged nasal intubation may also result in sinusitis.

Take-home points

- A normal small intestinal manometry may prove of critical value, in the appropriate context, in directing patient management.

- Studies of colon transit are easy to perform and can define slow-transit constipation.

- Anorectal manometry and an endoanal study of sphincter morphology provide valuable information in the context of fecal incontinence.

- A variety of techniques are available for the assessment of anorectal and pelvic floor function; the clinician should select tests based on both evidence of their impact and available local expertise.

References

1 Camilleri M, Bharucha AE, di Lorenzo C, *et al.* American Neurogastroenterology and Motility Society consensus statement on intraluminal measurement of gastrointestinal and colonic motility in clinical practice. *Neurogastroenterol Motil* 2008; **20**: 1269–82.

2 Camilleri M, Hasler WL, Parkman HP, *et al.* Measurement of gastrointestinal motility in the GI laboratory. *Gastroenterology* 1998; **115**: 747–62.

3 Romagnuolo J, Schiller D, Bailey RJ. Using breath tests wisely in a gastroenterology practice: an evidence-based review of indications and pitfalls in interpretation. *Am J Gastroenterol* 2002; **97**: 1113–26.

4 Bonapace ES, Maurer AH, Davidoff S, *et al.* Whole gut transit scintigraphy in the clinical evaluation of patients with upper and lower gastrointestinal symptoms. *Am J Gastroenterol* 2000; **95**: 2838–47.

5 Stanghellini V, Tosetti C, Corinaldesi R. Standards for non-invasive methods for gastrointestinal motility: scintigraphy. A position statement from the Gruppo Italiano di Studio Motilità Apparato Digerente (GISMAD). *Dig Liv Dis* 2000; **32**: 447–52.

6 Lin HC, Prather C, Fisher RS, *et al.* AMS Task Force Committee on Gastrointestinal Transit. Measurement of gastrointestinal transit. *Dig Dis Sci* 2005; **50**: 989–1004.

7 Camilleri M. New imaging in neurogastroenterology: an overview. *Neurogastroenterol Motil* 2006; **18**: 805–12.

8 Odunsi ST, Camilleri M. Selected interventions in nuclear medicine: gastrointestinal motor functions. *Semin Nucl Med* 2009; **39**: 186–94.

9 von der Ohe MR, Camilleri M. Measurement of small bowel and colonic transit: indications and methods. *Mayo Clin Proc* 1992; **67**: 1169–79.

10 Rao SSC, Kuo B, McCallum RW, *et al.* Investigation of colonic and whole-gut transit with wireless motility capsule and radiopaque markers in constipation. *Clin Gastroenterol Hepatol* 2009; **7**: 537–49.

11 Bharucha AE, Fletcher JG. Recent advances in assessing anorectal structure and functions. *Gastroenterology* 2007; **133**: 1069–74.

12 Fletcher JG, Busse RF, Riederer SJ, *et al.* Magnetic resonance imaging of anatomic and dynamic defects of the pelvic floor in defecatory disorders. *Am J Gastroenterol* 2003; **98**: 399–411.

13 Harewood GC, Coulie B, Camilleri M, *et al.* Descending perineum syndrome: audit of clinical and laboratory features and outcome of pelvic floor retraining. *Am J Gastroenterol* 1999; **94**: 126–30.

14 Barnett JL, Hasler WL, Camilleri M. American Gastroenterological Association medical position statement on anorectal testing techniques. American Gastroenterological Association. *Gastroenterology* 1999; **116**: 732–60.

15 Sun WM, Donnelly TC, Read NW. Utility of a combined test of anorectal manometry, electrogastrography, and sensation in determining the mechanism of "idiopathic" faecal incontinence. *Gut* 1992; **33**: 807–13.

16 Bharucha AE, Fletcher G, Harper CM, *et al.* Relationship between symptoms and disordered continence mechanisms in women with idiopathic faecal incontinence. *Gut* 2005; **54**: 540–55.

17 Kiff EG, Swash M. Normal proximal and delayed distal conduction in the pudendal nerves of patients with idiopathic (neurogenic) faecal incontinence. *J Neurol Neurosurg Psychiatr* 1984; **47**: 820–3.

18 Andrews C, Bharucha AE, Seide B, Zinsmeister AR. Rectal sensorimotor dysfunction in women with fecal incontinence. *Am J Physiol Gastrointest Liver Physiol* 2007; **292**: G282–9.

19 Quigley EMM, Deprez PH, Hellstrom P, *et al.* Ambulatory intestinal manometry: a consensus report on its clinical role. *Dig Dis Sci* 1997; **42**: 2395–400.

20 Metcalf AM, Phillips SF, Zinsmeister AR, *et al.* Simplified assessment of segmental colonic transit. *Gastroenterology* 1987; **92**: 40–7.

21 Martelli H, Devroede G, Arhan P, *et al.* Some parameters of large bowel motility in normal man. *Gastroenterology* 1978; **75**: 612–8.

22 Grybäck P, Jacobsson H, Blomquist L, *et al.* Scintigraphy of the small intestine: a simplified standard for study of transit with reference to normal values. *Eur J Nucl Med Mol Imaging* 2002; **29**: 39–45.

23 Cremonini F, Mullan BP, Camilleri M, *et al.* Performance characteristics of scintigraphic transit measurements for studies of experimental therapies. *Aliment Pharmacol Ther* 2002; **16**: 1781–90.

24 Bharucha AE. Pro: Anorectal testing is useful in fecal incontinence. *Am J Gastroenterol* 2006; **101**: 2679–81.

25 Tuteja AK, Rao SSC. Review article: recent trends in diagnosis and treatment of faecal incontinence. *Aliment Pharmacol Ther* 2004; **19**: 829–40.

CHAPTER 16

Pancreatic Function Testing

John G. Lieb II[1] and Christopher E. Forsmark[2]

[1] Division of Gastroenterology, University of Pennsylvania, Philadelphia, PA, USA
[2] Division of Gastroenterology, Hepatology, and Nutrition, University of Florida, Gainesville, FL, USA

Summary

The diagnosis of chronic pancreatitis, especially that of early or less-advanced chronic pancreatitis, is challenging. Diagnostic tests that measure changes of pancreatic function complement tests that measure changes of pancreatic structure. Some tests of pancreatic function can diagnose chronic pancreatitis after less cumulative damage to the pancreas than many routinely available tests of pancreatic structure, and hence have utility in making a diagnosis in early disease. More invasive pancreatic function tests are most accurate in the early diagnosis of chronic pancreatitis, but these tests are not widely available. Less-invasive function tests are more widely available but are generally more valuable in providing information on the severity of disease, rather than for diagnostic purposes. Several pancreatic function tests have been recently developed that may allow for more routine availability.

Case

A 22-year-old woman is seen for evaluation of abdominal pain. The pain was initially episodic but is now continuous with superimposed flares. The pain is described as epigastric, with radiation to the back and right scapula, and is associated with chronic nausea and occasional vomiting. The pain was severe enough on several occasions that she was evaluated in the emergency room. On two occasions, serum amylase was elevated to twice the upper limit of normal while liver chemistries and other laboratory tests have been normal. Several abdominal ultrasounds and abdominal computed tomography (CT) scans have been normal, as has an esophagogastroduodenoscopy (EGD). Family history is negative and the patient neither smokes or drinks. The patient has been labeled as having chronic pancreatitis and was recently denied health insurance due to an "pre-existing condition" of chronic pancreatitis. You perform an endoscopic ultrasound which reveals three features consistent with chronic pancreatitis. You remain unconvinced that the diagnosis of chronic pancreatitis has been firmly established and refer the patient for an invasive pancreatic function test, which reveals a peak bicarbonate concentration of 98 mEq/L.

Practical Gastroenterology and Hepatology: Small and Large Intestine and Pancreas, 1st edition. Edited by Nicholas J. Talley, Sunanda V. Kane and Michael B. Wallace. © 2010 Blackwell Publishing Ltd.

Normal Pancreatic Function and Principles of Pancreatic Function Testing

In order to appreciate the role of pancreatic function testing, one has to understand the normal functioning of the pancreas. During a meal, gastric distension and acid production stimulate the release of the hormone secretin, which signals the pancreatic ductal cells to secrete a large volume of bicarbonate-rich fluid. The postprandial increase in amino acids and fatty acids in the duodenum stimulates the release of cholecystokinin (CCK) which in turn signals the acinar cells to release digestive enzymes into the pancreatic duct. The effects of these two hormonal systems (secretin and CCK) on the pancreas are measurable. Absorption of nutrients requires the neutralization of gastric acid, the action of these enzymes, and bile acids (in the case of fat and fat-soluble vitamins).

Chronic pancreatitis is defined by the presence of irreversible damage to the pancreas. The process of damage is one which may occur over many years [1]. With enough accumulated damage, eventually there is failure of pancreatic function. In the exocrine pancreas, this leads to the development of maldigestion and steatorrhea; and in the endocrine pancreas, the development of diabetes. The pancreas has substantial reserves. Approximately 90% of the gland can to be destroyed or damaged before there is exocrine or endocrine failure. Prior to failure, however, there is a gradual drop in functional capacity which can be measured even though this may not lead to symptoms or signs of pancreatic insufficiency. Patients in this earlier stage of disease may not have features of pancreatic insufficiency, but may still suffer from substantial pain.

Pancreatic function tests may be divided into those that are direct or indirect. Direct tests are generally those that collect a sample of pancreatic juice, intestinal fluid, or stool and directly measure the output from the pancreas in these specimens. Indirect tests are those that attempt to measure pancreatic function by assessing the ability of pancreatic enzymes to digest a substrate. Pancreatic function tests may also be classified as invasive (utilizing a tube or endoscope to collect fluid) or non-invasive (collecting blood, urine, stool, or exhaled breath; or using some radiologic method of assessing function). Finally, these pancreatic function tests may be categorized by whether they are designed to determine the presence or absence of pancreatic functional failure (the end stage of disease) or whether they are attempting to assess for less-advanced damage. In the latter case, that generally means looking for a decrease in maximally stimulated pancreatic secretion, by administering a hormone and measuring output from the pancreas (an invasive direct pancreatic function test). The drop in maximum secretory capacity occurs before (in many cases years or even decades) the damage is so advanced as to cause functional failure. The pancreatic function tests currently available are presented in Table 16.1.

Importantly, pancreatic function tests do not stand alone but are used in conjunction with radiologic and endoscopic tests and clinical information to reach a diagnosis and determine severity. The challenges do not occur in patients with long-standing and advanced chronic pancreatitis, when most tests are likely to be abnormal. The diagnostic challenges are seen in those who may have severe symptoms of pain but do not have disease which is advanced enough to be easily identifiable on widely available diagnostic tests.

Table 16.1 Pancreatic function tests.

Invasive direct pancreatic function tests
  Secretin stimulation test utilizing an oroduodenal tube
  Secretin stimulation test utilizing an upper endoscope
  CCK or combined secretin and CCK tests utilizing either
    oroduodenal tube or endoscope
  Intraductal secretin test

Non-invasive direct pancreatic function tests
  Secretin-stimulated MRCP
  Fecal elastase
  Serum trypsin

Indirect pancreatic function tests
  72-h fecal fat
  Sudan stain of random specimen of stool
  Breath tests (various)
  Serum glucose

MRCP, magnetic retrograde cholangiopancreatography; CCK, cholecystokinin.

Direct Pancreatic Function Tests

These tests maximally stimulate pancreatic secretions and then collect and measure secretions to determine maximum secretory capacity.

Invasive Direct Pancreatic Function Tests

Secretin Stimulation Test (SST)
There are a few variations of this test. The method used at the University of Florida is described. A double-lumen, oroduodenal tube with both gastric and duodenal ports is introduced, utilizing only topical anesthesia. The weighted tip is advanced fluoroscopically to the ligament of Treitz. The gastric port is used to remove gastric secretions. A supraphysiologic intravenous bolus of synthetic human secretin at a dose of 0.2 mg/kg is administered. Duodenal fluid is collected under vacuum aspiration over 1 h in four 15-min aliquots. The fluid is analyzed for bicarbonate concentration in mEq/L. The highest concentration of bicarbonate obtained among the four 15-min aliquots is the peak bicarbonate concentration. The normal range for peak bicarbonate is greater than 80 mEq/L. The volume of secretions is also measured, for analysis in equivocal cases.

The SST is a sensitive test for chronic pancreatitis, and is best able to detect chronic pancreatitis in its earlier stages. The SST, when compared with the gold standard of pancreatic histology, is 75% sensitive in detecting early-stage chronic pancreatitis, and up to 97% for late-stage disease with a specificity of 90% [2]. Studies show a linear correlation with severity of histologic disease and peak bicarbonate concentration. Among patients with early disease (those without obvious calcific changes on routine imaging and without pancreatic insufficiency) with an abnormal SST, endoscopic retrograde cholangio-pancreatography (ERCP) is abnormal in only 66%, though ERCP is abnormal in almost all patients with late-stage disease [3].

The SST does have several important shortcomings, the most significant of which is that it is only available at a few tertiary-care centers. In addition, unsedated tube placement may be not well tolerated and false positives can be seen for several months after an attack of acute pancreatitis.

Cholecystokinin Stimulation Testing

The classical CCK stimulation test measures enzyme-rich secretion rather than bicarbonate secretion. The test is also only used at very few tertiary-care centers and is very similar to the SST, except that the CCK may be administered by continuous infusion or bolus infusion.

Combined Secretin–Cholecystokinin Stimulation Testing

This test allows measurement of both bicarbonate and enzyme production by the pancreas. In most studies, the accuracy of secretin-based pancreatic function testing is superior to CCK-based testing.

All of these traditional tests require a duodenal tube placement and so may be poorly tolerated, in addition to being unavailable to most clinicians and most patients.

Intraductal Secretin Stimulation Testing

One method to measure pancreatic function is to collect the fluid directly from the pancreatic duct at the time of ERCP. This could have theoretical advantages in allowing pure secretions to be collected. In the intraductal secretin stimulation test, the main pancreatic duct is cannulated at ERCP, secretin is administered, and pancreatic fluid is collected. Pancreatic secretions collected in this manner have a higher bicarbonate concentration than in the classical SST, with a normal range usually greater than 105 mEq/L. Disadvantages of this test include the complication rate of ERCP, the need for sedation, and the relatively short time periods of collection (usually 15 min,

as limited by sedation and fluoroscopy room time). This brief collection period makes the test relatively inaccurate. In one recent comparison of the intraductal secretin stimulation test and SST, the sensitivity of the intraductal secretin stimulation test compared to the conventional SST was 80%, with a specificity of 20% [4]. Based on these results, the intraductal secretin stimulation test should not be used for diagnostic purposes.

Endoscopic Secretin Stimulation Testing (eSST)

An alternative to traditional pancreatic function testing is to perform EGD and use a polyethylene tube passed through the biopsy channel to collect fluid after stimulation with secretin or the combination of secretin-CCK. This may offer the advantage of improved availability and patient comfort. The eSST usually employs a bolus injection of secretin (as in the SST), followed by EGD. At the time of EGD, all fluid is suctioned from the stomach and the scope is left in the duodenum and used to collect pancreatic secretions. Unlike the SST, aliquots of duodenal fluid are only collected every 15 min, rather than the continuous collection during the entire time period. Fluid is submitted to the central laboratory for bicarbonate measurement, with a normal result being at least one of the samples with a bicarbonate concentration above 80 mEq/L. The sedation used for endoscopy does not appear to have a major effect on pancreatic secretion, but this is incompletely studied. The eSST is slightly inferior in accuracy to the SST, but may be able to be utilized at more centers [5–7]. It may be difficult to keep a patient sedated for the entire 60 min of the test and this occupies an endoscopy room for a considerable period of time. Variations of the test attempting to shorten the time by administering the secretin before the procedure and collecting samples at fewer time points (only 30–45 min of collection time) show some loss of specificity but retain reasonable sensitivity [6,7].

Non-invasive Direct Pancreatic Function Tests

"Enhanced Imaging" Pancreatic Function Tests (S-MRCP)

Administering secretin at the time of a magnetic retro-grade cholangiopancreatography (MRCP) improves visualization of the pancreatic duct. The fluid which is produced after secretin stimulation fills the duodenum, and can be semiquantitated to measure volume output from the pancreas [8]. It should be noted that in traditional pancreatic function testing, it is the bicarbonate concentration rather than fluid volume that is used as the primary measure, largely because volume is less specific and sensitive. There are limited data on the accuracy of S-MRCP. Magnet resonance imaging (MRI) utilizing gadolinium infusion or diffusion weighting techniques are being studied but whether these improve upon the accuracy of MRI/MRCP is not known.

Fecal Elastase

Pancreatic elastase-1 is a pancreas-specific protease that is minimally degraded during intestinal transit. The concentration of fecal elastase in stool gives a rough estimation of the elastase output from the pancreas. The test utilizes only a spot collection of stool. A fecal elastase less than 100 µg/g of stool indicates severe pancreatic insufficiency. The test is most accurate in those with advanced and longstanding disease. A value between 100 and 200 µg/g of stool is indeterminant. Values over 200 µg/g of stool are normal. False positives occur by dilution in watery diarrhea.

In various studies, compared to conventional pancreatic function testing and ERCP, the sensitivity of fecal elastase varies from between 0 and 65% for mild disease to 33 and 100% for severe chronic pancreatitis, with reasonable specificity [1]. Fecal chymotrypsin can also be measured but is less accurate than fecal elastase.

Serum Trypsin

The serum trypsinogen (also known as trypsin) assay is unique among pancreatic function tests in being a serum sample. Levels less than 20 ng/mL, are specific for chronic pancreatitis but are sensitive only for advanced disease. Levels from 20 to 29 ng/mL are indeterminant. Sensitivities range from 33 to 65% but specificity is quite high. The test has high sensitivity once advanced chronic pancreatitis with exocrine insufficiency has developed, but like fecal elastase has poor sensitivity for less-advanced disease [1].

Indirect Pancreatic Function Tests

The general theme in these tests is to measure the effect of inadequate delivery of digestive enzymes to the intestine from the damaged pancreas. Generally these tests only detect advanced chronic pancreatitis with steatorrhea, but are fairly cheap and reliable in that setting.

72-h Fecal Fat

The 72-h fecal fat collection remains the gold standard for quantification of steatorrhea. However, it suffers from many drawbacks. The 72-h fecal fat is inaccurate when performed in the outpatient setting, for several reasons. First, it is unrealistic to expect the patient to refrigerate 72-h worth of stool. Second, adherence to a standardized, precise 100 g/24 h fat diet per day for a total of 6 days (the 3 days preceding the test and then the test itself) is difficult. A 72 h stool collection during a high-fat diet showing more than 7 g/24 h fat in the stool is abnormal. The levels of steatorrhea seen in chronic pancreatitis tends to be much higher (often >20 g/24 h) but interestingly they may not have diarrhea despite passing large amounts of fat.

Spot Fecal Fat

Sudan staining of a random stool sample for fecal fat is relatively insensitive for fat malabsorption. Generally, it detects steatorrhea only at 25 g/day or more. As a stool collection, it suffers many of the drawbacks of the 72-h fecal fat. Greater than six droplets of fat per high power field is indicative of steatorrhea. As in the case of the 72-h fecal fat analysis, fat substitutes in foods such as olestra (Olean©) or drugs such as orlistat or ezetimibe can give false-positive results.

Breath Tests

A radiolabeled substrate that requires digestion by pancreatic enzymes is administered, and the radioactive CO_2 which is produced through digestion is measured in the breath. A wide variety of these tests have been developed but none have entered clinical practice.

Serum Glucose

With the development of endocrine insufficiency, diabetes mellitus will develop. Hyperglycemia is neither sensitive nor specific for chronic pancreatitis.

Tests of Historical Interest Only

Two tests, the Bentiromide test and pancrealauryl test, administered oral substrates which underwent digestion by pancreatic enzymes, and the metabolites could be measured in the urine. They are no longer in clinical use.

Utilizing Pancreatic Function Tests

Chronic pancreatitis is a heterogeneous disease. Patients may have significant pain with preserved physiology and little direct imaging evidence of chronic pancreatitis (e.g., a normal CT scan of the pancreas). This type of pancreatitis is often called minimal change, or small duct chronic pancreatitis [3]. Patients with this early-stage chronic pancreatitis are very difficult to diagnose and distinguish from other causes of chronic abdominal pain. They are often misdiagnosed, with the most common mistake being to label a patient as having chronic pancreatitis without clear confirmatory evidence. The Case presented above poses just such a dilemma. Invasive direct pancreatic function tests are the best currently available method to more reliably diagnose these types of patients, although endoscopic ultrasound (EUS) is also quite helpful in these patients. As chronic pancreatitis progresses, the accumulated structural and functional damage becomes more obvious, and the wide variety of diagnostic tests (including the function tests described above but also the wide variety of structural tests such as CT, EUS, and MRI/MRCP) are accurate. In these patients with more advanced disease, the focus is on choosing the least costly and least invasive method, rather than on choosing the test with the highest sensitivity for chronic pancreatitis

Conclusions

Most pancreatic function tests have high sensitivity and specificity to accurately diagnose patients with advanced chronic pancreatitis. The indirect and non-invasive tests tend to perform poorly in patients with early, less-advanced disease. Some specialized invasive "tube" tests can most reliably detect mild, early chronic pancreatitis but are only available at a few referral centers. Endoscopic-based direct pancreatic function tests may eventually be more widely available.

Take-home points

- Tests of pancreatic function may be used both to diagnose chronic pancreatitis and to determine the severity of chronic pancreatitis.

- The most sensitive test to diagnose early or less-advanced chronic pancreatitis is an invasive direct pancreatic function test.

- Simpler indirect pancreatic function tests are best used to determine the severity of chronic pancreatitis, not to establish the diagnosis.

- Pancreatic function tests should be seen as complementary diagnostic tests to tests of pancreatic structure (CT, EUS, MRI).

References

1 Layer P, Yamamoto H, Kalthoff L, *et al.* The different courses of early- and late-onset idiopathic and alcoholic chronic pancreatitis. *Gastroenterology* 1994; **107**: 1481–7.

2 Chowdhury RS, Forsmark CE. Pancreatic function tests. *Aliment Pharmacol Ther* 2003; **17**: 733–50.

3 Forsmark CE, Toskes PP. What does an abnormal pancreatogram mean? *Gastrointest Endosc Clin N Am* 1995; **5**: 105–23.

4 Draganov P, Patel A, Fazel, *et al.* Prospective evaluation of the accuracy of the intraductal secretin stimulation test in the diagnosis of chronic pancreatitis. *Clin Gastroenterol Hepatol* 2005; **3**: 695–9.

5 Stevens T, Conwell DL, Zuccaro G Jr, *et al.* A prospective crossover study comparing secretin stimulated endoscopic and Dreiling tube pancreatic function testing in patients evaluated for chronic pancreatitis. *Gastrointest Endosc* 2008; **67**: 458–66.

6 Grendell JH. The endoscopic pancreatic function test-time to take a step back. *Gastrointest Endosc* 2008; **67**: 467–70.

7 Stevens T, Conwell DL, Zuccaro G Jr, *et al.* The efficiency of endoscopic pancreatic function testing is optimized using duodenal aspirates at 30 and 45 minutes after intravenous secretin. *Am J Gastroenterol* 2007; **102**: 297–301.

8 Sahni VA, Mortele KJ. Magnetic resonance cholangiopancreatography: current use and future applications. *Clin Gastroenterol Hepatol* 2008; **6**: 967–77.

PART 4

Problem-based Approach to Diagnosis and Differential Diagnosis

CHAPTER 17

General Approach to Relevant History Taking and Physical Examination

Sheryl A. Serbowicz[1] and Suzanne Rose[2]

[1] Department of Medical Education, Division of Gastroenterology, Mount Sinai School of Medicine, New York, NY, USA
[2] Department of Medical Education and Department of Medicine, Division of Gastroenterology, Mount Sinai School of Medicine, New York, NY, USA

Summary

In patients presenting with a gastrointestinal complaint, taking a comprehensive history and performing a thorough physical examination are key elements to target further evaluation and management. The line of questioning should focus on the complaint but be comprehensive enough to rule out non-gastrointestinal causes, gastrointestinal causes, as well as systemic problems. Superb communication skills will support a trusting patient–physician relationship and will facilitate in the care of the patient. This chapter offers strategies for lines of questioning that pertain to specific complaints and reviews the pertinent features of the physical examination.

Introduction to History Taking

The art of history taking is often the key to determining the correct diagnosis in a patient presenting with a specific complaint. In order to facilitate a meaningful exchange it is important for the health-care provider to introduce him or herself and identify his/her role. S/he should also facilitate the comfort of the patient in terms of assuring a private setting, making sure seating is comfortable, and making eye contact possible [1]. It is important to be aware of verbal and non-verbal cues. Questions should be open-ended, initially allowing the patient to freely express him or herself, but the perceptive history-taker will refine the line of questioning with more directed questions to characterize the chief complaint in an attempt to narrow the differential diagnosis. This will include questions designed to determine possible etiologies of the symptom. In considering the differential diagnosis during solicitation of the history, it is important to review the possible organ systems that may be involved and then the physiologic processes (e.g., inflammatory, infectious, neoplastic, congenital, etc.), narrowing the differential along the path of questioning as the answers are processed and clinical reasoning is employed. At the end of the interview, it is a good strategy to review the patient's story and ask the patient if there is anything that should have been asked but was not. This gives the patient an opportunity to contribute any other issue and to make sure the history taking has been comprehensive.

See Table 17.1 for general questioning strategies and an initial approach to diagnosing any patient complaint.

Common reasons for visiting a gastroenterologist include abdominal pain, bowel changes, nausea and vomiting, gastrointestinal bleeding, and jaundice. What follows is a guide to history taking and physical examinations appropriate to each of these symptoms.

Practical Gastroenterology and Hepatology: Small and Large Intestine and Pancreas, 1st edition. Edited by Nicholas J. Talley, Sunanda V. Kane and Michael B. Wallace. © 2010 Blackwell Publishing Ltd.

Table 17.1 General history taking.

What is the timing of the onset of the symptom?

Describe the character of onset—was it abrupt or gradual?

How frequently do you have this symptom?

Is there variation over a 24-h period?

Is there any association with eating, bowel movements, flatulence, or belching?

Have you had prior experience with similar symptoms?

Do you have close contacts with similar symptoms?

Name any precipitating factors.

List any palliating factors.

Have you taken anything to alleviate the symptom?

Can you identify any interference with daily activities?

Does this symptom cause disruption of sleep?

Patient Concern—Abdominal Pain

The quality of abdominal pain is determined through a detailed history and varies depending upon underlying pathophysiology. Visceral pain is the result of distension and spasm of an organ's lumen or covering. The pain is usually poorly localized and described as aching, dull, or cramping. Parietal pain is the result of peritoneal inflammation and is commonly described as severe, sharp, and well-localized. Referred pain is the result of crosstalk between visceral sensory nerves and somatic sensory nerves of the same vertebral level [2]. The pain is commonly felt along a dermatome at the skin surface and described as aching, burning, or gnawing. Causes of abdominal pain include gastrointestinal, neurological, musculoskeletal, psychological, gynecological, vascular, and renal disorders. The quality and severity of abdominal pain may vary between individuals based on clinical environment, culture, personality, mental status, medications, and past experiences with pain [2]. Take note of the patient's body position, as this may provide information about the severity of the pain.

Table 17.2 indicates abdominal anatomic regions with possible etiologies of pain in those regions and Table 17.3 provides questions to be asked to define abdominal pain.

Patient Concern—Bowel Complaints

Diarrhea and constipation can result from alterations in the balance of intestinal secretion, absorption, surface area, bacterial flora, transit time, and neurological and muscular function. Patients may describe bowel complaints in terms of stool consistency, frequency, volume, or sensation of stool passage [4–6]. A thorough history will elicit the time course and detailed characteristics of the stool changes.

Diarrhea or constipation may present acutely or it may be chronic. The knowledge of this time factor can help focus the line of questioning while taking the history. Both symptoms have many primary and secondary causes. The line of questioning should always include ruling out alarm signs or symptoms, which may differentiate a functional etiology from another possible cause, requiring further evaluation [5,6]. These alarm symptoms include: weight loss of more than 4.5 kg (10 pounds), blood in the stool or hemoccult-positive stool, anemia, a family history of colon cancer, fever, or extreme symptoms. An abrupt onset (or onset of these symptoms in the elderly) should prompt an exploration of additional causative factors.

It should be noted that there are some symptoms that patients do not openly describe due to embarrassment. Fecal incontinence is one such symptom, and it is a good strategy to ask directly about this problem, especially when pertaining to a presenting complaint. (It is also a good approach to include this symptom as part of a general survey of questions that should be asked of every patient.) For a patient with constipation, a question related to digitation or manual maneuvers should be asked explicitly. Dyschezia or difficulty defecating, as distinguished from constipation, may suggest pelvic floor dysfunction.

Table 17.4 includes questions to clarify the symptom of bowel complaints and Table 17.5 includes the Bristol Stool Form Scale.

Patient Concern—Nausea and Vomiting

The vomiting center in the medulla and the chemoreceptor trigger zone near the fourth ventricle coordinate vomiting in response to signals from the gastrointestinal

Table 17.2 Location of pain and possible etiologies. (Note: neoplasms and musculoskeletal pathology can also cause pain in any of the locations.)

Location of pain	Gastrointestinal causes					Non-gastrointestinal causes
	Inflammatory or infectious	**Vascular**	**Mechanical**	**Congenital**	**Functional**	
LUQ	Splenic infection Gastritis Gastric ulcer Pancreatitis	Splenic infarction	Volvulus		Gastroparesis	Myocardial infarction
RUQ	Hepatitis Cholecystitis Cholangitis Pancreatitis	Budd–Chiari	Biliary colic Volvulus		Irritable bowel syndrome	Subdiaphragmatic abscess Pneumonia Empyema Fitz-Hugh–Curtis
LLQ	Diverticulitis Inflammatory bowel disease	Ischemia	Inguinal hernia		Irritable bowel syndrome	Pelvic inflammatory disease Ectopic pregnancy Mittelschmerz Endometriosis Ovarian cysts Nephrolithiasis Pyelonephritis
RLQ	Late appendicitis Inflammatory bowel disease Pseudoappendicitis (Yersinia)		Inguinal hernia		Irritable bowel syndrome	Pelvic inflammatory disease Ectopic pregnancy Mittelschmerz Endometriosis Ovarian cysts Nephrolithiasis Pyelonephritis
Periumbilical	Early appendicitis Gastroenteritis	Aortic aneurysm or dissection	Intestinal obstruction Umbilical hernia			
Epigastric	Peptic ulcer disease Gastritis Pancreatitis Esophagitis	Aortic aneurysm or dissection			GERD Gastroparesis Non-ulcer dyspepsia	Myocardial infarction Pericarditis
Suprapubic					Irritable bowel syndrome	Cystitis Endometriosis
Diffuse	Gastroenteritis Malaria Peritonitis	Mesenteric ischemia	Intestinal obstruction Volvulus	Acute intermittent porphyria	Irritable bowel syndrome	

LUQ, left upper quadrant; RUQ, right upper quadrant; LLQ, left lower quadrant; RLQ, right lower quadrant; GERD, gastroesophageal reflux disease.

tract, blood and cerebrospinal fluid, and inner ear [10]. Pain, visual, gustatory, and olfactory stimuli, as well as memories, contribute to the individual experience of nausea and vomiting. A detailed history will help distinguish nausea and vomiting from rumination, regurgita-tion, and retching [11]. Although nausea and vomiting are gastrointestinal symptoms, their cause may or may not be of GI etiology. Other causes of nausea and vomiting include psychological (anorexia, bulimia), neurologi-cal (increased intracranial pressure), metabolic and

Table 17.3 Questions targeted to define abdominal pain.

Question	Indication
Where is the pain?	See Table 17.2
Has the pain radiated or moved since onset?	Appendicitis begins at umbilicus and later causes lower right quadrant pain Aortic dissection begins as chest pain and later causes abdominal or back pain Cholecystitis radiates to the right scapula Pancreatitis radiates to the back
How severe is the pain from 0–10?	Very severe pain with intestinal perforation, peritonitis, or volvulus
Describe the sensation of the pain	Differentiate between visceral, parietal, and referred pain Colicky pain often has a crescendo–decrescendo pattern
Is the pain associated with meals?	Worsens after fatty meals with biliary disease Worsens after meals with gastric peptic ulcers and mesenteric ischemia [3] Improves after meals with duodenal peptic ulcers [2,3]
Does the pain disrupt your sleep?	Duodenal peptic ulcers and GERD
Is the pain associated with nausea and vomiting?	Biliary disease, acute pancreatitis, appendicitis, peritonitis, intestinal obstruction, and ectopic pregnancy
Pain out of proportion to physical exam	Mesenteric ischemia

GERD, gastroesophageal reflux disease.

hormonal disturbances, infections (food-borne illness), pregnancy, and medications or other ingested substances.

Table 17.6 includes questions that may be asked to characterize a complaint of nausea or vomiting.

Patient Concern—Gastrointestinal Bleeding

Bleeding can occur from any location along the gastrointestinal tract. A detailed history can help characterize the bleeding in location and severity, but it should be remembered that manifestations of a GI bleed depend on the rate of bleeding in addition to the location of the bleed. Hematemesis is, by definition, the vomiting of bright red blood and indicates a source above the ligament of Treitz. Hematochezia, in contrast, is the passage of bloody bowel movements from the rectum. This may seem to indicate a lower GI bleed, but caution should be taken as a brisk upper GI bleed may present as hematochezia. Melena is black, tarry stool with a characteristic odor. Although the etiology is often an upper GI source, one must consider a small bowel or even right colon etiology. Occult GI bleeding may occur from anywhere in the GI tract and is usually detected with the presenta-

tion of chronic anemia or by testing the stool for occult blood. Patients with underlying ischemic cardiac disease are vulnerable to the development of angina or even an MI because of hypoperfusion in the setting of a GI bleed. Therefore the history must be comprehensive and simultaneous with physical observation and measurement of volume.

The following are among the more common causes of GI bleeding: esophageal varices, peptic ulcers, invasive infections, malignancy, arteriovenous malformations, vascular ectasia and other vascular abnormalities, diverticula, inflammatory bowel disease, internal and external hemorrhoids [13].

Table 17.7 provides a list of questions to ask a patient presenting with a GI bleed.

Patient Concern—Jaundice

By definition, jaundice is yellowing of the skin and sclera of the eyes due to excess of the pigment, bilirubin. Unlike jaundice, increased intake of carotene does not cause discoloration of the sclera. Jaundice is the disruption in either the uptake of bilirubin to the liver, the conjugation of bilirubin, or the excretion of bilirubin. Therefore jaundice may be the result of damage to liver cells or impaired

Table 17.4 Questions targeted to define bowel complaints.

Question	Indication
When was your most recent bowel movement?	
Describe the stool consistency and size	Utilize the Bristol Stool Form Scale (see Table 17.5) Thin stools with colon malignancy or with spasm Watery stool with infection or ingestion of indigestible particles [6] Greasy or floating stool with pancreatitis
Do you experience both diarrhea and constipation?	Irritable bowel syndrome, diverticulitis, and colon malignancy [3]
Have you experienced fecal incontinence?	A positive reply requires a comprehensive dietary history, gynecologic history, neurologic history
Are you passing more or less gas than usual?	Unable to pass gas with complete intestinal obstruction Excessive gas with malabsorption and maldigestion from pancreatitis or lactose intolerance
Is there blood and/or mucus in the stool?	Blood and mucus with ulcerative colitis, radiation colitis, pseudomembranous colitis, villous adenomas Blood with hemorrhoids, anal pathology, diverticula, malignancy, or vascular lesions Blood with invasive infections, such as *Shigella*, *E. coli*, *Salmonella*, *Yersinia*, and amoeba [7]
What is the color of the stool?	Black or tarry stool with proximal GI bleed Light brown or gray stool with biliary obstruction Red stool may indicate distal GI bleed or may occur after eating large amounts of beets or food dye
Does the stool have an usually foul odor?	Maldigestion of dietary fat with pancreatitis
Are the symptoms associated with eating certain types of food?	Wheat, barley, rye, and gluten-containing foods associated with celiac disease [7] Milk products with lactose intolerance Diarrhea after ingestion of caffeinated beverages, artificial sweeteners, or fruit products [6]
Do you experience rectal fullness or incomplete emptying?	Often a manifestation of visceral hypersensitivity and irritable bowel syndrome
Do you feel the need to strain or digitate to pass stool?	May indicate pelvic floor dysfunction

Table 17.5 Bristol Stool Form Scale [8,9].

Type	Stool description
1	Separate hard lumps, like nuts or pellets which are difficult to pass
2	Lumpy, but with a sausage-shape
3	Sausage-shaped with cracks on its surface
4	Smooth and soft, sausage-shaped
5	Soft pieces with clear cut edges which can be passed with ease
6	Ragged edges, fluffy pieces, "mushy"
7	Watery, entirely liquid stool with no solid pieces

liver cell function due to blockage of the bile ducts, either within the liver or extrinsic to this organ. It can also be due to excessive breakdown of red blood cells. Symptoms associated with jaundice are quite specific to the cause of the jaundice [15].

See Table 17.8 for specific questions that should be asked related to the presentation of jaundice.

Patient Concern—Other Symptoms

There are many other symptoms or primary complaints with which patients may present. These may include:

- Changes in weight
- Abdominal distension

Table 17.6 Questions targeted to define nausea and vomiting.

Question	Indication
How frequently are you vomiting?	Continuous vomiting with ingestion of toxic substances [3]
	Abrupt, forceful vomiting with increased intracranial pressure, or other CNS lesions [12]
	Early morning vomiting with metabolic disturbances or pregnancy
Have you taken recent steroids or pain medicines?	Nausea is an early sign of steroid, opioid, or sedative withdrawal
Do you have dizziness or difficulty with balance?	Vestibular or CNS lesion
Describe the color and consistency of the vomitus	Green or yellow vomitus with biliary disease
	Bloody vomitus with acute bleed of esophageal varices or peptic ulcer
	Coffee ground vomitus with upper GI bleed
	Feculent vomitus with ileus or intestinal obstruction
	Large volume vomitus with gastric outlet obstruction
	Undigested vomitus with achalasia and incompletely digested vomitus with gastroparesis
	Food particles on the pillow can be a sign of Zenker diverticulum
Has the color of your stool or urine changed?	Light stools and dark urine with biliary obstruction
Does anyone close to you have similar symptoms?	After meals with food-borne illness
	Gastroenteritis
Is the vomiting associated with abdominal pain?	Onset of pain occurs before onset of vomiting with appendicitis [3], can be a sign of early obstruction [11]
	Consider pancreatitis

Table 17.7 Questions targeted to define gastrointestinal bleeding.

Question	Indication
How did you first notice the blood?	Blood combined in with stool with ulcerative colitis, diverticula, infection [3], and malignancy
	Blood droplets or streaks on toilet paper with external hemorrhoids
	Blood on undergarments or bedsheets with a brisk bleed from malignancy
What color is the blood?	Dark red, maroon, or black blood usually with more proximal GI bleed [14]
	Bright red blood with hemorrhoids, diverticula, malignancy, ulcerative colitis, or brisk upper GI bleed
Do have constipation or diarrhea?	Diarrhea with infection and ulcerative colitis
	Chronic constipation associated with development of hemorrhoids and diverticula
Do you experience pain or itching when passing stool?	Presence of hemorrhoids or fissure [14]
Do you need to strain or digitate to pass stool?	Pelvic floor dysfunction
Do you experience rectal fullness or incomplete emptying?	Suggestive of functional problem with visceral hypersensitivity
Have you noticed lumps or flaps of tissue protruding from the anal opening?	External hemorrhoids, internal hemorrhoids, skin tags, prolapse, condyloma, or malignancy [14]

Table 17.8 Questions targeted to define jaundice.

Question	Indication
Is jaundice associated with abdominal pain?	Right upper quadrant pain with biliary obstruction or hepatitis
Do you have fever?	Biliary obstruction, hepatitis Fever, jaundice and RUQ abdominal pain is Charcot triad indicating ascending cholangitis [15]
Is jaundice associated with nausea, vomiting, or itching?	Severe itching with biliary obstruction, primary biliary cirrhosis
Has the color of your stool or urine changed?	Light brown or gray stool with biliary obstruction and liver, biliary, or pancreatic malignancy
Have you been feeling tired?	Fatigue with hemolytic anemia, malignancy, or hepatitis
Assess risk of infectious hepatitis	Intravenous or nasal drug use, unsafe sexual practices, tattoos, blood transfusions, and recent travel [3]
Assess risk of exposure to hepatotoxic substances	Exposure associated with occupation, recreation (solvents related to paints), accidents, or environment Use of alcohol or acetaminophen
A history of IBD?	Primary sclerosing cholangitis
Assess mental health status	Acetaminophen overdose (and other substance ingestion) can be a cause of acute fulminant liver failure

IBD, inflammatory bowel disease; RUQ, right upper quadrant.

- Perianal disease
- Fecal incontinence
- Gas or bloating
- Rectal pain
- Hiccups.

As part of any history a list of medications and allergies should be solicited. A family history should be documented, and a social history should be explored including tobacco use, alcohol and drug use, occupation, living environment, and sexual activity.

The elicitation of a history of abuse or domestic violence should be considered seriously in all patients. It is important to gain the trust of the patient; often this more personal history is obtained on a second or subsequent visit. It is crucial that the interviewer be non-judgmental and have resources available to help patients who have a positive response to this line of questioning (i.e., referral to a collaborative psychiatric support team). A history of abuse is more common in patients with functional GI complaints, but there is a high prevalence of abuse that spans the ages, socioeconomic lines and (although more common in women), gender [16].

Table 17.9 includes general history questions that should be asked of all patients.

Table 17.9 General history questions that should be asked of all patients.

Do you have any medical illnesses or chronic conditions?

Have you had any surgeries or other procedures in the abdomen or pelvis?

Do you take any prescriptions, over-the-counter medications, or herbal supplements?

Are symptoms associated with changes in your menstrual cycle?

Are there medical illnesses that run in your family?

Do you use alcohol, tobacco, illicit or recreational drugs?

Have you traveled recently?

Tell me about your diet

Assess risk of unsafe sexual practices

Have you ever had sexually transmitted infections?

Have you experienced recent life changes or stress?

Have you been feeling sad or anxious?

Have you ever witnessed or experienced physical, emotional, or sexual abuse?

Perform a Full Review of Systems/Symptoms

The review of systems should be comprehensive. In many cases it may be obtained by an assistant in the practice in the outpatient setting, or it may be obtained via a written questionnaire that the patient answers. Be sure to assess constitutional symptoms, such fever, chills, night sweats, weight loss, weight gain, and change in appetite. These symptoms may indicate the presence of infection, inflammation, malignancy, or other serious systemic process.

Physical Examination

This section will focus on the abdominal and rectal examination. However, given the specific complaint, it is important to consider performing detailed components of other parts of the physical examination. As an example, a comprehensive neurologic examination should be part of the evaluation of every patient presenting with fecal incontinence or constipation.

Abdominal Examination

- Inspection
  - Scars suggest prior procedures and increased risk for abdominal adhesions.
  - Striae may indicate exogenous or endogenous steroids, weight gain, or prior pregnancy.
  - Note rashes and abnormal skin color or texture.
  - Distended veins result from portal hypertension and perihepatic disease.
  - An enlarged abdomen may result from intestinal obstruction, constipation, hepatosplenomegaly, masses, and peritoneal fluid.
  - Excessive peritoneal fluid may develop with perihepatic disease, ovarian malignancy, and congestive heart failure.
  - Asymmetry and irregular shape may result from masses, hernias, or intestinal obstruction.
- Auscultation
  - Types of bowel sounds: normoactive, hyperactive, absent, hypoactive, rushes, borborygmi, and tinkling.
  - Normoactive bowel sounds are heard every 5–10 seconds [3].
  - Absent or hypoactive bowel sounds occur with intestinal perforation, peritonitis, impaired motility, and prolonged intestinal obstruction.

  - Hyperactive bowel sounds occur with the onset of intestinal obstruction, inflammatory bowel disease, infectious gastroenteritis, and bleeding.
- Percussion
  - Tympany suggests free air or intestinal gas.
  - Dullness suggests fluid, stool, or solid mass.
  - Assess for masses and hepatosplenomegaly.
- Palpation
  - Examine patient's facial expression to assess discomfort or pain during light and deep palpation in all four quadrants.
  - Assess for masses, hepatosplenomegaly, and texture of liver edge.
  - Always examine the painful or tender region of the abdomen last in order to optimize the patient's comfort level [3,17].

Table 17.10 indicates special maneuvers and signs on physical examination.

Digital Rectal Examination

- On external examination, assess for masses, fissures, scars, skin tags, condyloma, hemorrhoids, skin infections, mucus, and blood. Rectal prolapse may also be evident.
- Using a soft cotton tip, the external area adjacent to the anal opening can be "scratched" to elicit the "anal wink." This reflexive contraction of the external sphincter indicates an intact sacral reflex arc [18].
- On digital exam, assess the entire circumference of the rectum for masses, tenderness, impacted stool, and muscle tone and contractility. An assessment of the internal anal sphincter can be made with initial insertion of the finger, determining muscle strength at rest. The patient should then be asked to squeeze, so that the examiner may appreciate contraction strength. After the tone returns to a resting state, the examiner may ask the patient to bear down and try to expel the examining finger. A normal performance essentially excludes dyssynergic defecation (a pelvic floor disorder of failure of the muscle complex to relax with a defecatory effort). With this maneuver the degree of perineal descent may also be assessed (normal 1–3.5 cm) [5,18].
- In the male patient an assessment of the prostate gland should be part of the rectal examination.
- After withdrawing the gloved finger, assess the color of stool and presence of blood or mucus.

Table 17.11 lists GI disorders and the extraintestinal complaints and findings that may be associated with them.

Table 17.10 Special maneuvers and signs on physical examination.

Sign or special maneuver	Technique	Positive finding
McBurney point	Tenderness at location of appendix—one-third of way from anterior superior iliac crest to the umbilicus	Appendicitis
Rosving sign	Patient experiences RLQ pain as examiner applies pressure in LLQ	Appendicitis
Psoas sign	Patient flexes hip against resistance	Right—appendicitis Left—diverticulitis
Rebound tenderness	Apply deep, slow pressure to abdomen away from site of discomfort and then quickly remove the examining hand	Peritonitis
Guarding	Patient tenses abdominal muscles to protect the area	Peritonitis
Costovertebral tenderness	Tap the posterior thorax with a closed fist while stabilizing the patient	Kidney disease
Courvoisier sign	Palpation of RUQ of abdomen reveals an enlarged gall bladder	Gall-bladder mass or cancer
Murphy sign	Palpation of RUQ of abdomen during inspiration elicits pain and abrupt arrest of inspiration	Cholecystitis
Grey–Turner sign	Blue or purple color around the flanks	Pancreatitis
Cullen sign	Blue or purple color around the umbilicus	Peritoneal blood, as with pancreatitis
Shifting dullness	Percuss the abdomen with patient supine and then partially rolled toward the lateral position	Peritoneal fluid, as with liver disease
Succussion splash	Auscultate upper abdomen while gently moving patient from side to side	Gastric outlet obstruction
Carnett sign	Palpate abdomen at the site of discomfort while the patient engages the abdominal muscles and raises upper body from a horizontal position	Abdominal wall pathology

RLQ, right lower quadrant; LLQ, left lower quadrant; RUQ, right upper quadrant.

Table 17.11 Gastrointestinal disorders and the extraintestinal complaints and findings that may be associated with them [7,19].

Disease	Extraintestinal physical findings
Crohn disease	Erythema nodosum, pyoderma gangrenosum, axial arthritis
Ulcerative colitis	Erythema nodosum, pyoderma gangrenosum, axial arthritis, peripheral arthritis
Celiac disease	Dermatitis herpetiformis, polyarthralgia
Whipple disease	Polyarthralgia, lymphadenopathy
Enteric infections	Keratoderma blenorrhagica, reactive arthritis
Hepatitis B	Livedo reticularis, mononeuritis multiplex
Hepatitis C	Mixed cryoglobulinemia, palpable purpura
Henoch–Schönlein purpura	Palpable purpura, arthralgias
Neuroendocrine tumor or carcinoid	Flushing, wheezing, palpitations, right-sided heart murmur
Familial adenomatous polyposis	Thyroid and pancreatic cancer, hepatoblastomas, CNS tumors, various benign tumors, dental abnormalities
Gardner syndrome	Supernumerary teeth, osteomas, fibromas, epithelial cysts
Turcot syndrome	CNS tumors, café au lait spots, cutaneous port-wine stain, focal nodular hyperplasia
Peutz–Jegher syndrome	Genital tract tumors and other tumors, pigmented cutaneous manifestations
Cronkhite–Canada syndrome	Hyperpigmentation, nail and hair loss
Cowden disease	Craniomegaly, skin manifestations, breast and other cancers

Conclusions

The history and physical examination are the initial key factors in characterizing and determining the etiology of a patient's complaint. A careful and comprehensive history will help guide the focus of the physical examination. In addition to mastering the techniques of questioning and the skills of performing a physical examination, attention must be paid to other important factors including communication skills, professionalism, and appropriate sensitivity to gender-related problems and cultural differences [20]. Awareness of health-care disparities and health literacy, combined with a conscious effort to address such challenges, will promote the ideal patient–physician relationship and result in enhanced health care.

Take-home points

- Taking a history is a key component in determining a patient's problem and requires that the health-care provider:
  ○ Listens
  ○ Asks open ended questions
  ○ Focuses questions to elucidate the patient's symptoms.

- Physical examination can further define the etiology of a symptom. There are four key components of an effective and complete abdominal examination:
  ○ Inspection
  ○ Auscultation
  ○ Percussion
  ○ Palpation.

- Communication of findings procured from the history and physical examination is crucial in being able to participate in patient-centered, team-based care, especially for patients with complex problems or multiple complaints, and should include:
  ○ Oral presentation
  ○ Written record
  ○ Sensitivity to patient's needs.

References

1 Bickley LS. Interviewing and the health history. In: Bickley LS, Szilagyi PG, eds. *Bates' Guide to Physical Examination and History Taking*, 9th edn. Lippincott Williams & Wilkins, Philadelphia, 2007: 23–57.

2 Glasgow RE, Mulvihill SJ. Acute abdominal pain. In: Feldman M, *et al.*, eds. *Sleisenger and Fordtran's Gastrointestinal and Liver Disease: Pathophysiology/Diagnosis/Management*, 8th edn. Saunders, Philadelphia, 2006: 87–98.

3 Swartz MH. The abdomen. In: Swartz MH, ed. *Textbook of Physical Diagnosis History and Physical Exam*, 4th edn. WB Saunders Company, Philadelphia, 2002: 427–60.

4 Schiller L. Diarrhea. *Med Clin N Am* 2000; **84**: 1259–74.

5 Lembo A, Camilleri M. Chronic constipation. *N Engl J Med* 2003; **349**: 1360–8.

6 Longstreth GF, Thompson WG, Chey WD, *et al.* Functional bowel disorders. *Gastroenterology* 2006; **130**: 1480–91.

7 Karnath BM, Sunkureddi P, Nguyen-Oghalia TU. Extraintestinal manifestations of hepatogastrointestinal diseases. *Hospital Physician* 2006; **42** (July): 61–6.

8 Heaton KW, Ghosh S, Braddon FE. How bad are the symptoms and bowel dysfunction of patients with the irritable bowel syndrome? A prospective, controlled study with emphasis on stool form. *Gut* 1991; **32**: 73–9.

9 Lewis SJ, Heaton KW. Stool form scale as a useful guide to intestinal transit time. *Scand J Gastroenterol* 1997; **32**: 920–4.

10 Fraga XF, Malagelada J-R. Nausea and vomiting. *Curr Treat Options Gastroenterol* 2002; **5**: 241–50.

11 Quigley EM, Hasler WL, Parkman HP. AGA technical review on nausea and vomiting *Gastroenterol*, 2001; **120**: 263–86.

12 Malagelada J-R, Malagelada C. Nausea and vomiting. In: Feldman M, *et al.*, eds. *Sleisenger and Fordtran's Gastrointestinal and Liver Disease: Pathophysiology/Diagnosis/Management*, 8th edn. Saunders, Philadelphia, 2006: 143–158.

13 Marek TA. Gastrointestinal bleeding. *Endoscopy* 2007; **39**: 998–1004.

14 Madoff RD, Fleshman JW, Clinical Practice Committee, American Gastroenterological Association. American Gastroenterological Association technical review on the diagnosis and treatment of hemorrhoids. *Gastroenterology* 2004; **126**: 1463–73.

15 Roach SP, Kobos R. Jaundice in the adult patient. *Am Fam Physician* 2004; **69**: 299–304.

16 Drossman DA, Talley NJ, Leserman J, *et al.* Sexual and physical abuse and gastrointestinal illness: review and recommendations. *Ann Inter Med* 1995; **123**: 782–94.

17 Bickley LS. The abdomen. In: Bickley LS, Szilagyi PG, eds. *Bates' Guide to Physical Examination and History Taking*, 9th edn. Lippincott Williams & Wilkins, Philadelphia, 2007: 359–409.

18 Talley NJ. How to do and interpret a rectal examination in gastroenterology. *Am J Gastroenterol* 2008; **103**: 820–2.

19 Rustgi A. Hereditary polyposis and nonpolyposis syndromes. *N Engl J Med* 1994; **331**: 1694–702.

20 Talley NJ, O'Connor S. *Clinical Examination: A Systematic Guide to Physical Diagnosis*, 6th edn. Elsevier, 2010.

CHAPTER 18

Acute Abdominal Pain

Robert M. Penner[1] and Sumit R. Majumdar[2]

[1] Department of Medicine, University of Alberta, Edmonton, AB, Canada, and Department of Medicine, University of British Columbia, Vancouver, BC, Canada

[2] Department of Medicine, University of Alberta, Edmonton, AB, Canada

Summary

Acute abdominal pain has a very broad diagnosis, and therefore requires a stepwise approach to triage and subsequent management. The first step is assessing patient stability and the possibility of need for urgent surgery. Consideration should then be given to whether a serious non-abdominal source of pain exists. In stable patients, location and characteristics of the pain can be used to guide investigations.

Case

A 24-year-old presents to the local emergency department with a 2-day history of worsening abdominal pain. She states that it came on gradually but has progressively worsened. It does not appear to be localized to one specific area but rather diffuse. There is associated nausea and one episode of emesis. She has had a recent travel history and is taking antibiotics to treat topical acne. Blood work including a complete blood count, liver panel and lipase are normal, as are abdominal plain films. Her physicians contemplate the possibility of an abdominal ultrasound or gastroscopy, but decide that watchful waiting is reasonable for 24–48 h.

Definition

Acute abdominal pain is a common presentation in both emergency departments and ambulatory care facilities, but its triage, investigation, and management can be fraught with complications for two reasons.

First, its chronicity can be difficult to determine. Patients with chronic functional causes of abdominal pain, such as irritable bowel syndrome, will frequently

Practical Gastroenterology and Hepatology: Small and Large Intestine and Pancreas, 1st edition. Edited by Nicholas J. Talley, Sunanda V. Kane and Michael B. Wallace. © 2010 Blackwell Publishing Ltd.

describe flares of pain as new or acute pain. Conversely, many causes of acute abdominal pain, such as biliary colic, can produce a chronic intermittent pattern of pain. For these reasons, regardless of specific time course, any persistently worsening abdominal pain over a period from minutes to weeks can be considered acute, as can any pain resulting in destabilization of a patient's clinical status. In many cases, it may be impossible to clearly categorize pain as acute or chronic, and in this case, an initial workup tailored to acute pain is always reasonable.

Second, the differential diagnosis of abdominal pain is broad, and includes both intra- and extra-abdominal sources of pathology. A complete differential diagnosis of abdominal pain is beyond the scope of this chapter, which will focus instead on the triage of patients with abdominal pain, and the first steps in their investigation and treatment. Abdominal pain following trauma and pediatric abdominal pain will not be covered here.

Clinical Features

Assessment of patients with abdominal pain should begin with a focused history and physical examination that will determine whether emergent intervention is required, and whether proceeding to a broader workup of abdominal pain will be helpful (Figure 18.1). After assessment of

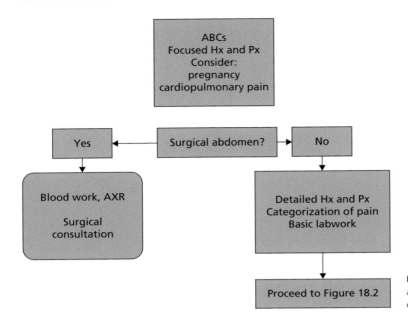

Figure 18.1 Initial approach to acute abdominal pain. Hx, history; Px, physical examination; AXR, abdominal X-ray.

the patient's airway, breathing, and circulation, an assessment should proceed to answering the following questions:

• Does this patient have a "surgical abdomen"?
• Could this be a serious presentation of non-abdominal (e.g., cardiac) pathology?
• In females, could the patient be pregnant or might the pain be pelvic in origin?

In patients where answers to the above questions are negative, the workup can then proceed to investigations for causes of abdominal pathology (Figure 18.2).

Surgical Abdomen

A "surgical abdomen" exists in any patient whose prognosis will rapidly worsen without surgical intervention. The diagnosis is clinical, and can mandate laparotomy without a specific diagnosis. Most surgical presentations will involve bowel obstruction or peritonitis. These generally present with severe acute abdominal pain, but a subacute presentation with rapid deterioration is not uncommon in bowel obstruction.

Patients with bowel obstruction have varying combinations of obstipation, vomiting, and abdominal distension. Physical examination can reveal high-pitched or absent bowel sounds. Patients with peritonitis tend to

avoid movement. Abdominal rigidity, percussion tenderness, and rebound tenderness are all signs of peritonitis.

All patients with a clinical diagnosis of a surgical abdomen should be assessed by a surgeon for consideration of immediate laparotomy versus further diagnostic testing. Appropriate analgesia, including use of parenteral narcotics, should never be withheld for fear of masking a surgical abdomen [1].

Among the most emergent of abdominal presentations is the ruptured abdominal aortic aneurysm. Patients at risk for atherosclerosis presenting with sudden abdominal pain radiating to the back and a pulsatile abdominal mass should undergo laparotomy without delay for any further diagnostic testing.

Non-Abdominal Sources of Abdominal Pain

Urgent non-abdominal pathology, most commonly cardiopulmonary or metabolic, must be considered early in the assessment of patients with abdominal pain. Features suggesting cardiopulmonary pain include exacerbation with exercise or inspiration, shortness of breath, or radiation of pain into the precordium. Any patients in whom a cardiopulmonary source of pain is being considered

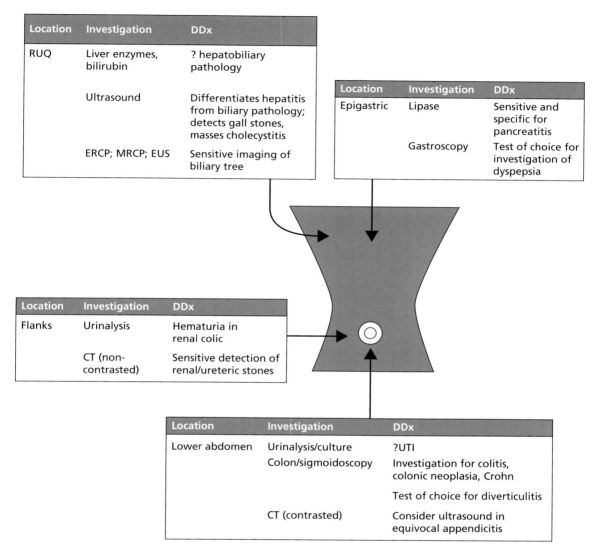

Figure 18.2 Examples of types of abdominal pain and their investigation. DDx, differential diagnosis; RUQ, right upper quadrant; ERCP, endoscopic retrograde cholangiopancreatography; MRCP, magnetic resonance cholangiopancreatography; EUS, endoscopic ultrasonography; CT, computed tomography; UTI, urinary tract infection.

should have their initial workup complemented by an electrocardiogram, chest radiograph, and serial cardiac enzyme measurements. Patients with profound metabolic abnormalities, such as uremia, hypercalcemia, or ketoacidosis, may also have non-specific nausea or malaise, and clues to the etiology of their presentation are often present in the initial blood work. Known diabetics and anyone in whom a new diagnosis of diabetes

is considered possible, such as young patients presenting with polyuria or weight loss preceding a vague abdominal presentation, should have a bedside blood sugar measurement performed early in their assessment.

Abdominal Pain in Women

The oft-repeated axiom that all female patients should be considered pregnant until proven otherwise remains crucial for formulation of differential diagnosis, for consideration of the safety of investigations employing ionizing radiation, and in consideration of treatments that may be teratogenic. Females of childbearing potential should be asked about pregnancy and a pregnancy test should be undertaken.

Lower abdominal versus pelvic pain has no clear line of delineation, but association of the pain with changes in bowel habit or eating are more suggestive of abdominal etiologies, whereas associations with the menstrual cycle or vaginal symptoms point to the reproductive tract.

Classification of Stable Patients with Abdominal Pain

Once a surgical abdomen is ruled out, and an intra-abdominal source of pain is considered most likely, time can be taken for a more complete history and physical examination, and subsequent workup can be directed appropriately. While there is overlap, classification of patients by location of their pain still helps direct investigation.

Right Upper Quadrant Pain

Hepatobiliary pain most commonly presents in the right upper quadrant, but pain associated with the liver itself is generally vague and ill-defined since pain receptors are present only in the liver's capsule. Supporting features for a biliary source of pain include:

- Jaundice
- Exacerbation of pain with food, particularly fatty food
- An intermittent paroxysmal course is typical for biliary colic or choledocholithiasis
- Right upper quadrant pain associated with fever and jaundice should be recognized as suspicious for ascending cholangitis requiring urgent therapy.

Epigastric Pain

Sudden onset of epigastric pain, with or without radiation to the back, is typical for pancreatitis. Epigastric pain associated with features such as belching, regurgitation, bloating, nausea (particularly in the morning), and heartburn is described as dyspepsia. Its main differential diagnosis includes reflux esophagitis and gastric or duodenal ulceration, but the clinical presentation is not accurate at distinguishing these underlying diagnoses [2], and

there can be significant overlap with presentations of right upper quadrant pain.

Lower Abdominal Pain

Pain associated with diarrhea and rectal bleeding suggests colitis. Diarrhea with right lower quadrant pain is the hallmark of Crohn disease. Some patients have vague pain that with time resolves itself into a surgical abdomen, such as patients with diverticulitis, who present with lower abdominal pain, more commonly on the left side, and often associated with fever, or patients with appendicitis, who classically have ill-defined periumbilical pain which migrates to the right lower quadrant.

Retroperitoneal pain can present in the lower abdomen, such as renal colic, which can begin in the flank and migrate to the groin. Cystitis can present as suprapubic pain with or without obvious urinary tract symptoms.

Investigation

General

Initial lab work reasonable in all patients with acute abdominal pain includes:

- Complete blood count
- Electrolytes, creatinine, blood urea nitrogen (BUN), glucose
- Aminotransferases, alkaline phosphatase, bilirubin
- Lipase
- Urinalysis
- Pregnancy test in women of childbearing potential.

This basic blood work often guides the differential diagnosis. Anemia may suggest GI blood loss. Elevation of the white blood cell count can be a marker of severity. Abnormal electrolytes or creatinine may point to dehydration, or to an underlying metabolic problem. A thyroid stimulating hormone (TSH) and ionized calcium can be helpful in patients with vague abdominal pain suggestive of an underlying metabolic derangement. Elevated liver enzymes point to hepatobiliary pathology. Elevation of lipase can be non-specific in patients with renal failure or in cases where there is only mild elevation, but levels over 1000 U/L are highly specific for pancreatitis [3], and the combination of elevated lipase and liver enzymes suggests gall-stone pancreatitis [4].

Plain abdominal films, including an upright abdomen and chest radiograph are widely available, non-invasive, and often informative. While they are not useful in detecting many causes of abdominal pain, distended bowel suggestive of obstruction and free air demonstrating hollow viscus perforation are key findings that can indicate necessity of surgical management, and intrathoracic pathology are indicative of cardiopulmonary causes.

When findings are equivocal for obstruction or perforation, or in cases such as suspected diverticulitis, where a localized perforation may be present, computed tomography (CT) scanning is a useful investigation with high sensitivity for obstruction, and imaging quality adequate to point to an obstructed level [5]. CT scans are also the test of choice for imaging retroperitoneal perforations. While CT scans are now widely used for assessment of unexplained abdominal pain, it is important for a clinician to have a good sense of which specific diagnoses the test is being used to distinguish. For example, a CT of the abdomen without contrast has poor sensitivity for most intra-abdominal pathology, while accurate for visualization of ureteric stones as a cause for renal colic [6]. The addition of oral contrast highlights intestinal abnormalities, but obscures visualization of kidney stones.

Right Upper Quadrant Pain

For most patients with right upper quadrant pain, an abdominal ultrasound to assess for biliary dilation or gall-bladder wall thickening is the initial imaging test of choice, since the sensitivity of ultrasound for biliary dilation exceeds that of CT scanning [7]. In patients with pancreatitis, ultrasound is the imaging test of choice initially to assess for findings suggestive of a biliary cause, while CT scanning is often used later in the course of illness to detect complications of pancreatitis, such as pseudocysts or pancreatic necrosis.

When a high level of suspicion exists for biliary obstruction, with or without ultrasound confirmation, endoscopic retrograde cholangiopancreatography (ERCP) is the intervention of choice for diagnosis and therapy. When biliary obstruction resolves spontaneously, such as from a passed common bile duct stone, or when the clinical picture is equivocal, endoscopic ultrasound [8] or magnetic resonance cholangiopancreatography [9] are less invasive alternatives to ERCP.

Dyspepsia

Young patients with dyspeptic pain may be candidates for empiric therapy with proton pump inhibitors but older patients, or those with alarm symptoms (vomiting, GI bleeding, weight loss, dysphagia), should be investigated with gastroscopy [10].

Lower Abdominal Pain

Patients with symptoms suggestive of colitis should all be investigated with stool cultures and testing for *Clostridium difficile*. A stool microscopy for ova and parasites is indicated in patients with symptoms of parasitic infection, such as the diarrhea and vomiting of giardiasis, but can also be useful when fecal leukocytes are observed as a non-specific indicator of intestinal inflammation. Additional history should focus on underlying causes (non-steroid anti-inflammatory drug use, risk factors for ischemia). In patients with a prolonged course or with no obvious cause after history and lab work, endoscopic evaluation confirms the diagnosis of colitis. Sigmoidoscopy is adequate to diagnose distal colitis and sometimes establish extent of disease, while a full colonoscopy is required to assess for ileitis or proximal colitis.

Observation of Suspected Benign Pathology

Abdominal pain is a common presentation of functional pathology or somatization, and can also be a symptom of self-limited illnesses such as viral gastroenteritis. Patients with severe constipation can present with abdominal pain, particularly those requiring narcotic analgesics for unrelated pain.

In these groups of patients, when initial investigations are normal or compatible with self-limited illness, a period of watchful waiting and symptomatic therapy may be reasonable before considering more invasive investigation or investigation with significant burden of ionizing radiation. Caution should be taken with this approach in groups of patients at risk of serious pathology with atypical or indolent presentations, such as elderly or immunosuppressed patients.

A classic example of pain whose presentation may be overlooked is mesenteric ischemia, in which recurrent postprandial pain occurs out of proportion to laboratory or physical findings. As this typically occurs in elderly patients at risk for atherosclerosis, consideration of the patient's demographic should lead to appropriate aggressive investigation with angiography or abdominal CT with appropriately contrasted protocol.

Take-home points

- Patients with abdominal pain should first be triaged for a "surgical abdomen."
- Consider cardiopulmonary sources of pain before proceeding to an intra-abdominal differential diagnosis.
- Pregnancy should be excluded in women of childbearing age.
- Ultrasonography exceeds CT scanning in sensitivity for biliary pathology.
- Use of CT scanning requires careful consideration of differential diagnosis to determine the appropriate use of contrast.

References

1 Manterola C, Astudillo P, Losada H, *et al.* Analgesia in patients with acute abdominal pain. *Cochrane Database Syst Rev* 2007: CD005660.

2 Thomson AB, Barkun AN, Armstrong D, *et al.* The prevalence of clinically significant endoscopic findings in primary care patients with uninvestigated dyspepsia: the Canadian Adult Dyspepsia Empiric Treatment–Prompt Endoscopy (CADET-PE) study. *Aliment Pharmacol Ther* 2003; **17**: 1481–1491.

3 Yadav D, Agarwal N, Pitchumoni CS. A critical evaluation of laboratory tests in acute pancreatitis. *Am J Gastroenterol* 2002; **97**: 1309–1318.

4 Tenner S, Dubner H, Steinberg W. Predicting gallstone pancreatitis with laboratory parameters: a meta-analysis. *Am J Gastroenterol* 1994; **89**: 1863–1866.

5 Obuz F, Terzi C, Sokmen S, *et al.* The efficacy of helical CT in the diagnosis of small bowel obstruction. *Eur J Radiol* 2003; **48**: 299–304.

6 Reddy S. State of the art trends in imaging of renal colic. *Emerg Radiol* 2008; **15**: 217–225.

7 Cooperberg PL, Gibney RG. Imaging the gallbladder, 1987. *Radiology* 1987; **163**: 605–613.

8 Garrow D, Miller S, Sinha D. Endoscopic ultrasound: a meta-analysis of test performance in suspected biliary obstruction. *Clin Gastroenterol Hepatol* 2007; **5**: 616–623.

9 Romagnuolo J, Bardou M, Rahme E, *et al.* Magnetic cholangiopancreatography: a meta-analysis of test performance in suspected biliary disease. *Ann Intern Med* 2003; **139**: 547–557.

10 Ford AC, Moayyedi P. Current guidelines for dyspepsia management. *Dig Dis* 2008; **26**: 225–230.

CHAPTER 19
Acute Diarrhea

John R. Cangemi

Division of Gastroenterology and Hepatology, Department of Internal Medicine, Mayo Clinic, Jacksonville, FL, USA

Summary

Acute diarrhea is a common, primarily self-limited illness which can be managed most often with supportive care. Stool cultures are rarely indicated early on unless the patient has severe or bloody diarrhea. The focus of treatment should be on replacement of fluid and electrolytes, especially in the extremely young and elderly who are at increased risk of excessive morbidity and mortality. Specific antibiotic therapy is determined by the organism identified, but empiric therapy may be indicated if the patient presents with symptoms of inflammatory diarrhea with co-morbidities or progressive disease. Any decision to treat must carefully weigh the potential risks and benefits particularly if the patient is at risk for Shiga-toxin-producing *E. coli*.

Case

A 62-year-old male presents with acute onset of diarrhea of 36 h duration associated with a low-grade fever and lower abdominal crampy pain. He has no significant prior history and reports onset 2 days after returning from a Caribbean cruise. He traveled with his wife who is not ill. He is complaining of feeling nauseated and weak with dizziness upon standing. He is asking for treatment to alleviate his symptoms. On physical exam, his heart rate is 88; blood pressure lying is 130/80 and 110/70 sitting. His abdomen is tender without mass, guarding, or rebound. On rectal exam, there is non-bloody liquid stool without a mass. Laboratory testing reveals a hemoglobin of 13.2, white cell count of 7.4, and creatinine of 1.1. Stool studies are negative for bacterial pathogens, *C. difficile* toxin, *Giardia* antigen, ova, and parasites.

Definition and Epidemiology

Acute diarrhea is defined as an increase in stool frequency (>3 loose bowel movements daily) or volume (>200 g daily) for less than 14 days. The majority of cases is of infectious origin, primarily bacterial or viral, but

Practical Gastroenterology and Hepatology: Small and Large Intestine and Pancreas, 1st edition. Edited by Nicholas J. Talley, Sunanda V. Kane and Michael B. Wallace. © 2010 Blackwell Publishing Ltd.

may also result from a drug reaction or an underlying systemic illness. In the United States up to 1.4 cases occur per person each year, accounting for up to 375 million cases annually and 6000 deaths [1]. Fortunately, the majority of cases are self limited with morbidity and mortality primarily seen in the immunocompromised or at extremes of age [2]. Fecal–oral transmission accounts for most cases through contaminated water, food, or direct person to person contact. The mechanism of diarrhea in each case varies with the specific pathogen, whether toxin mediated or through direct invasion.

History and Physical Examination

A careful history is essential to guide the diagnostic algorithm. In addition to travel history, food consumption, and recent medication use, it is helpful to describe the stool frequency, volume, and appearance (bloody, watery) [3], for example frequent, small-volume, urgent stools suggest colonic involvement. The patient's age and living environment (e.g., nursing home), as well as potential common outbreak exposure may further aide in the diagnosis. Was the onset acute and are the symptoms progressive? Does the patient report a fever, or is nausea with vomiting present? Is the diarrhea a manifestation of an underlying illness or is the patient immunocompromised? In addition to these questions, on physical exam, the patient must be evaluated for dehydration as an essential first step in assessment and management.

Differential Diagnosis

If vomiting is a predominant symptom associated with non-bloody loose stools, then either viral or toxin-induced food poisoning should be suspected. Viral illnesses are the most common cause of acute diarrhea in adults in the United States and the majority of infections are from norovirus [4]. Sixty to 90% of outbreaks which were not bacterial were caused by norovirus [5]. These outbreaks tend to occur more commonly during the winter months and are seen in institutional, cruise ship, social event, or vacation settings. The illness is generally self-limited, lasting 24 to 48 h after an incubation period of 1 to 3 days. Food-borne bacterial toxins have a shorter incubation phase (*Bacillus cereus* and *Staphylococcus aureus*: 2–7 hours; and *Clostridium perfringens*: 8–14 hours) and are less severe. More significant watery diarrhea is usually enterotoxin induced. Common pathogens include enterotoxigenic *E. coli*, enteropathogenic *E. coli*, *Vibrio cholera*, or early infection with *Vibrio parahemolyticus*, *Campylobacter jejuni*, *Salmonella*, *Clostridium difficile*, *Yersinia enterocolitica*, *Plesiomonas* spp., or *Aeromonas* spp. The later manifestations of these invasive organisms are fever associated with bloody diarrhea as seen in *E. coli* 0157:H7 and *Shigella* spp. Protozoal infections are less common and more often associated with chronic symptoms, but pathogens include *Giardia*, *Crytosporidium*, *Isospora belli*, and *Cyclospora*. Bloody diarrhea would be predictive of infection with *Entamoeba histolytica*.

Drug-induced diarrhea is an important aspect of the differential [6]. Over 700 drugs have been listed as a potential cause for diarrhea and it is essential that a careful history focuses on prescribed drugs as well as non-prescription drugs and supplements.

Diagnostic Evaluation

As the majority of episodes of acute diarrhea are of viral origin and self-limited, there is no evidence to support stool cultures in all patients in the acute setting. The diagnostic yield overall ranges from 1.5 to 5.6% [7] and the cost will then exceed $900 to $1000 per positive result [8]. Clinical assessment early on is the key. Stool cultures are warranted if the patient presents with fever, dehydration, blood or pus in the stool, or diarrhea of several days duration. Exceptions are made for those with significant co-morbidities or those who are elderly or immunocompromised where an early diagnosis has important implications for therapy. An alternative, early screening test for equivocal cases is the fecal lactoferrin. Lactoferrin is a marker for fecal leukocytes and has a sensitivity and specificity ranging from 79 to 92% for diarrhea of inflammatory etiology. If positive then stool cultures are warranted and should be guided by the clinical history (Table 19.1). Routine cultures will identify most organisms, but special stains may be required for specific pathogens (*Yersinia*, cold enrichment; *E. coli* 0157:H7, Sorbitol-MacConkey agar). Up to 20–40% of acute infectious diarrhea cases will escape diagnosis even with appropriate cultures.

There are only limited circumstances where ova and parasites are of value in the diagnostic algorithm of acute diarrhea. Travelers with exposure to untreated water (*Giardia*, *Cryptosporidium*, or *Cyclospora*) patients with persistent diarrhea, or immunocompromised patients should all be tested. Enzyme immunoassay is the preferred method of testing, with a sensitivity of better than 95%.

Lastly, there are few indications for endoscopic procedures. Sigmoidoscopy or colonoscopy could be considered in the patient with bloody diarrhea who does not respond to antibiotics. Biopsies should complement the procedure even with normal-appearing mucosa.

Treatment

Early management of the patient with acute diarrhea should focus on appropriate replacement of fluid and electrolytes. Oral rehydration is adequate in most settings unless the patient is incapable of retaining fluids (severe nausea and vomiting) or is severely dehydrated or comatose. This should consist of a glucose-based solution as glucose facilitates the absorption of sodium and water even in the face of a secretory process. The World Health Organization recommends an oral rehydration solution with 3.5 g sodium chloride, 2.5 g sodium bicarbonate,

Table 19.1 Common pathogens in acute diarrhea.

Pathogen	Source	Indicated therapy	Antibiotic (alternative)
Norovirus	Institutions, cruise ships, common outbreaks	Supportive	
Salmonella	Poultry, eggs, raw milk, beef, vegetables	Not indicated in healthy host with no risk of sepsis	Fluoroquinolones (trimethoprim-sulfamethoxazole)
Shigella	Person to person, vegetables	Indicated	Fluoroquinolones (trimethoprim-sulfamethoxazole)
Campylobacter	Poultry, raw milk	Only in severe cases	Erythromycin (fluoroquinolones?)
Vibrio parahemolyticus	Raw seafood, shellfish	Not indicated in healthy host	Tetracycline
Enterotoxigenic E. coli	Travelers	Not indicated in healthy host	Fluoroquinolones (trimethoprim-sulfamethoxazole)
Enteroinvasive E. coli	Milk, cheese	Indicated	Fluoroquinolones (trimethoprim-sulfamethoxazole)
Enterohemorrhagic E. coli	Beef, pork, lettuce, milk, cheese, raw seed sprouts	Avoid antibiotics—can induce Shiga-toxin (HUS)	
Yersinia	Beef, milk, cheese	Only in severe cases	Doxycycline (trimethoprim-sulfamethoxazole)
Giardia	Contaminated water	Indicated	Metronidazole (tinidazole, quinacrine HCL)
Cryptosporidium	Contaminated water	Not proven effective	Paromomycin plus azithromycin (nitazoxanide)
Cyclospora	Imported fruit	Indicated	Trimethoprim-sulfamethoxazole
Entamoeba histolytica	Travelers	Indicated	Metronidazole plus iodoquinol (paromomycin)

1.5 g of potassium chloride, and either 20 g of glucose or 40 g of sucrose per liter of fluid. This should be given at 1.5 times the volume of stool lost over 24 h. A number of effective commercial products are available. When intravenous hydration is required Ringer's lactate should be used and at least half the calculated deficit should be administered in the first 4 h. If tolerated, the diet should be continued as adequate nutrition is important. Early feeding may also be beneficial by decreasing intestinal permeability induced by the infection and decreasing the duration of the illness [8]. In an acute infection, secondary lactose intolerance may occur due to loss of brush border enzymes and can last up to several weeks, requiring a lactose restriction.

The use of antidiarrheal medications in patients with acute diarrhea is controversial. In a systematic review of adjunctive loperamide with antibiotics in traveler's diarrhea, antibiotic therapy plus loperamide was more effective than antibiotics alone in terms of decreasing the duration of illness and achieving an earlier cure [9]. However, these were not patients with severe inflammatory diarrhea nor bloody stools. In these patients, antimotility agents may enhance the severity of the illness by delaying excretion of the organism. Their use may result in prolonged fever plus increased risk of toxic megacolon or hemolytic-uremic syndrome (HUS) in patients infected with E. coli 0157:H7 and should be avoided. Bismuth subsalicylate is an alternative to loperamide yet is slower in onset and less effective in comparative trials [10].

Most cases of acute diarrhea resolve spontaneously and antibiotics are not required. Yet if treatment is

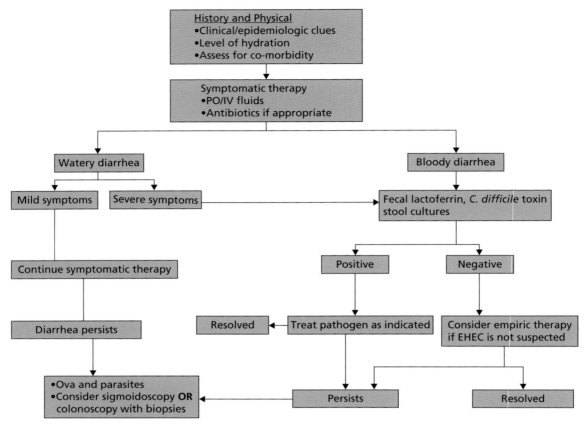

Figure 19.1 Approach and therapy of acute diarrhea. EHEC, enterohemorrhagic *E. coli.*

considered, often the decision is made prior to isolation of a specific pathogen. In this case it is important to weigh the risks, such as prolonged carriage of *Salmonella* or induction of Shiga-toxin versus the benefit of an earlier response in a susceptible organism. Empiric therapy, usually with a fluoroquinolone, is suggested in patients with inflammatory diarrhea when Shiga-toxin-producing *E. coli* seems less likely from the clinical history. This is also true for traveler's diarrhea, where antibiotics in adults have lead to a less severe illness of shorter duration [11]. The exception is in patients who have traveled to southern Asia where fluoroquinolone-resistant *Campylobacter* are endemic and azithromycin is the favored choice [12].

With identification of the pathogen, specific therapy can be initiated (Table 19.1). Antibiotic therapy is most

effective when given at the onset of symptoms. However, not all infections require treatment. Treatment of non-typhoidal *Salmonella* may actually prolong shedding of the organism and is rarely required unless the host is immunocompromised or at increased risk of sepsis. Treatment of Shiga-toxin producing *E. coli* may induce Shiga-toxin production and result in HUS. *Shigella*, on the other hand, responds well to therapy with a fluoro-quinolone and treatment will shorten the period of diarrhea by 2.4 days and is therefore recommended. *Campylobacter* will typically clear without therapy and should not be treated unless associated with a prolonged, severe illness or in an immunocompromised patient.

Special considerations need be given to the elderly patient with acute diarrhea [2]. Older patients are at increased risk secondary to achlorhydria, altered gut motility, frequent antibiotic exposure, and serious co-morbidities. Morbidity and mortality are significantly increased, which requires aggressive supportive care and early institution of therapeutic measures. An algorithm is presented in Figure 19.1 to outline the approach and therapy of acute diarrhea.

Case continued

The patient recovered over next 48 h with nothing but supportive therapy. No antibiotics were given for his presumed diagnosis of enterotoxigenic *E. coli* infection.

Take-home points

- Most cases of acute diarrhea are self-limited and require no therapy.
- The most common pathogens in acute diarrhea are viral (norovirus) and early stool cultures yield less than 6% and are not cost effective.
- The most important aspect of management early on is repletion of fluid and electrolytes. The majority of the time, this can be done with oral rehydration solution.
- Fecal lactoferrin is both sensitive and specific for identifying inflammatory diarrhea.
- It is essential to weigh the risks and benefits of therapy when managing a patient with acute infectious diarrhea.
- Elderly patients are at increased risk of morbidity and mortality from acute diarrhea and require special considerations.

References

1 Thielman NM, Guerrant RL. Acute infectious diarrhea. *N Engl J Med* 2004; **350**: 38–47.

2 Trinh C, Prabhakar K. Diarrheal diseases in the elderly. *Clin Geriat Med* 2007; **23**: 833–56.

3 Manatsathit S, Dupont HL, Farthing M, *et al.* Guideline for the management of acute diarrhea in adults. *J Gastroenterol Hepatol* 2002; **17**: S54–S71.

4 Marcos LA, DuPont HL. Advances in defining etiology and new therapeutic approaches in acute diarrhea. *J Infection* 2007; **55**: 385–93.

5 Goodgame R. Norovirus gastroenteritis. *Curr Gastroenterol Rep* 2006; **8**: 401–8.

6 Abraham B, Sellin JH. Drug-induced diarrhea. *Curr Gastroenterol Rep* 2007; **9**: 365–72.

7 Guerrant RL, Vangilder T, Steiner TS, *et al.* Practice guidelines for the management of infectious diarrhea. *Clin Infect Dis* 2001; **32**: 331–51.

8 Gadewar S, Fasano A. Current concepts in the evaluation, diagnosis and management of acute infectious diarrhea. *Curr Opin Pharmacol* 2005; **5**: 559–65.

9 Riddle M, Arnold S, Tribble DR. Effect of adjunctive loperamide in combination with antibiotics on treatment outcomes in traveler's diarrhea: a systematic review and meta-analysis. *Clin Infect Dis* 2008; **47**: 1007–14.

10 De Bruyn G. Diarrhea in adults (acute). *Am Fam Physician* 2008; **78**: 263–6.

11 Kamat D, Mathur A. Prevention and management of travelers' diarrhea. *Dis Mon* 2006; **52**: 289–302.

12 DuPont HL. What's new in enteric infectious diseases at home and abroad. *Clin Infect Dis* 2005; **18**: 407–12.

CHAPTER 20
Chronic Diarrhea

Lawrence R. Schiller

Division of Gastroenterology, Baylor University Medical Center, Dallas, TX, USA

Summary

Chronic diarrhea is a common clinical problem, most inclusively defined as frequent passage of fluid stools lasting more than 1 month. A comprehensive history is the best start to the evaluation. Probably the most important features to define are the onset (acute or gradual), pattern (continuous or intermittent), severity (causing dehydration or not), and type of stool produced (watery, fatty, or inflammatory). Coexisting symptoms, such as weight loss or abdominal pain, may be important clues to etiology. Patients with irritable bowel syndrome (IBS) should be identified by the presence of characteristic abdominal pain associated with variable stool form or frequency, and should be distinguished from others with chronic diarrhea. IBS patients may have definable problems with small bowel bacterial overgrowth, food sensitivities, or celiac disease, but usually no cause is identified. The differential diagnosis of continuing chronic diarrhea is broad, but targeted evaluation often is rewarded with a diagnosis that can be treated.

Case

A 78-year-old woman presents with a 3-year history of diarrhea. The problem began gradually and is now complicated by episodes of fecal incontinence. She has watery stools every day, moves her bowels up to five times a day and has lost about 2 kg (5 pounds). She has no abdominal pain, never sees blood in her stools and has never been hospitalized for dehydration. Occasional loperamide reduces stool frequency and urgency of defecation, but does not eliminate loose stools. She has taken non-steroidal anti-inflammatory drugs for arthritis, but uses no other scheduled medications. Physical examination is unremarkable except for reduced anal sphincter tone and squeeze.

Definition and Epidemiology

Chronic diarrhea is best described as frequent passage of liquid stools for more than 1 month. Some patients confuse fecal incontinence with diarrhea and a few consider frequent passage of formed stool to be diarrhea, but

Practical Gastroenterology and Hepatology: Small and Large Intestine and Pancreas, 1st edition. Edited by Nicholas J. Talley, Sunanda V. Kane and Michael B. Wallace. © 2010 Blackwell Publishing Ltd.

otherwise patient reports of diarrhea usually are valid. For clinical purposes it is best to distinguish chronic diarrhea from irritable bowel syndrome (IBS) with diarrhea in which abdominal pain is prominent [1,2]. IBS tends to have more variable stool frequency and form, typically runs a benign course without medical complications, and does not need an extensive diagnostic evaluation. In contrast, patients with chronic diarrhea typically always have loose stools, may have medical complications, and often have treatable causes for chronic diarrhea that can be discovered [3–5]. Therefore, efforts to make a diagnosis will be rewarded. Surveys suggest that 3–5% of the population have chronic diarrhea in any given year. It is unclear how many of these people have IBS as opposed to other causes of chronic diarrhea.

Pathophysiology

At a fundamental level diarrhea is due to excess water in stools because absorption of fluid from the lumen is reduced or secretion of fluid into the lumen is increased [5]. This may occur because of toxins, hormones, neurotransmitters, bile acids, or cytokines that affect mucosal absorption directly; because rapid motility hurries fluid past the absorptive surface; because absorptive surface area is reduced or bypassed; or because poorly absorbed substances are ingested and hold water within the lumen osmotically.

Clinical Features

Diarrhea is a symptom that most people experience transiently from time to time and so there is a universal appreciation of acute diarrhea. Chronic diarrhea is less common and patients often are bewildered when it does not go away spontaneously. Other symptoms may be present, such as weight loss, evidence of malnutrition, cramps, bleeding, fecal incontinence, and abdominal pain that produce substantial disability.

While most patients know diarrhea when they have it, few have a good idea about its severity. Many view the number of stools per day, coexisting urgency or incontinence, or the intensity of cramps as key measures. Researchers often consider stool weight (>200 g/24 h) to be critical—and in some ways it is—because stool weights greater than 1000 g may be associated with dehydration and electrolyte depletion. However, patients have no idea what their stool weights are and clinicians typically do not measure stool weight, depending instead upon weight loss, dehydration, and the intensity of patient complaints in deciding how severe diarrhea is.

Clinical signs associated with chronic diarrhea often are sparse although when present they may be helpful [4,5] (Figure 20.1).

Diagnosis and Differential Diagnosis

Chronic diarrhea can be a symptom of many different conditions that have multiple diagnostic pathways [5]. Given this complexity, even experienced clinicians worry about getting the diagnosis right. Three general approaches can be recommended, depending upon circumstances [6]:

• **Presumptive diagnosis:** when the temporal association of events and onset, course of the illness, and clinical features are characteristic thereby making the diagnosis likely, *and* definitive diagnostic tests are not readily available or are imprecise, *and* therapy is not risky, a pre-

sumptive diagnosis can be made and a therapeutic trial should be instituted.

• **Directed evaluation:** when the clinician has a good idea of the diagnosis or a limited differential diagnosis, *and* a definitive diagnostic test is available, that diagnostic test should be done to confirm the diagnosis and to direct further management.

• **Categorization and algorithmic evaluation:** when no particular diagnosis is especially likely, categorizing diarrhea as watery (with subtypes of secretory and osmotic), inflammatory, or fatty by simple tests can lead to a series of diagnostic tests that may yield a diagnosis.

Presumptive diagnosis might be used, for example, in a patient who developed chronic diarrhea shortly after a cholecystectomy. If the diarrhea had the expected characteristics of watery stools that were more numerous in the morning, a therapeutic trial of bile acid binding resin would be warranted since no definitive diagnostic test is available and the therapeutic trial would not be risky or expensive. If the patient improved, the diagnosis of postcholecystectomy diarrhea would be likely.

Directed evaluation might be employed in a patient who was likely to have celiac disease based on a characteristic history of weight loss, bloating, and fatty stools. Serological testing and small bowel biopsy have a very high true-positive rate and would confirm the diagnosis if positive [7]. The thoughtful clinician would obtain those tests early in the evaluation and proceed on to long-term treatment with confidence.

Categorization and algorithmic evaluation make sense when there is no dominant diagnosis [4]. In this scenario the extensive differential diagnosis of chronic diarrhea is limited by categorizing the type of stools produced as watery, inflammatory, or fatty, and then looking for the specific problems causing that type of diarrhea. This categorization is done by gross inspection of stools and by analyzing stools for blood, white blood cells (or a surrogate marker, such as lactoferrin or calprotectin), and fat (Figure 20.1). Watery stools are easily pourable, and have no blood or pus. Inflammatory stools have blood or pus. Fatty stools have excess fat or oil.

Watery stools can be subdivided into secretory diarrhea or osmotic diarrhea based on stool electrolyte analysis [8]. Secretory diarrhea is due to incomplete absorption of electrolytes and so the stools are electrolyte-rich.

Osmotic diarrhea is due to ingestion of a poorly absorbed substance that obligates water retention within

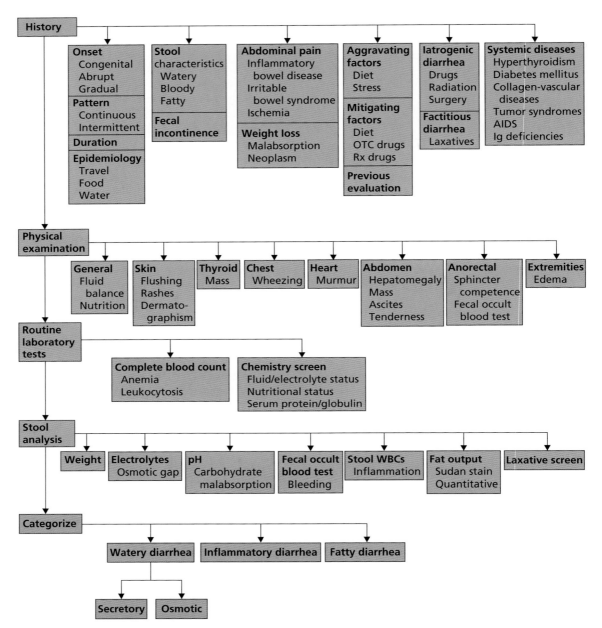

Figure 20.1 Initial diagnostic approach to chronic diarrhea. OTC drug, over-the-counter drug; Rx drug, prescription drug; WBC, white blood cell. Adapted from Fine KD, Schiller LR. AGA technical review on the evaluation and management of chronic diarrhea. *Gastroenterology* 1999; **116**: 1464–86.

the lumen to maintain osmotic equilibration with serum. (The intestine is too permeable to water to allow an osmotic gradient to develop between the lumen and serum.) Electrolyte absorption is unaffected and so stools have very low electrolyte concentrations. This distinction can be quantitated by calculating the fecal osmotic gap (FOG) which estimates the contribution of non-electrolytes to stool osmolality:

$$FOG = 290 - 2([Na^+] + [K^+]),$$

where 290 is the assumed luminal osmolality and $2([Na^+] + [K^+])$ represents an estimate of the total cations and anions present in stool water. A fecal osmotic gap above 100 mosm/kg suggests osmotic diarrhea and FOG below 25 mosm/kg suggests secretory diarrhea.

Once the diarrhea has been categorized, the differential diagnosis becomes more manageable (Table 20.1) and algorithmic approaches to each subtype are feasible (Figure 20.2).

Case continued

Because there is no dominant diagnosis, this patient is most appropriately evaluated by categorizing the diarrhea and using an algorithmic approach. Routine laboratory tests, including complete blood count, metabolic profile, and C-reactive protein, are unremarkable. A 48-h stool collection yielded 550 g/24 h of watery diarrhea. Fecal occult blood test was negative, fecal lactoferrin was negative, and stool fat excretion was 2 g/24 h. Fecal $[Na^+]$ was 40 mmol/L and fecal $[K^+]$ was 100 mmol/L, making the FOG = 10 mosm/kg, consistent with a secretory diarrhea. Flexible sigmoidoscopy revealed normal appearances, but biopsies were interpreted as showing collagenous colitis.

Table 20.1 Differential diagnosis of chronic diarrhea.

Osmotic diarrhea
Osmotic laxative abuse
  Mg^{++}, SO_4^{-2}, PO_4^{-3}, lactulose, mannitol, sorbitol, PEG
Carbohydrate malabsorption
  Lactose, fructose, others

Fatty diarrhea
Malabsorption syndromes
  Mucosal diseases
  Short bowel syndrome
  Postresection diarrhea
  Small bowel bacterial overgrowth
  Mesenteric ischemia
Maldigestion
  Pancreatic insufficiency
  Reduced luminal bile acid

Inflammatory diarrhea
Inflammatory bowel disease
  Ulcerative colitis
  Crohn disease
  Diverticulitis
  Ulcerative jejunoileitis
Infections
  Invasive bacterial infection
    Clostridium, E. coli, tuberculosis, others
  Ulcerating viral infection
    Cytomegalovirus, herpes simplex
  Invasive parasites
    Amebiasis
    Strongyloides
Ischemic colitis
Radiation enterocolitis
Neoplasia
  Carcinoma of colon
  Lymphoma

Secretory diarrhea
Congenital chloridorrhea
Chronic infections
Inflammatory bowel disease
  Ulcerative colitis
  Crohn disease (ileum)
  Microscopic colitis
    Lymphocytic colitis
    Collagenous colitis
  Diverticulitis
Drugs and poisons
  Stimulant laxative abuse
Disordered regulation
  Postvagotomy
  Postsympathectomy
  Diabetic neuropathy
  Irritable bowel syndrome
Ileal bile acid malabsorption
Endocrine diarrhea
  Hyperthyroidism
  Addison disease
Neuroendocrine tumors
  Gastrinoma
  VIPoma
  Somatostatinoma
  Mastocytosis
  Carcinoid syndrome
  Medullary carcinoma of the thyroid
Other neoplasia
  Colon carcinoma
  Lymphoma
  Villous adenoma
Idiopathic secretory diarrhea
  Epidemic (Brainerd)
  Sporadic

Adapted from Fine KD, Schiller LR. AGA technical review on the evaluation and management of chronic diarrhea. *Gastroenterology* 1999; **116**: 1464–86.

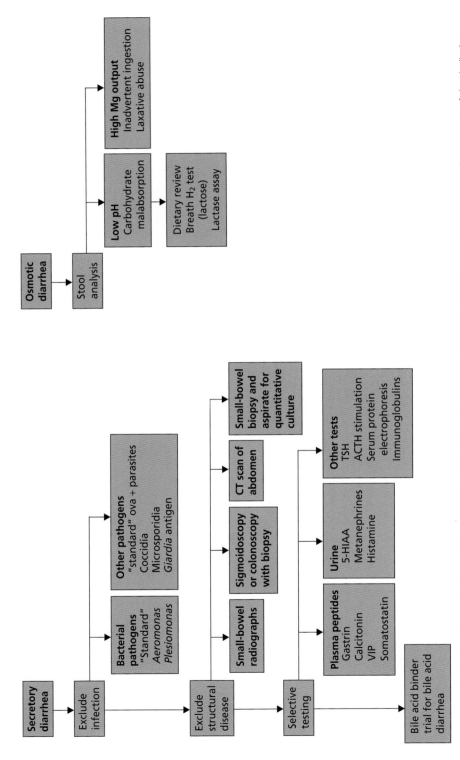

Figure 20.2 Algorithmic evaluation of subtypes of chronic diarrhea. Adapted from Fine KD, Schiller LR. AGA technical review on the evaluation and management of chronic diarrhea. *Gastroenterology* 1999; **116**: 1464–86.

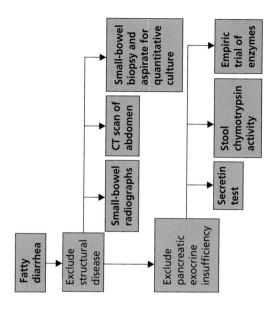

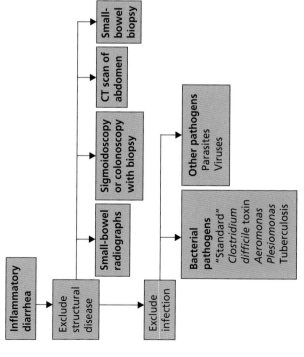

Figure 20.2 continued

Therapeutics

The treatment of chronic diarrhea ultimately depends on the underlying condition. For some conditions therapy can be *curative*, such as a gluten-free diet for celiac disease [7]. For relapsing conditions, such as collagenous colitis, appropriate therapy can *induce remission* [9]. For all the others *symptomatic therapy* can diminish the impact of diarrhea on quality of life, both while evaluation is ongoing and chronically (Table 20.2) [10].

The most important issue to address is rehydration. Intravenous fluid is used in hospitalized patients. Oral rehydration can correct even serious fluid depletion [11]. Intraluminal agents can modify stool texture, but may not reduce stool output.

The most effective and widely-applicable symptomatic therapies are antidiarrheal opiates [12]. Low-potency opiates include loperamide, and diphenoxylate combined with low-dose atropine (to reduce abuse potential). The key difference in using these agents to treat chronic diarrhea rather than acute diarrhea is to give the antidiarrheal on a scheduled basis (e.g., before each meal) instead of on an "as-needed" basis. Antidiarrheal drugs work best if given before meals, when they can blunt the physiological stimulus for defecation.

When low-potency opiate antidiarrheal drugs fail to control diarrhea, higher potency opiates, such as codeine, morphine, or deodorized tincture of opium, should be used [10]. These agents should be started at a low dose and titrated up slowly to allow tolerance to sedative effects to develop in the brain. Tolerance does not develop to the constipating effects of these agents and so an effective dose usually can be achieved that will control diarrhea, but not produce sedation.

Clonidine and octreotide have non-specific antidiarrheal activity, but should be reserved for special cases, such as those that fail opiate therapy [10].

> ### Case continued
>
> The patient was started on loperamide 4 mg three times per day as symptomatic therapy after the stool collection was completed. Stool frequency decreased from five to two bowel movements daily, but stools remained fluid. When the biopsy was reported as showing collagenous colitis, the patient was started on oral budesonide 9 mg daily, a drug shown to work well for this condition by meta-analysis [9]. Her diarrhea resolved and budesonide was tapered.

Prognosis

Diarrhea resolves or is controlled in most patients with chronic diarrhea. The prognosis depends on the underlying diagnosis and the availability of treatment for that condition.

Table 20.2 Non-specific treatment of diarrhea.

Category	Treatment	Typical adult dose
Rehydration	Intravenous fluid	1–5 L/24 h
	Oral rehydration solution	1–5 L/24 h
Intraluminal agents	Adsorbents (kaolin–pectin)	15–60 mL QID
	Bismuth subsalicylate	30 mL QID
	Texture modifiers (psyllium)	15–30 g/24 h
Drugs that inhibit transit		
Potent opiates	Deodorized tincture of opium (10 mg morphine/mL)	5–20 drops QID
	Morphine sulfate (20 mg/mL)	2–10 drops QID
	Codeine phosphate or sulfate	15–60 mg QID
Less potent opiates	Diphenoxylate with atropine	1–2 tablets QID
	Difenoxin with atropine	1–2 tablets QID
	Loperamide (2 mg)	1–2 tablets QID
Others	Clonidine	0.1–0.3 mg TID
	Octreotide injection	50–200 µg TID

QID, four times per day; TID, three times per day.

References

1 Ford AC, Talley NJ, Veldhuyzen van Zanten SJ, *et al.* Will the history and physical examination help establish that irritable bowel syndrome is causing this patient's lower gastrointestinal tract symptoms? *JAMA* 2008; **300**: 1793–805.

2 Longstreth GF, Thompson WG, Chey WD, *et al.* Functional bowel disorders. *Gastroenterology* 2006; **130**: 1480–91.

3 Talley NJ. Chronic unexplained diarrhea: what to do when the initial workup is negative? *Rev Gastroenterol Disord* 2008; **8**: 178–85.

4 Fine KD, Schiller LR. AGA technical review on the evaluation and management of chronic diarrhea. *Gastroenterology* 1999; **116**: 1464–86.

5 Schiller LR, Sellin JH. Diarrhea. In: Feldman M, Friedman L, Brandt LJ, eds. *Sleisenger & Fordtran's Gastrointestinal and Liver Disease*, 8th edn. Philadelphia: WB Saunders Co., 2006: 159–86.

6 Schiller LR. Management of diarrhea in clinical practice: strategies for primary care physicians. *Rev Gastroenterol Disord* 2007; **7** (Suppl. 3): S27–38.

7 Freeman HJ. Pearls and pitfalls in the diagnosis of adult celiac disease. *Can J Gastroenterol* 2008; **22**: 273–80.

8 Eherer AJ, Fordtran JS. Fecal osmotic gap and pH in experimental diarrhea of various causes. *Gastroenterology* 1992; **103**: 545–51.

9 Chande N, McDonald JW, MacDonald JK. Interventions for treating collagenous colitis. *Cochrane Database Syst Rev* 2008; **2**: CD003575.

10 Schiller LR. Chronic diarrhea. *Curr Treat Options Gastroenterol* 2005; **8**: 259–66.

11 Hartling L, Bellemare S, Wiebe N, *et al.* Oral versus intravenous rehydration for treating dehydration due to gastroenteritis in children. *Cochrane Database Syst Rev* 2006; **3**: CD004390.

12 Hanauer SB. The role of loperamide in gastrointestinal disorders. *Rev Gastroenterol Disord* 2008; **8**: 15–20.

CHAPTER 21

Loss of Appetite and Loss of Weight

Ronald L. Stone[1], Kanwar Rupinder S. Gill[2], and James S. Scolapio[3]

[1] Department of Dietetics, Mayo Clinic, Jacksonville, FL, USA
[2] Department of Gastroenterology, Sutter Gould Medical Foundation, Modesto, CA, USA
[3] Division of Gastroenterology and Hepatology, Mayo Clinic, Jacksonville, FL, USA

Summary

The evaluation of unintentional weight loss can be intriguing and challenging; therefore, a systematic approach is required to avoid lengthy workups, which can lead to over utilization of health resources, and to uncover the correct diagnosis. There are essentially three primary reasons for weight loss: (i) reduced caloric intake; (ii) increased caloric losses (i.e., malabsorption); and (iii) increased energy expenditure (organic illness). Non-organic causes of weight loss account for up to 33–46% of cases. Evaluation should include: (i) detailed history and physical examination; (ii) laboratory and imaging testing; (iii) radiographic studies; and (iv) gastrointestinal testing. In many cases weight loss can be treated by increasing nutrition orally to meet demand. Use of liquid nutritional supplements to supplement dietary intake are an effective way of increasing calories and reversing weight loss. In patients with anorexia, the use of appetite stimulants may need to be considered. Finally, for patients with functional deficits the use of enteral or parenteral nutrition maybe necessary.

Case

A 50-year-old female patient presents with a 10-kg weight loss over a period of 6 months. Her usual weight is 61 kg. A detailed history notes that the patient has a normal appetite and is eating an estimated 1800 calories per day. Her BMI is 27. On further review of systems she notes five to 10 liquid bowel movements a day. She has had no previous gastrointestinal surgeries and denies abdominal bloating or postprandial abdominal pain. Her physical examination is unremarkable. Routine laboratory blood testing is unremarkable, including normal thyroid function studies. Given her history a 72-fecal fat study was performed to exclude intestinal malabsorption. Her fecal fat level was elevated at 17 g. Upper endoscopy with a small bowel aspirate was done to exclude bacterial overgrowth and a small intestine biopsy taken to exclude celiac disease. Aspirate was normal; however, the small intestine biopsy revealed total villous atrophy consistent with celiac disease. The patient was referred to a registered dietician for instruction on a gluten-free diet. Two weeks after being placed on a gluten free diet the patient's diarrhea resolved and over a period of 12 weeks the patient returned to her usual weight.

Introduction

Unintentional weight loss is a powerful indicator of nutrition risk, nutrition-associated complications, and as an independent predictor of increased morbidity and mortality [1]. The prevalence of the different etiologies of weight loss varies among studies. In several studies the most common cause of weight loss was organic illness *without* cancer (30–50%), cancer alone (19–36%), and psychiatric illness (9–20%) [2–4]. In 24–26% of patients with unintentional weight loss no cause can be identified despite extensive testing. It is very important to carefully evaluate a patient with unintentional weight loss as significant weight loss carries a very high mortality. This chapter will present an overview of the evaluation and causes of patients with unintentional weight loss.

Practical Gastroenterology and Hepatology: Small and Large Intestine and Pancreas, 1st edition. Edited by Nicholas J. Talley, Sunanda V. Kane and Michael B. Wallace. © 2010 Blackwell Publishing Ltd.

Table 21.1 Body mass index (BMI).

BMI <18.5	Low body weight
BMI 18.6–24.9	Normal body weight
BMI 25–29.9	Preobese/overweight
BMI 30–34.9	Obese class I
BMI 35–39.9	Obese class II
BMI >40	Obese class III

History and Physical Exam

The first step when evaluating a patient with unintentional weight loss is to take a thorough medical history with focus on a patient's weight history. It is very important to ask a patient if they have been trying to lose weight (intentional) or if the weight loss has occurred without trying to lose weight (unintentional). Most studies suggest that an absolute weight loss of 4.5 kg (10 pounds) or more, or weight loss of greater than 5% in the past 6 months, is clinically significant. Weight loss greater than 10% is associated with protein–energy malnutrition, while weight loss of more than 20% from baseline usually indicates severe protein–energy malnutrition. Most physiological body functions will show some degree of impairment at this level of weight loss [5]. In addition to a history of weight loss, it is important to consider physical findings such as loss of subcutaneous fat and muscle mass. Physical assessment of lean muscle mass with triceps skin fold thickness using a caliper or body fat analysis by bioelectrical impedance are useful tools in determining overall nutrition stores.

The associated risk of weight loss depends greatly on the patient's overall stores, which may be defined in terms of body mass index (BMI). Patients with a low body mass index (<18.5) are at greater risk [6]. Body mass index can be calculated as follows:

$$\text{weight (kg)}/\text{height (m)}^2$$

or by

$$\text{weight (lbs)}/\text{height (in)}^2 \times 703$$

Refer to Table 21.1 for interpretation.

Causes of Unintentional Weight Loss

In obtaining the patient history the clinician needs to ask for clues that attempt to identify the cause of the weight loss. There are essentially three primary reasons for weight loss: (i) reduced caloric intake; (ii) increased caloric losses (i.e., malabsorption); and (iii) increased energy expenditure (organic illness). Patients usually have a good sense of what category they belong to, if appropriately asked. Once a category is determined the etiology and evaluation is greatly simplified.

Reduced Caloric Intake

An obvious but often overlooked component of weight loss is a decrease in the amount of food, and particularly the caloric value of the food the patient is consuming. Changes in caloric intake can take place gradually and patients may not be weighing themselves frequently enough to notice the impact immediately. It has been estimated that as adults age, caloric intake may decrease by as much as 30% between the ages of 20 and 80 years, and with weight loss of as much as 4% per year after age 65 [7]. A dietetic consult by a registered dietitian can be extremely helpful in determining deficits in patient's intake compared to estimated energy needs. A 250 calorie reduction per day can create significant changes in weight in as little as 6 months [8]. Over time, these seemingly small changes in intake can create more dramatic weight loss and overall health risk, especially in the elderly population.

Along with age come a number of functional disabilities that may impact the patient's ability to consume adequate calories. A decline in general oral health, including loss of teeth, ill fitting dentures, or pain while eating have been identified as strong predictors of weight loss [9]. Difficulty chewing and swallowing may limit the patient's choice of foods, making eating less pleasurable, especially if modified diets such as pureed or thickened liquids are used. Motor skill disabilities, visual impairment, and dementia may also be a factor.

Loss of appetite with early satiety is frequently described by patients as the primary cause of a decrease in caloric intake. Chronic illnesses such as HIV, chronic kidney disease, and cancer are all associated with anorexia. However, loss of appetite alone is not usually enough to result in significant weight loss as there is often other mechanisms associated with the chronic illness, such as altered metabolism, disruption in the gastrointestinal absorption, and side effects of treatment, causing the weight loss [10]. Clinical depression and medication side effects are very important and often overlooked causes of weight loss.

Dysgeusia may also result in a significant decrease in caloric intake through a decline in the patient's enjoyment for eating and increased food aversions. Dysguesia is a common side effect of cancer patients. For non-cancer patients, taste changes can occur with aging, and in various chronic illnesses, such as diabetes, this can be caused by medications used to treat the chronic illness [11]. Taste alterations may also occur with thrush.

An estimated 10% of unintentional weight loss cases can be traced to psychological causes [1]. Of these, depression is a major concern, considering symptoms of major depression affect as many as 12% of the population and symptoms of one or more elements of depression affect up to 23% of Americans [12]. Depression can result in apathy towards life as well as food and lead to a patient's gradual disinterest in their well-being. Many adults will never visit a mental health professional for their depression, leaving the diagnosis of these symptoms to the primary-care provider. Understanding the symptoms of depression and how they may be affecting eating habits and weight loss is essential for diagnosis. Depression may also lead to substance abuse, with use of the substance either acting as an anorexant or replacing the enjoyment of eating. Chronic anxiety may also cause weight loss as a result of increased basal metabolic rate and altered eating habits.

Increased Caloric Losses (Intestinal Malabsorption)

Various gastrointestinal illnesses that can result in intestinal malabsorption will be covered in detail in other chapters of this book. The authors have highlighted some of the more common gastrointestinal illnesses that may result in weight loss below. It is very important in the medical history to ask the patient if they are having diarrhea. If the patient admits to frequent stooling and has stool characteristics of steatorrhea, intestinal malabsorption is the most likely culprit of their weight loss.

Chronic pancreatitis can result in weight loss by exocrine function and subsequent malabsorption of all macronutrients and fat-soluble vitamins. The clinical manifestations include postprandial abdominal pain (which may limit oral intake of food), steatorrhea, and anorexia. The diagnosis may be late in the illness as 90% of the pancreatic exocrine function is usually lost before signs and symptoms are clinically observed. Chronic

alcoholism usually compounds the malnutrition in this group of patients.

Bacterial overgrowth of the small bowel can cause malabsorption of intraluminal nutrients and decreased oral intake of food due to bloating symptoms. Common causes of bacterial overgrowth may include small intestinal diverticulosis, surgically created blind loops, small bowel strictures, and small bowel motility disorders. The symptoms are non-specific, and the diagnosis is established by $[^{14}C]$-D-xylose breath test or small bowel aspirate.

Short bowel syndrome and disorders affecting the motor function of the stomach and small bowel can result in unintentional weight loss as well. A thorough history and review of surgical reposts is needed to make an appropriate diagnosis. Such disorders that may result in weight loss include gastric surgery (pyloroplasty, gastrojunostomy, subtotal gastric resection, total gastrectomy), and small bowel resections (short bowel syndrome). Short bowel syndrome usually becomes clinically significant when more than 200 cm of the small bowel has been removed. Review of operative reports is critical to determine a patient's prognosis and management.

Gastroparesis and chronic intestinal pseudo-obstruction may also result in significant weight loss. A history of diabetes and early satiety should provide the significant clues necessary to make a diagnosis of gastroparesis. Many of these patients will require dietary counseling, that is small frequent meals, and occasionally the use of an enteral feeding tube for nutritional delivery. Patients with scleroderma and amyloidosis frequently will have involvement of the intestinal system and have signs and symptoms of pseudo-obstruction. Often dietary counseling on an oral diet is not enough and these patients may require enteral feeding and occasionally parenteral nutrition.

Many diseases discussed in other chapters of this book may cause gastric and intestinal mucosal disruption and subsequent weight loss by immunological (Crohn disease, celiac disease, autoimmune enteritis, eosinophillic gastroenteritis), infectious (tropical sprue, AIDS, enteropathy), ischemic (chronic mesenteric ischemia), and radiation (radiation enteritis) induced injury. These diagnoses usually require a thorough medical history and examination and laboratory and endoscopic testing. Radiation enteritis and chronic mesenteric ischemia are two diagnoses that are frequently overlooked.

Radiation enteritis may not present with weight loss until 20 years following treatment. Frequently, this piece of information is not gathered during the history of a patient. These patients may present with diarrhea or obstructive symptoms. They usually are women that have been treated with radiation for ovarian cancer or men that have been treated with radiation for testicular cancer years prior. Chronic mesenteric ischemia should be suspected in patients with postprandial pain (30 min following a meal) in the *absence* of bloating. These patients are usually smokers that may have a history of peripheral vascular disease. An abdominal bruit may or may not be heard on physical examination.

Increased Energy Expenditure

When energy demand exceeds energy intake weight loss will occur over time in direct relation to the degree of deficit. Generally, a deficit of about 500 kilocalories per day equates to approximately 0.45 kg (one pound) of weight loss per week. Patients who develop hypermetabolism usually experience weight loss in the absence of reduced oral intake. In other words they have a good appetite. Common causes of unintentional weight loss in this category may include cancer, chronic infection, and hyperthyroidism. Use of illicit drugs, alternative non-prescribed medications, and weight loss stimulants should be questioned in select patients.

Evaluation of Unintentional Weight Loss

The evaluation of unintentional weight loss can be challenging; however, a systematic approach is required to avoid lengthy workups which can lead to over utilization of health resources. For purpose of this review we have divided the approach into four steps.

Step 1: Detailed history and physical examination. A detailed history and physical examination can identify the etiology of unintentional weight loss in majority of patients. As described above, the focus of history and physical examination should not be focused solely on the exploration of medical causes, but also on psychosocial and nutritional causes. The patient's history should begin with documentation of accurate weights over time and a diet diary or recall over the past month. As mentioned

above, it is helpful to place a patient in one of the three categories discussed. In select patients the flowing next steps should be followed.

Step 2: Laboratory and imaging testing. The laboratory testing may include complete blood cell (CBC) count with differential, comprehensive erythrocyte profile, thyroid-stimulating hormone along with T4 measurement, iron studies, fecal occult blood testing (FOBT), and urinalysis. Additional testing can be obtained based on the clinical history and may include: 48-h stool collection for fat, tissue transglutaminase antibodies (TTG) for celiac disease, prostatic specific antigen (PSA), protein electrophoresis for age-related occult cancer and amyloidosis, and HIV antibodies in high-risk patients.

Step 3: Radiographic studies. A chest X-ray is usually included in the initial evaluation. Additional testing should be based on the clinical situation, for example mammogram can be obtained in women with risk of breast cancer (abnormal breast examination, personal or family history of breast cancer, age >40 years), CT or MRI scan of the neck, chest, or abdomen for occult cancers.

Step 4: Gastrointestinal testing. If the diagnosis is not obvious after the steps 1 to 3, further testing including endoscopic procedures may be required. Usually, an esophagogastroduodenoscopy (EGD) and colonoscopy are done with biopsies. If routine endoscopies are negative, additional testing including capsule endoscopy and gastrointestinal motility studies may be required in select patients.

Patients with a negative evaluation are unlikely to have a serious organic explanation for weight loss. In one out of of four patients a cause is not indentified. These patients should have follow-up in 3 to 6 months. Additionally, a nutrition consult by a registered dietitian should be obtained to assess continued nutritional status, and protein and caloric intake.

Nutrition Management of Unintentional Weight Loss

Management of unintentional weight loss is largely dependent on the findings of evaluation. If there are deficits in caloric intake but no functional impairments, use of an oral calorie–protein supplement is the first line of intervention. Most over-the-counter oral supplements (e.g., Boost (Abbott Nutrition, Abbott Laboratories, Abbott Park, IL) or Ensure (Nestle HealthCare Nutrition, Inc. Florham Park, NJ)) provide 1 kcal/mL and 10 g of protein per 227 g unit. The standard supplement should be in addition to meals and not used as a meal replacement. For patients with severe early satiety or anorexia there are supplements that provide as high as 2 kcal/mL and 20 g of protein per unit. Evidence from two separate reviews demonstrate that use of supplements in addition to dietary counseling is more beneficial than dietary counseling alone, and that nutritional supplements can be used effectively to promote small but consistent weight gain [13,14]. In addition, patients found to have inadequate intakes should take a daily multivitamin.

In patients with inadequate intake the clinician may also consider an appetite stimulant. Megestrol acetate, dronabinol, and oxandrolone are options. While these have been investigated in patients with cancer cachexia and HIV, studies are lacking for their use to treat non-organic weight loss. There are significant side effects of each so determination for use should be on a case by case basis.

Patients with functional deficits most likely will require alternate nutrition such as tube feeds or parenteral nutrition. If the patient has a functional gastrointestinal tract placement of a feeding tube is the preferred route of feeding. The length of time the patient is expected to require the feeding should dictate whether to use a nasal tube or a percutaneous placed tube. If the feeding device is expected to be needed only on a short-term basis (generally <4 weeks) then a nasal tube is recommended. If therapy is expected to be greater than 4–6 weeks then an endoscopically or fluoroscopically placed gastrostomy or jejunostomy tube may be necessary [15]. When oral or enteral tube feeding cannot be achieved, total parenteral nutrition (TPN) has been shown to be an adequate and important source of nutrition. Patients with short bowel syndrome, intestinal disease, obstruction, and severely malnourished patients may require TPN. Given the risk of catheter sepsis, TPN should only be used when oral nutrition and tube feeds have failed or are not possible.

Take-home points

- The evaluation of unintentional weight loss can be intriguing and challenging, therefore a systematic approach is required to avoid lengthy workups which can lead to over utilization of health resources.
- There are essentially three primary reasons for weight loss: (i) reduced caloric intake; (ii) increased caloric losses (i.e. malabsorption); and (iii) increased energy expenditure (organic illness).
- Non-organic causes of weight loss account for up to 33–46% of cases.
- Evaluation should include: (i) detailed history and physical examination; (ii) laboratory and imaging testing; (iii) radiographic studies; and (iv) gastrointestinal testing.

References

1 Reife CM. Involuntary weight loss. *Med Clin N Am* 1995; **79**: 299–313.

2 Marton KI, Sox HC Jr, Krupp JR. Involuntary weight loss: diagnostic and prognostic significance. *Ann Intern Med* 1981; **95**: 568–74.

3 Rabinovitz M, Pitlik SD, Leifer M, *et al.* Unintentional weight loss. A retrospective analysis of 154 cases. *Arch Intern Med* 1986; **146**: 186–7.

4 Thompson MP, Morris LK. Unexplained weight loss in the ambulatory elderly. *J Am Geriatr Soc* 1991; **39**: 497–500.

5 Jeejeebhoy KN, Detsky AS, Baker JP. Assessment of nutritional status. *J Parenter Enteral Nutr* 1990; **15** (5 Suppl.): 193S–6S.

6 Nightingale JMD, Walsh N, Bullock ME, Wicks AC. Three simple methods of detecting malnutrition on medical wards. *J Royal Soc Med* 1996; **89**: 144–8.

7 Chapman IM. Nutritional disorders in the elderly. *Med Clin N Am* 2006; **90**: 887–907.

8 Gans KM, Wylie-Rosett J, Eaton CB. Treating and preventing obesity through diet: Practical approaches for family physicians. *Clin Fam Pract* 2002; **4**: 391.

9 Sullivan DH, Martin W, Flaxman N, *et al.* Oral health problems and involuntary weight loss in a population of frail elderly. *J Am Geriatr Soc* 1993; **41**: 725–31.

10 Delano MJ, Moldawer LL. The origins of cachexia and chronic inflammatory diseases. *Nutr Clin Pract* 2006; **21**: 68–81.

11 Dahlin C, Lynch M, Szmuilowicz E, Jackson V. Management of symptoms other than pain. *Anesthesiol Clin N Am* 2006; **24**: 39–60.

12 Coyne JC, Fechner-Bates S, Schwenk TL. Prevalence, nature, and comorbidity of depressive disorders in primary care. *Gen Hosp Psychiatry* 1994; **16**: 267–76.

13 Milne AC, Potter J, Avenall A. Protein and energy supplementation in elderly people at risk from malnutrition. Cochrane Metabolic and Endocrine Disorders Group. *Cochrane Database Systematic Reviews* 2008; **3**.

14 Baldwin C, Weekes CE. Dietary advice for illness-related malnutrition in adults. Cochrane Cystic Fibrosis and Genetic Disorders Group. *Cochrane Database of Systematic Reviews* 2008; **3**.

15 Bankhead RR, Fang JC. Enteral access devices. In: Gottschlich MM, ed. *The A.S.P.E.N. Nutrition Core Curriculum*, 2nd edn. A.S.P.E.N, 2007.

CHAPTER 22

Gastrointestinal Food Allergy and Intolerance

Sheila E. Crowe

Division of Gastroenterology and Hepatology, Department of Medicine, University of Virginia, Charlottesville, VA, USA

Summary

Adverse reactions to food (ARF) affect at least 20% of populations in developed countries. ARF are categorized as immune-mediated (food allergy (FA) or food hypersensitivity) or non-immunological (food intolerance). FA occurs in 4–8% of children and 1–4% of adults in the USA. Common food allergens in children include cow's milk, wheat, eggs, peanuts, and soy products and in adults, peanuts, tree nuts, seafood, and fish are most common. Most FA involves systems outside the GI tract but approximately 50% of presentations include GI complaints such as nausea, vomiting, abdominal cramping or pain, and diarrhea. Diagnosis of FA is based on clinical presentation, food diaries, response to elimination diets, and certain diagnostic tests (skin testing, radioallergoabsorbent test (RAST)). Management of FA centers on avoidance of the food(s) identified as causing symptoms although medications can play a role in minimizing reactions of inadvertent exposure to the antigen or modulating the immune response to foods.

Case

A 22-year-old Caucasian woman comes to see you for complaints of intermittent diarrhea and abdominal cramping after eating. She has tried a lactose free diet but it did not seem to help. The only food type that has caused a specific reaction was tomato, which led to oropharyngeal swelling and tightness in her throat and also some nausea and vomiting. She has a past history of recurrent otitis media and eczema as a child with skin testing that showed reactivity to cow's milk protein and wheat. Although she was told that she outgrew these food allergies, in recent years she gets nasal congestion and feels "wheezy" when she mows the grass. She denies weight loss, fevers, rash, and arthralgias but notes fatigue, decreased energy, and headaches. Her physical examination is unremarkable. She is concerned that she may have some type of food allergy, lactose intolerance, or celiac disease causing her current problems. Although you suspect the GI diagnosis may be functional bowel disease, you wonder how to best evaluate and treat for possible adverse reactions to foods that may be contributing to her clinical presentation.

Practical Gastroenterology and Hepatology: Small and Large Intestine and Pancreas, 1st edition. Edited by Nicholas J. Talley, Sunanda V. Kane and Michael B. Wallace. © 2010 Blackwell Publishing Ltd.

Overview of Food Allergy (Hypersensitivity) and Food Intolerances

Allergic reactions to food frequently occur in early childhood and disappear spontaneously within the first 4–6 years of life. Sometimes, these reactions are replaced by inhalant allergies to plant pollens, mites, or animal epithelia. Relatively few children retain their food allergies until adulthood. Some adults, however, develop food allergies without experiencing food allergy in childhood. The prevalence of food allergy decreases from 4–8% in children to 1–4% in adults. In contrast, at least 20% of the population in developed nations reports adverse reactions to food (ARF). ARF are caused by a variety of mechanisms with only about a third of the reactions in children and 10% of those in adults due to actual food allergy in which there is an abnormal immunological reaction to food (Table 22.1) [1]. The majority of ARF are non-immunologic in origin (Table 22.2) with lactose intolerance and physiological food reactions being the most common types of adverse reactions to food worldwide.

Table 22.1 Gastrointestinal disorders associated with food allergy or food intolerance.

Immediate GI hypersensitivity
   Oral allergy syndrome (OAS)
   Allergic gastritis
   Allergic enterocolitis

Eosinophilic gastroenteropathies
   Eosinophilic esophagitis
   Eosinophilic gastritis
   Eosinophilic enterocolitis
   Eosinophilic proctitis

Food protein-induced enterocolitis syndromes (FPIES)

Celiac disease

Conditions associated with non-immune mechanisms of food
      intolerance
   Gastroesophageal reflux disease (GERD)
   Functional dyspepsia
   Irritable bowel syndrome (IBS)
   Other functional GI disorders
   Inflammatory bowel disease (IBD)

Table 22.2 Types of food intolerances (non-immune adverse reactions to food).

Food toxicity (microorganisms or bacterial toxins)

Pseudoallergic reactions (non-immune mast cell activation by strawberries, chocolate, tomatoes, and other foods as well as additives such as salicylates, benzoates, and tartrazine)

Pharmacological reactions (histamine found in scombroid fish, and other foods—histamine intolerance in diamino-oxidase-deficient individuals; tyramine in chocolate, cheese, red wine, etc.; additives such as sulfites, tartrazine, and monosodium glutamate and other amines)

Metabolic reactions—lactose intolerance (hereditary or acquired)

Psychological food intolerance

Physiological food intolerance (e.g., starches found in legumes serve as substrate for gas production by colonic flora, and favoring histamine synthesis by fermentation)

The symptoms of allergy range from minor symptoms to life-threatening anaphylaxis [2]. Of the patients suffering from true food allergy, roughly a third complain predominantly of gastrointestinal (GI) symptoms (nausea, vomiting, cramps, bloating, diarrhea), with the others also reporting skin symptoms (urticaria, atopic dermatitis), respiratory complaints (rhinitis, asthma), or

less well-defined systemic complaints, which may not be related to food allergy (migraine headaches, fatigue, edema, arthritis). While dermatologic, respiratory, and systemic manifestations of food allergy are often easy to recognize, reactions manifesting primarily in the digestive tract can be difficult to diagnose and treat.

It appears that along with allergic reactions in general, allergic reactions to food are increasing in prevalence. However, data confirming this increase are lacking except for peanut allergy [3]. In addition, food allergy has become the most common cause of life-threatening anaphylaxis in industrialized countries [4]. The reasons for the increase of allergic diseases including food allergy are not entirely apparent although recent epidemiologic studies suggest that the greater level of hygiene in urbanized populations in industrialized countries might play a central role [5].

Immune-mediated Gastrointestinal Adverse Reactions to Food

Food allergy or food hypersensitivity can result in GI symptoms (nausea, vomiting, abdominal pain, and diarrhea) that can occur in conjunction with allergic manifestations in other target organs (skin, respiratory tract). The reactions are self-limited and do not lead to chronic damage to the GI tract, unlike other immune-mediated types of ARF. The foods primarily responsible for this type of GI food allergy include cow's milk, eggs, peanuts, seafood, and fish [2]. The oral allergy syndrome is the most common manifestation of food allergy in adults with triggering allergens that are plant proteins, which cross-react with certain inhalant antigens [6]. Examples include birch pollen cross-reacting with apple, peach, pear, almond, hazelnut, potato, and carrot; ragweed cross-reacting with melons, banana, and the gourd family; mugwort cross-reacting with celery, carrot, and various herbs and spices; and grass cross-reacting with tomato. Exposure to the cross-reacting foods may lead to pruritis, tingling and/or swelling of the tongue, lips, palate, or oropharynx, and occasionally to bronchospasm or more systemic reactions, occurring a few minutes after ingestion of the allergen. Latex-food allergy syndrome is a form of food allergy of increasing prevalence throughout the world with banana, avocado, chestnut, and kiwi the most common causes of food-induced symptoms associated with latex allergy [7]. In latex-sensitive individuals exposure to these cross-reacting foods can result in the same symptoms as if exposed to latex, ranging from pruritis, eczema, oral–facial swelling, asthma, GI complaints, and anaphylaxis. The most important manifestation of food allergy is systemic anaphylaxis. Food allergy is now the major cause of anaphylactic reactions in industrialized societies with peanuts the main antigen responsible for anaphylaxis and anaphylactic death [8]. Cofactors such as ingestion of acetyl-salicylic acid ASA or non-steroidal anti-inflammatory drugs or exercising at the time of eating a specific food such as wheat are important to identify since recurrence of anaphylaxis due to exercise and/or ingestion of wheat was identified a s a major cause of recurrent anaphylaxis in one study [9].

Eosinophilic gastroenteritis is an uncommon disorder characterized by eosinophilic inflammation of the gastrointestinal tissues [10]. Abdominal pain, vomiting, and diarrhea occur together in nearly 50% of cases and peripheral eosinophilia is seen in up to two-thirds of patients with eosinophilic gastroenteritis. Eosinophilic gastroenteritis is associated with food allergies, and concomitant atopic diseases or a family history of allergies in 50–70% of cases. Eosinophilic esophagitis is being increasingly recognized and presents most often in males in childhood through to adult life with symptoms of heartburn, dysphagia, and odynophagia [11]. Food allergies appear to play a significant role in this disorder and the elimination of offending antigens from the diet can be beneficial as are swallowed steroids formulated as inhalants.

Celiac disease results from chronic stimulation of T lymphocytes by a food protein (gluten), which results in chronic intestinal damage in genetically predisposed individuals. It is readily recognized in its classical form with diarrhea, bloating, flatulence, weight loss, and evidence of malabsorption. Withdrawal of gluten from the diet results in a rapid clinical and serological improvement and a slower but corresponding improvement of small bowel histology. Celiac disease can present in many other ways including anemia, chronic fatigue, osteopenic bone disease, recurrent miscarriages, and a wide variety of GI presentations including irritable bowel syndrome (IBS)-like symptoms, and even constipation. Celiac disease may complicate other disorders, particularly autoimmune endocrine and connective tissue diseases.

Food protein-induced enterocolitis syndromes (FPIES) typically affect young children and can arise from various foods including cow's milk proteins and soy protein [12]. The immunological mechanisms leading to chronic GI mucosal inflammation are complex and can lead to diarrhea, failure to thrive, anemia, and protein-losing enteropathy. The illness resolves with removal of the offending antigen(s) from the diet and, typically, afflicted children outgrow this condition.

Non-immune Gastrointestinal Adverse Reactions to Food

Lactose intolerance produces symptoms (bloating, cramping, diarrhea, flatulence) resulting from ingestion of foods containing lactose (milk, ice cream, butter) that is broken down by colonic flora in individuals with low levels of small intestinal lactase activity. It is important to note that most yogurts and firm cheeses do not cause GI symptoms on the basis of lactose intolerance since bacteria used to produce these dairy products break down lactose so that lactose levels are very low or zero in these products. Lactose intolerant patients should continue to eat naturally lactose-free dairy products as these are excellent sources of bioavailable calcium. Intolerance to fat and other components of such dairy products or, more rarely, extreme sensitivity to very low amounts of lactose, should be considered as a cause of symptoms in truly lactose intolerant patients.

Physiological reactions to food components or additives are perhaps the most common form of GI adverse reaction to food. For example, it is well known that starches found in legumes serve as substrate for gas production by colonic flora. Many other foods are associated with "gas", including cabbage, bran fiber, and other vegetables and grains. Other foods and food additives affect the lower esophageal sphincter, while foods high in fat delay gastric emptying, all with the potential to cause symptoms of heartburn and dyspepsia. IBS with sensitivity to dietary factors is very common and typically these patients do not report specific food intolerances but rather symptoms due to large meals, fatty foods, restaurant meals, and other more general forms of food intolerance are characteristic. However, it is important to determine whether specific food intolerances exist in this group of patients, since some studies have suggested elimination of the offending food(s) can provide some benefit [13]. Psychological reactions to food are another non-immune category of adverse reactions to food [14], although studies suggest that one can condition immune reactions to food and other antigens without the antigen being present [15].

Anaphylactoid or pseudoallergic reactions to food result from foods that mimic the effects of mast cell degranulation but do not involve IgE antibodies [16]. As with true food allergy, patients exhibiting such reactions should be instructed to avoid the offending food substance if identifiable. Pharmacological reactions to food or food additives represent a relatively common type of adverse reaction to food although most of these reactions cause symptoms outside of the GI tract, such as migraine headaches, asthma, and urticaria. Food toxicity or food poisoning due to staphylococcal enterotoxins, Gram-negative enteric pathogens, hepatitis A virus, and other infectious agents carried in food are not usually considered in the differential diagnosis of most cases of food-induced GI symptoms. However, these acute illnesses may lead to post-infectious IBS with intolerance to food similar to idiopathic forms of IBS. Recent reports from the CDC estimate that 25% of Americans get food poisoning every year.

Evaluation for GI Food Allergy and Intolerances

The medical history can provide clues that help with determining whether food allergy or specific food intolerances may be playing a role in the patient's complaints. Factors that suggest food allergy include other atopic presentations (hay fever, asthma, eczema), family history of atopy, specific food reactions, relatively acute reactions including oropharyngeal symptoms, nausea, vomiting, diarrhea, and abdominal pain that is self-limited and may be associated with urticaria, wheezing, and other non-GI manifestations of allergy. Eosinophilic esophagitis is suggested by a history with primarily esophageal symptoms occurring in young males. Features pointing more to celiac disease include associated autoimmune disorders (type I diabetes mellitus, thyroid disease), certain non-GI presentations (skin lesions of dermatitis herpetiformis, osteopenic bone disease, iron-deficiency anemia, fatigue, depression) and a family history of celiac disease and associated autoimmune conditions. Lactose intolerance is suggested by an acute reaction to foods containing lactose such as milk, ice cream, and butter. Symptoms are typically cramping and diarrhea. There may be a family history and this condition is very common in individuals of Mediterranean, African, Asian, and Native American heritage.

After taking a history to determine if specific foods can be correlated with specific GI symptoms, the next step in the author's practice for patients in whom culprit foods cannot be identified is to have the patient keep a record of their food intake and symptoms (food diary) for a minimum of several weeks before returning for follow up. If the initial history or the food diary suggest food allergy then further testing by skin prick tests and/or laboratory assays to detect food-specific antibodies (IgE) that can degranulate mast cells and basophils can be checked. Skin prick testing is quite sensitive but not very specific. Unless there is a clinical correlation to a positive skin prick tests, or there is an associated high level of specific IgE to that food, the response to a skin prick test alone may be insufficient to recommend avoiding that food. Allergy specialists should be involved in evaluating and managing such patients. Atopy patch testing can be used when immune reactions to foods other than those mediated by IgE are being considered [17].

More often, the food diary fails to identify specific foods that trigger symptoms but instead reveals that food in general is a factor. The diary may identify fatty foods, large meals, restaurant meals, meals eaten close to bedtime, and other associations as giving rise to GI complaints. In this setting, lifestyle changes including eating habits should be advised. In cases where certain foods seem to be a factor a trial of removing the offending item(s) from the diet can be tried for 3 to 4 weeks. For those who cannot be sure what is causing the problem but are still concerned that certain foods are an issue, a trial of an elimination or hypoallergenic diet is the next step recommend by the author (Table 22.3). This can prove helpful for patients without allergies who realize that no matter what they eat, there is a tendency to get symptoms. At the same time, it may help a few individuals ascertain that a certain food is causing the problems.

Laboratory tests to check when considering the gamut of food allergies and intolerances include a

Table 22.3 Elimination diet (also referred to as an exclusion or hypoallergenic diet).

Food category	Allowed	Avoid
Meat and meat alternatives	Lamb Chicken Turkey	Pork Beef Fish Eggs Milk and milk products Seafood
Grains	Rice (Barley) Tapioca Arrowroot	Wheat Oats Corn Rye
Legumes and nuts		Avoid all dried peas, beans, nuts
Vegetables	All except corn and peas	
Fruits	All except citrus fruits, strawberries, and tomatoes	
Sweeteners	Sugar (cane or beet) Maple syrup Honey	
Fats and oils	Olive oil Safflower oil Crisco	Soy, corn, peanut oils Butter Margarine
Miscellaneous	White vinegar Water (Ginger ale) Salt (Pepper) Fruit juices	Coffee, tea Alcohol Chocolate Colas Spices Chewing gum

Foods in parentheses may cause adverse reactions in some individuals. These may be omitted from the trial elimination diet. If an allowed food is one that has caused a reaction in the past it should also be omitted. While on the trial elimination diet, symptoms are recorded and note should be made if there is any change from ones on the previous regular diet. If there are symptoms, determine if there is any relationship to particular foods. (Reproduced from Gastrointestinal food allergy: new insights into pathophysiology and clinical perspectives. Crowe SE, Bischoff SC. *Gastroenterology* 2005; **128**: 1089–113.)

complete blood count, differential with a total eosinophil count, tissue transglutaminase (TTG) IgA and possibly other celiac disease-associated antibodies, and in some settings HLA DQ2 and DQ8 screening by polymerase chain reaction (PCR) (usually in the setting of excluding the possibility of celiac disease by demonstrating they do not have HLA celiac disease susceptibility genes.) Lactose hydrogen breath testing does not need to be checked in everyone with suspected lactose intolerance since the history is often helpful in making the diagnosis, as is the response to a lactose-free diet. However, this test can play a role in patients reporting many different dietary associations with their complaints or those who wish to have a diagnostic test confirm the diagnosis. Unlike hydrogen breath tests for other sugar intolerances, the lactose hydrogen breath test is very sensitive and specific when compared to the gold standard of intestinal lactase enzyme activity.

Esophagogastroduodenoscopy (EGD) or lower GI endoscopy with mucosal biopsies help confirm or refute the diagnosis of several food-associated GI disorders, including eosinophilic esophagitis, eosinophilic gastroenteritis, celiac disease, and cow's milk enteropathy and other FPIES. Radiological tests do not play much of a role in evaluating food-related GI illnesses.

Management of Adverse Reactions to Foods

The main advice to give someone suffering from food-induced GI complaints is to avoid the offending agent [2,18]. Surprisingly, this can be hardest for the person who overeats and gets dyspepsia and GERD. Individuals with IBS and other functional GI disorders also find this difficult to do since they cannot identify specific foods to avoid. However, the individuals for whom this is most difficult and potentially the most dangerous are highly atopic children have several key foods that cannot easily be avoided such as wheat, eggs, peanut, and cow's milk allergies. The author advocates that patients and their families with food allergies, including those with eosinophilic GI conditions associated with food allergies and those with celiac disease, become aware of cross-reacting food groups, learn to read labels, get nutrition counseling, and join appropriate support groups. An important resource for food allergy is the Allergy and Anaphylaxis Network (www.foodallergy.org). Food allergic individuals and their families should have injectable epinephrine available, particularly if there is a history of asthma or anaphylaxis, or any progression of symptoms toward more serious reactions. Certain allergens are more likely to induce severe reactions, including peanuts, tree nuts, and seafood. Antihistamines and, sometimes, oral sodium cromoglycate can help reduce GI symptoms to food allergies. Corticosteroids play a role in eosinophilic esophagitis (swallowed inhaled formulations), for some cases of eosinophilic gastroenteritis, and in truly refractory celiac disease. Desensitization to food antigens does not work as it does for inhalant antigens and insect venoms. New approaches are being developed for managing food allergies [19] but none are ready to be included in a practical approach for managing these problems at this time.

Take-home points

- Adverse reactions to food (ARF) are common with at least 20% of populations in developed countries reporting ARF.
- ARF are categorized as immune-mediated (food allergy or food hypersensitivity) or non-immunological (food intolerance).

- Food allergy occurs in 4–8% of children and 1–4% of adults in the USA.
- Common food allergens in children include cow's milk, wheat, eggs, peanuts, and soy products.
- Common food allergens in adults are peanuts, tree nuts, seafood, and fish.
- Food allergies and intolerances manifest in different ways. Most food allergies involve systems outside the GI tract but approximately 50% of presentations include GI complaints, including nausea, vomiting, abdominal cramping or pain, and diarrhea.
- Diagnosis of food allergies is based on clinical presentation, food diaries, response to elimination diets, and certain diagnostic tests (skin testing, RAST).
- Management of food allergy is primarily based on avoidance of the food antigen(s) identified as causing symptoms, although medications can play a role in minimizing reactions of inadvertent exposure to the antigen or to modulate the immune response to foods.
- A good resource for patients and families with food allergies is the Food Allergy and Anaphylaxis Network (www.foodallergy.org).

References

1 Bischoff SC, Crowe SE. Gastrointestinal food allergy: New insights into pathophysiology and clinical perspectives. *Gastroenterology* 2005; **128**: 1089–113.

2 Lack G. Clinical practice. Food allergy. *N Engl J Med* 2008; **359**: 1252–60.

3 Burks W. Peanut allergy: a growing phenomenon. *J Clin Invest* 2003; **111**: 950–2.

4 Yocum MW, Butterfield JH, Klein JS, *et al.* Epidemiology of anaphylaxis in Olmsted County: A population-based study. *J Allergy Clin Immunol* 1999; **104**: 452–6.

5 Warner JO. The hygiene hypothesis. *Pediatr Allergy Immunol* 2003; **14**: 145–6.

6 Hofmann A, Burks AW. Pollen food syndrome: update on the allergens. *Curr Allergy Asthma Rep* 2008; **8**: 413–7.

7 Blanco C. Latex-fruit syndrome. *Curr Allergy Asthma Rep* 2003; **3**: 47–53.

8 Burks AW. Peanut allergy. *Lancet* 2008; **371**: 1538–46.

9 Mullins RJ. Anaphylaxis: risk factors for recurrence. *Clin Exp Allergy* 2003; **33**: 1033–40.

10 DeBrosse CW, Rothenberg ME. Allergy and eosinophil-associated gastrointestinal disorders (EGID). *Curr Opin Immunol* 2008; **20**: 703–8.

11 Furuta GT, Liacouras CA, Collins MH, *et al.* Eosinophilic esophagitis in children and adults: a systematic review and

consensus recommendations for diagnosis and treatment. *Gastroenterology* 2007; **133**: 1342–63.

12 Sicherer SH, Eigenmann PA, Sampson HA. Clinical features of food protein-induced enterocolitis syndrome. *J Pediatr* 1998; **133**: 214–9.

13 Atkinson W, Sheldon TA, Shaath N, Whorwell PJ. Food elimination based on IgG antibodies in irritable bowel syndrome: a randomised controlled trial. *Gut* 2004; **53**: 1459–64.

14 Kelsay K. Psychological aspects of food allergy. *Curr Allergy Asthma Rep* 2003; **3**: 41–6.

15 Crowe SE, Perdue MH. Gastrointestinal food hypersensitivity: Basic mechanisms of pathophysiology. *Gastroenterology* 1992; **103**: 1075–95.

16 Shah U, Walker WA. Pathophysiology of intestinal food allergy. *Adv Pediatr* 2002; **49**: 299–316.

17 Niggemann B. The role of the atopy patch test (APT) in diagnosis of food allergy in infants and children with atopic dermatitis. *Pediatr Allergy Immunol* 2001; **12** (Suppl. 14): 37–40.

18 Sicherer SH, Leung DY. Advances in allergic skin disease, anaphylaxis, and hypersensitivity reactions to foods, drugs, and insects in 2008. *J Allergy Clin Immunol* 2009; **123**: 319–27.

19 Burks W, Kulis M, Pons L. Food allergies and hypersensitivity: a review of pharmacotherapy and therapeutic strategies. *Expert Opin Pharmacother* 2008; **9**: 1145–52.

CHAPTER 23
Abdominal Bloating and Visible Distension

Laura Hwang and Mark Pimentel

GI Motility Program, Cedars-Sinai Medical Center, Los Angeles, CA, USA

Summary

Bloating and distension are two symptoms commonly encountered in the gastrointestinal clinic. As these symptoms could be either a result of dietary factors or a sign of a more serious gastrointestinal disease, a comprehensive evaluation is necessary in order to determine the proper course of treatment. This review summarizes features of gas-related symptoms and outlines several possible causes and treatments that can be utilized in the clinical setting.

Case

This is the case of a 36-year-old female who presented with significant postprandial gas, bloating, and distension. She had stated that 18 months prior to consultation, she began having a dramatic increase in postprandial gas and bloating. There was associated abdominal distension. There was mild nausea on occasion but no vomiting. In addition to the bloating, there were some changes in stool consistency including alternating soft and normal stool consistency. The patient had no red flag symptoms, including no blood in her stool and no weight loss. There was essentially no past medical history and patient was taking oral contraceptives.

She had seen three previous gastroenterologists and was given a diagnosis of functional bloating and possible bacterial overgrowth. To arrive at this conclusion the previous consultants had conducted a colonoscopy, upper GI series, celiac serologic testing, and a lactulose breath test. At this point, her most recent consultant had noted a clinical improvement with antibiotic therapy. However, the improvement was short lived (less than 2 weeks) after each of two course of treatment. This prompted the referral.

On examination, the patient had clear bloating and distension with mild right lower quadrant tenderness to deep palpation.

The clinical feeling was that despite a previously negative upper GI series, that the distension was too great for simple functional bowel disease. After reviewing the three images provided by the outside centers upper GI small bowel follow through, it was decided that the patient needed a more comprehensive barium. This second barium test reveal mild to moderate dilation of the ileum and a normal-caliber 20 cm of ileum. Based on this finding, a laparoscopy was conducted. This demonstrated an noose-like adhesion band tethering the ileum in an angulated fashion in the right lower quadrant. Lysis of this band resulted in resolution of the patient's complaint of gas and bloating.

The lesson in this case is that the clinician needs to recognize that causes of gas and bloating can be multi-factorial. While bacterial overgrowth may have been a factor in producing symptoms, the cause of the overgrowth and the clinical presentation was an adhesion. Ironically, the patient had never had abdominal surgery or trauma.

Introduction

The average human digestive tract produces many liters of gas per day through digestion of nutrients and bacterial fermentation. This gas is mainly composed of nitrogen, carbon dioxide, methane, and hydrogen. The smell that is associated with flatulence comes not from the

Practical Gastroenterology and Hepatology: Small and Large Intestine and Pancreas, 1st edition. Edited by Nicholas J. Talley, Sunanda V. Kane and Michael B. Wallace. © 2010 Blackwell Publishing Ltd.

methane (which is odorless), but from traces of gases containing sulfur, including hydrogen sulfide, methanethiol, dimethyl disulfide, and dimethyl trisulfide [1,2]. Surveys suggest that gas-related symptoms are common. In fact, 16% of apparently healthy individuals experience bloating at least once a month, and 30% within the previous 3 months [3,4].

One of the most challenging areas in gastroenterology is treating the patient with gas and bloating. A large proportion of patients in a gastroenterological clinic present with symptoms related to gas and bloating, for which no underlying cause can be detected [5]. As there is an incomplete understanding of the mechanisms by which patients experience those symptoms, the lack of adequate therapies is most frustrating for the clinician.

In this chapter, the concepts of what is gas and bloating to the patient, clinician, and scientist will be discussed. Furthermore, this chapter will review the latest treatment options for this clinical situation.

Definitions of Gas, Bloating, and Distension

The first challenge is to understand what gas and bloating are. For example, when a patient presents to their clinician with a complaint of "gas", this could have many meanings. Some interpretations could be excessive flatus, bloating, belching, dyspepsia, or even just foul smelling but normal gas frequency.

Bloating involves four main factors: the sensation of bloating, actual physical distension, volume of intra-abdominal contents, and muscular activity of the abdominal wall [6]. Intra-abdominal contents include solid, liquid, and gaseous components, however, for the purposes of this chapter we will focus primarily on gaseous contents.

Since the body is equipped to naturally handle enteric gas production, the simple presence of excess gas does not automatically translate into the sensation of bloating [7] or visible distension [8]. Further complicating the issue is that the perception of bloating is different from the physical manifestation of abdominal distension. In fact, 25% of patients with bloating report no visible abdominal distension [9]. A study by Serra *et al.* showed that perception of symptoms depends on the responsiveness of the intestinal motor mechanism, whereas objec-

tive physical distension is more directly related to pooling of excess gas in the gut [7].

Pathophysiology

The pathophysiology of gas and bloating can be divided into to a number of categories (Table 23.1). However, in some cases the cause is multifactorial.

Excessive Fermentation

Flatus consists of nitrogen, carbon dioxide, hydrogen, methane, and hydrogen sulfide. While some of these component gases could have originated from the environment, such as nitrogen and carbon dioxide, most of the gases originate from bacterial byproducts of fermentation. The production of these gases is a complex process.

Malabsorption

Food ingested by humans contains both digestible and indigestible products. In a normal human, readily available nutrients are absorbed in the small intestine. All

Table 23.1 Causes of gas and bloating.

Category	Specific cause
Excessive fermentation	Lactose maldigestion
	Fructose maldigestion
	Small intestinal bacterial overgrowth
	Irritable bowel syndrome
	Functional bloating
	Ingestion of non-digestible carbohydrates (e.g., sucralose)
	Malabsorption (e.g., gastric bypass, celiac disease, small bowel Crohn)
	Excessive probiotic use
Poor gas clearance	Medications (e.g., narcotics)
	Pseudo-obstruction
	Scleroderma
	Adhesions/mechanical obstruction
	Irritable bowel syndrome
	Fundoplication (gas bloat syndrome)
Increased gas ingestion	Air swallowing
	Carbonated beverages
Altered sensation	Visceral hypersensitivity/functional bloating
Other	High altitude (e.g., flying)

remaining material is then passed into the colon where bacteria begin to ferment the contents (particularly undigested carbohydrates), producing carbon dioxide and hydrogen [1]. However, this material has a low potential for fermentation, as colonic bacteria require simple substrates for metabolism, and those have usually already been absorbed by the small intestine.

There are essentially two ways to increase the production of fermentation in the gut: gas production in the colon depends on presence of fermentable food and composition of colonic flora [10]. For example, a common cause of gas and bloating is chewing sugar free gum. Often this gum contains a vast range of simple carbohydrates that reach the colon since they are not digested or absorbed by humans. They are subsequently available for colonic bacterial fermentation and gas production.

There are several commonly malabsorbed substrates. Lactose malabsorption, arising from the inability to enzymatically hydrolyze lactose completely in the small intestine, is the most common of these conditions. Studies have shown that a majority of people, even those with some degree of lactose intolerance, can digest at least 240 mL (12 g) of lactose normally [11–13]. When this capacity is exceeded by over-ingestion or if there is a genetic lactase deficiency, lactose will arrive in the colon and will ferment, producing an excess of short-chain fatty acids and hydrogen gas. Since discrepancies can arise between the patient's perception of lactose intolerance and their actual capacity to digest lactose normally, diagnosing lactose intolerance is challenging [12].

Fructose malabsorption is a more recently described phenomenon. The concept is similar, but the human capacity to digest fructose is higher than lactose, at 25 g in healthy individuals [14]. The most recent addition to the malabsorption list is sucralose. The rate of fermentation with the addition of these simpler carbohydrates is much higher and this can result in excessive flatus and the sensation of bloating.

Diseases that cause malabsorption have a similar issue. They result in arrival of nutrients to the colon that failed to be digested and absorbed in the small bowel. These simpler nutrients are better substrates for rapid fermentation.

Other causes of global maldigestion also cause gas and bloating through excessive fermentation. Celiac disease is probably the most common example of this method of

causing gas and bloating. Other examples are listed in Table 23.1.

Small Intestinal Bacterial Overgrowth

Another cause of excessive fermentation is an expansion of the normal flora. In small intestinal bacterial overgrowth, the normal colonic bacteria expand into the small bowel. In this case, the substrate does not need to reach the colon to produce fermentation. In addition, since food is being digested and absorbed in the small intestine, the bacteria are now exposed to simpler and more readily fermentable substrates. This leads to gas and bloating.

However, bacterial overgrowth is a special case since overgrowth is often a manifestation of other physiologic problems. Bacterial overgrowth could be caused by both motility and mechanical issues and the specific etiology of gas and bloating in these cases can be multifactorial.

Methane Production

Some patients have also been found to have an increase in methane producing bacteria. Methane has been shown to slow intestinal transit and detection on breath testing has been consistently shown to coincide with symptoms of constipation [15,16]. Methane production in healthy individuals seems to be limited to colonic anaerobic conditions [10,17]. Methanogenic bacteria are estimated to be present in at least 30% of the population [1,17,18]. Methane levels in flatus can range widely between individuals [1]. Interestingly, methanogenic species produce methane but only in the presence of hydrogen [1] and this metabolic process actually produces energy for the methanogen [19].

Poor Gas Clearance

Poor gas clearance is another means of producing gas and bloating. Under normal circumstances, the bowel is able to handle a very broad range of gas loads, increasing evacuation volumes to adjust for larger infusion volumes [8] in healthy individuals. This is achieved through flatulence, belching, and, to some extent, absorption into the blood stream. In a healthy individual intraluminal gases tend to diffuse into and equilibrate with the gases in venous blood via partial pressure, diffusibility, and speed of gas transit [20,21].

Obvious examples of poor gas clearance are mechanical issues of the bowel. Adhesions in the small bowel should always be sought, especially if there is a history of multiple surgical procedures.

Two types of impaired gas handling that have been studied are self-restrained anal gas evacuation and impaired intestinal propulsion [7]. Incomplete anal relaxation during straining may lead to gas retention in some patients.

Changes in Abdominal Wall Activity

The shape of the abdominal cavity is defined by the vertebral column, the diaphragm, and the anterolateral musculature [6]. Whorwell *et al.* studied changes in abdominal distension extensively, using the technology of abdominal inductance plethysmography [22,23] and found that posture effects abdominal girth. Sullivan found that patients whose primary complaint was abdominal distension tend to have weak abdominal muscles [24]. Alternatively, changes in the relative positioning of the walls can change the shape of the abdomen (causing distension), even in the absence of changes in intra-abdominal contents.

Increased Gas Ingestion

Swallowing air, or aerophagia, is another means of having excessive gas in the gastrointestinal tract. Swallowing small amounts air occurs regularly when eating or drinking; however, in some patients, excessive air intake may lead to symptoms of belching, bloating, and abdominal distension. A link between some anxiety conditions and aerophagia has been suggested and must be further explored [25]. Ingestion of carbonated beverages is another method of adding increased amounts of gas into the intestinal tract. In some patients, attempts to alleviate upper abdominal bloating through belching actually results in aspiration of additional air, causing a vicious cycle [26].

Altered Sensation

A very challenging problem in the case of gas and bloating is visceral hyperalgesia. In this situation, the patient may have normal amounts of gas dynamics in the gut, but the patient interprets events in the gut in an abnormal fashion so they have the sensation of excessive gas or distension. In patients with irritable bowel syndrome (IBS), gas infusion into the small intestine produce sensations at an earlier volume compared to controls [27].

Relationship to Functional GI Disorders

High percentages of patients with functional disorders report bloating as a symptom. Furthermore, patients suffering from more than one functional disorder are more likely to report bloating as a symptom. A majority of patients complaining of bloating are ultimately diagnosed with a functional GI disorder [3]. For instance, 75–96% of patients with IBS report bloating as a symptom [24,28].

Often, the area and type of abdominal discomfort/bloating relates to the type of functional bowel disease. As would be expected, in patients suffering from functional dyspepsia, bloating tends to be more situated in the upper abdominal area [29]. This is in contrast to the periumbilical bloating that a patient with IBS might experience.

Diagnostic Evaluation for Gas and Bloating Patients (Table 23.2)

Radiographic

A non-invasive procedure to test for high gas volume is plain abdominal radiographs using computed radiography. In a study by Koide *et al.*, IBS patients had consistently higher gas volume scores (GVS) than the normal control group [30]. Furthermore, longer colonic transit times were observed in constipated patients in the GVS high score group, versus patients with diarrhea or alternating symptoms.

Table 23.2 Diagnostic workup for gas and bloating.

Category	Diagnostic testing
Excessive fermentation	Lactose breath test/tolerance test
	Fructose breath test
	Lactulose/glucose breath test
	Small bowel culture?
Poor gas clearance	Radiographic studies
	Motility studies (e.g., gastric emptying, small bowel motility)
	Scleroderma
Aerophagia	Video-fluoroscopic assessment
	Evaluation of postnasal drip
	Investigation of rhinolaryngeal problems
Altered sensation	Rectal barostat (not routine clinical test)

Breath Test/Small Bowel Culture

Small bowel culture has been suggested to be the best method to evaluating bacterial overgrowth. The current standard ($>10^5$ cfu) was derived from a study of Billroth II patients, who cannot truly be considered "normal" patients in this context. A much debated, recent study by Posserud et al. demonstrated through small bowel culture of aspirates that, though below the commonly utilized definition of small intestinal bacterial overgrowth (SIBO) as more than 10^5 colonic bacteria/mL, patients with irritable bowel syndrome have elevated coliform counts when compared to healthy controls [31]. A gold standard test for SIBO is necessary, but has been yet to be developed. Difficulties in quantification arise from the large variety of enteric bacteria, many of which are obligate anaerobes and cannot be cultured with current methods.

Breath tests are an indirect, non-invasive method of testing a patient for SIBO. They are based on the assumption that higher bacterial levels result in a greater volume of certain gases, mainly hydrogen and methane. Debates around breath testing revolve around the lack of a uniform testing methods as well as the inability to specify a gold standard to distinguish normal subjects from those with overgrowth [32].

Approximately half of the hydrogen evacuated is via breath excretion [33], allowing for breath testing. The two most commonly used types of breath tests for small intestinal bacterial overgrowth are the glucose and lactulose breath tests. Patients with positive breath tests have been found to respond to antibiotic treatment, particularly when accompanied by a normalization of breath test results [34], further correlating breath testing and bacterial agents although the relationship remains controversial.

The glucose test is based on the fact that glucose is mostly absorbed in the small bowel, so all gas production can be assumed to be from small bowel flora. On the other hand, the lactulose breath test uses specific time points to distinguish small bowel and colonic fermentation. As a result, the glucose breath test is highly specific for the small bowel, while the lactulose breath test is highly sensitive for overgrowth.

Lactose and Fructose Breath Testing

Lactose and fructose intolerances can be detected non-invasively by administering the substrates to the patients and then measuring breath hydrogen. For instance, lactose breath tests traditionally use 25–50 mg of lactose [35]. High volumes of hydrogen (>20 parts per million) 2–3 h following ingestion are usually indicative of fermentation of incompletely absorbed substrates by colonic bacteria.

Serologic Testing for Celiac

Celiac disease is another cause of bloating and abdominal distension. Serologic testing as well as small bowel biopsy are important tools in its diagnosis.

Aerophagia

The diagnosis of aerophagia involves observation of actual air swallowing [36].

Treatment

The treatment options for gas and bloating are listed in Table 23.3, and several are discussed below.

Antigas Agents

Conflicting evidence exists on the efficacy of activated charcoal and simethicone in the treatment of gas and bloating. Simethicone works by breaking mucus-embedded bubbles in the gastrointestinal tract, making it easier for the gas inside to clear from the patient [37]. Simethicone has been shown to improve gas-related complaints of the upper gastrointestinal tract at significantly higher rates than placebo [37]. Interestingly, in some patients with gas-related symptoms associated with

Table 23.3 Treatment for gas and bloating.

Category	Treatment
Excessive fermentation	Food avoidance (lactose, fructose)
	Antibiotics (neomycin, rifaximin)
	Discontinue probiotics
	Gluten free diet (celiac disease)
Poor gas clearance	Surgery in cases of mechanical causes
	Prokinetics (erythromycin)
Increased gas ingestion	Avoid carbonated beverages
	Biofeedback for air swallowing
Altered sensation	Tricyclic antidepressants
Reduce existing gas	Simethicone
	Activated charcoal

acute diarrhea, a combination treatment of loperamide (a commonly used antidiarrheal agent) and simethicone resulted in faster relief of both diarrheal and gas-related symptoms than either agent taken separately [38].

The over-the-counter antigas agent Beano (α-galactosidase) has been shown to reduce flatus volume and frequency in patients with high-fiber diets, but as it does not resolve intestinal mechanical issues it has no effect on bloating or abdominal pain [39].

Dietary Changes

Eliminating or reducing intake of foods that can lead to bloating may also be recommended for some patients. Particularly, reducing intake of foods that can be digested by colonic flora such as lactose, sugar free gum, wheat fiber, fat, and artificial sweeteners should be considered. Cutting down on soda or other carbonated beverages may also be beneficial to some patients suffering mainly from upper gastrointestinal bloating and excess gas.

Prokinetics and Spasmolytics

Though mild exercise has been found to improve gas transit, resulting in alleviation of some bloating and distension [40], treatments targeting movement of the gut musculature produce more consistently effective results.

Prokinetics operate by stimulating gut propulsion. In a study observing patients with functional bowel disorders (functional bloating and IBS) versus controls, Caldarella et al. found that increased gas retention in functional bowel patients resolved with the administration of neostigmine, a prokinetic. Furthermore, this passage of retained gas correlated with improvement of abdominal distension and bloating-related symptoms [41].

Tegaserod, a 5-HT$_4$ receptor partial agonist, has been shown to be effective in treating symptoms of abdominal pain and bloating, especially in patients with constipation-predominant irritable bowel syndrome [42]. Unfortunately, due to potential, rare cardiovascular events, the product was discontinued by regulatory agencies in many countries around the world in 2007.

Antibiotics

Antibiotics have been shown to facilitate improvement of bloating and symptoms of IBS. Particularly, rifaximin [43] and neomycin [34] have been shown to correlate with symptom improvement in non-constipation predominant and constipation-predominant IBS. In addition, symptom improvement correlated with normalization of breath testing.

Erythromycin, a macrolide antibiotic, has been shown to facilitate gastric emptying and alleviate postprandial bloating in patients with functional dyspepsia [44].

Probiotics

Probiotics are live or attenuated bacterial products that are purported to improve the host's intestinal microbial balance. The challenge with probiotics is the lack of convincing data in the treatment of bloating. In fact, some argue that bloating is a side effect of probiotics. Due to the complexities of population variety of gut microbiota, each probiotic strain must be evaluated individually.

To date, the best-described probiotic in the treatment of functional bowel disease is using a particular strain of Bifidobacterium. While two studies have been conducted in double blind fashion, only one study utilized an encapsulated version of the organism which is available commercially. In this study Whorwell et al. demonstrated that Bifidobacterium at a dose of 1×10^8 was the most effective for relief of IBS and bloating [45].

Conclusion

The pathophysiologies behind gas, bloating, and distension are multifactorial. Further complicating the establishing the underlying cause of gas and bloating in a particular patient is the relationship of these symptoms to the balance of enteric flora. An understanding of the relationships between structure, function, and the constituent bacteria of the gut is needed in order to establish a diagnosis. While there are empiric therapies for gas and bloating, a better approach is to seek an underlying mechanism for the symptoms. Treating the underlying mechanism for these symptoms is likely to lead to greater patient satisfaction and long-term benefits.

Take-home points

Diagnosis:
- The diagnosis of the underlying causes of bloating and distension is difficult since causes can be multifactorial.
- It is important to rule out celiac disease and other serious GI conditions, especially in high-risk subgroups.

Therapy:

- Ultimately, the underlying cause of the symptoms will determine the correct course of treatment.
- If environmental factors appear to be the cause, over-the-counter antigas agents can be used to temporarily alleviate symptoms. Dietary changes will have to be instituted to avoid recurrence of symptoms.
- Prokinetics and spasmolytics aid in stimulating gut propulsion, which may accelerate evacuation of excess gas.
- Antibiotic treatment has been shown to alleviate bloating symptoms. Probiotics are another method of regulating intestinal flora, but much evaluation still has to be conducted as to their efficacy.

References

1 Suarez F, Furne J, Springfield J, Levitt M. Insights into human colonic physiology obtained from the study of flatus composition. *Am J Physiol* 1997; **272**: G1028–33.

2 Moore JG, Jessop LD, Osborne DN. Gas-chromatographic and mass-spectrometric analysis of the odor of human feces. *Gastroenterology* 1987; **93**: 1321–9.

3 Lea R, Whorwell PJ. Expert commentary—bloating, distension, and the irritable bowel syndrome. *Med Gen Med* 2005; **7**: 18.

4 Drossman DA, Li Z, Andruzzi E, *et al.* US Householder survey of functional gastrointestinal disorders. *Dig Dis Sci* 1993; **38**: 1569–80.

5 Thompson WG, Longstreth GF, Drossman DA, *et al.* Functional bowel disorders and functional abdominal pain. *Gut* 1999; **45**: ii43–7.

6 Azpiroz F, Malagelada JR. Abdominal bloating. *Gastroenterology* 2005; **129**: 1060–78.

7 Serra J, Azpiroz F, Malagelada JR. Mechanisms of intestinal gas retention in humans: impaired propulsion versus obstructed evacuation. *Am J Physiol Gastrointest Liver Physiol* 2001; **281**: G138–43.

8 Serra J, Azpiroz F, Malagelada JR. Intestinal gas dynamics and tolerance in humans. *Gastroenterology* 1998; **115**: 542–50.

9 Chang L, Lee OY, Naliboff B, *et al.* Sensation of bloating and visible abdominal distension in patients with irritable bowel syndrome. *Am J Gastroenterol* 2001; **96**: 3341–7.

10 Levitt MD, Ingelfinger FJ. Hydrogen and methane production in man. *Ann NY Acad Sci* 1968; **150**: 75–81.

11 Scrimshaw NS, Murray EB. The acceptability of milk and milk products in populations with a high prevalence of lactose intolerance. *Am J Clin Nutr* 1988; **48** (4 Suppl.): 1079–159.

12 Suarez FL, Savaiano DA, Levitt M. A comparison of symptoms after the consumption of milk or lactose-hydrolyzed milk by people with self-reported severe lactose intolerance. *N Engl J Med* 1995; **333**: 1–4.

13 Suarez FL, Savaiano D, Arbisi P, Levitt MD. Tolerance to the daily ingestion of two cups of milk by individuals claiming lactose intolerance. *Am J Clin Nutr* 1997; **65**: 1502–6.

14 Skoog SM, Bharucha AE. Dietary fructose and gastrointestinal symptoms: a review. *Am J Gastroenterol* 2004; **99**: 2046–50.

15 Pimentel M, Mayer AG, Park S, *et al.* Methane production during lactulose breath test is associated with gastrointestinal disease presentation. *Dig Dis Sci* 2003; **48**: 86–92.

16 Lin HC, Pimentel M, Chen JH. Intestinal transit is slowed by luminal methane. *Neurogastroenterol Motil* 2002; **4**: 437.

17 Flourie B, Pellier P, Florent C, *et al.* Site and substrates for methane production in human colon. *Am J Physiol* 1991; **260**: G752–7.

18 Kajs TM, Fitzgerald JA, Buckner RY, *et al.* Influence of a methanogenic flora on the breath H2 and symptom response to ingestion of sorbitol or oat fiber. *Am J Gastroenterol* 1997; **92**: 89–94.

19 Oelgeschlager E, Rother M. Carbon monoxide-dependent energy metabolism in anaerobic bacteria and archaea. *Arch Microbiol* 2008; **190**: 257–69.

20 Forster RE. Physiological basis of gas exchange in the gut. *Ann N Y Acad Sci* 1968; **150**: 4–12.

21 Pogrund RS, Steggerda FR. Influence of gaseous transfer between the colon and blood stream on percentage gas compositions of intestinal flatus in man. *Am J Physiol* 1948; **153**: 475–82.

22 Lewis MJV, Reilly B, Houghton LA, Whorwell PJ. Ambulatory abdominal inductance plethysmography: towards objective assessment of abdominal distension in irritable bowel syndrome. *Gut* 2001; **48**: 216–20.

23 Houghton LA, Lea R, Agrawal A, Reilly B, Whorwell PJ. Relationship of abdominal bloating to distention in irritable bowel syndrome and effect of bowel habit. *Gastroenterology* 2006; **131**: 1003–10.

24 Sullivan SN. A prospective study of unexplained visible abdominal bloating. *N Z Med J* 1994; **107**: 428–30.

25 Chitkara DK, Bredenoord AJ, Rucker MJ, Talley NJ. Aerophagia in adults: a comparison with functional dyspepsia. *Ailment Pharmacol Ther* 2005; **22**: 855–8.

26 Bond JH, Levitt MD. Gaseousness and intestinal gas. *Med Clin North Am* 1978; **62**: 155–64.

27 Agrawal A, Houghton LA, Lea R, *et al.* Bloating and distention in the irritable bowel syndrome: the role of visceral sensation. *Gastroenterology* 2008; **134**: 1882–9.

28 Lembo T, Naliboff B, Munakata J, *et al.* Symptoms and visceral perception in patients with pain-predominant irritable bowel syndrome. *Am J of Gastoenterol* 1999; **94**: 1320–6.

29 Jiang X, Locke III, GR, Choung RS, *et al.* Prevalence and risk factors for abdominal bloating and visible distention: a population-based study. *Gut* 2008; **57**: 756–63.

30 Koide A, Yamaguchi T, Odaka T, *et al.* Quantitative analysis of bowel gas using plain abdominal radiograph in patients with irritable bowel syndrome. *Am J Gastoenterol* 2000; **95**: 1735–41.

31 Posserud I, Stotzer PO, Bjornsson ES, *et al.* Small intestinal bacterial overgrowth in patients with irritable bowel syndrome. *Gut* 2007; **56**: 802–8.

32 Khoshini R, Dai SC, Lezcano S, Pimentel M. A systematic review of diagnostic tests for small intestinal bacterial overgrowth. *Dig Dis Sci* 2008; **53**: 1443–54.

33 King TS, Elia M, Hunger JO. Abnormal colonic fermentation in irritable bowel syndrome. *Lancet* 1998; **352**: 1187–9.

34 Pimentel M, Chow EJ, Lin HC. Normalization of lactulose breath testing correlates with symptom improvement in irritable bowel syndrome: a double-blind, randomized, placebo-controlled study. *Am J Gastoenterol* 2003; **98**: 412–9.

35 Romagnuolo J, Schiller D, Bailey RJ. Using breath tests wisely in a gastroenterology practice: An evidence-based review of indications and pitfalls in interpretation. *Am J Gastoenterol* 2002; **97**: 1113–26.

36 Tack J, Talley NJ, Camiller M *et al.* Functional gastroduodenal disorders. *Gastroenterology* 2006; **130**: 1466–79.

37 Bernstein JE, Kasich AM. A double-blind trial of simethicone in functional disease of the upper gastrointestinal tract. *J Clin Pharmacol* 1974; **14**: 617–23.

38 Kaplan MA, Prior MJ, Ash RR, *et al.* Loperamide-simethicone vs loperamide alone, simethicone alone, and placebo in the treatment of acute diarrhea with gas-related abdominal discomfort. *Arch Fam Med* 1999; **8**: 243–8.

39 Ganiats TG, Norcross WA, Halverson AL, *et al.* Does Beano prevent gas? A double-blind crossover study of oral alpha-galactosidase to treat dietary oligosaccharide tolerance. *J Fam Pract* 1994; **39**: 441–5.

40 Villoria A, Serra J, Azpiroz F, Malagelada JR. Physical activity and intestinal gas clearance in patients with bloating. *Am J Gastroenterol* 2006; **101**: 2552–7.

41 Caldarella MP, Serra J, Azpiroz F, Malagelada J-R. Prokinetic effects in patients with intestinal gas retention. *Gastroenterology* 2002; **122**: 1748–55.

42 Muller-Lissner SA, Fumagalli I, Bardhan KD, *et al.* Tegaserod, a 5-HT$_4$ receptor partial agonist, relieves symptoms in irritable bowel syndrome patients with abdominal pain, bloating and constipation. *Ailment Pharmacol Ther* 2001; **15**: 1655–66.

43 Pimentel M, Park S, Mirocha J, *et al.* The effect of a nonabsorbed oral antibiotic (rifaximin) on the symptoms of the irritable bowel syndrome. *Ann Intern Med* 2006; **145**: 557–63.

44 Arts J, Caenepeel P, Verbeke K, Tack J. Influence of erythromycin on gastric emptying and meal related symptoms in functional dyspepsia with delayed gastric emptying. *Gut* 2005; **54**: 455–60.

45 Whorwell PJ, Altringer L, Morel J, *et al.* Efficacy of an encapsulated probiotic *Bifidobacterium infantis* 35624 in women with irritable bowel syndrome. *Am J Gastroenterol* 2006; **101**: 1581–90.

CHAPTER 24

Obesity and Presentations after Anti-obesity Surgery

Patrick Gatmaitan, Stacy A. Brethauer, and Philip R. Schauer

Bariatric and Metabolic Institute, Cleveland Clinic, Cleveland, OH, USA

Summary

Over one-third of the US population is obese and this public health problem has reached epidemic proportions in industrialized countries throughout the world. The prevalence of type 2 diabetes and other obesity-related co-morbidities has increased dramatically over the last decade as well. Medical and behavioral therapies are not effective long-term treatments for patient with severe obesity and, currently, bariatric surgery is the only therapy that provides the massive weight loss that is durable.

There has been a dramatic increase in the number of bariatric procedures performed worldwide over the last decade. Despite the high-risk nature of this patient population, the risk–benefit analysis for surgery is favorable for the majority of patients who seek bariatric surgery. This review will discuss the indications for bariatric surgery and outcomes of commonly performed procedures.

Case

A 48-year-old female presents with morbid obesity with a body mass index of 45 kg/m² (height 5 foot 1 inch, weight 238 lbs). She has been obese since adolescence and has failed multiple attempts at weight loss with supervised diets and exercise. She also has diabetes mellitus, hypertension on two medications, hyperlipidemia, gastroesophageal reflux disease, and sleep apnea. She was evaluated at a bariatric center of excellence program and underwent laparoscopic Roux-en-Y gastric bypass. Two months after surgery, she developed progressive dysphagia and was diagnosed with a stricture at her gastrojejunostomy that was successfully treated with a single endoscopic balloon dilation. No other complications occurred. One year after surgery, she has lost a total of 36 kg (80 lbs) (corresponding to 60% excess weight loss, BMI 30), is euglycemic off medication with a glycosylated hemoglobin of 5.9, no longer requires continuous positive airway pressure (CPAP) machine, has no heartburn, and is only on a single agent for hypertension.

Practical Gastroenterology and Hepatology: Small and Large Intestine and Pancreas, 1st edition. Edited by Nicholas J. Talley, Sunanda V. Kane and Michael B. Wallace. © 2010 Blackwell Publishing Ltd.

Introduction

Obesity can be defined as a body mass index (BMI, calculated as weight in kilograms divided by the square of height in meters) of above 30 kg/m². It has become a major global health problem with 1.6 billion adults overweight and at least 400 million obese. The latest National Health and Nutrition Examination Survey (NHANES) reported that one-third of the adult American population is obese. The problem can be expected to worsen with the increasing incidence of childhood and adolescent obesity [1].

Obesity affects almost every organ system in the body and increases the risk of numerous diseases including type 2 diabetes mellitus, hypertension, dyslipidemia, cardiovascular disease, and cancer (Table 24.1). Increased severity of obesity correlates with a higher prevalence of the associated co-morbidities [2]. Likewise, obesity increases the risk of premature mortality [3]. It is estimated that a man in his twenties with a BMI over 45 will have a 22% reduction (13 years) in life expectancy [4].

Table 24.1 Co-morbidities associated with obesity.

Cardiovascular
    hypertension, hyperlipidemia, coronary artery disease, left ventricular
        hypertrophy, heart failure, venous stasis, thrombophlebitis
	Genitourinary
	    stress urinary incontinence, urinary tract infections

Pulmonary
    obstructive sleep apnea, asthma, obesity hypoventilation syndrome
	Obstetric/gynecologic
	    infertility, miscarriage, fetal abnormalities

Endocrine
    insulin resistance, type 2 diabetes, polycystic ovarian syndrome
	Musculoskeletal
	    degenerative joint disease, gout, plantar fasciitis, carpal tunnel
	        syndrome

Hematopoietic
    deep venous thrombosis, pulmonary embolism
	Neurologic/psychiatric
	    stroke, pseudotumor cerebri, migraine headaches, depression,
	        anxiety

Gastrointestinal
    gall stones, gastroesophageal reflux disease, abdominal hernia
	Increased cancer risk
	    endometrial, ovarian, breast, prostate, kidney, liver, esophagus,
	        colon, pancreas

Management Options

Non-surgical strategies for weight loss include diet, physical activity, behavior therapy, and pharmacotherapy with the initial goal of 10% weight loss over a 6-month period (calorie deficit of 500–1000 kcal/day for weight loss of 0.5–1 kg/week (1–2 lb/week)). This 5–10% weight loss affords some short-term benefit but the results are not durable. Currently, bariatric surgery is the only effective and durable treatment for morbid obesity [5].

In 1991, the National Institutes of Health set forth the guidelines for weight loss surgery to treat morbid obesity [6,7]. Bariatric surgery is appropriate for the carefully selected patients with clinically severe obesity (BMI $\geq$ 40 or $\geq$35 with co-morbid conditions) when less invasive methods of weight loss have failed and the patient is at high risk for obesity-associated morbidity or mortality.

Weight-loss Procedures

The two most commonly performed weight-loss procedures today in the United States are laparoscopic Roux-en-Y gastric bypass (LRYGB) and laparoscopic adjustable gastric banding (LAGB). Other bariatric operations include vertical banded gastroplasty (VBG), sleeve gastrectomy, biliopancreatic diversion (BPD), and duodenal switch (DS) (Figure 24.1).

Restrictive procedures such as LAGB create a small gastric pouch with a narrow outlet that restricts the amount of food that the patient can eat at one time. Approved for use in the United States in 2001, the LAGB is a silastic ring with an inflatable inner balloon. The size of the inner diameter is adjusted by adding or removing fluid through a subcutaneous port. The adjustable nature of the LAGB is a major advantage over previous non-adjustable bands and the degree of gastric restriction can be titrated to minimize side effects and maximize weight loss. Vertical banded gastroplasty was developed in 1980 but is now rarely performed. Long-term weight loss was generally poor and many patients developed complications such as staple line failure or band stenosis that required re-operation [8–12].

Malabsorptive procedures bypass a long segment of the small intestine to limit caloric absorption. Biliopancreatic diversion and its modification, duodenal switch, are technically demanding to perform and have a higher incidence of nutritional deficiencies compared to other procedures. As such, they only account for about 5% of the bariatric procedures performed in the United States.

Roux-en-Y gastric bypass creates a small gastric pouch (15–30 mL) that limits food intake. The proximal intestine is bypassed with a Roux limb (typically 75–150 cm long). More than 90% of the small bowel is left intact so malabsorptive side effects such as diarrhea and protein malnutrition are rare. RYGB accounts for approximately 80% of all bariatric surgeries in the United States.

Open gastric bypass was first performed by Mason in 1967 [13] and has been modified over the past four decades to eliminate bile gastritis and reduce the inci-

Restrictive procedures

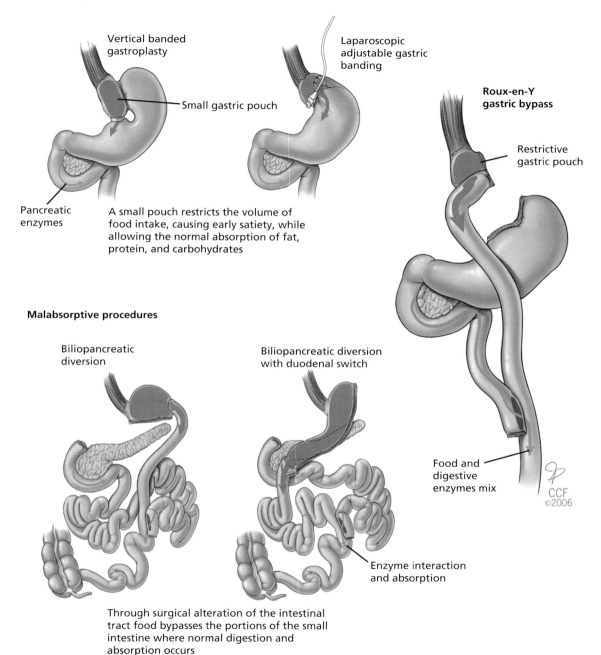

Vertical banded gastroplasty

Small gastric pouch

Laparoscopic adjustable gastric banding

Roux-en-Y gastric bypass

Restrictive gastric pouch

Pancreatic enzymes

A small pouch restricts the volume of food intake, causing early satiety, while allowing the normal absorption of fat, protein, and carbohydrates

Malabsorptive procedures

Biliopancreatic diversion

Biliopancreatic diversion with duodenal switch

Food and digestive enzymes mix

Enzyme interaction and absorption

Through surgical alteration of the intestinal tract food bypasses the portions of the small intestine where normal digestion and absorption occurs

Figure 24.1 Different weight-loss operations. Reprinted with the permission of The Cleveland Clinic Center for Medical Art & Photography © 2008. All rights reserved.

dence of marginal ulcers and staple-line disruption. LRYGB was introduced in 1994 [14] and since then, several studies have been published comparing open and laparoscopic gastric bypass [15–23]. Laparoscopic surgery results in less postoperative pain, earlier return of normal pulmonary function, faster return to normal daily activities, and fewer incisional wound infections and hernias.

Complications of Laparoscopic Gastric Bypass

Postoperative complications following LRYGB can be categorized into early and late postoperative complications. Early postoperative complications include anastomotic leak, hemorrhage, thromboembolic events, and wound infection. Late postoperative complications include anastomotic stricture, marginal ulcer, bowel obstruction, abdominal hernia, and micronutrient and vitamin deficiency.

Anastomotic leaks occur less than 5% of the time after LRYGB. Most large series report leak rates of 1–2%. The most common site is at the gastrojejunostomy followed by the jejunojejunostomy. Persistent tachycardia (>120 bpm), tachypnea, or hypoxia should alert the clinician to look for a leak even when other symptoms or laboratory abnormalities are absent.

Pulmonary embolism after LRYGB occurs 1% of the time but is highly lethal when it occurs in these patients with little pulmonary reserve. The complication accounts for 30–50% of all deaths after gastric bypass.

Bleeding complications occur in fewer than 4% of patients. Postoperative bleeding can be from mesenteric or omental vessels within the peritoneal cavity or from an anastomosis or staple line.

Marginal ulceration occurs at the gastrojejunostomy less than 5% of the time after laparoscopic gastric bypass and is associated with ischemia at the anastomosis, smoking, excessive acid exposure (gastrogastric fistula), non-steroidal anti-inflammatory use, foreign material at the anastomosis such as non-absorbable suture, and *H. pylori* infection. This complication typically occurs within 2 months after surgery but can occur years later. Treatment includes removing the inciting factor, sucralfate, and acid suppression.

Other late complications of RYGB include bowel obstruction and anastomotic stricture. Bowel obstruc-

tion after LRYGB is most commonly secondary to an internal hernia. Patients who develop internal hernias may not present with the typical symptoms of abdominal bloating and vomiting seen with an adhesive obstruction and may only report intermittent crampy abdominal pain. The incidence of gastrojejunal stricture is 5–10% and varies with the technique used to create the anastomosis [24]. The use of a circular stapler, particularly the 21-mm size, is associated with higher stricture rates than other techniques [25,26]. This complication is easily managed with endoscopic dilation [27,28].

Weight loss following gastric bypass is accompanied by increased incidence of cholelithiasis: 38–52% of patients develop stones within 1 year of surgery [29]. Between 15 and 28% of all patients require urgent cholecystectomy within 3 years. This incidence can be reduced by using ursodiol for 6 months postoperatively.

Complications of Laparoscopic Adjustable Gastric Banding

Early, major postoperative complications following LAGB are rare and include bleeding (0.1%), iatrogenic bowel perforation (0.5%), deep venous thrombosis (0.1%), and pulmonary embolism (0.1%) [30,31].

Band-related complications can occur in the early or late postoperative period. Among 8504 patients studied by Chapman *et al.* [32] tube or port malfunction requiring reoperation occurred in 1.7% of cases, band erosion into the gastric lumen occurred in 0.6% of patients, and pouch dilation or band slippage occurred in 5.6%. Overall, complications requiring an operation can occur in up to 18% of patients.

Mortality Risk

In Buchwald's recent systematic review of 85 048 patients [33], overall 30-day perioperative mortality rate after bariatric surgery was 0.28% while total mortality at later than 30 days was 0.35%. Laparoscopic restrictive procedures carried a 0.07% 30-day mortality rate compared to 0.16% for laparoscopic restrictive/malabsorptive (gastric bypass), and 1.11% for laparoscopic malabsorptive procedures.

Weight Loss

Weight loss after bariatric surgery is typically expressed as the percentage of excess weight lost (excess weight defined as the number of pounds above the patient's ideal body weight). In Buchwald's meta-analysis [5], excess weight loss for all bariatric procedures combined was 61%. Excess weight loss was greatest with BPD (70%), followed by gastric bypass (62%), and gastric banding (48%).

Resolution of Co-morbidities

In Buchwald's meta-analysis of 22094 patients in 2004 [5], diabetes was completely resolved in 77% of patients, hyperlipidemia improved in 70% or more of patients, hypertension resolved in 62%, and obstructive sleep apnea resolved in 86% of patients. Several co-morbidities are likewise dramatically improved or resolved (Figure 24.2). Remission of diabetes occurred more frequently after bypass procedures compared to restrictive procedures.

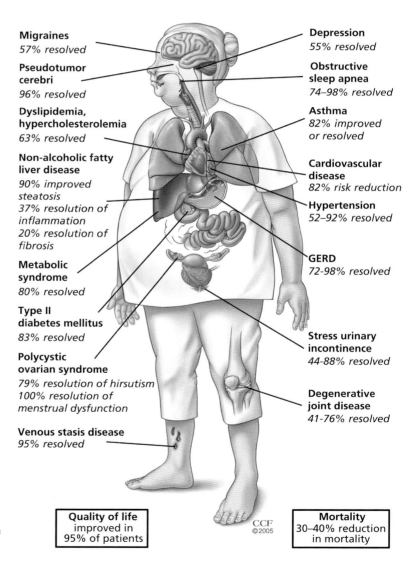

Migraines
57% resolved

Pseudotumor cerebri
96% resolved

Dyslipidemia, hypercholesterolemia
63% resolved

Non-alcoholic fatty liver disease
90% improved steatosis
37% resolution of inflammation
20% resolution of fibrosis

Metabolic syndrome
80% resolved

Type II diabetes mellitus
83% resolved

Polycystic ovarian syndrome
79% resolution of hirsutism
100% resolution of menstrual dysfunction

Venous stasis disease
95% resolved

Depression
55% resolved

Obstructive sleep apnea
74–98% resolved

Asthma
82% improved or resolved

Cardiovascular disease
82% risk reduction

Hypertension
52–92% resolved

GERD
72-98% resolved

Stress urinary incontinence
44-88% resolved

Degenerative joint disease
41-76% resolved

Quality of life improved in 95% of patients

CCF
©2005

Mortality 30–40% reduction in mortality

Figure 24.2 Benefits of bariatric surgery [16,19,20,34–40]. GERD, gastroesophageal reflux disease. Reprinted with the permission of The Cleveland Clinic Center for Medical Art & Photography © 2008. All rights reserved.

Mortality Reduction

In 2007, two separate studies reported a significant reduction in the long-term mortality after bariatric surgery. The prospective, controlled Swedish Obese Subjects study involving 4047 obese subjects (2010 surgery patients vs. 2037 matched control subjects), with a mean follow-up of 10.9 years and 99.9% follow-up rate, demonstrated a 29% reduction in the adjusted mortality rate following bariatric surgery [34]. Adams *et al.* performed a retrospective cohort study of 7925 surgical patients matched with 7925 severely obese control subjects with a mean follow-up of 7.1 years. The adjusted long-term mortality from any cause decreased by 40% following gastric bypass whereas cause-specific mortality decreased by 56% for coronary artery disease, by 92% for diabetes, and by 60% for cancer [35].

Conclusion

The prevalence of obesity and diabetes is increasing dramatically in the United States and worldwide. Bariatric surgery is currently the only effective and durable therapy for obesity and results in complete remission or improvement in all major obesity-related co-morbidities. The majority of bariatric procedures are performed laparoscopically and the two most commonly performed, laparoscopic adjustable gastric banding and gastric bypass, can be performed with low complication rates.

Take-home points

- The prevalence of obesity has markedly increased in the United States and worldwide; one-third of adult Americans are obese.

- Bariatric surgery remains the only therapy that affords significant and durable weight loss.

- Weight loss following bariatric surgery is associated with improvement and resolution of multiple co-morbidities and reduction in long-term mortality.

- When performed in experienced centers bariatric surgery is associated with low complication rates.

- Perioperative mortality rates after laparoscopic bariatric procedures have declined significantly in the last decade and are comparable to many other elective operations.

References

1 Hedley AA, Ogden CL, Johnson CL, *et al.* Prevalence of overweight and obesity among US children, adolescents, and adults, 1999–2002. *JAMA* 2004; **291**: 2847–50.

2 Must A, Spadano J, Coakley EH, *et al.* The disease burden associated with overweight and obesity. *JAMA* 1999; **282**: 1523–9.

3 Hensrud DD, Klein S. Extreme obesity: a new medical crisis in the United States. *Mayo Clin Proc* 2006; **81**: S5–10.

4 Fontaine KR, Redden DT, Wang C, *et al.* Years of life lost due to obesity. *JAMA* 2003; **289**: 187–93.

5 Buchwald H, Avidor Y, Braunwald E, *et al.* Bariatric surgery: a systematic review and meta-analysis. *JAMA* 2004; **292**: 1724–37.

6 NIH conference. Gastrointestinal surgery for severe obesity. Consensus Development Conference Panel. *Ann Intern Med* 1991; **115**: 956–61.

7 Gastrointestinal surgery for severe obesity: National Institutes of Health Consensus Development Conference Statement. *Am J Clin Nutr* 1992; **55**: 615S–9S.

8 Kim CH, Sarr MG. Severe reflux esophagitis after vertical banded gastroplasty for treatment of morbid obesity. *Mayo Clin Proc* 1992; **67**: 33–5.

9 Nightengale ML, Sarr MG, Kelly KA, *et al.* Prospective evaluation of vertical banded gastroplasty as the primary operation for morbid obesity. *Mayo Clin Proc* 1991; **66**: 773–82.

10 MacLean LD, Rhode BM, Forse RA. Late results of vertical banded gastroplasty for morbid and super obesity. *Surgery* 1990; **107**: 20–7.

11 Ramsey-Stewart G. Vertical banded gastroplasty for morbid obesity: weight loss at short and long-term follow up. *Aust N Z J Surg* 1995; **65**: 4–7.

12 Balsiger BM, Poggio JL, Mai J, *et al.* Ten and more years after vertical banded gastroplasty as primary operation for morbid obesity. *J Gastrointest Surg* 2000; **4**: 598–605.

13 Mason EE, Ito C. Gastric bypass in obesity. *Surg Clin North Am* 1967; **47**: 1345–51.

14 Wittgrove AC, Clark GW, Tremblay LJ. Laparoscopic gastric bypass, Roux-en-Y: preliminary report of five cases. *Obes Surg* 1994; **4**: 353–7.

15 Abdel-Galil E, Sabry AA. Laparoscopic Roux-en-Y gastric bypass—evaluation of three different techniques. *Obes Surg* 2002; **12**: 639–42.

16 DeMaria EJ, Sugerman HJ, Kellum JM, *et al.* Results of 281 consecutive total laparoscopic Roux-en-Y gastric bypasses to treat morbid obesity. *Ann Surg* 2002; **235**: 640–5; discussion 645–7.

17 Higa KD, Ho T, Boone KB. Laparoscopic Roux-en-Y gastric bypass: technique and 3-year follow-up. *J Laparoendosc Adv Surg Tech A* 2001; **11**: 377–82.

18 Papasavas PK, Hayetian FD, Caushaj PF, *et al.* Outcome analysis of laparoscopic Roux-en-Y gastric bypass for morbid obesity. The first 116 cases. *Surg Endosc* 2002; **16**: 1653–7.

19 Schauer PR, Ikramuddin S, Gourash W, *et al.* Outcomes after laparoscopic Roux-en-Y gastric bypass for morbid obesity. *Am J Physiol Endocrinol Metab* 2000; **232**: 515–29.

20 Wittgrove AC, Clark GW. Laparoscopic gastric bypass, Roux-en-Y- 500 patients: technique and results, with 3–60 month follow-up. *Obes Surg* 2000; **10**: 233–9.

21 Lujan JA, Frutos MD, Hernandez Q, *et al.* Laparoscopic versus open gastric bypass in the treatment of morbid obesity: a randomized prospective study. *Ann Surg* 2004; **239**: 433–7.

22 Nguyen NT, Goldman C, Rosenquist CJ, *et al.* Laparoscopic versus open gastric bypass: a randomized study of outcomes, quality of life, and costs. *Ann Surg* 2001; **234**: 279–89; discussion 289–91.

23 Westling A, Gustavsson S. Laparoscopic vs open Roux-en-Y gastric bypass: a prospective, randomized trial. *Obes Surg* 2001; **11**: 284–92.

24 Podnos YD, Jimenez JC, Wilson SE, *et al.* Complications after laparoscopic gastric bypass: a review of 3464 cases. *Arch Surg* 2003; **138**: 957–61.

25 Suggs WJ, Kouli W, Lupovici M, *et al.* Complications at gastrojejunostomy after laparoscopic Roux-en-Y gastric bypass: comparison between 21- and 25-mm circular staplers. *Surg Obes Relat Dis* 2007; **3**: 508–14.

26 Fisher BL, Atkinson JD, Cottam D. Incidence of gastroenterostomy stenosis in laparoscopic Roux-en-Y gastric bypass using 21- or 25-mm circular stapler: a randomized prospective blinded study. *Surg Obes Relat Dis* 2007; **3**: 176–9.

27 Peifer KJ, Shiels AJ, Azar R, *et al.* Successful endoscopic management of gastrojejunal anastomotic strictures after Roux-en-Y gastric bypass. *Gastrointest Endosc* 2007; **66**: 248–52.

28 Escalona A, Devaud N, Boza C, *et al.* Gastrojejunal anastomotic stricture after Roux-en-Y gastric bypass: ambulatory management with the Savary-Gilliard dilator. *Surg Endosc* 2007; **21**: 765–8.

29 Sugerman HJ, Brewer WH, Shiffman ML, *et al.* A multicenter, placebo-controlled, randomized, double-blind, prospective trial of prophylactic ursodiol for the prevention of gallstone formation following gastric-bypass-induced rapid weight loss. *Am J Surg* 1995; **169**: 91–6; discussion 96–7.

30 Belachew M, Belva PH, Desaive C. Long-term results of laparoscopic adjustable gastric banding for the treatment of morbid obesity. *Obes Surg* 2002; **12**: 564–8.

31 Biertho L, Steffen R, Ricklin T, *et al.* Laparoscopic gastric bypass versus laparoscopic adjustable gastric banding: a comparative study of 1,200 cases. *J Am Coll Surg* 2003; **197**: 536–44; discussion 544–53.

32 Chapman AE, Kiroff G, Game P, *et al.* Laparoscopic adjustable gastric banding in the treatment of obesity: a systematic literature review. *Surgery* 2004; **135**: 326–51.

33 Buchwald H, Estok R, Fahrbach K, *et al.* Trends in mortality in bariatric surgery: a systematic review and meta-analysis. *Surgery* 2007; **142**: 621–32; discussion 632–5.

34 Sjostrom L, Narbro K, Sjostrom CD, *et al.* Effects of bariatric surgery on mortality in Swedish obese subjects. *N Engl J Med* 2007; **357**: 741–52.

35 Adams TD, Gress RE, Smith SC, *et al.* Long-term mortality after gastric bypass surgery. *N Engl J Med* 2007; **357**: 753–61.

36 Christou NV, Sampalis JS, Liberman M, *et al.* Surgery decreases long-term mortality, morbidity, and health care use in morbidly obese patients. *Ann Surg* 2004; **240**: 416–23; discussion 423–4.

37 Mattar SG, Velcu LM, Rabinovitz M, *et al.* Surgically-induced weight loss significantly improves nonalcoholic fatty liver disease and the metabolic syndrome. *Ann Surg* 2005; **242**: 610–17; discussion 618–20.

38 Schauer PR, Burguera B, Ikramuddin S, *et al.* Effect of laparoscopic Roux-en Y gastric bypass on type 2 diabetes mellitus. *Ann Surg* 2003; **238**: 467–84; discussion 484–5.

39 Sugerman HJ, Felton WL, 3rd, Sismanis A, *et al.* Gastric surgery for pseudotumor cerebri associated with severe obesity. *Ann Surg* 1999; **229**: 634–40; discussion 640–2.

40 Sugerman HJ, Sugerman EL, Wolfe L, *et al.* Risks and benefits of gastric bypass in morbidly obese patients with severe venous stasis disease. *Ann Surg* 2001; **234**: 41–6.

CHAPTER 25

Assessment of Nutritional Status

English F. Barbour and Mark DeLegge

Digestive Disease Center, Medical University of South Carolina, Charleston, SC, USA

Summary

Many gastrointestinal diseases have significant nutritional consequences related to anorexia, nausea and vomiting, malabsorption, and increased metabolic demand. Proper identification of patients at nutritional risk is imperative to improve their overall clinical outcomes. The most reliable component of a proper nutritional assessment is a medical history and physical. There is no serum protein marker of malnutrition. In general, bedside, validated scoring systems are the most reliable tool for identifying patients at nutritional risk.

Definition and Epidemiology

Nutrition assessment is an important component of a patient's medical therapy. The goals of nutrition assessment include: (i) identification of patients who are malnourished or at risk of developing malnutrition; (ii) identification of a patient's degree of malnutrition; and (iii) monitoring the adequacy of nutrition therapy.

A traditional nutrition assessment will often include a dietary, medical, and body weight history. Measurements of current body weight, height, serum proteins levels, body anthropometrics measurements, and functional measurements of muscle strength may be incorporated into the overall final assessment.

Studies have consistently revealed the inadequacy of any single assessment method or tool to assess a patient's nutritional state. As a result, combinations of diverse measurements have been developed into scoring systems designed to increase the sensitivity and specificity of determining nutritional status [1]. In general, global approaches to nutrition assessment of the hospitalized patient can provide a much more definitive picture of a patient's true nutrition risk.

Practical Gastroenterology and Hepatology: Small and Large Intestine and Pancreas, 1st edition. Edited by Nicholas J. Talley, Sunanda V. Kane and Michael B. Wallace. © 2010 Blackwell Publishing Ltd.

Pathophysiology

Malnutrition is important clinically when it is severe enough to impact a patient's physiologic function, inhibit their response to medical therapy, impair protein-related metabolic functions, and/or prolong time to recovery. The physiologic devastation seen with protein–calorie malnutrition (PCM) is secondary to loss of total body protein and muscle function [2]. When more than 20% of a person's usual body weight is lost, most physiologic body functions become significantly impaired [3].

Protein malnutrition can be divided academically into two generalized categories: marasmus and kwashiorkor. Patients with marasmus have a significant deficit of total body fat and body protein with a slight increase in extracellular water. Clinically, this presents as obvious body wasting, including sunken eyes and prominent skull and cheekbones [4]. The plasma albumin is often in the low normal range. Resting energy expenditure is not increased despite any concurrent, severe physiologic dysfunction. In contrast, while patients with kwashiorkor have similar deficits of body protein and fat, they also have markedly increased extracellular fluid, low plasma albumin levels, and an accelerated metabolic rate [4].

Organ function is affected by malnutrition, as muscle strength and protein stores decrease over time. Respiratory function, including forced expiratory volume, vital capacity, and peak expiratory flow, all decline.

Malnutrition can also reduce cardiac output, impair wound healing, and depress immune function [5]. Nutritional repletion, however, can often reverse these processes and significantly improve patient outcomes.

Clinical Features

Weight History

Recent weight loss is a very sensitive marker of a patient's nutritional status. Weight loss of more than 5% in 1 month or 10% in 6 months prior to hospitalization has been shown to be clinically significant [6]. When 20% of usual body weight has been lost in 6 months or less, severe physiologic dysfunction occurs. Patient's who are obese, or those with edema, may be very difficult to nutritionally assess solely relying upon their body size or body weight.

Obtaining a patient's weight in the inpatient or outpatient setting should be a common and easily performed process. It is important that clinicians obtain a measured weight as recalled weights are much less accurate. Numerous studies have documented huge variances in reported weights when a patient's own weight recall is used as the sole determining factor, with sensitivities as low as 65% [7].

Anthropometrics

Anthropometrics is the scientific study of measurements of the human body. Estimates of body energy stores can be obtained by measurement of body compartments. Anthropometrics is used as a bedside method of estimating body fat and protein stores using two bedside instruments: a Lange caliper and a tape measure (Figure 25.1). The measurements obtained from anthropometrics are compared to reference ranges for the normal population and also followed in the same patient over time. A drawback of anthropometrics is its reliance on age-, sex- and race-matched reference values. Additionally, because muscle mass is somewhat dependent on exercise, bedridden patients can have decreased muscle mass without a corresponding reduction in body protein stores.

Inaccurate measurements of body protein and fat stores using anthropometric methods are common in certain patient populations. For example, critically ill patients, or those with liver and/or renal disease often present with total body water increase and significant

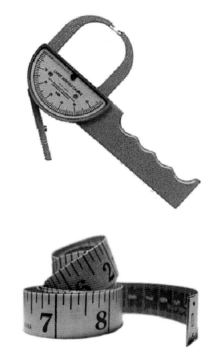

Figure 25.1 Bedside anthropometric tools: Lange calipers and tape measure.

edema. There is also significant variance among clinicians measuring anthropometrics in the same patient.

The measurement of the triceps skinfold (TSF) with a Lange caliper has been recognized as an indirect marker of body fat stores. The measurement of the circumference of the mid-point of the upper arm using a tape measure or mid-arm muscle circumference (MAMC) has also been recognized as an indirect marker of body protein stores. From the MAMC the mid-arm muscle area (MAMA) can be calculated with the following equation

$$MAMA = \left\{ \left(MAMC - (3.14 \times TSF)^2 \right) / 4 \times 3.14 \right) \right\}$$
$$(\text{in millimeters})$$

The minimum MAMA known to be compatible with survival is between $900\,mm^2$ and $1200\,mm^2$ [8].

Plasma Proteins

Plasma proteins, such as albumin, prealbumin, transferrin, ferritin, and retinol binding protein, have all been used as nutritional markers. The serum concentrations of albumin and other plasma proteins are affected by a patient's total body water status, liver function, physiologic status, and renal losses; therefore they should be considered markers of a patient's overall health status rather than a true nutritional marker.

Direct Measurements of Body Physiologic Function

Direct measurements of body functions can be used as markers of the degree and significance of malnutrition. For example, skeletal muscle function can be rapidly affected by malnutrition regardless of other major disease processes such as sepsis, trauma, or renal failure [9].

In the patient who is able to follow commands, handgrip strength can be measured by the use of a bedside tool known as a handgrip dynamometer (Figure 25.2). Hospitalized patients with poor grip strength have been shown to have an increase in hospital length of stay, reduced ability to return home, and increased mortality [11]. Patients with upper arm and/or hand injuries or other abnormalities can not produce a reliable grip strength analysis. In critically ill patients who are not able to follow commands, bedside muscle function can still

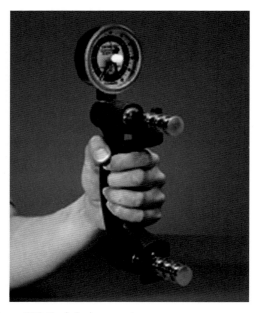

Figure 25.2 Handgrip dynamometer.

be tested. Stimulation of the ulnar nerve at the wrist with measurement of contraction of the abductor pollicus longus has been standardized [10].

Scoring Systems

There is no one test or marker which exists to accurately identify all patients who are malnourished or at nutritional risk. Therefore scoring systems have been developed that combine history, physical, and laboratory information.

The Subjective Global Assessment (SGA) is practical and reliable tool used for nutrition assessment. It includes a dietary and medical history, a functional assessment, and a physical examination (Figure 25.3) [12]. An SGA (A) level is designated as a minimal change in food intake, a minimal change in body function, and a steady body weight. An SGA (B) level consists of clear evidence of decreased food intake with some physiologic functional changes, but no significant change in body weight. An SGA (C) level consists of a significant decrease in body weight and food intake along with a reduction in physiologic function.

Other well used scoring systems or tools include the Mini-Nutritional Assessment [13], Nutrition Risk Score [14], Nutritional Risk Index [15], Malnutrition Universal Screening Tool [16], Geriatric Nutritional Risk Index [17], and the Instant Nutritional Assessment [18].

Bioelectric Impedance

Bioelectric impedance (BIA) is a non-invasive method to determine body composition by using the difference in electrical conductivity of various body tissue components It is inexpensive, easy to perform, and reproducible. However, it may be inaccurate for patients with edema or dehydration [19].

Research Laboratory Methods of Nutritional Assessment

Various tools found in the research laboratory are available to determine body composition. These tools serve as gold standards against which bedside clinical body composition tests are compared [20]. These tools can include dual energy absorptiometry (DEXA), whole body counting/ nuclear activation, computerized axial tomography (CT) and magnetic resonance imaging (MRI), hydrodensitometry, and near-infrared

Scored Patient-Generated Subjective Global Assessment (PG-SGA)

Patient ID Information

History (Boxes 1–4 are designed to be completed by the patient.)

1. Weight (See Worksheet 1)

In summary of my current and recent weight:

I currently weight about _____ pounds
I am about _____ feet _____ tall

One month ago I weighed about _____ pounds
Six months ago I weighed about _____ pounds

During the past two weeks my weight has:

☐ Decreased (1)   ☐ Not changed (0)   ☐ Increased (0)

Box 1 _____

2. Food Intake: As compared to my normal intake, I would rate my food intake during the past month as:

☐ Unchanged (0)
☐ More than usual (0)
☐ Less than usual (1)
I am now taking:

☐ Normal food but less than normal amount (1)
☐ Little solid food (2)
☐ Only liquids (3)
☐ Only nutritonal supplements (3)
☐ Very little of anything (4)
☐ Only tube feedings or only nutrition by vein (0)

Box 2 _____

3. Symptoms: I have had the following problems that have kept me from eating enough during the past two weeks (check all that apply):

☐ No problems eating (0)
☐ No appetite, just did not feel like eating (3)
☐ Nausea (1)   ☐ Vomiting (3)
☐ Constipation (1)   ☐ Diarrhea (3)
☐ Mouth sores (2)   ☐ Dry mouth (1)
☐ Things taste funny or have no taste (1) ☐ Smells bother me (1)
☐ Problems swallowing (2)   ☐ Feel full quickly (1)
☐ Pain; where? (3) _____
☐ Other** (1) _____

** Examples: depression, money, or dental problems

Box 3 _____

4. Activities and Function: Over the past month, I would generally rate my activity as:

☐ Normal with no limitations (0)

☐ Not my normal self, but able to be up and about with fairly normal activities (1)

☐ Not feeling up to most things, but in bed or chair less than half the day (2)

☐ Able to do little activity and spend most of the day in bed or chair (3)

☐ Pretty much bedridden, rarely out of bed (3)

Box 4 _____

Additive score of the boxes 1–4 _____ A

The remainder of this form will be completed by your doctor, nurse, or therapist. Thank you.

5. Disease and its relation to nutritional requirements (see Worksheet 2)

All relevant diagnoses (specify) _____
Primary disease stage (circle if known or appropriate)   I   II   III   IV   other _____
Age _____

Numerical score from Worksheet 2 _____ B

6. Metabolic Demand (see Worksheet 3)

Numerical score from Worksheet 3 _____ C

7. Physical (see Worksheet 4)

Numerical score from Worksheet 4 _____ D

Global Assessment (see Worksheet 5)

☐ Well-nourished or anabolic (SGA-A)
☐ Moderate or suspected malnutrition (SGA-B)
☐ Severely malnourished (SGA-C)

Total PG-SGA score

(Total numerical score of A + B + C + D above) _____

(See triage recommendations below)

Clinician signature _____   RD RN PA MD DO Other___   Date _____

Nutritional Triage Recommendation: Additive score is used to define specific nutritional interventions including patient & family education, symptom management including pharmacologic intervention, and appropriate nutrient intervention (food, nutritional supplements, enteral, or parenteral triage). First line nutrition intervention includes optimal symptom management.

0–1   No intervention required at this time. Re-assessment on routine and regular basis during treatment.
2–3   Patient & family education by dietitian, nurse, or other clinician with pharmacologic intervention as indicated by symptom survey (Box 3) and laboratory values as appropriate.
4–8   Requires intervention by dietitian, in conjunction with nurse or physician as indicated by symptoms survey (Box 3).
≥9   Indicates a critical need for improved symptom management and/ or nutrient intervention options.

© FD Ottery, 2001

Figure 25.3 Subjective Global Assessment.

interactance (NIR). These tools are generally not condu-
cive to daily patient care.

Calorimetry

Direct calorimetry, or the measure of total heat loss from
the body, has served as the gold standard for studying
metabolism. This is performed in a closed, specialized
room and not practical for routine patient use. Alternatively indirect calorimetry (IC), or the measure of total
energy production by the body, is utilized more extensively today. Indirect calorimetry is accomplished by a
device that measures a patient's oxygen inhalation and
carbon dioxide excretion under specific conditions. Indirect calorimetry is able to quantify energy expenditure by
measuring O_2 consumption and CO_2 production. The
calculation of the resting energy expenditure (REE) is
estimated to be approximately 10% greater than the basal
energy expenditure (BEE) which can only be measured
in deep sleep [21].

IC also provides a measure of substrate utilization by
calculation of the respiratory quotient (RQ). The RQ is
an indicator of current body substrate metabolism. An
RQ greater than 1.0 is considered to be consistent with
overfeeding and an RQ less than 0.80 is considered to be
consistent with underfeeding. An RQ within normal biological range (0.67–1.3) can serve as a marker of test
reliability and validity (an acceptable energy measurement) [22].

A hand-held device (MedGem®, Microlife USA Inc.,
Duniden, FL) can be used to measure resting metabolic
rate (RMR) in spontaneously breathing patients. Advantages include convenience and decreased expense.
However, limitations make the product most useable for
only certain populations, usually excluding ICU patients.
With the hand-held device only an energy expenditure
can be calculated, not an RQ.

Therapeutics

Nutritional intervention can include a variety of
approaches including dietary counseling or instruction,
oral supplementation, appetite stimulation, enteral and/
or parenteral nutrition. Specialized nutritional intervention may include the use of anabolic agents, immune
enhancing enteral formulations, medium-chain triglycerides, probiotics, or other novel approaches. Prior to

intervention, clinicians must first assess the patient's
caloric, protein and water needs.

Calorie Needs

There are multiple equations used to determine a
patient's calorie needs. The most commonly used formula
is the Harris–Benedict equation [23]. This equation estimates a patient's basal energy expenditure (BEE) using
the following formulas and then is multiplied by a stress
factor to determine the actual daily calorie needs:

$$BEE \text{ men} = 66 + \{(13.7 \times \text{weight (kg)}) \\ + (5.0 \times \text{height (cm)})\} \\ - (6.8 \times \text{age}) \text{ kcal/day}$$

$$BEE \text{ women} = 655 + \{(9.6 \times \text{weight (kg)}) \\ + (1.8 \times \text{height (cm)})\} \\ - (4.7 \times \text{age}) \text{ kcal/day}$$

Stress factors:
Maintenance–mild stress 1–1.2
Moderate stress 1.3–1.4
Severe stress 1.5

If a patent is less than 80% or more than 125% of their
ideal body weight, an adjusted body weight should be
calculated. The Hamwi equation, given below, can be
used to determine ideal body weight (IBW) and therefore
determine adjusted body weight as needed [24]:

$$IBW \text{ men} = 48 \text{ kg} + (48.1 \text{ kg for the first } 1.52 \text{ m plus} \\ 1.1 \text{ kg for every cm} > 1.52 \text{ m})$$

$$IBW \text{ women} = 45 \text{ kg} + (45.5 \text{ kg of the first } 1.52 \text{ m plus} \\ 0.9 \text{ kg for every cm} > 1.52 \text{ m})$$

$$\text{Adjusted body weight} = IBW + 0.25 \,(\text{Actual Body} \\ \text{Weight} - IBW)$$

There are other calorie calculation formulas, including
the Ireton–Jones equation and the Mifflin–St Jeor equation (Table 25.1).

Protein/Nitrogen Needs

A positive nitrogen balance is known as anabolism
and is important for wound healing, recovery from
illness, and growth. A positive nitrogen balance
consists of a greater daily nitrogen intake as compared
to nitrogen excretion. On the contrary, a negative
nitrogen balance is known as catabolism. This is commonly seen in critically ill patients and is the result of a

Table 25.1 Calorie needs equations.

Ireton–Jones equation

Ventilator-dependant: 1784 − 11(age) + 5 (weight in kg) + 244 (male = 1, female = 0) + 239 (if trauma) + 804 (if burn) = kcal/day

Spontaneously breathing: 629 − 11 (age) + 25 (weight in kg) − 609 (obesity, if present = 1, absent = 0) = kcal/day

Mifflin–St Jeor

Men: 5 + 10 (weight in kg) + 6.25 (height in cm) − 5 (age) = kcal/day

Women: −161 + 10 (weight in kg) + 6.25 (height in cm) − 5 (age) = kcal/day

Table 25.2 Quick formulas for protein and calorie needs.

	Protein needs (g/kg/day)	Calorie needs (kcal/kg/day)
Minimal severity of illness	0.8–1.0	20–25
Moderate severity of illness	1.0–1.4	26–30
Severe severity of illness	1.5–2.5	31–35

greater daily nitrogen excretion as compared to nitrogen intake.

Daily nitrogen needs can be converted to daily protein needs by using the following formula:

$$\text{Total grams of nitrogen} \times 6.25 = \text{Total grams of protein required/day}$$

Nitrogen balance can be calculated using the formula below. The goal is zero for maintenance or 2–4 g for repletion.

$$\text{Nitrogen balance (g/day)} = (\text{protein intake}/6.25) - (\text{urinary nitrogen} + \text{fecal losses} + \text{obligatory losses})$$

Quick Formulas for Protein and Calorie Needs

There are more-rapid methods available to determine a patient's daily calorie and protein needs, as given in Table 25.2. These formulas have been shown to be reliable in most patients.

Daily Fluid Needs

Daily fluid needs for patients are based on maintenance needs plus losses through urine, stool, emesis, and wound output. A quick method for determining fluid needs that is considered reliable for most patients is:

30 cc H_2O/kg body weight/day or 1 mL H_2O/kcal of tube feeding delivered.

Conclusion

Nutrition assessment is a critical part of the overall clinical evaluation of patients. Familiarity with appropriate nutrition assessment can help identify patients requiring a nutrition intervention and ultimately help determine the efficacy of the intervention.

Take-home points

- Nutrition assessment helps to identify patients who would benefit from nutritional intervention.
- Organ function becomes impaired with protein–calorie malnutrition.
- Recent body weight loss (5% at 1 month, 10% at 6 months) is the most sensitive nutrition assessment measurement in patients without edema/ascites.
- Patient's recall of their own weight is poor.
- Serum protein markers (e.g., albumin) are poor markers of malnutrition.
- Global scoring systems provide a very good nutritional assessment tool.
- Calorie needs can be determined by calorie equations or a quick formula.
- Protein needs can be determined by urine urea nitrogen excretion or a quick formula.

References

1 Schneider SM, Hebuterne X. Use of nutritional scores to predict clinical outcomes in chronic diseases. *Nutr Rev* 2000; **1**: 31–8.

2 Windsor JA, Hill GL. Weight loss with physiologic impairment: a basic indicator of surgical risk. *Ann Surg* 1988; **207**: 290–9.

3 Jeejeebhoy KN, Detsky AS, Baker JP. Assessment of nutritional status. *JPEN J Parenter Enteral Nutr* 1990; **14**: 193S–9S.

4 Hill GL, Jonathan E. Rhoads lecture. Body composition research: implications for the practice of clinical nutrition. *JPEN J Parenter Enteral Nutr* 1992; **16**: 197–217.

5 Rasmussen HH, Kondrup J, Staun M, *et al.* Prevalence of patients at nutritional risk in Danish hospitals. *Clin Nutr* 2004; **23**: 1009–115.

6 Blackburn GL, Bistrian BR, Maini BS, *et al.* Nutritional and metabolic assessment of the hospitalized patient. *JPEN J Parenter Enteral Nutr* 1977; **1**: 11–22.

7 Campbell SE, Avenell A, Walker AE. Assessment of nutritional status in hospital in-patients. *QJM* 2002; **95**: 63–7.

8 Heymsfield SB, McManus C, Stevens V, Smith J. Muscle mass: reliable indicator of protein-energy malnutrition severity and outcome. *Am J Clin Nutr* 1982; **35**: 1192–9.

9 Brough W, Horne G, Blount A, *et al.* Effects of nutrient intake, surgery, sepsis and long-term administration of steroids on muscle function. *BMJ* 1986; **293**: 983–8.

10 Menton PA. Voluntary strength and disease. *J Physiol* 1954; **123**: 533–64.

11 Webb AR, Newman LA, Taylor M, Decosta BR. Handgrip dynamometry as a predictor of postoperative complications reappraisal using age standardized grip strengths. *JPEN J Parenter Enteral Nutr* 1989; **13**: 30–3.

12 Detsky AS, McLauhlin JR, Baker JP, *et al.* What is subjective global assessment of nutritional status. *JPEN J Parenter Enteral Nutr* 1987; **11**: 8–13.

13 Guigoz Y, Vellas B, Garry PJ. Mini-Nutritional Assessment, a practical assessment tool for grading the nutritional status of elderly patients. *Facts Res Gerontol* 1994; **4** (Suppl. 2): 15–19.

14 Reilly HM. Screening for nutritional risk. *Proc Nutr Soc* 1996; **55**: 841–53.

15 Veterans Affairs Total Parenteral Nutrition Cooperative Study Group. Perioperative total parenteral nutrition in surgical patients. *N Engl J Med* 1992; **325**: 525–32.

16 Stratton JS, Hackston A, Longmore D, *et al.* Malnutrition in hospital outpatients and inpatients: prevalence, concurrent validity, and ease of use of the "malnutrition universal screening tool" (MUST) for adults. *Br J Nutr* 2004; **92**: 799–808.

17 Pablo AM, Izaga MA, Alday LA. Assessment of nutritional status on hospital admission: nutritional scores. *Eur J Clin Nutr* 2003; **57**: 824–31.

18 Seltzer MH, Bastidas A, Cooper DM, *et al.* Instant nutritional assessment. *JPEN J Parenter Enteral Nutr* 1979; **3**: 157–9.

19 Khaled MP, McCutcheon MJ, Reddy S. Electrical impedance is assessing human body composition by the BIA method. *Am J Clin Nutr* 1988; **47**: 789–92.

20 Hill GL. Body composition research: implications for the practice of clinical nutrition. *JPEN J Parenter Enteral Nutr* 1992; **16**: 197–218.

21 McClave SA, Snider HL. Use of indirect calorimetry in nutrition. *Nutr Clin Pract* 1992; **7**: 207–22.

22 McClave SA, Lowen CC, Kebler MJ. Is the respiratory quotient a useful indicator of over or underfeeding? [abstract]. *JPEN J Parenter Enteral Nutr* 1997; **21**: S11.

23 Harris JA, Benedict FG. *Standard Basal Monitoring Constants for Physiologists and Clinicians: a Biometric Study of Basal Metabolism in Man.* Philadelphia: JB Lippincott, 1919.

24 Hamwi GJ. Changing dietary concepts. In: Danowski TS, ed. *Diabetes Mellitus: Diagnosis and Treatment*, Vol. 1. New York, NY: American Diabetes Association, 1964: 73–8.

CHAPTER 26
Hematochezia

Lisa L. Strate

Division of Gastroenterology, University of Washington School of Medicine, Harborview Medical Center, Seattle, WA, USA

Summary

Hematochezia is a very common gastrointestinal problem, especially among the elderly. Most patients with hematochezia have colonic sources of bleeding such as diverticular bleeding, ischemic colitis, and hemorrhoids. However, it is important to exclude an upper gastrointestinal source in patients with significant blood loss. Colonoscopy is the best strategy for most patients with acute hematochezia because of its diagnostic and therapeutic possibilities and safety. Colonoscopy should generally be performed within 12–24h of presentation or close to the onset of bleeding and after a good bowel preparation. Radiographic interventions, including angiography, radionuclide scintigraphy, and multidetector CT scanning, are useful for patients who cannot be stabilized or who have failed endoscopic diagnosis or treatment. Aggressive resuscitation and management of other co-morbid illnesses is important.

Case

An 80-year-old female is admitted to the hospital with 2 days of hematochezia and lightheadedness. She has a history of arthritis and hypertension and reports a normal colonoscopy 5 years previously. She takes a daily aspirin (81 mg), an angiotensin converting enzyme inhibitor, and acetaminophen as needed for pain. She lives independently. On physical examination she is an elderly woman in no distress. Her blood pressure is 118/80 mmHg and her heart rate is 105 beats per min. She has no abdominal tenderness. There is maroon stool on rectal exam. The remainder of the exam is unremarkable. Her admission hematocrit is 25%, a drop of 14% from her recent baseline. Her platelets and prothrombin time are normal. Her creatinine is 1.8 mg/dL an increase from 1.1 mg/dL and her blood urea nitrogen is 7 mg/dL. She passes another bloody stool in the emergency department.

Definition and Epidemiology

Hematochezia is defined as the passage of red or maroon blood per rectum. Hematochezia is most often associated

Practical Gastroenterology and Hepatology: Small and Large Intestine and Pancreas, 1st edition. Edited by Nicholas J. Talley, Sunanda V. Kane and Michael B. Wallace. © 2010 Blackwell Publishing Ltd.

with lower intestinal bleeding (bleeding beyond the ligament of Treitz) but can represent bleeding from any source, depending on the amount of bleeding and transit time. Five to fifteen percent of individuals with hematochezia have an upper gastrointestinal source of bleeding, and 5–10% have small bowel sources [1]. It can be difficult to determine whether hematochezia is from the upper gastrointestinal tract, the mid-bowel, or the colon based on the initial presentation. This review will focus on hematochezia from a colonic source or lower intestinal bleeding.

The annual incidence of hospitalization for lower intestinal bleeding is estimated to be 20 per 100 000 individuals [2]. However, the incidence reaches 200 per 100 000 individuals by the ninth decade of life [2]. Therefore, although not formally documented, lower intestinal bleeding is likely to be an increasingly common clinical problem. The majority of patients with lower intestinal bleeding have at least one co-morbid condition, which adds to the complexity of this disorder.

Clinical Features

There are a number of clinical features that can guide the diagnosis and management of hematochezia. The character, volume, frequency, and duration of the bleeding can help determine the source and severity of bleeding. Typically, small amounts of bright red blood indicate an anal or rectal source, whereas larger amounts of maroon stool signify a brisk bleed from a more proximal source. Rectal symptoms such as pain with the passage of stool, presence of hemorrhoids, and tenesmus are also clues to a rectal source. However, symptoms and clinical features alone cannot be used to exclude lesions in the proximal colon [3]. The presence of abdominal pain and tenderness usually reflect diffuse mucosal injury such as inflammatory bowel disease (IBD) or ischemic colitis. A prior or family history of intestinal disorders (IBD, cancer), radiation treatment (radiation colitis), or abdominal surgeries (aortoenteric fistula, anastomotic bleeding) may also allude to specific sources.

Four risk models or scores have been developed for prediction of poor outcome in lower intestinal bleeding [4–7]. Predictors common to each of these studies include indicators of hemodynamic instability (hypotension, tachycardia, syncope, and orthostasis), ongoing rectal bleeding, and the presence of co-morbid illness. Older age, the use of aspirin or anticoagulants, a non-tender abdominal exam, and a past history of bleeding from diverticulosis or angiodysplasia were also predictive in one or more of the studies. In one study, the number of risk factors correlated with the risk of poor outcome [6]. These risk factors can assistant in decision making, particularly at the point of first medical contact to help determine which patients would benefit from intensive care and urgent interventions.

Case continued

Given the patient's high-risk features, an emergent EGD is performed and is negative. After the procedure, she passes more blood per rectum and is briefly hypotensive. It is now 7 PM. A colon preparation with 4 liters of polyethylene glycol is started. She remains stable overnight and a colonoscopy is performed the next morning. There is a large diverticulum with ulceration and adherent clot in the sigmoid.

Diagnosis

There are a number of strategies available for the diagnosis of hematochezia (Figure 26.1). In patients with brisk hematochezia and/or hemodynamic instability, the first step is exclusion of an upper GI source with a nasogastric lavage or preferably an esophagogastroduodenoscopy (EGD). Colonoscopy is the preferred test for most patients presenting with hematochezia because of its diagnostic and therapeutic capabilities as well as its safety (Table 26.1). Studies suggest that performing colonoscopy within 12–24 h of presentation improves diagnostic and therapeutic yield and reduces hospital length of stay [8–11]. However, bowel preparation is probably as important as urgent timing. In studies with exemplary results, 4–6 liters of polyethylene glycol are given over 3–4 h (often via a nasogastric tube) until the effluent is clear [9]. Aspiration precautions should be followed during rapid colon cleansing. Flexible sigmoidoscopy is an alternative intervention in patients with a very high likelihood of a left-sided source who have had a recent

	Diagnosis* (%)	Definite diagnosis (%)	Therapeutic intervention (%)	Complications (%)
Colonoscopy within 24 h	75–100	65–75	10–35	0–2
Colonoscopy (no time frame)	50–90	40–75	10–15	0–2
Angiography	20–70	–	15–55	2–30
Radionuclide scintigraphy	25–70	–	–	–
Multidetector CT scan	25–80	–	–	0–2

Table 26.1 Diagnostic and therapeutic modalities for the evaluation of hematochezia.

*For radiographic studies diagnosis refers to the presence of bleeding or a "positive" exam.

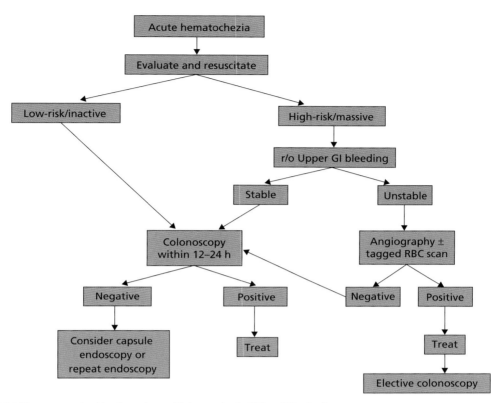

Figure 26.1 Management algorithm for patients with hematochezia. RBC, red blood cell.

full colonoscopy, or as an initial test prior to preparation for colonoscopy. However, the yield of this approach in the literature has been low, and a full colonoscopy to rule out proximal lesions is necessary in most patients. Angiography is an option in patients with very brisk bleeding who cannot be stabilized. However, the need for active bleeding at the time of examination, highly skilled operators, and a confirmatory colonoscopy are disadvantages of this approach. Angiography can also be associated with serious complications such as renal failure and bowel infarction. The use of radionuclide scintigraphy or tagged red blood cell scanning prior to angiography is controversial because of variable bleeding localization and potential delays in other therapeutic interventions [12]. Multidetector-row CT scanning is a newer diagnostic modality that is potentially more accurate and widely available than radionuclide scintigraphy. Advantages of radiographic tests in the management of hematochezia

are the absence of a bowel preparation and the ability to detect bleeding anywhere in the gastrointestinal tract.

Literature comparing management strategies is limited. In a prospective trial, 100 patients were randomized to colonoscopy in less than 8 h from admission or tagged scan followed by angiography if positive and colonoscopy if negative [8]. A definitive source of bleeding was found in statistically significantly more patients in the colonoscopy arm than in the radiology arm (42 vs. 22%). The study was underpowered to assess other outcomes, but there was a trend in favor of colonoscopy, particularly with regards to treatment (34 vs. 20%).

Differential Diagnosis

The differential diagnosis for hematochezia is very broad, but can generally be broken down into three main cate-

Table 26.2 Differential diagnosis of hematochezia.

Diverticulosis	30–40%
Ischemic colitis	10–20%
Hemorrhoids	10–15%
Upper gastrointestinal source	5–15%
Colitis*	5–25%
Unknown†	5–20%
Neoplasia	5–10%
Small bowel source	5–10%
Postpolypectomy	3–10%
Angiodysplasia	1–5%
Other	1–10%
Rectal varices	
Solitary rectal ulcer	
Dieulafoy	

*Inflammatory bowel disease, infectious colitis, radiation enteritis.
†Unknown sources are most likely in the small bowel.

gories: vascular (e.g., diverticular bleeding, angiodysplasia), mucosal (infectious, ischemic, or inflammatory colitis), or neoplastic (Table 26.2). The management of vascular sources focuses on bleeding control, whereas treatment of the underlying condition and not the bleeding itself is usually the primary concern for mucosal or neoplastic lesions.

Case continued

Eight cubic centimeters of dilute epinephrine (1 : 10 000) is injected in four quadrants around the diverticulum. A large clot is expelled. Three endoclips are placed across the ulcer. The patient has no further bleeding.

Therapeutics

Resuscitation is the initial priority in patients with significant hematochezia. A surgical consultation should be obtained in unstable patients with massive hematochezia. Endoscopic therapy can be used to treat a variety of bleeding sources in the colon. Treatment modalities are largely the same as in upper gastrointestinal bleeding, including thermal contact methods, epinephrine injection, endoclips, banding, and argon plasma coagulation except that lower power settings (10–15 watts), pressure

(light to moderate), and treatment duration (1–2 seconds) are used to reduce the risk of perforation [13]. The efficacy of endoscopic treatment with bimodal therapy (epinephrine injection and bipolar coagulation) for diverticular bleeding was demonstrated in a prospective study of 48 patients [9]. Endoscopic therapy was used in the 10 patients (21%) with stigmata of recent hemorrhage. No patient had recurrent bleeding or required surgery and there were no complications. In comparison, in 17 historical controls with stigmata who received no endoscopic treatment, 53% experienced rebleeding and 35% required surgery. There are no studies comparing endoscopic treatment modalities in the colon. The choice of treatment modality depends on the location and source of bleeding and the experience of the endoscopist. Endoclips in combination with epinephrine injection may be safer than thermal methods especially in the cecum and the base of diverticula where the colon is particularly thin (Video 12 and 13). Overall, complications of colonoscopy in the setting of acute hematochezia are rare (1.3% in a summary of 13 studies) [14], and include heart failure, bowel perforation, postcoagulation syndrome and aspiration pneumonia. Newer angiographic super-selective embolization techniques decrease the risk of bowel ischemia and achieve hemostasis in up to 100% of patients but with rebleeding rates of 15–50% [15].

Prognosis

The prognosis for patients with lower intestinal bleed is good, despite an older demographic with co-morbid illness. As in upper GI bleeding, 20–25% will stop bleeding spontaneously. Recent studies indicate that approximately 5% of patients who continue to bleed will require surgery. Death in the setting of lower intestinal bleeding is uncommon (less than 5%) and is usually due to co-morbid illness rather than uncontrolled bleeding [16]. Therefore, aggressive supportive care and management of co-morbid conditions are central tenets of management. Recurrent bleeding is a significant problem for patients with bleeding from diverticulosis or angiodysplasia [2]. Preventative measures are not well-defined but avoidance of non-steroidal anti-inflammatory drugs (NSAIDs) including aspirin is a prudent measure.

Take-home points

- Rule out upper GI bleeding in all patients with severe hematochezia.

- Hemodynamic instability, ongoing bleeding, and co-morbid illness are risk factors consistently shown to predict poor outcome in lower intestinal bleeding. Patients with these risk factors benefit from aggressive supportive care and urgent interventions.

- Colonoscopy is the test of choice for the diagnosis and treatment of hematochezia.

- Performance of colonoscopy within 12–24 h of admission may improve diagnostic and therapeutic opportunities and shorten length of hospital stay.

- A good bowel preparation is critical. Aim for 4–6 liters of polyethylene glycol over 3–4 h and perform colonoscopy when effluent is clear.

- Endoscopic hemostasis can be used successfully in the colon.

- Injection and hemoclips may be safer than thermal methods, especially in the cecum and within diverticula.

- Radiographic strategies should be reserved for patients who cannot be stabilized for endoscopy and are likely to have active bleeding at the time of the examination.

- Aggressive supportive care and management of co-morbid illness are keys to reducing poor outcomes in lower intestinal bleeding.

References

1 Jensen DM, Machicado GA. Diagnosis and treatment of severe hematochezia. The role of urgent colonoscopy after purge. *Gastroenterology* 1988; **95**: 1569–74.

2 Longstreth GF. Epidemiology and outcome of patients hospitalized with acute lower gastrointestinal hemorrhage: a population-based study. *Am J Gastroenterol* 1997; **92**: 419–24.

3 Fine KD, Nelson AC, Ellington RT, Mossburg A. Comparison of the color of fecal blood with the anatomical location of gastrointestinal bleeding lesions: potential misdiagnosis using only flexible sigmoidoscopy for bright red blood per rectum. *Am J Gastroenterol* 1999; **94**: 3202–10.

4 Das A, Ben-Menachem T, Cooper GS, *et al*. Prediction of outcome in acute lower-gastrointestinal haemorrhage based on an artificial neural network: internal and external validation of a predictive model. *Lancet* 2003; **362**: 1261–6.

5 Kollef MH, O'Brien JD, Zuckerman GR, Shannon W. BLEED: a classification tool to predict outcomes in patients with acute upper and lower gastrointestinal hemorrhage. *Crit Care Med* 1997; **25**: 1125–32.

6 Strate LL, Saltzman JR, Ookubo R, *et al*. Validation of a clinical prediction rule for severe acute lower intestinal bleeding. *Am J Gastroenterol* 2005; **100**: 1821–7.

7 Velayos FS, Williamson A, Sousa KH, *et al*. Early predictors of severe lower gastrointestinal bleeding and adverse outcomes: a prospective study. *Clin Gastroenterol Hepatol* 2004; **2**: 485–90.

8 Green BT, Rockey DC, Portwood G, *et al*. Urgent colonoscopy for evaluation and management of acute lower gastrointestinal hemorrhage: a randomized controlled trial. *Am J Gastroenterol* 2005; **100**: 2395–402.

9 Jensen DM, Machicado GA, Jutabha R, Kovacs TO. Urgent colonoscopy for the diagnosis and treatment of severe diverticular hemorrhage. *N Engl J Med* 2000; **342**: 78–82.

10 Schmulewitz N, Fisher DA, Rockey DC. Early colonoscopy for acute lower GI bleeding predicts shorter hospital stay: a retrospective study of experience in a single center. *Gastrointest Endosc* 2003; **58**: 841–6.

11 Strate LL, Syngal S. Timing of colonoscopy: impact on length of hospital stay in patients with acute lower intestinal bleeding. *Am J Gastroenterol* 2003; **98**: 317–22.

12 Hunter JM, Pezim ME. Limited value of technetium 99m-labeled red cell scintigraphy in localization of lower gastrointestinal bleeding. *Am J Surg* 1990; **159**: 504–6.

13 Jensen DM, Machicado GA. Colonoscopy for diagnosis and treatment of severe lower gastrointestinal bleeding. Routine outcomes and cost analysis. *Gastrointest Endosc Clin N Am* 1997; **7**: 477–98.

14 Zuckerman GR, Prakash C. Acute lower intestinal bleeding: part I: clinical presentation and diagnosis. *Gastrointest Endosc* 1998; **48**: 606–17.

15 Kuo WT, Lee DE, Saad WE, *et al*. Superselective microcoil embolization for the treatment of lower gastrointestinal hemorrhage. *J Vasc Interv Radiol* 2003; **14**: 1503–9.

16 Strate LL, Ayanian JZ, Kotler G, Syngal S. Risk factors for mortality in lower intestinal bleeding. *Clin Gastroenterol Hepatol* 2008; **6**: 1004–10.

CHAPTER 27
Obscure Gastrointestinal Bleeding

Lisa L. Strate

Division of Gastroenterology, University of Washington School of Medicine, Harborview Medical Center, Seattle, WA, USA

Summary

Patients with obscure bleeding make up 5% of patients with gastrointestinal bleeding and most have bleeding from lesions in the small bowel. Angioectasias are a common cause in older patients while small bowel tumors are the most frequently seen lesions in younger age groups. Improved access to the small bowel has revolutionized the management of obscure gastrointestinal bleeding. Capsule endoscopy is generally the test of choice after standard EGD and colonoscopy are unrevealing. Push enteroscopy and double-balloon enteroscopy are subsequent therapeutic strategies. Patients with obscure bleeding tend to require more interventions and have a poorer prognosis than patients with blood loss from the stomach or colon.

Case

A 66-year-old male presents to clinic with recurrent melena and iron-deficiency anemia. He has approximately one melanotic stool per month and complains of fatigue. He has a history of hypertension, GERD, and osteoarthritis. His medications include a beta blocker, a proton pump inhibitor, iron, and acetaminophen. He stopped taking aspirin recently. Physical examination is unremarkable except for heme-positive stool on rectal exam. His hematocrit is 33%, iron 50 µg/dL, transferrin saturation 10%, ferritin 12 µg/L. He had an EGD with gastric and small bowel biopsies and a colonoscopy that were reported as normal at an outside hospital.

Definition and Epidemiology

Obscure gastrointestinal (GI) bleeding is defined as continuous or recurrent bleeding from the gastrointestinal tract without a clear source after evaluation with esophagogastroduodenoscopy (EGD), colonoscopy, and radiologic evaluation of the small bowel [1]. Obscure bleeding

Practical Gastroenterology and Hepatology: Small and Large Intestine and Pancreas, 1st edition. Edited by Nicholas J. Talley, Sunanda V. Kane and Michael B. Wallace. © 2010 Blackwell Publishing Ltd.

is further classified as overt (clinically evident blood loss) or obscure (evident only on fecal occult blood testing). Obscure bleeding makes up 5% of patients with GI bleeding. The small bowel is the source in 75% of cases. The incidence of obscure GI bleeding has not been defined in population-based studies.

Clinical Features

Hematemesis generally indicates a bleeding source proximal to the ligament of Treitz. Hematochezia and melena can represent an upper, small bowel, or colon source, although melena is an uncommon presentation of blood loss from the colon. A history of non-steroidal anti-inflammatory drug (NSAID) use raises the possibility of small bowel ulcerations. Obstructive symptoms and weight loss suggest a small bowel etiology. Patients with aortic stenosis, renal failure, or von Willebrand disease may be predisposed to bleeding from angioectasias.

Case continued

The patient undergoes a capsule endoscopy. This finds several scattered angioectasias in the proximal small bowel.

Diagnosis

Clinical factors and the availability of interventions guide the approach to patients with obscure GI bleeding (Figure 27.1). Evaluation beyond colonoscopy, and EGD if there are localizing symptoms, is generally not necessary in patients with occult blood loss who do not have iron-deficiency anemia. In patients with overt bleeding or occult bleeding with iron-deficiency anemia, repeat standard endoscopy can be valuable especially if there is suspicion of a missed lesion (e.g., hematemesis, poor-quality colon preparation). Repeat EGD reveals a previously missed source in up to 64% of patients [2]. Repeat colonoscopy has a much lower yield. Capsule endoscopy (CE) is generally the next step after initial or repeat standard endoscopy [3,4]. The diagnostic yield of capsule endoscopy is about twice that of push enteroscopy (PE) and small bowel imaging (60–75% vs. 20–40%) (Table 27.1) [5]. In a randomized controlled trial of CE versus PE as the initial investigation, CE was more sensitive (80 vs. 40%) but the performance of the tests was otherwise

Table 27.1 Diagnostic and therapeutic modalities for the evaluation of obscure overt gastrointestinal bleeding.

	Diagnosis (%)	Treatment (%)	Complications (%)
Capsule endoscopy	55–75	—	<1
Double-balloon enteroscopy	40–80	40–75	0–4
Intraoperative enteroscopy	60–85	70–85	3–42*
Push enteroscopy	20–60	15–30	<2
Small bowel series	10–30	—	—
Radionuclide scintigraphy†	15–70	—	—
Angiography†	30–80	50–70	3–10

*Complications of intraoperative enteroscopy include death which is reported in up to 17% of patients.
†In patients with massive blood loss.

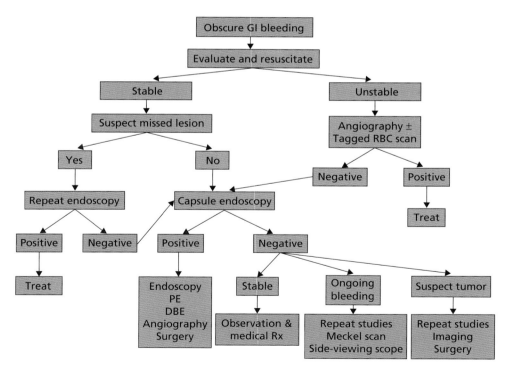

Figure 27.1 Management algorithm for patients with obscure gastrointestinal bleeding.

similar (specificity 90 vs. 100%, positive predictive value 90 vs.100% and negative predictive value 80 vs. 60%, respectively) [6]. Experience and diligence in the review of the capsule images is critical for accurate diagnosis [7]. Capsule endoscopy has the highest yield in patients with recent overt bleeding. Studies indicate that capsule endoscopy guides subsequent management, and may improve bleeding outcomes and treatment costs [8,9]. Patients with a negative capsule endoscopy have a low risk of subsequent bleeding and the evaluation can usually stop in patients with obscure bleeding. However, if a small bowel tumor is suspected further work is usually required. Small bowel obstruction is a contraindication for capsule endoscopy, and in this situation, small bowel imaging may be necessary. Patients with pacemakers or defibrillators should be carefully monitored during the capsule examination.

Double-balloon endoscopy (DBE) is a new method that enables examination and endoscopic treatment of lesions in the small bowel [10,11]. Studies comparing DBE to CE are limited but a recent meta-analysis suggests equivalent diagnostic yields [8]. Cost-minimization analyses indicate that the optimal strategy may be initial DBE, particularly if treatment or a definitive diagnosis is necessary [12,13]. However, CE remains the initial test of choice for most patients because it is non-invasive, more widely available, and more reliably visualizes the entire small bowel. Capsule endoscopy and DBE have largely replaced the need for intraoperative enteroscopy and Sonde enteroscopy. Radionuclide scintigraphy and angiography require active bleeding at the time of examination and are therefore reserved for patients with massive, ongoing bleeding [14,15]. Provocative angiography with intra-arterial administration of vasodilators, anticoagulants or thrombolytics has been utilized to localize bleeding of obscure origin but poses additional risks [16]. Other diagnostic tests such as endoscopy with a side-viewing endoscope and Meckel scanning may be revealing in patients with suspicion of bleeding in the duodenal sweep (e.g., hemobilia) or a Meckel diverticulum, respectively.

Table 27.2 Differential diagnosis of obscure bleeding.

Source	Comment
Angiodysplasia	Can be missed on routine endoscopy, possible association with aortic stenosis, renal insufficiency
NSAID enteropathy or ulcers	Common source in older patients
Small bowel tumors	Most common source in patients <40 years
Crohn disease	More common in young patients
Meckel diverticulum	More common in patients <25 years old
Hemobilia	Patients after liver biopsy or biliary trauma
Hemosuccus pancreatiticus	Patients with pancreatitis and pseudocysts
Aortoenteric fistula	Patients with prior vascular graft; herald bleed
Celiac disease	Can be missed on routine endoscopy
Dieulafoy lesion	Can be missed on routine endoscopy
Peptic ulcer disease	Can be missed on routine endoscopy
Cameron ulcers	Can be missed on routine endoscopy

NSAID, non-steroidal anti-inflammatory drug.

the small bowel (Table 27.2). Cameron erosions, Dieulafoy lesions, and angioectasias are lesions commonly missed on standard endoscopy. In patients younger than 40 years of age, tumors are the most common cause of obscure bleeding and careful evaluation and follow-up is necessary [4]. Meckel diverticula and Crohn disease must also be considered in young patients. Older patients are more likely to have angioectasias and NSAID-related ulcerations [4].

Case continued

A push enteroscopy is performed with electrocoagulation of five angioectasias in the distal duodenum and jejunum. He remains off aspirin. His melena stops and his iron deficiency resolves after several months.

Differential Diagnosis

The differential diagnosis of obscure GI bleeding includes lesions not seen on EGD or colonoscopy and lesions in

Therapy

Therapy of obscure GI bleeding is guided by the diagnosis, the degree of bleeding, and the presence of co-morbid illness. Patients with acute bleeding require resuscitation. Endoscopic therapy is often possible using standard, push, or balloon enteroscopy. Angiography with endovascular therapy may be necessary for very brisk bleeding and surgery for tumors. Iron supplementation and blood transfusions should be used to treat iron-deficiency anemia, and medical therapy alone may be appropriate for patients with diffuse lesions or significant co-morbid illness. There are few data to suggest a benefit of medical therapy with hormonal agents, somatostatin, or thalidomide.

Prognosis

Patients with small bowel bleeding tend to require more diagnostic examinations and blood transfusions and have longer, costlier hospitalizations than patients with colonic sources of bleeding [17]. The mortality rate may also be higher. Recurrent bleeding is a common problem particularly with vascular ectasias [18].

Take-home points

- Capsule endoscopy (CE) is the best initial strategy for most patients with overt obscure GI bleeding.

- Vigilance and experience are important for accurate interpretation of CE images.

- Repeat standard endoscopy is useful when a missed lesion is suspected such as in patients with hematemesis (EGD), or a prior poor colon preparation (colonoscopy).

- The diagnostic yield of double-balloon endoscopy (DBE) is equivalent to CE. DBE may be the best initial strategy if treatment is very likely.

- Careful evaluation and follow-up is necessary in young patients (<50 years) with obscure bleeding because small bowel tumors are the most common source in this age group.

- Patients with diffuse lesions or severe co-morbidity may be managed supportively.

- In patients with occult bleeding without iron-deficiency anemia, no work up is needed beyond colonoscopy with or without EGD if localizing symptoms.

References

1 American Gastroenterological Association. American Gastroenterological Association medical position statement: evaluation and management of occult and obscure gastrointestinal bleeding. *Gastroenterology* 2000; **118**: 197–201.

2 Zaman A, Katon RM. Push enteroscopy for obscure gastrointestinal bleeding yields a high incidence of proximal lesions within reach of a standard endoscope. *Gastrointest Endosc* 1998; **47**: 372–6.

3 Pennazio M, Eisen G, Goldfarb N. ICCE consensus for obscure gastrointestinal bleeding. *Endoscopy* 2005; **37**: 1046–50.

4 Raju GS, Gerson L, Das A, Lewis B. American Gastroenterological Association (AGA) Institute technical review on obscure gastrointestinal bleeding. *Gastroenterology* 2007; **133**: 1697–717.

5 Triester SL, Leighton JA, Leontiadis GI, *et al.* A meta-analysis of the yield of capsule endoscopy compared to other diagnostic modalities in patients with obscure gastrointestinal bleeding. *Am J Gastroenterol* 2005; **100**: 2407–18.

6 de Leusse A, Vahedi K, Edery J, *et al.* Capsule endoscopy or push enteroscopy for first-line exploration of obscure gastrointestinal bleeding? *Gastroenterology* 2007; **132**: 855–62; quiz 1164–5.

7 Lewis BS. How to read wireless capsule endoscopic images: tips of the trade. *Gastrointest Endosc Clin N Am* 2004; **14**: 11–6.

8 Pasha SF, Leighton JA, Das A, *et al.* Double-balloon enteroscopy and capsule endoscopy have comparable diagnostic yield in small-bowel disease: a meta-analysis. *Clin Gastroenterol Hepatol* 2008; **6**: 671–6.

9 Pennazio M, Santucci R, Rondonotti E, *et al.* Outcome of patients with obscure gastrointestinal bleeding after capsule endoscopy: report of 100 consecutive cases. *Gastroenterology* 2004; **126**: 643–53.

10 Yamamoto H, Sekine Y, Sato Y, *et al.* Total enteroscopy with a nonsurgical steerable double-balloon method. *Gastrointest Endosc* 2001; **53**: 216–20.

11 Yamamoto H, Yano T, Kita H, *et al.* New system of double-balloon enteroscopy for diagnosis and treatment of small intestinal disorders. *Gastroenterology* 2003; **125**: 1556; author reply 7.

12 Gerson L, Kamal A. Cost-effectiveness analysis of management strategies for obscure GI bleeding. *Gastrointest Endosc* 2008; **68**: 920–36.

13 Somsouk M, Gralnek IM, Inadomi JM. Management of obscure occult gastrointestinal bleeding: a cost-minimization analysis. *Clin Gastroenterol Hepatol* 2008; **6**: 661–70.

14 Lau WY, Ngan H, Chu KW, Yuen WK. Repeat selective visceral angiography in patients with gastrointestinal bleeding of obscure origin. *Br J Surg* 1989; **76**: 226–9.

15 Wang CS, Tzen KY, Huang MJ, *et al.* Localization of obscure gastrointestinal bleeding by technetium 99m-labeled red blood cell scintigraphy. *J Formos Med Assoc* 1992; **91**: 63–8.

16 Bloomfeld RS, Smith TP, Schneider AM, Rockey DC. Provocative angiography in patients with gastrointestinal hemorrhage of obscure origin. *Am J Gastroenterol* 2000; **95**: 2807–12.

17 Prakash C, Zuckerman GR. Acute small bowel bleeding: a distinct entity with significantly different economic implications compared with GI bleeding from other locations. *Gastrointest Endosc* 2003; **58**: 330–5.

18 Landi B, Cellier C, Gaudric M, *et al*. Long-term outcome of patients with gastrointestinal bleeding of obscure origin explored by push enteroscopy. *Endoscopy* 2002; **34**: 355–9.

CHAPTER 28

Constipation

Erica N. Roberson and Arnold Wald

Section of Gastroenterology and Hepatology, University of Wisconsin School of Medicine and Public Health, Madison, WI, USA

Summary

Constipation is a common complaint that can be primary (idiopathic or functional) or associated with a number of disorders or medications. Symptomatic treatment such as fiber supplements and laxatives is often effective. Functional constipation that fails to respond to symptomatic treatment should be investigated with a colon transit study, anorectal manometry, and balloon expulsion to assess colonic and anorectal functions. Slow-transit constipation ("colonic inertia") is defined by an abnormal transit study and normal manometry and balloon expulsion; it is often difficult to treat and sometimes requires surgery. Subtotal colectomy with ileorectal anastomosis should be reserved for those few patients with intractable slow-transit constipation without disordered defecation or generalized gastrointestinal dysmotility. Defecation disorders may be due to poor relaxation or inappropriate contraction of the pelvic floor muscles, with or without inadequate propulsion. It is best treated with biofeedback therapy which teaches the patient to better control the muscles used in defecation.

Case

A 36-year-old woman consults with a gastroenterologist for chronic constipation. She has had one to two bowel movements weekly for the past 6 years, often with straining and a sense of incomplete evacuation. She denies abdominal pain, blood per rectum, nausea, weight change, diarrhea, fecal or urinary incontinence, dry skin, cold intolerance, or neuromuscular symptoms. Except for mild hypertension, for which she takes a β-blocker, she is otherwise healthy and takes no other medications. She has had no abdominal surgeries. On the advice of her primary-care physician she has increased fiber intake and exercise, to no avail. She has also tried over-the-counter laxatives such as senna, milk of magnesia, and polyethylene glycol, which helped only temporarily.

Practical Gastroenterology and Hepatology: Small and Large Intestine and Pancreas, 1st edition. Edited by Nicholas J. Talley, Sunanda V. Kane and Michael B. Wallace. © 2010 Blackwell Publishing Ltd.

Definition and Epidemiology

Although most individuals have a bowel movement at least three times per week, infrequent defecation alone is very uncommon among constipated persons. Most constipated patients have other symptoms such as straining or stools which are too hard or too small. Consensus guidelines [1] define functional constipation as a combination of symptoms (Table 28.1). Prevalence in many studies ranges from 5% to as high as 28%. Constipation is more common in women and the elderly and accounts for 2.5 million physician visits each year in the US, mainly to primary-care physicians and gastroenterologists [2].

Pathophysiology

Constipation may be associated with a systemic disorder, such as hypothyroidism, neurologic diseases, and collagen vascular diseases, and is associated with many drugs

Table 28.1 Rome III Diagnostic Criteria for functional constipation*[1].

Must include 2 or more of the following:
  Straining during at least 25% of defecations
  Lumpy or hard stools in at least 25% of defecations
  Sensation of incomplete evacuation for at least 25% of
    defecations
  Sensation of anorectal obstruction/blockage for at least 25% of
    defecations
  Manual maneuvers to facilitate at least 25% of defecations
    (e.g., digital evacuation, support of the pelvic floor)
  Fewer than 3 defecations per week
  Loose stools are rarely present without the use of laxatives
  There are insufficient criteria for IBS

*Criteria fulfilled for the last 3 months with symptom onset at least 6 months prior to diagnosis.

Table 28.2 Some common medications associated with constipation.

Opiates
Antipsychotics
Anticholinergics
Tricyclic antidepressants
Calcium channel blockers
Iron
5-HT$_3$ antagonists (i.e., ondansetron)
Anticonvulsants
Diuretics
Antineoplastic agents

(Table 28.2). It may be precipitated or exacerbated by physical or mental disorders interfering with toileting. Low income, low education, physical inactivity, depression, and low calorie intake are known risk factors for constipation. Two subgroups of constipation require special attention.

Slow-Transit Constipation ("Colonic Inertia")

Patients with slow-transit constipation often have unremitting constipation characterized by infrequent defecation without a defecation disorder. These individuals lack the increase in colonic motility ordinarily promoted by stimulants, such as eating, cholinergic agents, and stimulant laxatives. Colonic inertia refers to patients with delayed passage of radiopaque markers in the proximal colon. Histologic studies in severe cases have shown a

decrease in enteric "pacemaker" neurons (interstitial cells of Cajal), and support cells that form myelin sheaths and modulate neurotransmitter concentrations (enteric glial cells). This may account for the often poor response to laxatives and dietary measures [3].

Defecation Disorders

Normal defecation involves coordinated actions including: (i) increase in intra-abdominal pressure; (ii) relaxation of the anal sphincters to reduce resistance to elimination; and (iii) relaxation of the puborectalis muscle to widen the anorectal angle. Constipation may result when this process is disordered. Disordered defecation can be divided into: (i) dyssynergic defecation which results from poor relaxation or inappropriate contraction of the pelvic floor muscles; and (ii) inadequate propulsive forces. Both lead to ineffective evacuation of the rectum and distal colon [4].

Clinical Features

Most patients with constipation respond to over-the-counter medications. When a patient consults with a physician for problematic symptoms, a detailed history and focused examination are important. This includes characterizing the frequency and nature of the patient's bowel movements, including what the patient means by "constipation" and what is the major concern. A 2-week prospective diary detailing food and beverage intake and frequency and characteristics of bowel movements may be useful in refractory cases. The assessment should explore for possible underlying disorders by inquiring about abdominal pain, weight gain or loss, eating disorders, and clues to disorders associated with constipation. Review of symptoms should also inquire about "alarm symptoms": anorexia, blood in stools, recent change in bowel habit, nausea, and vomiting. Other important aspects of the history include previous abdominal surgeries, medications, and a family history of colon cancer.

Physical exam should include a neurologic exam; an abdominal exam to assess for distension, hernias, abdominal muscle strength and integrity, and masses; and an anorectal exam to assess for fissures, mass, sphincter tone, rectocele, prolapse, and occult blood. The rectal exam should also assess for puborectalis muscle and anal sphincter responses when bearing down as if to defecate.

Diagnosis

Patients with chronic constipation and without alarm symptoms may be treated empirically and generally do not require further diagnostic tests. In those who do not respond to conservative therapy, history alone does not often distinguish the etiology of constipation [5]. Abdominal X-rays may confirm the presence of excessive stool in the colon whereas colonoscopy or barium radiograph may identify an anatomic cause of constipation. These tests are not recommended routinely unless alarm features are present or a patient is eligible for routine colon cancer screening [6,7]. This is because colon polyps and cancers are no more common in constipated patients than the normal population [8]. Useful diagnostic tests to assess anorectal and colonic function include a colon transit study, balloon expulsion, and anorectal manometry which allow differentiation into colonic or anorectal dysfunction (Figure 28.1). These tests are indicated only when patients do not respond to conservative measures. Characterizing these disorders is important as management differs [9].

Diagnosis of Colonic Inertia

To perform a colon transit study, patients ingest radiopaque markers and X-rays are obtained at various time points according to different protocols. The Hinton technique involves ingestion of 24 markers on day 0 and an abdominal X-ray (110 keV) on day 5 [10]. Slow transit is defined as the presence of greater than 20% (five) markers on day 5. Colon transit studies are normal in many patients with constipation. An abnormal colon transit study cannot reliably differentiate between colonic inertia and a defecation disorder; however, patients with disordered defecation may exhibit a predominance of markers in the left or rectosigmoid colons. Further studies are needed to assess if disordered defecation is present [11].

Diagnosis of Disordered Defecation

Disordered defecation has also been called outlet obstruction or pelvic floor dyssynergia. It is suspected when a patient contracts or fails to relax the external anal sphincter and puborectalis muscle on digital rectal exam when

asked to bear down. A colon transit study may be normal or show markers retained on the left and or rectosigmoid colon. Anorectal manometry demonstrates inadequate expulsion effort, inappropriate anal sphincter contraction, or no sphincter relaxation. However, many patients with abnormal manometry have normal defecation due to the artificial setting of the manometry study. Abnormal expulsion of a 50-mL water-filled balloon from the rectum (>60 seconds) supports the diagnosis of disordered defecation [12]. If only manometry or balloon expulsion is abnormal, defecography should be performed to establish or exclude the diagnosis.

Case continued

On physical exam, blood pressure and pulse are normal as are cardiac, pulmonary, thyroid, skin, and neurologic exams. Abdominal exam reveals normal bowel sounds with no tenderness or guarding, masses, or hepatosplenomegaly. Rectal exam reveals no perianal disease, prolapse, or rectocele. Stool is brown and hemoccult negative. During the rectal exam, there is an increase in both the external anal sphincter and puborectalis muscle tone when the patient is asked to bear down as if to defecate.

You suspect dyssynergic defecation and a Hinton transit study shows that 10 markers are present 5 days after administration of 24 markers; eight are on the left side (the descending colon). Anorectal manometry shows inappropriate anal sphincter contraction during straining. She is unable to expel a 50-mL water balloon within 60 seconds. You make a diagnosis of dyssynergic defecation and refer her for biofeedback therapy.

Differential Diagnosis

Irritable Bowel Syndrome

Constipation occurs in some patients with irritable bowel syndrome (IBS). However, IBS is differentiated from functional constipation by the predominance of abdominal pain.

Megarectum and Megacolon

Some patients with constipation have chronic megacolon or megarectum. These disorders are often seen in patients with psychosis, dementia, the institutionalized elderly, and diseases such as Parkinsonism. Megacolon and megarectum are associated with myogenic dysfunction, increased colonic or rectal compliance, and blunted

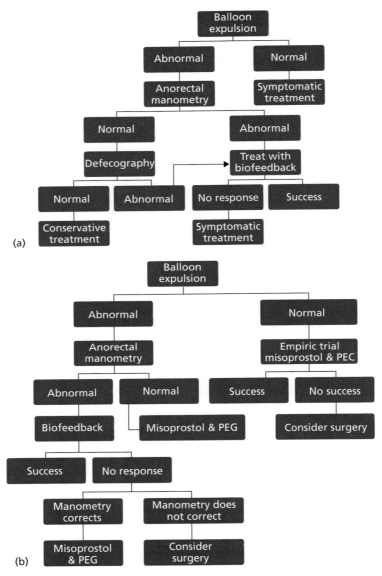

Figure 28.1 Management algorithm for refractory constipation. (a) Normal transit constipation. (b) Slow colonic transit.

rectal sensation. The diagnosis is usually made by radiographic studies.

Hirschsprung Disease (Aganglionic Megacolon)

This is a rare congenital disease that often presents with severe constipation, most often in male infants. Manometry shows no relaxation of the internal anal sphincter in response to rectal distension, the result of a congenital absence of enteric neurons in the distal bowel. Deep rectal biopsies are needed to confirm the diagnosis.

Therapy

Initial therapy includes alteration of lifestyle, such as regular exercise and increased dietary fiber. Patients who do not improve should be started on a laxative (Table

Table 28.3 Older medications for constipation.

Medication	Grade*[14]	Dose (daily)	Cost ($)†	Notes and side effects
Bulking agents				
Psyllium	B	20–30 g	7.80–15.60	Avoid in patients with IBS, megacolon, colonic inertia
Methylcellulose	C	19 g	9.33–21.00	
Stool softener				
Docusate	C	200 mg	5.87	Abdominal cramps
Stimulant laxatives				
Senna	C	17.2 mg	3.99	Melanosis coli
Bisacodyl	C	10 mg	7.19	
Osmotic laxatives				
Polyethylene glycol	A	17 g	12.00–48.00	Nausea, abdominal cramps
Milk of magnesia	C	5 mL	2.75	Avoid in renal failure
Lactulose	B	10 g (15 mL)	20.01	Bloating, gas
Sorbitol	C	21 g (30 mL)	25.92	Bloating, gas

*Based on strength of evidence and grading of recommendations as utilized by the US Preventive Services Task Force. Grade A: good evidence in support of the use of a modality in the treatment of constipation. Grade B: moderate evidence in support of the use of a modality in the treatment of constipation. Grade C: poor evidence to support a recommendation for or against the use of modality. Grade D: moderate evidence against the use of the modality. Grade E: good evidence to support a recommendation against the use of a modality.
†Dollar amount obtained from www.drugstore.com. February 2010 and based on a 30 day supply.

Table 28.4 Newer prescription drugs for constipation.

Medication	Evidence	Grade*	Dose	Cost ($)†	Side effects
Tegaserod	5 RCT (n = 3341) Duration = 4–12 weeks	A	4–6 mg twice daily	N/A	Headache, nausea
Lubiprostone	2 RCT (n = 371), Duration = 3–4 weeks	A	24 µg twice daily	253.30	Headache, nausea
Linaclotide	Phase 3 trials in progress	N/A	75–600 µg daily	N/A	

*Please see Table 28.3 for explanation of strength of evidence and grading.
†Dollar amount obtained from www.drugstore.com. February 2010 and based on a 30 day supply.
RCT, randomized placebo controlled, double blinded trial; N/A, not applicable.

28.3). A good first choice is polyethylene glycol (PEG) as side effects are minimal whereas lactulose and sorbitol often result in undesirable gas and bloating. Stimulant laxatives such are senna or bisacodyl are also inexpensive options. Senna and other anthraquinones are associated with melanosis coli, a benign dark pigmentation of the colonic mucosa. Magnesium salts may be used episodically but should be avoided in the presence of renal insufficiency. Many of these medications work well and should be used as first-line agents, either alone or together [13]. Lubiprostone, which stimulates intestinal chloride-2 channels to increase intraluminal fluid, has been recently approved for chronic constipation. Tegaserod, a partial 5-HT$_4$ agonist used for chronic constipation, was withdrawn from the market in 2007 after reports of increased cardiovascular events; it is now approved as an investigational drug for women less than age 55 years who have no cardiovascular risk factors and who have failed all other agents. No trials have compared established agents with lubiprostone. One trial showed that polyethylene glycol significantly improved symptoms of constipation and increased bowel movements compared to tegaserod, a moot point now that tegaserod is no longer available [14]. These more expensive agents are best used when other laxatives have failed [15]. Linaclotide is a promising new agent currently in phase 3 trials [16]. A guanylate cyclase-C receptor agonist, it increases intestinal intracellular cyclic guanosine monophosphate to increase secretion of chloride, bicarbonate, and fluid into the gastrointestinal lumen (Table 28.4).

Slow-Transit Constipation (Colonic Inertia)

Misoprostol can be very effective for slow-transit constipation, often combined with small doses of PEG, with titration of doses as tolerated. It should be used with caution in women of child bearing age as it is an abortifacient. In severe, refractory cases of colonic inertia, subtotal colectomy with ileorectostomy should be considered. Ideal candidates for this surgery should have normal anorectal function and absence of gastrointestinal dysmotility as established with esophageal, gastric, and small bowel motility studies. Pain should not be a major complaint as there is a high incidence of pain after surgery. If a patient has a co-existent defecation disorder not responsive to treatment, a diverting ileostomy may be considered.

Disordered Defecation

At least four studies have convincingly shown that biofeedback of pelvic floor dyscoordination by muscle retraining is effective in many patients. Patients undergo 30-min sessions up to several times a week to enhance rectal perception to rectal distension and relax the pelvic floor using instrumental feedback by manometry or electromyographic recordings [17,18].

Case continued

The patient undergoes biofeedback training with supplemental education regarding diet, exercise, pelvic floor exercises, and toileting habits. Her biofeedback sessions are twice weekly for 4 weeks. After training, her bowel movements increase to three to four times weekly. On a follow-up visit 6 months later, she continues to be satisfied with her bowel habit and uses laxatives only once to twice monthly.

Prognosis

Constipation is often controlled with change in diet, lifestyle, and medications such as bulking agents, stimulant laxatives, and osmotic laxatives. Newer agents may sometimes be helpful, either alone or in combination with established over-the-counter laxatives. Biofeedback is often effective in selected patients with dyssynergic defecation, and many colonic inertia patients may be treated with misoprostol and small amounts of PEG. In relatively

few and carefully selected patients is surgical intervention required.

Take-home points

- Constipation is a common disorder and may be functional or associated with systemic disorders or medications.
- Constipation is usually treated symptomatically with available laxatives and occasionally with newer agents.
- Patients with chronic constipation unresponsive to laxatives should undergo diagnostic testing with colon transit study, anorectal manometry, and balloon expulsion study.
- Colonoscopy is not part of the routine workup for constipation unless a patient has alarm symptoms or needs colon cancer screening.
- Slow-transit constipation ("colonic inertia") is diagnosed by colon transit study and the exclusion of defecation disorders.
- Defecation disorders are characterized by balloon expulsion study and anorectal manometry.
- Biofeedback therapy is effective in treatment of disordered defecation.

References

1 Longstreth GF, Thompson WG, Chey WD, *et al.* Functional bowel disorders. *Gastroenterology* 2006; **130**: 1480–91.

2 Higgins PD, Johanson JF. Epidemiology of constipation in North America: a systematic review. *Am J Gastroenterol* 2004; **99**: 750–9.

3 Wald A. Pathophysiology, diagnosis and current management of chronic constipation. *Nat Clin Pract Gastroenterol Hepatol* 2006; **3**: 90–100.

4 Bharucha AE, Wald A, Enck P, Rao S. Functional anorectal disorders. *Gastroenterology* 2006; **130**: 1510–8.

5 Rao SS, Ozturk R, Laine L. Clinical utility of diagnostic tests for constipation in adults: a systematic review. *Am J Gastroenterol* 2005; **100**: 1605–15.

6 Qureshi W, Adler DG, Davila RE, *et al.* ASGE guideline: guideline on the use of endoscopy in the management of constipation. *Gastrointest Endosc* 2005; **62**: 199–201.

7 Winawer S, Fletcher R, Rex D, *et al.* Colorectal cancer screening and surveillance: clinical guidelines and rationale-Update based on new evidence. *Gastroenterology* 2003; **124**: 544–60.

8 Halder SL, Locke GR, 3rd, Schleck CD, *et al.* Natural history of functional gastrointestinal disorders: a 12-year longitudi-

nal population-based study. *Gastroenterology* 2007; **133**: 799–807.

9 Bassotti G, de Roberto G, Sediari L, Morelli A. Colonic motility studies in severe chronic constipation: an organic approach to a functional problem. *Tech Coloproctol* 2004; **8**: 147–50.

10 Hinton JM, Lennard-Jones JE, Young AC. A new method for studying gut transit times using radioopaque markers. *Gut* 1969; **10**: 842–7.

11 Rao SS, Mudipalli RS, Stessman M, Zimmerman B. Investigation of the utility of colorectal function tests and Rome II criteria in dyssynergic defecation (anismus). *Neurogastroenterol Motil* 2004; **16**: 589–96.

12 Minguez M, Herreros B, Sanchiz V, *et al.* Predictive value of the balloon expulsion test for excluding the diagnosis of pelvic floor dyssynergia in constipation. *Gastroenterology* 2004; **126**: 57–62.

13 Muller-Lissner SA, Kamm MA, Scarpignato C, Wald A. Myths and misconceptions about chronic constipation. *Am J Gastroenterol* 2005; **100**: 232–42.

14 DiPalma JA, Cleveland M vB, McGowan BS, *et al.* A randomized, multicenter comparison of polyethylene glycol laxative and tegaserod in treatment of patients with chronic constipation. *Am J Gastroenterol* 2007; **102**: 232–42.

15 Ramkumar D, Rao SS. Efficacy and safety of traditional medical therapies for chronic constipation: systematic review. *Am J Gastroenterol* 2005; **100**: 936–71.

16 Harris LA, Crowell MD. Linaclotide, a new direction in the treatment of irritable bowel syndrome and chronic constipation. *Curr Opin Mol Ther* 2007; **9**: 403–10.

17 Heymen S, Scarlett Y, Jones K, *et al.* Randomized, controlled trial shows biofeedback to be superior to alternative treatments for patients with pelvic floor dyssynergia-type constipation. *Dis Colon Rectum* 2007; **50**: 428–41.

18 Rao SS, Seaton K, Miller M, *et al.* Randomized controlled trial of biofeedback, sham feedback, and standard therapy for dyssynergic defecation. *Clin Gastroenterol Hepatol* 2007; **5**: 331–8.

CHAPTER 29
Perianal Disease

David A. Schwartz and Brad E. Maltz

Division of Gastroenterology, Vanderbilt University, Nashville, TN, USA

Summary

Perianal disease is a common manifestation of Crohn disease. Perianal fistulae occur frequently and often are a major detriment to quality of life. Fistulae may be associated with active inflammation or quiescent disease. The diagnosis of fistula is made clinically and confirmed by exam under anesthesia and/or some imaging modality (either endoscopic ultrasound or magnetic resonance imaging). Treatment depends on severity of disease and complexity of the fistula. A combined medical and surgical treatment is typically the preferred approach. Anti-TNF drugs are the most efficacious medical therapy available. There are many studies underway to determine the long-term effectiveness of current therapies in maintaining cessation of fistula drainage over time.

Case

A 38-year-old woman presents with history of colonic Crohn disease of 5 years' duration. Her main symptoms include diarrhea and occasional blood in stool. She is currently on 5-aminosalicylic acid therapy alone. She presents to the office with stool "incontinence." She describes staining of her undergarments every day with small amounts of yellowish discharge, without the sensation of defecation. She has some discomfort when she defecates, and has no fevers or chills.

Definition and Epidemiology

Crohn disease can lead to a variety of perianal complications including skin tags, hemorrhoids, anal fissure, anal ulcer, anorectal stricture, or perirectal ulcers. In this section, we will focus on perianal fistulae. Fistulae are abnormal connections between two epithelium-lined organs that normally do not connect, in this case the colon/rectum and the perianal skin.

Practical Gastroenterology and Hepatology: Small and Large Intestine and Pancreas, 1st edition. Edited by Nicholas J. Talley, Sunanda V. Kane and Michael B. Wallace. © 2010 Blackwell Publishing Ltd.

Fistulae can be grouped into two categories: simple or complex. A simple fistula is superficial, intersphincteric, or low trans-sphincteric with only one external opening and it is not associated with an abscess nor connected to an adjacent structure. A complex fistula involves more of the anal sphincters (i.e., high trans-sphincteric, extrasphincteric, or suprasphincteric), has multiple openings, "horseshoes" (crossing the midline either anteriorly or posteriorly), is associated with a perianal abscess, and/or connects to an adjacent structure such as the vagina or bladder [1] (Figure 29.1).

The frequency of perianal fistulae in Crohn disease has been estimated to be 20% [2]. Distal disease is more likely to result in perianal fistula, for example colonic disease with rectal involvement (92% have fistulae) versus isolated disease of ileum (12% have fistulae) [3].

Pathophysiology

There are two proposed mechanisms for fistula development (Figures 29.2 and 29.3). Fistulae may develop as ulcers that extend over time as stool is forced into the ulcer with the pressure of defecation. Fistulae may also begin as anal gland abscesses that originate from the intersphincteric space.

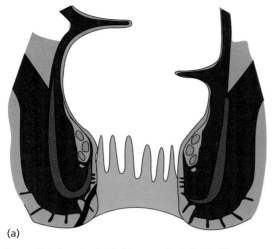 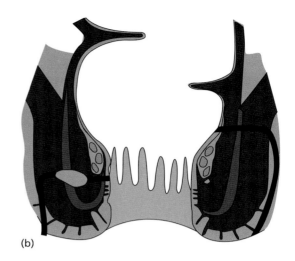

Figure 29.1 Complex fistula (a) versus simple fistula (b).

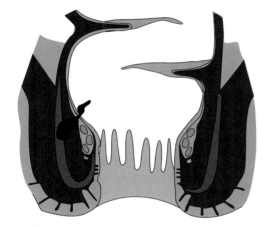 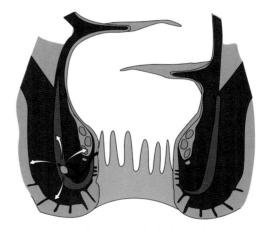

Figure 29.2 Proposed mechanism for fistula development: fistula beginning as an abscess.

Figure 29.3 Proposed mechanism for fistula development: fistula beginning as an ulcer.

Clinical Features

Perianal Crohn disease may present often as anorectal abscess, fistulae, or fissures. This is usually associated with pain, fluctuance, and/or drainage of stool or purulent material. It is common for fistulae to be more actively draining during periods of increased disease activity, that is diarrhea. Occasionally, perianal fistula may be the initial or only manifestation of a patient's Crohn disease.

Diagnosis

Great care should be taken to fully define the disease process prior to starting therapy. The type of fistula (simple vs. complex) and the degree of inflammation present will determine the initial choice of therapy (Figure 29.4). Because of the scarring and induration present, digital rectal examination or exam under anesthesia is not always an accurate way to assess fistulae.

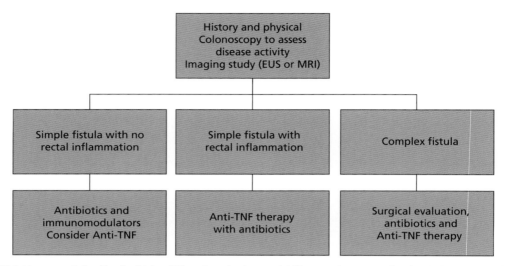

Figure 29.4 Management algorithm for fistulae. EUS, endoscopic ultrasound; MRI, magnetic resonance imaging; TNF, tumor necrosis factor.

Therefore, some imaging should be performed in nearly all situations.

Magnetic resonance imaging (MRI) and endoscopic ultrasound (EUS) have been studied extensively and have been shown to be very accurate for evaluating Crohn disease fistulae [4,5]. When EUS or MRI is combined with exam under anesthesia, the accuracy in diagnosing fistulae is 100% [6].

> **Case continued**
>
> On exam she has an obvious draining perirectal fistula. Colonoscopy was performed as well, revealing pan colitis of moderate intensity. Rectal EUS was then performed and revealed a complex fistula (high trans-sphincteric fistula without associated abscess) (Video 14).

Therapeutics

A number of medical options exist for the treatment of Crohn disease perianal fistula (Table 29.1). The therapies frequently used include antibiotics, immunomodulators, cyclosporine, tacrolimus, and antitumor necrosis factor-α antibodies (anti-TNF-α).

Antibiotics such as metronidazole 750–1000 mg/day or ciprofloxacin 1000–1500 mg/day are most commonly used. Several open-label studies support the observation that metronidazole may lead to cessation of fistula drainage in 34–50% of patients [7,8]. Typically, patients will have clinical improvement after 6–8 weeks of therapy, but reoccurrence is frequently noted after cessation of therapy. Ciprofloxacin has been used as an alternative to metronidazole for perianal disease although no controlled trials have been performed to support its use in this setting.

Immunomodulators, specifically 6-mercaptopurine and azathioprine, have been studied for perianal disease. Pearson *et al.* published a meta-analysis demonstrating that 22 of 41 (54%) of patients with perianal Crohn disease who received azathioprine responded versus only six of 29 (21%) who received placebo. The pooled odds ratio was 4.44 in favor of fistula healing [9].

Tacrolimus has been studied for fistulizing Crohn disease in a randomized, double-blinded, placebo-controlled trial [10]. In this trial, 43% of patients treated with 0.20 mg/kg/day of tacrolimus improved compared with 8% of placebo-treated patients. However, only 10% of tacrolimus-treated patients had complete fistula closure versus 8% of placebo-treated patients.

The Anti-TNF-α drugs have really changed perianal fistula management. The most extensive studies have been with infliximab. The initial short-term infliximab

Table 29.1 Evidenced-based therapeutics.

Reference	Year	Therapy	No of patients	Response (%)	Comment
Present *et al.* [15]	1980	Mercaptopurine	36	Therapy 31 Placebo 6	Daily 6-mercaptopurine or placebo for 1 year then crossed over to other arm of study for additional year
Sandborn *et al.* [10]	2003	Tacrolimus	48	Therapy 43 Placebo 8	Fistula remission similar between groups 10 vs. 8%
Present *et al.* [11]	1999	Infliximab	94	Therapy 68 Placebo 26	55% had closure of all fistulae, as compared with 13% in placebo
ACCENT II [12]	2004	Infliximab	195	Therapy 36 Placebo 19	Maintenance of fistula closure at 54 weeks
CHARM [13]	2007	Adalimumab	117	Therapy 33 Placebo 13	Durable response, all who had response at week 26 had continued response at week 56

fistula trial showed a 68% response rate for those that received the induction sequence of infliximab of 5 mg/kg at weeks 0, 2, and 6 compared to 26% response in the placebo cohort [11].

The ACCENT II trial investigated whether cessation of fistula drainage could be preserved with infliximab maintenance therapy given every 8 weeks. Patients who had active fistulae who responded to the induction sequence of infliximab of 5 mg/kg at weeks 0, 2, and 6 were randomized to receive infliximab or placebo every 8 weeks. After 54 weeks, 36% of patients in the infliximab group maintained complete fistula closure compared with 19% in the placebo arm (p = 0.009) [12].

The adalimumab maintenance trial (CHARM) looked at fistula healing as a secondary end point [13]. Complete fistula closure at 56 weeks was 33% versus 13% in the placebo arm (p = 0.016).

Although a thorough discussion of surgical options are beyond the scope of this chapter, conservative surgical procedures such as the placement of draining seton, fistulotomy, or incision and drainage of abscess are necessary components of fistula management and allow the for control fistula/abscess healing during medical treatment. This helps the medications to be more effective and optimizes outcomes. A retrospective study of patients with Crohn disease perianal fistulae treated with infliximab demonstrated that patients who underwent exam under anesthesia with seton placement prior to receiving infliximab had nearly half the recurrence rate of those treated with infliximab alone (44% vs. 79%, p = 0.001) [14].

Case continued

She was sent for exam under anesthesia and seton placement and started on infliximab. Drainage stopped in 4 weeks, then after 8 weeks no material could be expressed from fistula on exam. Twelve weeks later, EUS revealed fistula inactivity and the seton was removed.

Take-home points

- Perianal fistulae are a frequent manifestation in Crohn disease.
- Fistulae result in significant morbidity and often lead to a need for surgical intervention.
- Exam and imaging with EUS or MRI are recommended modalities to evaluate fistulae.
- Patients should be stratified into one of three groups: simple fistula and no proctitis; simple fistula and concomitant proctitis; and complex fistula.
- Simple fistulae and no proctitis can be treated with antibiotics and immunomodulators.
- Simple fistulae in the setting of proctitis can be treated with biologic agents.
- Complex fistulae require surgical intervention.
- In general, a combined medical and surgical approach is the preferred management strategy.

References

1 American Gastroenterological Association. American Gastroenterological Association medical position statement:

perianal Crohn's disease. *Gastroenterology* 2003; **125**: 1503–7.

2 Schwartz DA, Loftus EV, Jr., Tremaine WJ, *et al.* The natural history of fistulizing Crohn's disease in Olmsted County, Minnesota. *Gastroenterology* 2002; **122**: 875–80.

3 Hellers G, Bergstrand O, Ewerth S, *et al.* Occurrence and outcome after primary treatment of anal fistulae in Crohn's disease. *Gut* 1980; **21**: 525–7.

4 Haggett PJ, Moore NR, Shearman JD, *et al.* Pelvic and perineal complications of Crohn's disease: assessment using magnetic resonance imaging. *Gut* 1995; **36**: 407–10.

5 Tio TL, Mulder CJ, Wijers OB, *et al.* Endosonography of peri-anal and peri-colorectal fistula and/or abscess in Crohn's disease. *Gastrointest Endosc* 1990; **36**: 331–6.

6 Schwartz DA, Wiersema MJ, Dudiak KM, *et al.* A comparison of endoscopic ultrasound, magnetic resonance imaging, and exam under anesthesia for evaluation of Crohn's perianal fistulas. *Gastroenterology* 2001; **121**: 1064–72.

7 Jakobovits J, Schuster MM. Metronidazole therapy for Crohn's disease and associated fistulae. *Am J Gastroenterol* 1984; **79**: 533–40.

8 Brandt LJ, Bernstein LH, Boley SJ, *et al.* Metronidazole therapy for perineal Crohn's disease: a follow-up study. *Gastroenterology* 1982; **83**: 383–7.

9 Pearson DC, May GR, Fick GH, *et al.* Azathioprine and 6-mercaptopurine in Crohn disease. A meta-analysis. *Ann Intern Med* 1995; **123**: 132–42.

10 Sandborn WJ, Present DH, Isaacs KL, *et al.* Tacrolimus for the treatment of fistulas in patients with Crohn's disease: a randomized, placebo-controlled trial. *Gastroenterology* 2003; **125**: 380–8.

11 Present DH, Rutgeerts P, Targan S, *et al.* Infliximab for the treatment of fistulas in patients with Crohn's disease. *N Engl J Med* 1999; **340**: 1398–405.

12 Sands BE, Anderson FH, Bernstein CN, *et al.* Infliximab maintenance therapy for fistulizing Crohn's disease. *N Engl J Med* 2004; **350**: 876–85.

13 Colombel JF, Sandborn WJ, Rutgeerts P, *et al.* Adalimumab for maintenance of clinical response and remission in patients with Crohn's disease: the CHARM trial. *Gastroenterology* 2007; **132**: 52–65.

14 Regueiro M, Mardini H. Treatment of perianal fistulizing Crohn's disease with infliximab alone or as an adjunct to exam under anesthesia with seton placement. *Inflamm Bowel Dis* 2003; **9**: 98–103.

15 Present DH, Korelitz BI, Wisch N, *et al.* Treatment of Crohn's disease with 6-mercaptopurine. A long-term, randomized, double-blind study. *N Engl J Med* 1980; **302**: 981–7.

CHAPTER 30
Fecal Incontinence

Adil E. Bharucha and Karthik Ravi

Division of Gastroenterology and Hepatology, Mayo Clinic, Rochester, MN, USA

Summary

Fecal incontinence (FI) is commonly defined as the involuntary loss of feces, and has significant psychosocial consequences. Several factors, and in particular anal sphincter trauma secondary to obstetric injury, have been implicated as a cause of FI. The clinical evaluation is very useful for assessing symptom severity and for guiding management. Testing is guided by clinical features and the response to therapy and generally begins with anorectal manometry. Additional tests (e.g., endoanal ultrasound, defecography, pelvic MRI, and anal electromyography) are useful in selected cases. In many patients, patient education and management of disordered bowel habits are very useful for improving fecal continence; pelvic floor retraining may be useful for patients who do not respond to these measures. Although anal sphincteroplasty improves fecal continence in the short term, the beneficial effects wane over time.

Case

A 67-year-old female presented with incontinence for small amounts of formed stool on an average of 3 days a week for 6 months. This leakage was not associated with urgency and often occurred shortly after defecation. She used a protective panty liner, and changed this once daily. The rectal examination was notable for reduced anal resting tone, an impaired puborectalis lift during voluntary contraction of pelvic floor muscles, reduced perineal descent during simulated evacuation, a moderate-sized rectocele, normal perianal sensation, and an absent anal wink reflex.

Anal manometry demonstrated reduced anal resting and squeeze pressures with normal thresholds for sensation, desire to defecate, and urgency. The rectoanal inhibitory reflex was present. The rectal balloon expulsion test was abnormal. Anal surface electromyography disclosed increased resting activity, appropriate activation of pelvic floor and accessory muscles, and a tendency to paradoxically co-contract abdominal and pelvic floor muscles during simulated evacuation.

In addition to fiber supplementation, nine sessions of pelvic floor retraining by biofeedback therapy were provided over 1 week. Three months thereafter, she was passing an average of two large formed bowel movements daily and had less incontinence, that is an average of two episodes every month.

Introduction

Definition and Epidemiology

Fecal incontinence (FI) is the involuntary loss of feces— solid or liquid. FI occurs in a variety of disorders associated with pelvic floor weakness and/or altered bowel habits and can impact nearly every aspect of daily life.

The prevalence of FI in the community is variable and ranges from 2.2 to 15% [1]. Although most attention on FI has focused on women, prevalence maybe similar in men and is related to age, and increases from 7% in the third decade to 22% in the sixth decade, plateauing thereafter . The median age of onset is the seventh decade [2]. A majority of people with FI in the community have symptoms which are of mild (50%) or moderate (45%) severity.

Etiology

FI is attributable to anorectal sensorimotor dysfunctions and/or altered bowel habits, which may be caused by a

Practical Gastroenterology and Hepatology: Small and Large Intestine and Pancreas, 1st edition. Edited by Nicholas J. Talley, Sunanda V. Kane and Michael B. Wallace. © 2010 Blackwell Publishing Ltd.

Table 30.1 Etiology of fecal incontinence.

Anal sphincter weakness
  Injury: obstetric trauma, related to surgical procedures, e.g., hemorrhoidectomy internal sphincterotomy, fistulotomy, anorectal infection
  Non-traumatic: scleroderma, internal sphincter thinning of unknown etiology

Neuropathy: stretch injury, obstetric trauma, diabetes mellitus

Anatomical disturbances of pelvic floor: fistula, rectal prolapse, descending perineum syndrome

Inflammatory conditions: Crohn disease, ulcerative colitis, radiation proctitis

Central nervous system disease: dementia, stroke, brain tumors, spinal cord lesions, multiple system atrophy (Shy–Drager syndrome), multiple sclerosis

Diarrhea: irritable bowel syndrome, postcholecystectomy diarrhea

Reproduced with permission from Bharucha A. *Gastroenterology* 2003; 124: 1672–85.

Table 30.2 Relationship between obstetric history, anorectal injury, and incontinence.

Ultrasound reveals anal sphincter defects, which are often clinically occult, in 25–50% of women after a vaginal delivery

External sphincter defects are more likely to cause anal weakness than injury to the longitudinal muscle and transverse perinei

Incident postpartum FI is uncommon (i.e., 10% or less of all vaginal deliveries) and is more likely (15–59%) in women who sustain a 3rd or 4th degree anal sphincter tear during vaginal delivery

A higher body mass index (BMI), white race, antenatal urinary incontinence, and older age at delivery are risk factors for FI in women with anal sphincter tears

Obstetric risk factors for anal sphincter tears vary among studies

The use of forceps is a consistent risk factor

There is no difference between restrictive episiotomy practices versus midline versus mediolateral episiotomies

The risk of FI is not lower after cesarean section than after vaginal delivery

Reproduced with permission from Bharucha AE. Fecal incontinence. In: Parkman H, McCallum R, Rao S, eds. *The Handbook of Gastrointestinal Motility Testing*. Cambridge University Press. In Press.

variety of conditions (Table 30.1) [3]. In women, FI is generally attributed to pelvic floor trauma resulting from obstetric injury. While women with severe obstetric trauma (e.g., third or fourth-degree lacerations) may develop FI shortly after vaginal delivery, most women present with FI two to three decades after vaginal delivery [2]. Therefore, the contribution of obstetric injury to FI in many women is unclear (Table 30.2) [4].

Age, female gender, poor general health, physical limitations, obesity, loose stools, urgency, perianal injury, and surgery have all been identified as risk factors for FI; with some suggestion that rectal urgency is the single most important risk factor [5]. In people aged 65 years and older, self-reported diabetes mellitus, self-reported stroke, and certain medications (i.e., antiparkinsonian, hypnotic, and antipsychotic medications) are also risk factors for FI [6].

Pathophysiology of Fecal Incontinence

Mechanisms of Normal Fecal Continence

Fecal continence is maintained by anatomical factors, rectoanal sensation, and rectal compliance [7]. The internal anal sphincter, which is made of circular smooth muscle, maintains approximately 70% of anal resting tone. The external anal sphincter, comprised of striated muscle, accounts for the remaining component of resting tone. The puborectalis is a U-shaped component of the levator ani complex which also helps maintain the recto-anal angle at rest. The external sphincter, puborectalis, and levator ani contract further when necessary to preserve continence.

Rectal distension by stool induces rectal contraction, the sensation of urgency, reflex relaxation of the internal anal sphincter, and semivoluntary relaxation of pelvic floor muscles, prompting defecation if socially convenient. If not, rectal contractions and the sensation of urgency generally subside as the rectum accommodates to continued distension. This, together with voluntary contraction of the external anal sphincter and puborectalis muscles, permits defecation to be postponed when necessary.

Pathophysiology of Fecal Incontinence
Anal Sphincter Weakness

A majority of women with FI have reduced anal resting and/or squeeze pressures, reflecting weakness of the

Table 30.3 Symptom-Severity Scale in fecal incontinence.

Symptoms	Symptom Severity Score			
	1	2	3	4
Frequency	<1/month	>1/month to several times/week	Daily	
Composition	Mucus/liquid stool	Solid stool	Liquid and solid stool	
Amount	Small (i.e., staining only)	Moderate (i.e., requiring change of underwear)	Large (i.e. requiring change of all clothes)	
Urgency or passive incontinence	Neither	Passive incontinence	Urge incontinence	Combined (i.e., passive and urge) incontinence

The symptom severity score was derived by using a physician-assigned score (i.e., the symptom-severity score) to each of the four self-reported symptoms of FI [3]. Maximum total score = 13. Scores of 1–6, 7–10, and 11–13 were categorized as mild, moderate, and severe fecal incontinence, respectively. (Reproduced from Bharucha AE, *et al.* [12], with permission.)

internal and/or external anal sphincters respectively [8]. In addition to anal sphincter injury, FI is also associated with atrophy, denervation, and impaired function of the puborectalis muscle. Generalized pelvic floor weakness is often associated with pelvic organ prolapse affecting the anterior and/or middle compartments. Additionally, excessive straining may cause increased perineal descent, which can stretch and thereby damage the pudendal nerve and also make the anorectal angle more obtuse.

Rectal Sensorimotor Dysfunctions

Patients with FI may have normal, reduced, or increased rectal sensation [8]. When rectal sensation is reduced, the external anal sphincter may not contract promptly when the rectum is distended by stool. Conversely, rectal hypersensitivity in FI may be partly secondary to an exaggerated contractile response to distension, and/or increased rectal tone with reduced capacity.

Impaired Rectal Evacuation

Fecal incontinence may be associated with features of disordered evacuation [8]. Such patients may benefit from biofeedback retraining not only to improve rectal sensation and rectal coordination, but also to improve abdominopelvic coordination during defecation.

Clinical Features

In patients with FI, a detailed history is imperative for determining the etiology and severity and for guiding diagnostic testing and treatment (Table 30.3). Bowel habits, stool form, and consistency should preferably be characterized by pictorial stool scales (e.g., Bristol scale). Staining, soiling, seepage, and leakage are terms used to indicate the severity of incontinence [9]. Soiling indicates more leakage than staining of underwear; soiling can be specified further, that is of underwear, outer clothing, or furnishing/bedding. Seepage refers to leakage of small amounts of stool. Leakage of solid stool probably reflects more severe anal weakness than isolated leakage of liquid stool. Patients who report that they "leak liquid or solid stool without any warning" often (>25% of time) or usually (>75% of time) are considered to have passive incontinence [8]. Patients who report experiencing an "urgent need to empty their bowels" often or more, are considered to have rectal urgency. Patients can present with urgency incontinence, passive incontinence, or a combination [8]. The impact on quality of life should be ascertained [10]. The severity of FI can be scored by standardized scoring systems [2,11,12].

After anal inspection, a digital rectal examination is very useful for gauging anal sphincter and puborectalis functions. The resistance to anal digital insertion provides a measure of anal resting pressure. Voluntary contraction should lift the examining finger anteriosuperiorly (i.e., toward the umbilicus). Conversely, simulated defecation should be accompanied by 2–4 cm of perineal descent and puborectalis relaxation. Finally, examination in the seated position on a commode may reveal rectal prolapse or excessive perineal descent, which may not be evident when supine.

Diagnostic Testing

The extent of diagnostic testing is tailored to the patient's age, probable etiological factors, symptom severity, impact on quality of life, response to conservative medical management, and availability of tests.

Endoscopy

Endoscopic assessment of the rectosigmoid mucosa should be considered in most patients, particularly those with constipation and/or diarrhea.

Anal Manometry

Assessment of anal pressures by manometry is a starting point for diagnostic testing in FI. Manometry should be interpreted with reference to normal values in age- and gender-matched subjects. Anal resting and squeeze pressures are frequently reduced in FI. Anorectal testing (i.e., anal manometry, rectal balloon expulsion test) can also identify a rectal evacuation disorder, which may coexist with FI.

Rectal Sensation and Compliance

Rectal sensation is assessed by distending a balloon manually, or with a barostat. Volume thresholds for first perception, desire to defecate, and severe urgency are measured during distension. Thresholds for rectal sensation may be normal, reduced, or increased in FI, as discussed above.

Rectal compliance is optimally measured by assessing rectal pressure–volume relationships with a barostat [8]. Reduced compliance may cause symptoms of rectal urgency and frequent defecation.

Endoanal Ultrasound

Endoanal ultrasound identifies anal sphincter thinning and defects, which are often clinically unrecognized and may be amenable to surgical repair. Whereas endoanal ultrasound reliably identifies anatomic defects or thinning of the internal sphincter, interpretation of external sphincter images is much more subjective, operator-dependent, and confounded by normal anatomical variations in the external sphincter.

Dynamic Proctography (Defecography)

Dynamic proctography is useful when clinical features suggest excessive perineal descent, internal rectal intus-susception, rectoceles, sigmoidoceles, or enteroceles. Puborectalis dysfunction during squeeze and evacuation can also be characterized. Contrast retention and evacuation, the anorectal angle, and position of the anorectal junction are tracked at rest and while patients squeeze and subsequently strain to expel barium paste from the rectum.

Pelvic Magnetic Resonance Imaging

Pelvic magnetic resonance imaging (MRI) is the only imaging modality that can visualize both anal sphincter anatomy and global pelvic floor motion in real-time without radiation exposure. MRI performs the same or better than ultrasound for assessing the external sphincter [8]. Endoanal MRI also reveals puborectalis atrophy in FI [8]. Dynamic MRI provides a unique appreciation of global pelvic floor motion because the bladder and genital organs are also visualized.

Needle Electromyography (EMG) of the External Sphincter

Needle EMG provides a sensitive measure of denervation and can usually identify myopathic damage, neurogenic damage, or mixed injury affecting the external anal sphincter. Anal EMG should be considered in patients with clinically suspected neurogenic sphincter weakness.

Management

Dietary and Pharmacological Approaches

Modifying irregular bowel habits is the cornerstone to effectively managing FI (Figure 30.1). A detailed dietary history is useful for identifying excessive ingestion of foods, such as those that contain fructose and sorbitol, which might cause or aggravate diarrhea. Loperamide reduces diarrhea and slightly increases internal sphincter tone, thereby reducing FI [3]. Adequate doses are essential (i.e., 2–4 mg, 30 min before meals; up to 16 mg daily). Taking loperamide before social occasions may reduce the risk of having an accident outside the home. Diphenoxylate and amitriptyline are alternative options for diarrhea; amitriptyline may also reduce rectal urgency. The 5-HT_3 antagonist alosetron is useful for managing refractory functional diarrhea. Patients with constipa-

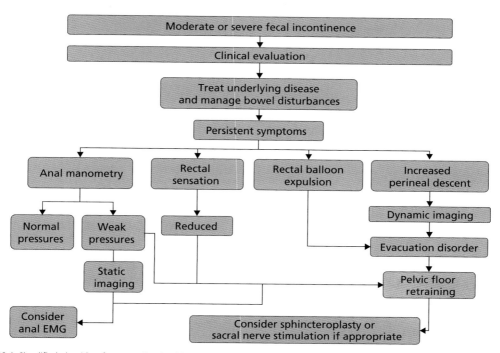

Figure 30.1 Simplified algorithm for managing fecal incontinence. The choice of investigations is guided by the clinical features as detailed in the text, and by the response to conservative measures, particularly management of bowel disturbances. Thereafter, further measures (e.g., pelvic floor retraining) may be necessary. Reprinted with permission from Bharucha AE, Fletcher JG. Investigation of fecal incontinence. In: Stoker J, Taylor SA, DeLancey JOL, eds. *Medical Radiology: Diagnostic Imaging and Radiation Oncology; Imaging and Pelvic Floor Disorders*, 2nd revised edn. Springer, 2008: 229–43.

tion, fecal impaction, and overflow incontinence might benefit from an evacuation program and may include one or more of the following measures: using timed evacuation by bisacodyl or glycerol suppositories, fiber supplementation, and judicious use of oral laxatives.

Pelvic Floor Exercises and Biofeedback Therapy

Pelvic floor exercises entail contraction of the sphincter, anal and pelvic floor muscles but not the abdominal wall. Biofeedback therapy is generally performed by providing patients, usually with visual, feedback anal manometric or surface EMG sensors. Patients learn to coordinate sphincter contraction during rectal distension. If rectal sensation is reduced, patients are taught to recognize rectal distension with progressively smaller volumes, generally beginning with 50 mL and declining to 10 mL or lower. In general, biofeedback is more effective than pelvic floor exercises alone for patients with FI who do

not respond to routine medications, and educational and behavioral strategies [13].

Incontinence Products

Perineal protective devices include disposable and reusable body worn products (diaper-type garments or pads), and disposable and reusable under pads (also called bed pads). Many patients wear panty liners and often line them with toilet paper. Anal plugs are available in Europe but not in the United States.

Surgical Approaches

Anal Sphincteroplasty

Consideration should be given to repairing external sphincter defects in women with postpartum FI. The benefit of repairing defects with overlapping anterior sphincteroplasty is not clear because the initial improvement in fecal continence is not often sustained, with a 50% failure rate after 40–60 months [14].

Other Surgical Approaches

Dynamic graciloplasty involves continuous electrical stimulation of the gracilis muscle, which is surgically transposed around the anal canal [3]. Although fecal continence may improve, this procedure and artificial sphincter are often complicated by mortality and significant morbidity. Therefore, these procedures are not widely used in the United States. A colostomy is the last resort for patients with severe fecal incontinence.

Sacral Nerve Stimulation

Several uncontrolled studies and more recently, a North American multicenter study of 120 patients with fecal incontinence, suggest that sacral nerve stimulation (SNS) is safe; 83% of subjects achieved therapeutic success (95% confidence interval: 74–90%), defined as a 50% or greater reduction in the number of weekly incontinent episodes at 12 months. While patients had not responded to conservative therapy, this was not standardized. Moreover, the mechanisms of action for SNS are not understood since effects on anal pressures and rectal sensation are inconsistent across studies [15,16].

Conclusions

Fecal incontinence is a common and often devastating symptom. Because people with FI are often reluctant to acknowledge the symptom, it behooves physicians to ask patients with risk factors for FI (e.g., diarrhea, urinary incontinence) whether they have FI. The clinical assessment is extremely useful for understanding the circumstances and severity surrounding FI. It also provides considerable information about the pathophysiology of FI. Diagnostic testing should be guided by the clinical features and the response to previous therapy. The management should focus on regulation of bowel disturbances. Pelvic floor retraining and surgery are also helpful in selected patients.

Take-home points

Diagnosis:
- It is imperative to ask patients if they have fecal incontinence (FI) and to obtain a detailed history.
- A careful digital rectal examination is useful for assessing anal sphincter functions and rectal evacuation.

- Assessment of anal resting and squeeze pressures by manometry is a starting point for diagnostic testing in FI.
- Depending on the clinical features, anorectal imaging (ultrasound, defecography, and pelvic MRI) and electromyography may also be useful.

Therapy:
- Modifying irregular bowel habits is the cornerstone to effectively managing FI in most patients.
- Biofeedback therapy should be considered in patients who do not respond to conservative management.
- Although anal sphincteroplasty improves fecal continence in the short term, these beneficial effects decline over time.

References

1 Nelson RL. Epidemiology of fecal incontinence. *Gastroenterology* 2004; **126** (Suppl. 1): S3–7.

2 Bharucha AE, Zinsmeister AR, Locke GR, *et al.* Prevalence and burden of fecal incontinence: A population based study in women. *Gastroenterology* 2005; **129**: 42–9.

3 Andrews CN, Bharucha AE. The etiology, assessment, and treatment of fecal incontinence. *Nat Clin Pract Gastroenterol Hepatol* 2005; **2**: 516–25.

4 Wheeler TL, 2nd, Richter HE. Delivery method, anal sphincter tears and fecal incontinence: new information on a persistent problem. *Curr Opin Obstet Gynecol* 2007; **19**: 474–9.

5 Bharucha AE, Zinsmeister AR, Locke GR, *et al.* Risk factors for fecal incontinence: a population based study in women. *Am J Gastroenterol* 2006; **101**: 1305–12.

6 Quander CR, Morris MC, Melson J, *et al.* Prevalence of and factors associated with fecal incontinence in a large community study of older individuals. *Am J Gastroenterol* 2005; **100**: 905–9.

7 Bharucha AE. Pelvic floor: anatomy and function. *Neurogastroenterol Motil* 2006; **18**: 507–19.

8 Bharucha AE, Fletcher JG, Harper CM, *et al.* Relationship between symptoms and disordered continence mechanisms in women with idiopathic fecal incontinence. *Gut* 2005; **54**: 546–55.

9 Perry S, Shaw C, McGrother C, *et al.* Prevalence of faecal incontinence in adults aged 40 years or more living in the community. *Gut* 2002; **50**: 480–4.

10 Norton NJ. The perspective of the patient. *Gastroenterology* 2004; **126** (Suppl. 1): S175–9.

11 Rockwood TH. Incontinence severity and QOL scales for fecal incontinence. *Gastroenterology* 2004; **126**: S106–13.

12 Bharucha AE, Zinsmeister AR, Locke GR, *et al.* Symptoms and quality of life in community women with fecal incontinence. *Clin Gastroenterol Hepatol* 2006; **4**: 1004–9.

13 Heymen S, Scarlett Y, Jones K, *et al.* AGA Institute Abstracts: Randomized controlled trial shows biofeedback to be superior to alternative treatments for patients with fecal incontinence. *Gastroenterology* 2007; **132** (Suppl. 2): A–83.

14 Brown SR, Nelson RL. Surgery for faecal incontinence in adults. [update of *Cochrane Database Syst Rev* 2000; **2**: CD001757; PMID: 10796816]. *Cochrane Database System Rev* 2007; **2**: CD001757.

15 Rosen HR, Urbarz C, Holzer B, *et al.* Sacral nerve stimulation as a treatment for fecal incontinence. *Gastroenterology* 2001; **121**: 536–41.

16 Wexner SD, Coller JA, Devroede G, *et al.* Sacral nerve stimulation for fecal incontinence. Results of a 120-patient prospective multicenter study. *Ann Surg* 2010; **51**: 441–9.

31

CHAPTER 31
Colorectal Cancer Screening

Katherine S. Garman[1] and Dawn Provenzale[2]

[1] Division of Gastroenterology and Institute for Genome Sciences and Policy, Veterans Affairs Medical Center, Duke University Medical Center, Durham, NC, USA
[2] Veterans Affairs Medical Center, Division of Gastroenterology, Duke University Medical Center, Durham, NC, USA

Summary

Colorectal cancer screening is an important mission for a practicing gastroenterologist. Several different screening modalities are available: fecal occult blood test, flexible sigmoidoscopy, colonoscopy, barium enema, and, more recently, CT-colonography and stool DNA tests. The physician is charged with weighing the pros and cons of the different screening methods and selecting the most appropriate method for each patient.

Case

A 35-year-old man with positive family history of colorectal cancer, diagnosed in his father at age 53, presents for information about colorectal cancer screening. He is in good health with hypertension controlled on hydrochlorothiazide. What recommendations should be provided in terms of screening? What other information should be gathered from the patient?

Introduction

Prior to embarking upon a discussion of colorectal cancer screening, some definitions are warranted. Screening applies to healthy, asymptomatic individuals and should improve the life expectancy of those screened. Surveillance applies to the follow-up of patients at increased risk for colorectal cancer including patients with a personal or family history of colorectal cancer or polyps, or with a history of inflammatory bowel disease.

Formal recommendations for colorectal screening began in 1980 with the first guidelines for screening issued by the American Cancer Society, initiating a series of society-issued guidelines with the goal of reducing

Practical Gastroenterology and Hepatology: Small and Large Intestine and Pancreas, 1st edition. Edited by Nicholas J. Talley, Sunanda V. Kane and Michael B. Wallace. © 2010 Blackwell Publishing Ltd.

colorectal cancer mortality [1]. Since then, the guidelines have become numerous and more complex, culminating in two recent guidelines: a Joint Guideline by the US Multi-Society Task Force on Colorectal Cancer and the American College of Radiology [2] released in 2008, and the updated National Comprehensive Cancer Network Guidelines in 2010 [3].

Review of Screening Methods

The current Joint Guidelines suggest that all screening tests should detect the majority (>50%) of prevalent or incident cancers at the time of testing. Colorectal cancer screening modalities are divided into two groups: tests that detect primarily cancer and those that detect either polyps or cancer.

Stool-Based Tests

The studies that primarily detect cancer are stool-based. The two tests designed to detect blood in the stool are the guaiac-based fecal occult blood test (gFOBT) and the immunochemical test for globin (iFOBT). DNA-based stool tests are designed to test for the presence of DNA carrying some of the common genetic mutations in colorectal cancer.

The gFOBT was the first screening test shown to decrease mortality from colorectal cancer [4–6]. The tests are inexpensive and easy to perform, making them ideal for population-based screening programs. It is important to note that there is no role for office-based gFOBT in colorectal cancer screening; these tests should be sent home with the patient and completed using two samples from each of three consecutive bowel movements. Sensitivity for cancer in the gFOBT ranges from 37.1 to 79.4% [7] and it is recommended that the gFOBT be repeated annually. Specificity for detection of cancer ranges from 86.7 to 97.7% [7].

The iFOBT for globin represents a variation on the FOBT and has not been studied in randomized controlled trials. Rather, the iFOBT has been compared to the gFOBT with the assumption that mortality reduction will be similar or better [8]. One limitation with the iFOBT is the lack of data regarding the optimal number of stool samples needed for screening. The Joint Guidelines [2] indicate that two samples may be better than one, but the ideal regimen has not been established. As with gFOBT, immunochemical stool tests should be repeated annually, and a positive test should always be followed with a colonoscopy.

The stool DNA test considers that most colorectal cancers acquire a series of mutations that can be detected by the presence of abnormal DNA in stool [9]. One stool DNA test is commercially available that examines mutations in *APC*, K-*ras*, *TP53*, and *BAT26*. A stool specimen is collected and mailed to a central lab. In a large prospective study using stool DNA in average risk individuals for screening [10], it detected 51.6% of invasive cancers, 32.5% of adenomas with high grade dysplasia, and 18.2% of all advanced adenomas. Specificity was high at 94.4%. There is no clearly specified interval for repeating the stool DNA test and it is expensive, limiting its general application as a clinically useful screening tool. The Joint Guidelines [2] include the stool DNA test as an acceptable screening test, but the US Preventive Services Task Force (USPSTF) Guidelines do not include it, citing lack of evidence [11].

Endoscopic Screening Tests

Flexible sigmoidoscopy has been associated with a significantly decreased risk of colorectal cancer. The exam can be performed in an office setting by a broad set of providers. Guidelines recommend a 5-year follow-up after a normal flexible sigmoidoscopy. The combination of flexible sigmoidoscopy and one-time FOBT increases the sensitivity of advanced adenoma detection from 70.3% for screening flexible sigmoidoscopy alone to 75.8% for both tests combined [12].

Colonoscopy has become the gold standard to which other colorectal cancer screening tests are compared, yet direct evidence for colonoscopy as a screening tool is limited. Colonoscopy is the screening test of choice for most gastroenterologists because it provides a complete exam of the colon with the opportunity for polypectomy and diagnostic biopsy of any suspicious lesion. There have been no prospective randomized controlled trials demonstrating a reduced cancer incidence or mortality benefit from screening colonoscopy.

Several studies have evaluated colonoscopy miss rates. For large adenomas, the colonoscopy miss rate has been estimated at 6–12% [2,13], and for colorectal cancers as high as 4% [14,15].

Recent data suggest that the colonoscopy miss rate may be higher for lesions in the proximal colon compared to the distal colon. In a cohort of Ontario residents, while the relative risk of colorectal cancer after colonoscopy was 0.21 (95% CI 0.05–0.36), colorectal cancers diagnosed after a negative colonoscopy were more likely to be located in the proximal colon compared with the control group [16]. In this same cohort, colonoscopy performed by a non-gastroenterologist was more likely to be associated with finding colorectal cancer after negative colonoscopy [17]. In a cross-sectional German cohort, the prevalence of colorectal cancer in patients who had undergone colonoscopy in the past ten years was decreased compared to those without previous colonoscopy with an adjusted prevalence ratio 0.54 (95% CI 0.39–0.75) [3]. However, the adjusted prevalence ratio for right-sided lesions was 1.05 (95% CI 0.63–1.76), indicating no protective effect in the proximal colon after colonoscopy [18]. There are many potential reasons for higher miss-rates in the proximal colon including: quality of right-sided bowel preparation, different tumor biology in proximal and distal colon, increased likelihood of flat lesions in the proximal colon, and factors related to the endoscopist [19].

Compared to the other available screening tests, colonoscopy carries a higher burden of complications. Bleeding is a risk after polypectomy and the risk of perforation is 1/1000 in the Medicare population [20]. Additional adverse events, including cardiac arrhythmias, may result from the use of sedation for colonoscopy.

Most guidelines recommend a 10-year interval for follow-up after a normal colonoscopy. This interval is based on reports that suggest a slow growth rate of adenomatous polyps, some of which will eventually develop into cancers, but there are few data to support this interval.

Imaging Tests

Imaging tests have been recommended as a primary screening modality by some [2,21], but the recent USPSTF Guideline concluded that there is insufficient evidence to recommend computed tomography (CT) colonography for screening for colorectal cancer [22].

A double contrast barium enema (DCBE) can be a primary screening modality or used to complete a failed colonoscopy. The data are limited on the use of this modality for cancer screening. With the advent of other imaging techniques, DCBE is being performed less frequently. While DCBE is still included as a potential screening modality by most guidelines, its use is likely to continue to decline, as reflected by the recent omission of DCBE from the USPSTF guidelines [11]. It may be more appropriate to consider DCBE as a means of completely examining the colon when a complete colonoscopy is indicated but cannot be performed.

CT colonography is a new and minimally invasive method of examining the colon and the rectum. It has only recently been incorporated into the Joint Guidelines [2] as an acceptable form of colorectal cancer screening. However, the USPSTF Guidelines do not include CT colonography as a recommended screening method due to lack of evidence [11].

As with DCBE, the patient requires colon preparation. In addition, the patient consumes an oral contrast agent to tag the stool. The interpretation of CT colonography is time consuming, and this may limit use in clinical settings. The National Comprehensive Cancer Network (NCCN) Guidelines for colorectal screening suggest that if colonoscopy is incomplete, colon exam should be completed with DCBE or CT colonography.

Like with colonoscopy, there have not been randomized controlled trials demonstrating that CT colonography can reduce morbidity and mortality from colorectal cancer. A recent multisite American College of Radiology Imaging Network (ACRIN) study of asymptomatic people undergoing routine colorectal cancer screening via CT colonography demonstrated 65% sensitivity for detection of polyps of size 5 mm or larger with 89% speci-

ficity; for polyps of 9 mm or larger, sensitivity improved to 90% with 86% specificity [23]. One cancer was missed by CT colonography in 2531 participants.

At this time, several factors limit CT colonography. The optimal interval between screening CT colonography exams has not yet been established, but the Joint Guidelines suggest 5 years. This is particularly important as small polyps less than 5 mm are not reported and sensitivity for 5 mm polyps is only 65%.

Finally, the radiation-related risks from repeat CT scans have not been established.

Discussion of the Guidelines

Several different organizations and professional societies have created guidelines for colorectal screening and surveillance. Table 31.1 reviews the different screening modalities as recommended in the different guidelines. In general, the Joint Guidelines [2] include many different screening modalities, including newer options such as CT colonography and stool DNA, while the USPSTF [11,22,24,25] and NCCN Colorectal Cancer Screening [3] favor better-studied screening methods such as FOBT and colonoscopy.

The guidelines vary slightly as to when to initiate colorectal cancer screening, although for most asymptomatic individuals with a negative family history, screening should begin at age 50. The American College of Gastroenterology recommends beginning screening at age 45 for African Americans [26]. The screening guidelines also differ in the management of patients who are at increased risk of colorectal cancer due to a personal history of inflammatory bowel disease (IBD) or due to a positive family history for colorectal cancer. It is important to recall that 35% of colorectal cancer is associated with some hereditary factor even if it is not part of an established familial colorectal cancer syndrome [27]. A thorough family history including age of diagnosis and type of cancer for each affected family member should be considered an important part of cancer screening for every individual; those with significant family histories may warrant more aggressive screening. The NCCN guidelines for colorectal cancer screening provide information on collection and integration of a family history into colorectal cancer screening [3].

The 2008 USPSTF guidelines recommend against routine screening in persons age 75–85 and they

Table 31.1 Choice of colorectal screening modality by guideline.

Guideline	Year	FOBT	Stool DNA	DCBE	Flexible sigmoidoscopy	Combination FS and FOBT	Colonoscopy	CT-colonography
Joint Guideline [2]	2008	Annually using guaiac-based test or immunochemical test	Interval uncertain	Every 5 years	Every 5 years		Every 10 years	Every 5 years
USPSTF [11]	2008	Annually	Insufficient evidence	No longer recommended		FS every 5 years with high-sensitivity FOBT every 3 years	Every 10 years	
NCCN [3]	2010	Annually using guaiac-based test or immunochemical test	Not considered first line screening test except in specific circumstances	Every 5 years Reserved for those who are unable to undergo complete colonoscopy or colonoscopy is technically incomplete	Every 5 years	FOBT annually with FS every 5 years	Preferred test Every 10 years if no risk factors	No consensus on use as a primary screening modality

USPSTF, US Preventive Services Task Force; NCCN, National Comprehensive Cancer Network; FOBT, fecal occult blood test; DCBE, double contrast barium enema; CT, computed tomography.

recommend against screening for those older than age 85 [11].

Once polyps or cancer have been diagnosed, the patient enters into a program of surveillance by colonoscopy. The guidelines for surveillance are included in Table 31.2 for comparison.

Case continued

For a 35-year-old man with a positive family history for colorectal cancer in his father at age 53, cancer screening by colonoscopy should begin at age 40 or 10 years younger than the youngest family member with colorectal cancer. If normal, it should be repeated in 5 years. Otherwise, follow-up is indicated by the findings at colonoscopy. It would be helpful to obtain a more detailed family history, asking about any family members with high polyp burden, other family members with colorectal cancer, or any of the hereditary non-polyposis colorectal cancer (HNPCC) associated tumors (colorectal, endometrial, stomach, ovarian, pancreas, ureter, renal pelvis, biliary tract, brain, small intestine, sebaceous gland adenomas, and keratoacanthomas [3]). If suspicion is raised for a familial syndrome, then genetic counseling should be offered.

Conclusion

Colorectal cancer screening has assumed two goals: reduction of mortality due to colorectal cancer and prevention of colorectal cancer through the removal of polyps. The best mortality data are for the simple annual FOBT starting at age 50 with colonoscopy to follow-up any positive test. Colonoscopy has long been considered the gold standard for polyp detection and removal although miss rates for even the detection of cancer have been reported as high as 4% [14,15]. In addition, emerging evidence suggests that the effectiveness of colonoscopy as a colorectal cancer prevention tool is reduced, particularly in the right colon [16–19]. Newer, less-invasive tests, such as stool DNA and CT colonography, represent additional modes of screening and we can expect more debate regarding the role of these new modalities in the coming years. Average-risk individuals age 50 and older should be encouraged to participate in colorectal cancer screening. High-risk patients due to family history of cancer or polyps, or personal history of longstanding

Table 31.2 Colonoscopy surveillance by guideline.

Guideline	Hyperplastic polyps	1-2 Small adenomas	Advanced adenomas	>10 Adenomas at a single exam	Sessile polyps removed piecemeal	Personal history of CRC
Joint Guideline [2]	Small rectal hyperplastic polyps: follow average screening guidelines	1-2 small tubular adenomas: 5-10 years after initial polypectomy	3-10 adenomas or 1 adenoma >1 cm or any adenoma with villous features or high-grade dysplasia: 3 years after initial polypectomy; if polyps removed and follow-up is normal or with 1-2 small polyps, repeat in 5 years	<3 years after initial polypectomy: consider familial syndrome	2-6 months	3-6 months after surgery or intraoperatively for perioperative clearing and then 1 year after surgical resection or the perioperative clearing exam
ACG [28]		1 or 2 adenomas <1 cm in size and no family history: repeat in 5 years	>2 adenomas, adenoma ≥1 cm, high grade dysplasia, villous histology, high grade dysplasia or positive family history: repeat in 3 years and if normal, repeat in 5 years		3-6 months	Malignant polyps: 3 months after endoscopic resection
NCCN [3]	Hyperplastic: 10 years	≤2 polyps <1 cm: repeat in 5 years and if normal, repeat every 5-10 years	3-10 adenomas, adenoma ≥1 cm, high grade dysplasia, villous features: repeat within 3 years and if normal, repeat in 5 years	>10 adenomas in a single exam or >15 cumulative adenomas: consider polyposis syndrome and genetic screening	2-6 months	Colonoscopy within 1 year (or within 3-6 months if no complete preoperative colonoscopy)
SSAT [29]		2 small <1cm polyps: repeat in 3 years				

ACG, American College of Gastroenterology; NCCN, National Comprehensive Cancer Network; SSAT, Society for Surgery of the Alimentary Tract; CRC, colorectal cancer.

inflammatory bowel disease, should be encouraged to adhere to a regular program of surveillance through colonoscopy.

There are a variety of recommended modalities for colorectal cancer screening. Some are more acceptable to patients and feasible for health-care systems. Ideally, the choice of screening modalities should be screenee and provider based. In systems where resources are limited, any of the approved modalities is preferable to the alternative of no screening. Future research should focus on interventions to implement appropriate screening, and identify ways to reduce the need for more invasive and expensive tests [30].

Take-home points

- Colorectal cancer is the second leading cause of cancer death in the US.
- Colorectal cancer screening has been shown to reduce mortality from colorectal cancer.
- There are multiple recommended screening modalities including, fecal occult blood testing (FOBT), stool DNA tests, flexible sigmoidoscopy, CT colonography, colonoscopy, and barium enema. There are different levels of evidence supporting the efficacy of each of these tests. In addition, the tests need to be repeated at their suggested intervals for screening to be effective.
- The choice of screening modality should be based on risk assessment by the provider. Risk assessment will determine if the individual is eligible for screening, e.g., does not have life-limiting co-morbidities that would diminish the effectiveness of screening. Furthermore, risk assessment is critical to determine if the individual to be screened is at average risk for developing colorectal cancer or at high risk based on personal or family history.
- Once an assessment of the individual's risk for colorectal cancer has been performed, the choice of screening modality should be based on a shared decision between the provider and the individual to be screened.
- Population-based colorectal cancer screening requires a substantial investment of patient, provider and health-system time and resources. Screening must be offered to the patient. The patient must accept screening and comply with appropriate instructions for the screening test. Positive tests must be followed up in a timely manner to diagnose colorectal cancer in an early and treatable stage. Some colorectal cancer screening tests are more acceptable to patients and feasible for health-care systems. In systems or settings where resources are limited, any of the approved modalities is preferable to the alternative of no screening.

References

1 Eddy DM. *Screening for Cancer: Theory, Analysis, and Design.* Englewood Cliffs, NJ: Prentice-Hall, 1980: xii, 308.

2 Levin B, Lieberman DA, McFarland B, *et al.* Screening and surveillance for the early detection of colorectal cancer and adenomatous polyps, 2008: a joint guideline from the American Cancer Society, the US Multi-Society Task Force on Colorectal Cancer, and the American College of Radiology. *CA Cancer J Clin* 2008; **58**: 130–60.

3 National Comprehensive Cancer Network. *Colorectal Cancer Screening. NCCN Clinical Practice Guidelines in Oncology* V.1.2010: 1–69.

4 Scholefield JH, Moss S, Sufi F, *et al.* Effect of faecal occult blood screening on mortality from colorectal cancer: results from a randomised controlled trial. *Gut* 2002; **50**: 840–4.

5 Jorgensen OD, Kronborg O, Fenger C. A randomised study of screening for colorectal cancer using faecal occult blood testing: results after 13 years and seven biennial screening rounds. *Gut* 2002; **50**: 29–32.

6 Vernon SW, Meissner H, Klabunde C, *et al.* Measures for ascertaining use of colorectal cancer screening in behavioral, health services, and epidemiologic research. *Cancer Epidemiol Biomarkers Prev* 2004; **13**: 898–905.

7 Allison JE, Tekawa IS, Ransom LJ, *et al.* A comparison of fecal occult-blood tests for colorectal-cancer screening. *N Engl J Med* 1996; **334**: 155–9.

8 Morikawa T, Kato J, Yamaji Y, *et al.* A comparison of the immunochemical fecal occult blood test and total colonoscopy in the asymptomatic population. *Gastroenterology* 2005; **129**: 422–8.

9 Osborn NK, Ahlquist DA. Stool screening for colorectal cancer: molecular approaches. *Gastroenterology* 2005; **128**: 192–206.

10 Imperiale TF, Wagner DR, Lin CY, *et al.* Risk of advanced proximal neoplasms in asymptomatic adults according to the distal colorectal findings. *N Engl J Med* 2000; **343**: 169–74.

11 U.S. Preventive Services Task Force. Screening for Colorectal Cancer: U.S. Preventive Services Task Force Recommendation. *Ann Intern Med* 2008; **149**: 627–37.

12 Rex DK, Lieberman DA. Feasibility of colonoscopy screening: discussion of issues and recommendations regarding implementation. *Gastrointest Endosc* 2001; **54**: 662–7.

13 Rex DK, Cutler CS, Lemmel GT, *et al.* Colonoscopic miss rates of adenomas determined by back-to-back colonoscopies. *Gastroenterology* 1997; **112**: 24–8.

14 Bressler B, Paszat LF, Vinden C, *et al.* Colonoscopic miss rates for right-sided colon cancer: a population-based analysis. *Gastroenterology* 2004; **127**: 452–6.

15 Rex DK, Rahmani EY, Haserman JH, *et al.* Relative sensitivity of colonoscopy and barium enema for detection of colorectal cancer in clinical practice. *Gastroenterology* 1997; **112**: 17–23.

16 Lakoff J, Paszat LF, Saskin R, Rabeneck L. Risk of developing proximal versus distal colorectal cancer after a negative colonoscopy: a population-based study. *Clin Gastroenterol Hepatol* 2008; **6**: 1117–21; quiz 1064.

17 Rabeneck L, Paszat LF, Saskin R. Endoscopist specialty is associated with incident colorectal cancer after a negative colonoscopy. *Clin Gastroenterol Hepatol* 2010; **8**: 275–9.

18 Brenner H, Hoffmeister M, Arndt V, *et al.* Protection from right- and left-sided colorectal neoplasms after colonoscopy: population-based study. *J Natl Cancer Inst* 2010; **102**: 89–95.

19 Hewett DG, Kahi CJ, Rex DK. Does colonoscopy work? *J Natl Compr Canc Netw* 2010; **8**: 67–76; quiz 77.

20 Gatto NM, Frucht H, Sundararajan V, *et al.* Risk of perforation after colonoscopy and sigmoidoscopy: a population-based study. *J Nat Cancer Instit* 2003; **95**: 230–6.

21 Heiken JP, Bree RL, Foley WD, *et al.* Colorectal cancer screening. [online publication] Reston (VA), American College of Radiology (ACR); 2006. 7p. http://www.acr.org/SecondaryMainMenuCategories/quality_safety/guidelines/dx/gastro/ct_colonography.aspx

22 Whitlock EP, Lin JS, Liles E, *et al.* Screening for Colorectal Cancer: U.S. Preventive Services Task Force Recommendation Statement. *Ann Intern Med* 2008; **149**: 639–58.

23 Johnson CD, Chen M, Toledo AY, *et al.* Accuracy of CT colonosgraphy for detection of large adenomas and cancers. *N Engl J Med* 2008; **359**: 1207–1217.

24 U.S. Preventive Services Task Force. Screening for colorectal cancer: recommendation and rationale. *Ann Intern Med* 2002; **137**: 129–31.

25 Pignone M, Rich M, Teutsch SM, *et al.* Screening for colorectal cancer in adults at average risk: a summary of the evidence for the U.S. Preventive Services Task Force. *Ann Intern Med* 2002; **137**: 132–41.

26 Agrawal S, Bhupinderjit A, Bhutani MS, *et al.* Colorectal cancer in African Americans. *Am J Gastroenterol* 2005; **100**: 515–23; discussion 514.

27 Lichtenstein P, Holm NV, Verkasalo PK, *et al.* Environmental and heritable factors in the causation of cancer—analyses of cohorts of twins from Sweden, Denmark, and Finland. *N Engl J Med* 2000; **343**: 78–85.

28 Bond JH. Polyp guideline: diagnosis, treatment, and surveillance for patients with colorectal polyps. Practice Parameters Committee of the American College of Gastroenterology. *Am J Gastroenterol* 2000; **95**: 3053–63.

29 Society for Surgery of the Alimentary Tract. SSAT patient care guidelines. Management of colonic polyps and adenomas. *J Gastrointest Surg* 2007; **11**: 1197–9.

30 Enhancing use and Quality of Colorectal Cancer Screening. Evidence Report (Publication No. 10-E002) www.ahrq.gov/clinic/tp/crcprotp.htm (12k, accessed 2010-03-04)

CHAPTER 32

Endoscopic Palliation of Malignant Obstruction

Todd H. Baron

Division of Gastroenterology and Hepatology, Mayo Clinic, Rochester, MN, USA

Summary

Endoscopy plays a major role in the palliation of malignant obstruction, both luminal and biliary. Endoscopic palliation of malignant biliary obstruction is discussed in another chapter. There are a variety of endoscopic methods for endoscopic palliation of esophageal obstruction, including simple dilation, expandable stent placement, photodynamic therapy, argon plasma coagulation, and brachytherapy. However, palliation of lumenal obstruction beyond the esophagus and in the colon is achieved through the use of self-expandable metal stents. Finally, endoscopic placement of gastrostomy tubes for supplemental nutrition and/or decompression can be used for palliation of obstruction.

Case

A 75-year-old man presents with progressive dysphagia and now can only swallow liquids. An esophagogastro-duodenoscopy (EGD) reveals a malignant-appearing mass at the gastroesophageal junction. Biopsies reveal adenocarcinoma. Computed tomography scan of the abdomen reveals a large, locally invasive mass at the gastroesophageal junction with liver metastases. A self-expandable metal stent is placed for palliation of dysphagia, after which he can swallow semisolid food until death 12 weeks later.

Equipment and Review of Technology

Endoscopic palliation of luminal obstruction is primarily achieved using self-expandable metal stents (SEMS). There are a variety of types, particularly for use within in the esophagus [1]. SEMS are composed of alloys, most commonly composed of Nitinol, a nickel–titanium alloy.

Practical Gastroenterology and Hepatology: Small and Large Intestine and Pancreas, 1st edition. Edited by Nicholas J. Talley, Sunanda V. Kane and Michael B. Wallace. © 2010 Blackwell Publishing Ltd.

The stents have a lattice configuration and are pre-loaded onto a delivery system in a constrained fashion. When the constraining system is released, the stent expands. Almost all esophageal SEMS have a covering to allow closure of fistula and prevention of tissue ingrowth through the lattice of the stent. A removable, expandable, fully covered plastic esophageal stent is available. SEMS used outside the esophagus do not have a covering because of a high rate of migration. Non-esophageal SEMS are also available in a pre-deployed diameter small enough to pass through the endoscope channel.

Photodynamic therapy (PDT) requires the use of a photosensitizing agent and a laser fiber which emits a wavelength of light that activates the drug. This results in release of cytotoxic oxygen radicals which kill tumors cells in the areas where light exposure occurred.

Argon plasma coagulation palliation involves a specialized electrosurgical generator equipped with argon gas. A probe is available that passes through the endoscope channel to allow necrosis and ablation of tissue at high power settings.

Endoscopic placement of brachytherapy catheters have been described to delivery radiation therapy to the esophagus and provide palliation of malignant dysphagia [2].

How to Place Self-expanding Metallic Stents

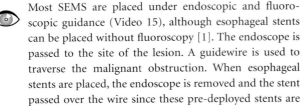

Most SEMS are placed under endoscopic and fluoroscopic guidance (Video 15), although esophageal stents can be placed without fluoroscopy [1]. The endoscope is passed to the site of the lesion. A guidewire is used to traverse the malignant obstruction. When esophageal stents are placed, the endoscope is removed and the stent passed over the wire since these pre-deployed stents are not small enough to pass through the endoscope. The endoscope can be passed alongside the stent so that it is deployed under direct endoscopic visualization. Alternatively, the stent can be deployed under fluoroscopic guidance alone. The approach to malignant obstruction outside the esophagus is similar, though the endoscope is not usually removed; the pre-deployed stent is passed through the channel of the endoscope and deployed under endoscopic view. Currently, deployment of stents through the endoscope can only done with uncovered stents as the covering makes the constrainable size too large for standard endoscopic channels.

PDT is performed at 48–72 h following infusion of a photosensitizing agent. The endoscope is passed into the esophagus to the level of the tumor. A laser diffusion fiber is inserted through the endoscope and positioned across the stricture for a defined period of time.

Argon beam coagulation has replaced laser in most endoscopy units and is applied by passing the probe into the esophagus. At high power setting and in close proximity to the lesion the tissue is coagulated to induce necrosis of the tumor [3].

Brachytherapy is performed by endoscopically placing a guidewire into the stomach and positioning the catheter fluoroscopically. The catheter remains in place for a defined period of time [2].

Malignant Dysphagia

In patients with advanced disease, palliation of dysphagia is performed to improve quality of life, nutritional status, and to prevent aspiration pneumonia (Table 32.1). Simple dilation using balloon or bougie can allow brief relief of dysphagia. Endoscopically placed stents apply internal radial forces to the esophagus, mechanically widening the esophageal lumen (Figure 32.1). Stents are

Table 32.1 Methods of palliation of esophageal cancer.

Simple dilation (balloon or bougie)
Expandable stent placement (plastic or metal)
Photodynamic therapy
Argon beam plasma coagulation
Gastrostomy tube placement

useful for palliating malignant dysphagia from both intrinsic tumors of the esophagus and from malignant extrinsic compression. Unlike feeding tubes, stents can result in palliation of dysphagia allowing peroral nutrition. Covered metal stents and an expandable plastic stent allow closure of tracheoesophageal fistulae. Dysphagia has been shown to be effectively and reliably relieved after insertion of SEMS [1]. Early complications after esophageal stent placement may include perforation, aspiration, chest pain, malpositioning of the stent, and acute airway obstruction (Table 32.2). Late stent complications may occur as a result of SEMS placement (Table 32.2). These may include gastroesophageal reflux and aspiration if the stent traverses the gastroesophageal junction. Stent occlusion may result from an impacted food bolus, and tumor ingrowth or tissue hyperplasia (through uncovered portions of metal stents). Additional stents can be placed to restore luminal patency through the previous stent (or after removal of self-expandable plastic stents). Covered metal stents placed across the gastroesophageal junction as well as plastic stents placed in any location are more prone to migration [4,5]. Major bleeding can result from erosion of the stent through the esophagus and into the aorta. Tracheoesophageal fistula can result from stent erosion into the respiratory tree.

Placement of SEMS after prior administration of radiation and/or chemotherapy may result in a higher complication rate [6,7]. There is little information about the effect of concomitant radiation and stent placement [8].

PDT allows successful palliation in the majority of patients with intrinsic esophageal lesions [9], although chest pain and fever are common. Ambient light photosensitivity occurs for up to 8 weeks. Mediastinitis is an uncommon complication.

Single-dose brachytherapy allows successful palliation of malignant dysphagia. Compared to stent placement, the effects are delayed but more durable palliation can be achieved [2].

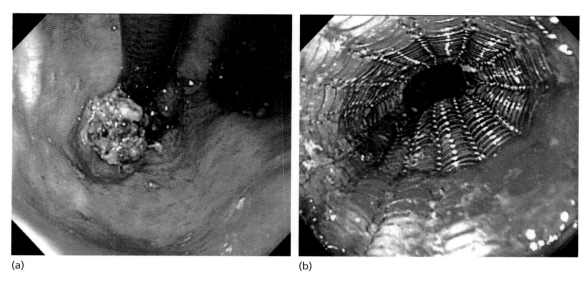

(a)   (b)

Figure 32.1 Expandable esophageal stent placement for unresectable tumor at the gastroesophageal junction. (a) Endoscopic retroflexed view in the stomach shows obstructing mass. (b) Endoscopic view from the esophagus immediately after placement of a covered self-expandable metal stent.

Table 32.2 Complications of expandable stents (early and delayed).

Esophageal stents
  Airway obstruction
  Aspiration
  Tracheoesophageal fistula
  Chest pain
  Reflux with aspiration, esophagitis
  Food impaction

All stents
  Obstruction: tumor ingrowth, overgrowth, tissue hyperplasia
  Bleeding
  Migration
  Perforation

Colonic stents
  Tenesmus, incontinence (rectal stent placement)

Malignant Gastric Outlet Obstruction

Malignant gastric outlet obstruction (GOO) produces postprandial abdominal pain, early satiety, vomiting, and intolerability of oral intake. SEMS for malignant GOO is usually due to pancreatic cancer (in the United States).

Other malignancies include gastric cancer, cholangiocarcinoma, gall bladder cancer, and metastatic disease. Technical success, defined as successful stent placement and deployment can be achieved in up to 97% [10]. Clinical success, defined as relief of symptoms and improved oral intake, occurs in about 90%. Stent occlusion occurs in about 20% due to tumor ingrowth. Migration occurs in 5% of patients. Compared to surgical bypass (gastroenterostomy) for palliation of malignant GOO, SEMS results in a shorter time to oral intake and a shorter initial hospital stay than surgery [11]. However, patients who live longer experience a higher recurrence of obstruction and need for reintervention.

Many patients with GOO may also need biliary stent placement (Figure 32.2), which should be done prior to gastroduodenal stent placement, since the duodenal portion of the stent can cover the papilla and make it inaccessible.

Colonic Obstruction

Patients with malignant colonic obstruction may present with minimal symptoms, or subtotal or complete obstruction. Mortality associated with acute malignant colonic obstruction is high. Endoscopic stent placement can be used for palliation of widespread, obstructive colorectal malignancy and in patients who are poor can-

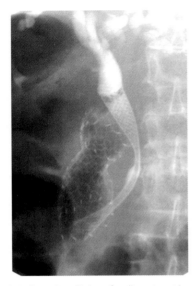

Figure 32.2 Endoscopic palliation of malignant gastric outlet obstruction and malignant biliary obstruction. Radiographic image shows a duodenal stent and biliary stent. Contrast is still visible in the biliary tree.

didates for surgery and can allow avoidance of a colostomy (Figure 32.3). Extrinsic compression from pelvic malignancies and lymphadenopathy may also be palliated with stents. Use of a covered stent in the rectum can allow closure of fistulas to the vagina and bladder [12].

Technical success rate for stent placement can be achieved in 93% and clinical success in 91% [13]. Perforation during or after stent placement usually requires emergency surgery. Re-obstruction due to tumor ingrowth occurs in about 8% of patients at a median time of 24 weeks. Other causes of obstruction include fecal impaction, tumor overgrowth, and peritoneal metastasis in other areas of the gastrointestinal tract. Stent placement in the right colon is also effective [14].

Complications of expandable enteral stents are listed in Table 32.2.

Enteral Tubes

Enteral tubes can be used to palliate obstruction [15]. Percutaneous endoscopic gastrostomy (PEG) tubes can be used to supplement nutrition in patients with esophageal cancer. Simultaneous endoscopic placement of jejunal feeding tubes and gastric decompression tubes can be used to palliate malignant gastroduodenal obstruc-

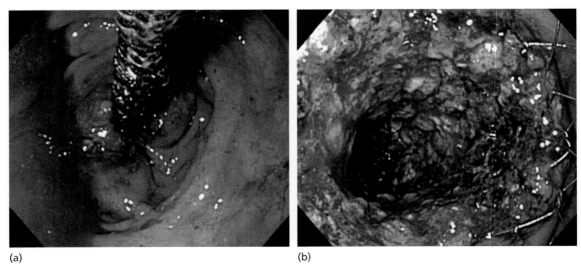

(a)   (b)

Figure 32.3 Palliation of malignant rectal stricture. (a) Endoscopic view of obstructive mass with predeployed stent visible. (b) Endoscopic view taken immediately after stent placement. Widely patent lumen inside the stent is seen.

tion. Finally, in patients with extensive peritoneal carcinomatosis, PEG tubes can be used as a final measure for comfort care as an alternative to nasogastric decompression.

Take-home points

- Palliation of malignant esophageal obstruction can be achieved endoscopically using a variety of techniques.

- Self-expandable esophageal stents are used as the primary modality for palliation of malignant esophagorespiratory fistulae.

- Esophageal stents are effective for the palliation of malignant dysphagia due to extrinsic compression of the esophagus.

- Expandable metal stents allow effective palliation of malignant gastroduodenal obstruction with an efficacy similar to surgical bypass.

- Colonic stents are useful for palliation of malignant colonic obstruction and can allow avoidance of a permanent colostomy.

- Endoscopically placed feeding and decompression tubes can be used as stand alone or supplemental measures for palliation of malignancy.

References

1 Papachristou GI, Baron TH. Use of stents in benign and malignant esophageal disease. *Rev Gastroenterol Disord* 2007; **7**: 74–88.

2 Homs MY, Steyerberg EW, Eijkenboom WM, *et al.* Single-dose brachytherapy versus metal stent placement for the palliation of dysphagia from oesophageal cancer: multicentre randomised trial. *Lancet* 2004; **364**: 1497–504.

3 Eriksen JR. Palliation of non-resectable carcinoma of the cardia and oesophagus by argon beam coagulation. *Dan Med Bull* 2002; **49**: 346–9.

4 Vakil N, Morris AI, Marcon N, *et al.* A prospective, randomized, controlled trial of covered expandable metal stents in the palliation of malignant esophageal obstruction at the gastroesophageal junction. *Am J Gastroenterol* 2001; **96**: 1791–6.

5 Conio M, Repici A, Battaglia G, *et al.* A randomized prospective comparison of self-expandable plastic stents and partially covered self-expandable metal stents in the palliation of malignant esophageal dysphagia. *Am J Gastroenterol* 2007; **102**: 2667–77.

6 Kinsman KJ, DeGregorio BT, Katon RM, *et al.* Prior radiation and chemotherapy increase the risk of life-threatening complications after insertion of metallic stents for esophagogastric malignancy. *Gastrointest Endosc* 1996; **43**: 196–203.

7 Lecleire S, Di Fiore F, Ben-Soussan E, *et al.* Prior chemoradiotherapy is associated with a higher life-threatening complication rate after palliative insertion of metal stents in patients with oesophageal cancer. *Aliment Pharmacol Ther* 2006; **23**: 1693–702.

8 Ludwig D, Dehne A, Burmester E, *et al.* Treatment of unresectable carcinoma of the esophagus or the gastroesophageal junction by mesh stents with or without radiochemotherapy. *Int J Oncol* 1998; **13**: 583–8.

9 Litle VR, Luketich JD, Christie NA, *et al.* Photodynamic therapy as palliation for esophageal cancer: experience in 215 patients. *Ann Thorac Surg* 2003; **76**: 1687–92.

10 Dormann A, Meisner S, Verin N, Wenk Lang A. Self-expanding metal stents for gastroduodenal malignancies: systematic review of their clinical effectiveness. *Endoscopy* 2004; **36**: 543–50.

11 Jeurnink SM, Steyerberg EW, Hof G, *et al.* Gastrojejunostomy versus stent placement in patients with malignant gastric outlet obstruction: a comparison in 95 patients. *J Surg Oncol* 2007; **96**: 389–96.

12 Repici A, Reggio D, Saracco G, *et al.* Self-expanding covered esophageal ultraflex stent for palliation of malignant colorectal anastomotic obstruction complicated by multiple fistulas. *Gastrointest Endosc* 2000; **51**: 346–8.

13 Sebastian S, Johnston S, Geoghegan T, *et al.* Pooled analysis of the efficacy and safety of self-expanding metal stenting in malignant colorectal obstruction. *Am J Gastroenterol* 2004; **99**: 2051–7.

14 Repici A, Adler DG, Gibbs CM, *et al.* Stenting of the proximal colon in patients with malignant large bowel obstruction: techniques and outcomes. *Gastrointest Endosc* 2007; **66**: 940–4.

15 Holm AN, Baron TH. Palliative use of percutaneous endoscopic gastrostomy and percutaneous endoscopic cecostomy tubes. *Gastrointest Endosc Clin N Am* 2007; **17**: 795–803.

PART 5

Diseases of the Small Intestine

CHAPTER 33
Crohn Disease

Faten N. Aberra and Gary R. Lichtenstein

Division of Gastroenterology, Hospital of the University of Pennsylvania, Philadelphia, PA, USA

Summary

Crohn disease is a chronic idiopathic inflammatory condition that affects the mucosa from mouth to anus. The presenting signs and symptoms can mimic a variety of other conditions and a thorough work up, including complete history and physical examination, blood tests, pertinent radiology, and endoscopy with biopsies, needs to be performed to make the diagnosis. Treatment is based on disease location, type (inflammatory or fistulizing), and severity. Most therapies are aimed at controlling inflammation with the intent to prevent complications.

Case

JH is a 30-year-old male who presented with a history of diarrhea for the past 6 weeks. He has 8–10 non-bloody bowel movements per day and has mild crampy left lower quadrant abdominal pain. He denies nausea, vomiting, fever, or chills. He has lost about 2.27 kg (5 lbs) and has bilateral lower back pain and denies any other symptoms. He is otherwise healthy, takes no medications, and has no medication allergies. He smokes a half pack of cigarettes per day, drinks alcohol occasionally, and denies illicit drug use. He has no family history of gastrointestinal diseases. His physical exam is remarkable for mild tenderness in the left lower quadrant of the abdomen and tenderness of bilateral sacroiliac joints with palpation.

Definition and Epidemiology

Inflammatory bowel disease (IBD) refers to two specific diseases, ulcerative colitis (UC) and Crohn disease (CD). Crohn disease was first described in 1932 in the *Journal of the American Medical Association* by Drs Crohn, Ginzberg, and Oppenheimer and was termed "regional enteritis" and "terminal ileitis". Crohn disease is a disorder of

Practical Gastroenterology and Hepatology: Small and Large Intestine and Pancreas, 1st edition. Edited by Nicholas J. Talley, Sunanda V. Kane and Michael B. Wallace. © 2010 Blackwell Publishing Ltd.

the immune system leading to persistent inflammation and ulceration that can occur anywhere in the gastrointestinal tract.

The highest incidence of CD occurs in the developed regions of the world: North America, United Kingdom, and Northern Europe. The incidence of CD in North America is estimated to be 3.1–14.6/100 000. The incidence of CD in United States is estimated to be 4–7/100 000 per year and the prevalence to be 100–200/100 000 [1]. The peak incidence of CD occurs between age 15 and 30 years of age with a second peak in the seventh decade. There is a slight female predominance with a 1.2 : 1 female to male ratio. Crohn disease affects all ethnic groups. Although traditionally a disease primarily affecting Caucasians in North America and the United Kingdom, the incidence of CD in African Americans and African Caribbeans has risen and matched Caucasians in those regions. Data are limited in other ethnic minority groups in these countries.

Pathophysiology

The etiology of CD is unknown but the disease is believed to manifest from genetic predisposition, immune dysregulation, and the environment triggers leading to persistent gastrointestinal mucosal ulceration.

Genetics play a significant role in developing CD. Familial studies reveal a genetic predilection for developing disease with identical twins having the highest concordance rate (50%) of disease, siblings (0–3%), and first-degree relatives 5–10%. The first gene identified to be associated with CD was *NOD2/CARD15* which is expressed in intestinal epithelial Paneth cells, macrophages, and dendritic cells [2]. This gene is involved in the expression of an intracellular receptor that senses muramyl dipeptide, a peptidoglycan component of Gram-positive bacteria. Activation of NOD2 leads to activation of NF-κB which mediates transcription of numerous proinflammatory cytokines. A mutation in NOD2 in the leucine-rich domain of the protein, which interacts with bacterial lipopolysaccharide, leads to failure in activation of NF-κB; this mutation is associated with the development of CD. Since the identification of this gene, there have been several other disease susceptibility loci identified which correlate with disease phenotype and surgical recurrence, including the organic cation transporter gene, interleukin -23 (IL-23) gene, and others. The practical clinical application of these gene mutations has yet to be determined.

Several findings over time have pointed to microbes playing a role in the development of CD. Several different animal models of colitis tend to show no active disease in a sterile environment and development of active colitis in the setting of commensal bacteria. Diverting the fecal stream has shown to help heal CD. Additionally, antibiotics, particularly broad-spectrum anaerobic coverage, seem to be helpful in the treatment of CD. Most importantly, the identification of the *NOD2/CARD15* genetic mutation has solidified the intricate interplay between the intestinal microbial environment and immune system.

It is believed that the innate immune system's inability to clear microbial antigens leads to an overactive adaptive immune response. The alteration in the immune system associated with CD was traditionally viewed as a preponderance of T helper-1 response. It has been more recently understood that the alterations in the immune system in CD are heterogeneous and this has lead to the finding of a new line of proinflammatory T cells, T_{IL-17}. IL-23, produced by antigen presenting cells, triggers T_{IL-17} cells which stimulates the immune system. Variations in single nucleotide polymorphisms of the gene encoding the receptor for IL-23 have been found to be associated with CD [3].

Clinical Features

Symptoms of CD are varied and may be a consequence of the location of the disease, type of disease behavior (non-penetrating/non-stricturing, stricturing, and penetrating/fistulizing disease), and duration. The most common location of CD is the terminal ileum and right colon (ileocolonic), occurring in half of all patients with CD, with symptoms which may include diarrhea, hematochezia, and abdominal pain.

Upper gastrointestinal CD is rare. Esophageal CD occurs in less than 2% of patients [4]. Symptoms may include dysphagia, odynophagia, chest pain, or heartburn. Gastroduodenal disease occurs in 0.5 to 4% of patients and commonly occurs along with distal disease [5]. Symptoms and signs may include upper abdominal pain and iron-deficiency anemia. Isolated jejunal disease is rare and when the jejunum is involved there is also distal small bowel involvement.

Primary ileal disease occurs in 30% of patients, whereas ileocolonic disease occurs in 40%. Symptoms may include abdominal pain, typically in the right lower quadrant, and may include diarrhea, hematochezia, and fatigue. With more severe disease, fever may be present as well as weight loss and anemia. In some patients disease may present with obstructive-type symptoms in the setting of insidious structuring disease such as abdominal pain, nausea, and abdominal distension. On examination, findings may include abdominal tenderness, classically in the right lower quadrant, and may include fullness or mass depending on the severity of inflammation.

Isolated colonic disease occurs in 25% of patients and 60% will have rectal involvement, making it at times difficult to differentiate from UC. Symptoms classically include diarrhea, hematochezia, and abdominal pain.

Up to 30% of patients will develop perianal disease, which may include development of fistula/abscesses, fissures, and skin tags. Symptoms of perianal disease include pain and discharge. Fever may be present if there is an abscess.

Penetrating/fistulizing disease occurs in 20–40% of CD patients. Fistulae are internal connections that can occur anywhere in the gastrointestinal tract and connect to various sites. Fistulae can occur internally, such as enteroenteric or enterocolonic, or present externally, such as enterocutaneous, rectovaginal, or perianal. Penetrating disease may also cause intra-abdominal and perianal abscesses and, in rare scenarios, perforation.

Subjects may also have extraintestinal manifestations of disease which include arthropathy, the most common, and affects up to 22% of subjects [6]. Peripheral arthropathy (arthralgias to arthritis), ankylosing spondylitis, and sacroiliitis may develop with peripheral arthropathy exacerbating along with gastrointestinal symptoms. Rash may develop in up to 14%, specifically erythema nodosum and pyoderma gangrenosum. Eye symptoms from uveitis or episcleritis may occur. Crohn disease subjects are also at risk, as high as 9%, for renal calculi, more commonly calcium oxalate stones. Although not as frequent as in UC, CD subjects are at risk for developing primary sclerosing cholangitis.

Diagnosis

During an evaluation for possible CD and when diarrhea is the predominant symptom the differential diagnosis is broad. The initial evaluation for diarrhea should include a thorough medical history, testing for infectious colitis, and screening for endocrine-metabolic disorders such as hyperthyroidism and hypocalcemia.

Endoscopic Findings
Diagnostic testing performed for a suspicion of IBD entails endoscopic evaluation. Colonoscopy is usually the initial endoscopic test for patients presenting with lower gastrointestinal symptoms such as diarrhea and hematochezia. Colonoscopy performed with intubation of the terminal ileum is important if a diagnosis of inflammatory bowel disease is suspected. Small bowel imaging (such as small bowel follow through or computed tomography (CT) enterography) may also be needed to determine if there is small bowel disease or to determine the extent of disease. Capsule endoscopy may be needed if all other testing is non-diagnostic and CD of the small bowel is still suspected. Endoscopic findings early in the disease process include superficial mucosal ulcers (aphthous ulcers). As CD progresses the ulceration becomes deeper, typically transmural, discrete, may occur in a serpiginous pattern, and may occur anywhere from esophagus to anus in a skipped pattern (Figure 33.1 and Table 33.1).

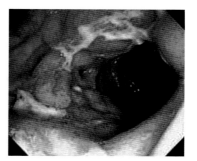

Figure 33.1 Endoscopic photographs of Crohn ileitis.

Histopathology
The diagnosis of IBD hinges on histopathology and therefore biopsies from the affected as well as unaffected areas is critical. In early CD the histopathology is characterized by an acute inflammatory infiltrate and crypt abscesses. Later in the disease process, there is distortion of mucosal crypt architecture, lymphocytic inflammatory infiltrate, crypt abscesses, and in some subjects noncaseating granulomas are present (Figure 33.2). Noncaseating granulomas are not unique to CD but help confirm a diagnosis of CD when other manifestations that are classic features are present. Granulomas are present in up to 15% of subjects based on endoscopic biopsy specimens and as high as 70% of surgical specimens.

The most common method of diagnosing CD is based on a combination of information from histopathology, colonoscopy, and small bowel imaging. In the absence of granulomas, the pattern of ulceration helps determine if someone may have CD. Skipped pattern of ulceration, ulceration in small bowel or upper gastrointestinal tract, or the presence of a fistula support a diagnosis of CD.

Laboratory Measures
Serologic markers for IBD are supportive but are not diagnostic alone. Anti-*Saccharomyces cerevisiae* antibodies (ASCA) are antibodies to yeast, and present in 40–70% of CD patients and in less than 15% of patients with UC. The combination of ASCA IgA and IgG titers is highly specific for CD, ranging from 89 to 100%. Perinuclear antineutrophil cytoplasmic antibody (pANCA) is present in 20% of Crohn patients who have colon-predominant disease. Based on a meta-analysis of 60 studies, ASCA positive and pANCA negative disease is associated

Table 33.1 Differential diagnosis of ileitis/colitis.

Infections
    Bacterial
        Aeromonas spp.
        Campylobacter jejuni
        Chlamydia (proctitis)
        Clostridium difficile
        Mycobacterium tuberculosis
        Salmonella
        Shigella
        Enterohemorrhagic *E. coli*
        Yersinia
    Viral
        Cytomegalovirus
        Herpes simplex virus (proctitis)
        HIV
    Fungal
        Histoplasma capsulatum
    Parasites
        Entamoeba histolytica
        Helminths

Vascular
    Collagen vascular disease
    Behçet disease
    Churg–Strauss syndrome
    Henoch–Schönlein purpura
    Systemic lupus erythematosus
    Polyarteritis nodosa
    Ischemia

Neoplasia
    Carcinoid
    Carcinoma primary or metastatic
    Lymphoma
    Mycosis fungoides
    Malignant histiocytosis

Medications/toxins
    Non-steroidal anti-inflammatory drugs (NSAIDs)
    Pancreatic enzyme supplements—"Fibrosing colopathy"
    Phosphosoda bowel preparations
    Radiation

Inflammatory
    Appendicitis
    Diverticular disease
    Eosinophilic gastroenteritis
    Non-granulomatous ulcerative jejunoileiitis (celiac disease)

Miscellaneous
    Amyloidosis
    Sarcoidosis
    Endometriosis
    Tubo-ovarian abscesses

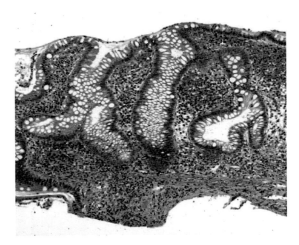

Figure 33.2 Colonic biopsy demonstrating crypt architectural distortion.

with a sensitivity of 55% and specificity of 93% for Crohn disease [7]. The antimicrobial antibodies anti-I2 (Crohn related protein from *Pseudomonas fluorescens*), anti-Cbir1 (flagellin-like antigen), and anti-OmpC (*Escherichia coli* outer membrane porin C), are also associated with CD but the utility of these additional markers has yet to be determined.

Both erythrocyte sedimentation rate (ESR) and C-reactive protein (CRP) are non-specific measures of inflammation which may be elevated in the setting of active Crohn disease.

Case continued

JH had stool sent for stool culture, ova and parasites, and *Clostridium difficile* to evaluate for infectious colitis were negative. Blood work was also completed revealed a hemoglobin of 10 g/dL with a mean corpuscular volume of 85 fL. A colonoscopy was performed and revealed serpiginous ulcerations in an irregular pattern in the colon and distal terminal ileum (Figure 33.1). Biopsies were obtained and revealed crypt distortion with inflammatory infiltration of the lamina propria (Figure 33.2). The findings were suggestive of Crohn disease.

Disease Activity

Indices

The most widely used disease activity index for CD is the Crohn disease activity index (CDAI), however it is not

Table 33.2 Crohn disease activity index.

Variable	Descriptor	Score	Multiplier
Number of liquid stools	Sum of 7 days		2
Abdominal pain	Sum of 7 days ratings	0 = none 1 = mild 2 = moderate 3 = severe	5
General well being	Sum of 7 days ratings	0 = generally well 1 = slightly under par 2 = poor 3 = very poor 4 = terrible	7
Extraintestinal complications	Number of listed complications	Arthritis/arthralgia, iritis/uveitis, erythema nodosum, pyoderma gangrenosum, apthous stomatitis, anal fissure/fistula/abscess, fever >37.8°C	20
Antidiarrheal drugs	Use in the previous 7 days	0 = no 1 = yes	30
Abdominal mass		0 = no 2 = questionable 5 = definite	10
Hematocrit	Expected–observed hematocrit	Males: 47–observed Females: 42–observed	6
Body weight	Ideal/observed ratio	[1–(ideal/observed)] × 100	1 (Not <–10)

useful in a purely clinical setting. Eight variables are in the index and based on a 7-day patient diary. The Harvey Bradshaw index was created to simplify the CDAI. The Harvey Bradshaw Index (HBI) utilizes same-day measurements (Table 33.2 and 33.3).

Risk Factors

Cigarette smoking and the use of non-steroidal anti-inflammatory drugs have been associated with disease exacerbation. No specific diets have been associated with developing CD or exacerbation of disease. Low-fiber diets are recommended if a patient has stricturing CD to avoid obstruction or moderate–severe flare to avoid symptom exacerbation.

Therapeutics

Medical Therapy

The aim with medical therapy is to induce and maintain a remission of CD. Medications include topical anti-

Table 33.3 Harvey Bradshaw index.

Variable	Score
General well being	0 = very well 1 = slightly below par 2 = poor 3 = very poor 4 = terrible
Abdominal pain	0 = none 1 = mild 2 = moderate 3 = severe
Number of liquid stools daily	N
Abdominal mass	0 = none 1 = dubious 2 = definite 3 = definite and tender
Complications	1 point for each item = arthralgia, uveitis, erythema nodosum, aphthous ulcer, pyoderma gangrenosum, anal fissure, new fistula, abscess

Table 33.4 Common medications for treatment of Crohn disease.

Drug	Dose	Release site
5-aminosalicylates		
Sulfasalazine (Azulfidine)	2–6 g/day	Colon
Mesalamine (Asacol, Lialda)	2.4–4.8 g/day	Distal ileum, colon
Olsalazine (Dipentum)	1–3 g/day	Colon
Balsalazide (Colazal)	6.25 g/day	Colon
Mesalamine (Pentasa)	2–4 g/day	Duodenum, jejunum, ileum, colon
Mesalamine (Rowasa) enema, suppository	4 enema g/day	Rectum/sigmoid
	1 suppository g/day	Rectum
Mesalamine (Canasa) suppository	1 g/day	Rectum
Corticosteroids		
Budesonide (Entocort)	Induction: 9 mg/day orally	Small intestine
	Maintenance: 6 mg/day orally	
Prednisone	0.25–0.75 mg/kg/day orally	Systemic
Methylprednisolone (Solumedrol)	40–60 mg/day IV	Systemic
Immunomodulators		
6-Mercaptopurine	1.5 mg/kg	
Azathioprine	2.5 mg/kg	
Methotrexate	Induction: 25 mg SC every week × 4 months	
	Maintenance: 15 mg SC every week	
Biologics		
Infliximab	Induction: 5 mg/kg IV weeks 0, 2, 6	Systemic
	Maintenance: 5 mg/kg IV every 8 weeks	
Adalimumab	Induction: 160 mg SC week 0, 80 mg week 2	Systemic
	Maintenance: 40 mg SC every other week	
Certolizumab pegol	Induction: 400 mg SC week 0, 2, 4	Systemic
	Maintenance: 400 mg SC every 4 weeks	
Natalizumab	300 mg IV every 4 weeks	Systemic

inflammatory agents (5-aminosalicylates (5-ASA)), antibiotics, and systemic immunosuppressants, (corticosteroids), budesonide, azathioprine (AZA), 6-mercaptopurine (6MP), methotrexate, and biologics (infliximab, adalimumab, certolizumab pegol, and natalizumab) (Table 33.4). The medical therapy chosen is based on the disease location, behavior (non-penetrating/non-stricturing, sticturing, and penetrating/fistulizing disease) and severity.

5-Aminosalicylates

5-Aminosalicylic acid preparations are indicated for mild to moderate non-penetrating CD. Sulfasalazine (sulphapyridine and 5-ASA) is the first compound of 5-ASA developed, initially used for the treatment of rheumatoid arthritis. It was shown that 5-ASA was responsible for the anti-inflammatory property of this drug whereas sulphapyridine was found to be a carrier for 5-ASA, allowing for its delivery into the colon. 5-ASA functions as a topical anti-inflammatory within the lumen of the intestine [8]. Several oral formulations of 5-ASA have been developed, mesalamine (Pentasa®, Asacol®, Lialda®, Apriso®), olsalazine (Dipentum®), and balsalazide (Colazal®). For distal disease 5-ASA suppository and enema preparations are also available. Response rates to 5-ASAs range from 43 to 64% for induction of remission with better response in colonic disease than for small bowel disease. Based on a systematic review, 5-ASAs are not effective in maintaining remission [8].

Adverse events associated with 5-ASAs are rare and may include nausea, dyspepsia, hair loss, headache, worsening diarrhea, and rare hypersensitivity reactions [8].

Corticosteroids

Systemic Corticosteroids. Oral systemic corticosteroids have been shown to be effective in the treatment of active

CD. Corticosteroids such as prednisone and methylprednisolone are used for treating moderate to severe disease. Dosing of prednisone ranges from 0.25 mg to 0.75 mg/kg per day. Maintenance with systemic corticosteroids is not recommended due to the numerous side effects. The use of systemic corticosteroids is associated with significant dose-dependent side effects such as increase in body weight, fat redistribution, changes in mood, insomnia, osteoporosis and osteonecrosis, myopathy, cataracts, hypokalemia, hypertriglyceridemia, growth retardation in children, arterial hypertension, edema of lower extremities, hyperglycemia, and acne.

Budesonide. An alternative to prednisone is budesonide, a corticosteroid which demonstrates high topical activity and low-systemic bioavailability (10%) and associated with a reduced risk of systemic complications. Controlled-ileal release and pH-dependent release formulations of budesonide are used for treatment of active mild to moderate CD. Budesonide 9 mg/day orally for 8–10 weeks is more effective than mesalamine for induction of remission of disease located in the terminal ileum and ascending colon and it may be used for maintenance for 3 additional months at 6 mg/day. Treatment with budesonide for up to 6 months is more effective than placebo, but treatment out to 1 year with budesonide has not been found to be more effective than placebo.

Azathioprine/6-mercaptopurine

For patients that have failed 5-ASA therapy or whose disease is more than mild, the thiopurine analogs, 6-mercaptopurine (6MP) and azathioprine (AZA), are options for treatment. Azathioprine is the pro-drug of 6MP. 6MP is metabolized to 6-thioisonine 5′-monophosphate (TIMP) by the enzyme hypoxanthine–guanine phosphoribosyl transferase (HPRT). TIMP is eventually metabolized to 6-thioguanine nucleotides, the active metabolite causing inhibition of deoxyribonucleic acid (DNA) and ribonucleic acid (RNA) synthesis and likely T-cell apoptosis. A meta-analysis of eight studies revealed a response rate (defined as clinical improvement or remission) of 54% for those treated with AZA (2–3 mg/kg per day) or 6MP (50 mg/day or 1.5 mg/kg per day) compared to 33% in those receiving placebo [9]. Benefit has also been shown for maintaining remission at the same dose range. AZA and 6MP are also used to treat fistulizing disease. The disadvantage of the thiopurine analogs is the long

onset of action, up to 12 weeks. Several side effects have been associated with 6MP and AZA use and include allergic reactions, pancreatitis, myelosuppression, nausea, infections, hepatotoxicity, and malignancy, in particular lymphoma. Labs such as complete blood cell count and liver enzymes need to be routinely monitored due to potential leukopenia and drug-induced hepatitis.

Methotrexate

Methotrexate is a folic acid antagonist that leads to the inhibition of purine synthesis, DNA and RNA formation, and eventually inhibition of the S phase of the cell cycle. It also has inhibits proinflammatory cytokine. Methotrexate 25 mg IM or SC once per week for 16 weeks is used for active CD [10]. For maintenance of remission methotrexate 15 mg once per week has been shown to be effective compared to placebo out to 40 weeks [11]. Studies with oral methotrexate have not yet been shown to be effective and may be related to the low doses studied and poor bioavailability. Methotrexate is also used to treat fistulizing disease.

Antibiotics

Several mechanisms have been proposed to explain the mechanism of action of antibiotics for the treatment of active inflammatory bowel disease. One theory is that changing the intestinal microbial flora prevents inhabitation of pathogenic bacteria. Another potential mechanism is that in genetically susceptible individuals, there is a lack of tolerance to commensal bacteria in the gastrointestinal tract leading to activation of the gut immune system. Suppression of bacterial flora may lead to down regulation of the immune system. Antibiotics such as metronidazole also may have direct anti-inflammatory effects independent of their antimicrobial activity. Many studies have shown a benefit for the treatment of active CD with sparse data examining the role of antibiotics in preventing relapse of CD in non-surgically treated patients. Metronidazole and ciprofloxacin are indicated for CD complicated by perianal fistula and metronidazole may be a helpful adjunctive treatment for colonic CD.

Biologics

Anti-TNF- Agents. The first class of biologics developed were antibodies to tumor necrosis factor-α (anti-TNF-α) and includes infliximab, adalimumab, and certolizumab pegol. Infliximab, a chimeric mouse–human IgG₁ monoclonal antibody, was the first anti-TNF-α approved in the United States for the treatment of CD. Infliximab is administered as an infusion and approved by the FDA for induction and maintenance therapy in patients with moderate to severe active or fistulizing CD refractory to conventional therapies [12,13].

Over the past 2 years, there have been a number of other anti-TNF-α therapies approved for the treatment of moderate to severe CD and fistulizing disease [14]. Adalimumab is fully humanized IgG₁ antibody which is self-administered subcutaneously. The most recent anti-TNF-α approved is certolizumab pegol, a chimeric pegylated Fab fragment to TNF-α, which is also administered subcutaneously [15,16].

Antiadhesion Molecules. Natalizumab, a humanized IgG₄ monoclonal antibody, binds to the α4 subunit of α4β1 and α4β7 integrins expressed on all leukocytes except neutrophils. Natalizumab inhibits the interactions between a4 integrins on the surface of leukocytes and adhesion molecules on vascular endothelial cells in the gastrointestinal tract, preventing adhesion and recruitment of leukocytes. Natalizumab is approved for the treatment of moderate to severe CD refractory to standard therapy [17]. Due to three cases of progressive multifocal leukoencephalopathy (PML), in one CD patient and two multiple sclerosis patients during the clinical trials for natalizumab, there are strict guidelines for prescribing.

Case continued

JH was treated with sulfasalazine 1 g orally four times per day which alleviated his diarrhea and joint symptoms. Three months later he developed a nodular, tender pretibial rash bilaterally with a flare of his gastrointestinal symptoms. He was treated with prednisone and developed recurrence of symptoms once the prednisone was tapered to 20 mg a day. Treatment was initiated with azathioprine 2.5 mg/kg per day and by the third month of therapy prednisone was discontinued and he remained in remission.

Surgery

Surgery will eventually be required in most patients with CD, as high as 70% based on a population cohort over 25 years [18]. Indications for surgery include disease refractory to medical therapy, obstruction, abscess, colonic dysplasia or colon cancer, and significant gastrointestinal hemorrhage. Disease refractory to medical therapy may include persistent symptoms such as diarrhea and/or abdominal pain, persistent fistulizing disease, or a toxic megacolon presentation.

Take-home points

- Infectious colitis may mimic early Crohn disease and infection should be excluded.
- Histopathology is critical in establishing a diagnosis of inflammatory bowel disease.
- Endoscopic and radiologic patterns of disease help to differentiate Crohn from ulcerative colitis.
- Smoking exacerbates Crohn disease and increases the risk for flare.
- Maintenance medication therapy reduces the risk of relapse.

References

1 Loftus EV Jr. Clinical epidemiology of inflammatory bowel disease: Incidence, prevalence, and environmental influences. *Gastroenterology* 2004; **126**: 1504–17.

2 Cho JH. Significant role of genetics in IBD: The NOD2 gene. *Rev Gastroenterol Disord* 2003; **3** (Suppl. 1): S18–22.

3 Duerr RH, Taylor KD, Brant SR, *et al.* A genome-wide association study identifies IL23R as an inflammatory bowel disease gene. *Science* 2006; **314**: 1461–3.

4 Decker GA, Loftus EV Jr, Pasha TM, *et al.* Crohn's disease of the esophagus: Clinical features and outcomes. *Inflamm Bowel Dis* 2001; **7**: 113–9.

5 Nugent FW, Roy MA. Duodenal Crohn's disease: An analysis of 89 cases. *Am J Gastroenterol* 1989; **84**: 249–54.

6 Shashidhar H, *et al.* In: Kirsner JB, Shorter RG, eds. *Inflammatory Bowel Disease*, 5th edn. Baltimore: Williams and Wilkins, 2000.

7 Nikolaus S, Schreiber S. Diagnostics of inflammatory bowel disease. *Gastroenterology* 2007; **133**: 1670–89.

8 Akobeng AK, Gardener E. Oral 5-aminosalicylic acid for maintenance of medically-induced remission in crohn's disease. *Cochrane Database Syst Rev* 2005; **1**: CD003715.

9 Sandborn W, Sutherland L, Pearson D, *et al.* Azathioprine or 6-mercaptopurine for inducing remission of Crohn's disease. *Cochrane Database Syst Rev* 2000; **2**: CD000545.

10 Feagan BG, Rochon J, Fedorak RN, *et al.* Methotrexate for the treatment of Crohn's disease. the north american crohn's study group investigators. *N Engl J Med* 1995; **332**: 292–7.

11 Feagan BG, Fedorak RN, Irvine EJ, *et al*. A comparison of methotrexate with placebo for the maintenance of remission in Crohn's disease. North American Crohn's study group investigators. *N Engl J Med* 2000; **342**: 1627–32.

12 Hanauer SB, Feagan BG, Lichtenstein GR, *et al*., ACCENT I Study Group. Maintenance infliximab for Crohn's disease: The ACCENT I randomised trial. *Lancet* 2002; **359**: 1541–9.

13 Sands BE, Anderson FH, Bernstein CN, *et al*. Infliximab maintenance therapy for fistulizing Crohn's disease. *N Engl J Med* 2004; **350**: 876–85.

14 Sandborn WJ, Hanauer SB, Rutgeerts P, *et al*. Adalimumab for maintenance treatment of crohn's disease: Results of the CLASSIC II trial. *Gut* 2007; **56**: 1232–9.

15 Sandborn WJ, Feagan BG, Stoinov S, *et al*., PRECISE 1 Study Investigators. Certolizumab pegol for the treatment of crohn's disease. *N Engl J Med* 2007; **357**: 228–38.

16 Schreiber S, Khaliq-Kareemi M, Lawrance IC, *et al*., PRECISE 2 Study Investigators. Maintenance therapy with certolizumab pegol for crohn's disease. *N Engl J Med* 2007; **357**: 239–50.

17 Targan SR, Feagan BG, Fedorak RN, *et al*. International Efficacy of Natalizumab in Crohn's Disease Response and Remission (ENCORE) Trial Group. Natalizumab for the treatment of active Crohn's disease: Results of the ENCORE trial. *Gastroenterology* 2007; **132**: 1672–83.

18 Munkholm P, Langholz E, Davidsen M, Binder V. Intestinal cancer risk and mortality in patients with Crohn's disease. *Gastroenterology* 1993; **105**: 1716–23.

CHAPTER 34
Small Bowel Tumors

Nadir Arber and Menachem Moshkowitz

Tel-Aviv Sourasky Medical Center, Sackler Faculty of Medicine, Tel-Aviv University, Tel Aviv, Israel

Summary

Tumors of the small bowel, both benign and malignant, are relatively uncommon but may cause significant morbidity and mortality if undetected. These tumors present a diagnostic challenge as their symptoms are often vague. Small bowel tumors have a poor prognosis because most patients present with advanced disease. Surgical resection remains the cornerstone of therapy for these malignancies. New endoscopic modalities such as capsule endoscopy and double balloon enteroscopy allow full examination of the small bowel with improved diagnosis. Advanced endoscopic interventions are likely to broaden the endoscopic management of small bowel tumors.

Case

A 51-year-old woman presented with general malaise, loss of weight, and vomiting. At 18 years of age she had first presented with abdominal pain, diarrhea, and general malaise. Barium follow-through examination showed Crohn disease of the terminal ileum. She was treated with sulfasalazine and corticosteroids. In the following years, the patient experienced repeated episodes of abdominal pain without diarrhea.

Two years ago, the severity of the abdominal pain increased and she underwent ileocolonoscopy, which yielded no suspicious macroscopic or histopathologic findings. Blood tests showed mild iron deficiency and hypoalbuminemia. C-reactive protein (CRP) and erythrocyte sedimentation rate (ESR) were within normal limits. The recommended enteroclysis of the small bowel was not performed. In order to taper her steroids, azathioprine was initiated (3 mg/kg/day). Recently, she presented again with abdominal pain, vomiting, and distended abdomen. Enteroclysis revealed a dilated intestinal loop of the ileum and a pseudotumor in the right abdomen with two stenotic areas. Prednisone was increased to 50 mg/day, in addition to metronidazole and ciprofloxacin. Three weeks later due to signs of intestinal obstruction, the patient underwent exploratory laparotomy.

The resected small intestinal specimen showed multiple strictures and sacculation with superficial ulceration and fissures, mucosal edema, and fibrosis. There was an ulcerated lesion (3 x 2 cm) 3 cm from the distal end of the resected specimen. Histologic examination showed adenocarcinoma of the small intestine complicating Crohn disease.

Introduction

Small bowel tumors are extremely rare and account for only 1–2% of all gastrointestinal malignancies [1,2]. It was estimated that there will be 5640 new cases and 1090 deaths in the USA in 2007, making it one of the most uncommon types of cancer. This low incidence is intriguing, considering the fact that the small bowel comprises 75% of the length and 90% of the mucosal surface area of the alimentary tract. Various theories have been proposed to explain this resistance to carcinogenesis, among them the short contact time with potential carcinogens, reduced intestinal concentrations of inherent potential carcinogens, high concentrations of biliary and pancreatic secretions, low concentration of bacteria, and well-developed local immunoglobulin A antibody (IgA)-mediated immune and lymphatic systems [3].

Practical Gastroenterology and Hepatology: Small and Large Intestine and Pancreas, 1st edition. Edited by Nicholas J. Talley, Sunanda V. Kane and Michael B. Wallace. © 2010 Blackwell Publishing Ltd.

The non-specific symptoms and the lack of typical laboratory and physical signs serve to explain the long latency period before establishing the diagnosis. This delay in identifying the pathology contributes to the poor prognosis and presence of metastases in 50% of the subjects at the time of diagnosis. Approximately two-thirds of all small bowel tumors are malignant, although benign tumors are detected in up to 0.3% of all primary tumors of the small intestine [4].

Benign Tumors of the Small Intestine

Benign tumors of the small intestine include adenomas, leiomyomas, lipomas, hamartomas, desmoid tumors, hemangiomas, lymphangiomas, neurofibromas, and ganglioneuromas, depending on their cell of origin [5].

Adenomas usually appear in the duodenum, mostly on the medial wall, around the ampulla of Vater. A more distal location is rather unusual. Similar to colonic polyps, they are classified as tubular, villous, or tubulovillous. They follow the adenoma–carcinoma sequence, as is seen in colorectal cancer (CRC) [6]. Tubular adenomas bear a relatively low malignant potential, while villous adenomas carry a significant risk of malignant transformation. A focus of carcinoma *in situ* can be detected in 40% of these villous adenomas [7], and synchronous colonic polyps are frequently detected as well. A colonoscopy is a must in these patients. Duodenal adenomas often develop in familial adenomatous polyposis (FAP) syndrome, in which there is a greater risk for malignant transformation than in sporadic cases.

Leiomyomas are true smooth muscle cell tumors arising from the muscularis propria. They are usually small and well-circumscribed. The peak incidence is seen in the sixth decade. Malignant transformation is unusual when they are less than 4 cm in diameter. They need to be differentiated from gastrointestinal stromal tumors (GISTs).

Brunner gland hyperplasia is defined as benign hyperplasia of the exocrine glandular structures in the postpyloric part of the duodenum. It carries no malignant risk.

Systemic neurofibromatosis (von Recklinghausen disease) involves the small bowel in up to 25% of the patients. The submucosal neurofibromas tend mostly to be asymptomatic, but ulceration of the overlying mucosa may be a cause of gastrointestinal bleeding.

Hamartomas are found in Peutz–Jeghers syndrome (PJS), a rare autosomal dominant disorder characterized by multiple hamartomatous (non-neoplastic) gastrointestinal polyps that are spread throughout the entire gastrointestinal tract and which have characteristic mucocutaneous melanin pigmentation. These hamartomatous polyps arise in the stromal tissue of the muscularis mucosae and vary in size from a few millimeters up to 5 cm. They have normal overlying mucosa, and develop as early as the first decade of life. They become symptomatic by the age of 10–30 years, and are characterized by signs of intussusception, intestinal obstruction, or ulceration with bleeding. A germline mutation in the *LKB1/STK11* gene can be found in 50% of the families. Hamartomas *per se* do not harbor any cancer risk, but adenomatous tissue can be formed in 5% of them. Up to 90% of patients with PJS carry a lifetime risk for cancer, including colon, small bowel, pancreatic, cervical, uterine, ovarian, breast, testicular, and lung cancers [8].

Malignant Small Bowel Tumors

Small bowel cancer has four major histologic subtypes: adenocarcinoma is the most common malignancy (accounting for 40–50% of all primary small bowel neoplasm) [3], followed by neuroendocrine tumors (20–40%, mostly carcinoids that are located in the ileum), lymphomas (14%) and GISTs (11–13%).

The mean age at diagnosis is 57 years (median 67 years), males are slightly more affected, and African Americans have almost twice the incidence compared to caucasians [2].

Adenocarcinoma of the Small Bowel

This malignancy occurs most frequently within the duodenum (49%), particularly around the ampulla of Vater, and with decreasing frequency in the jejunum (21%) and ileum (15%) [9]. It is more common in men than in women and twice as common in African Americans. In Crohn-associated cases, 70% of adenocarcinomas are found in the ileum [10]. Risk factors for this type of tumor include: Crohn disease [11], FAP [12], and hereditary non-polyposis colorectal cancer syndrome. Smoking, alcohol use, high intake of sugar, red meat, salt cured/ smoked foods or low intake of fish, fruit, and vegetables, and environmental factors, such as radiation therapy, have all been associated with increased risk for small bowel tumors [13,14].

Neuroendocrine Tumors

The term "neuroendocrine tumor (NET)" (also called carcinoid and APUDoma) is used for all endocrine tumors of the digestive system that derive from the intestinal neuroendocrine system [15]. The mucosa of the gastrointestinal tract contains at least 15 different endocrine cell types that produce hormonal peptides and/or biogenic amines [16]. NETs are more common in the ileum (mostly located within 60 cm of the ileocecal valve). The clinical picture is characterized by sluggish biologic behavior. The vast majority of the tumors are carcinoids with some gastrinomas located in the duodenum. Other types of NETs are quite rare in the small bowel. Most of the cases are sporadic, but some are associated with inherited syndromes, with multiple endocrine neoplasia type 1 being the most significant among them. Diagnostic strategies include ultrasonography (US), computerized tomography (CT), magnetic resonance imaging (MRI), bone scanning, angiography, and, in rare cases, selective venous sampling for hormonal gradients. Somatostatin receptor scintigraphy has begun to play a central role as well [17].

Gastrointestinal Stromal Tumors

Mesenchymal tumors of the small bowel comprise a widely diverse group of neoplasms (leiomyoma, schwannoma, neurofibroma, sarcoma, and others). GISTs are the most common subtype of mesenchymal neoplasm, and they are derived from the interstitial cells of Cajal. They occur anywhere within the gastrointestinal tract, but are most common in the stomach (60–70%) and small bowel (20–25%) [18]. GISTs may be benign or malignant, depending on their size and mitotic index. They are submucosal, highly vascular tumors ranging in size from 1 to 40 cm. Ulceration of these lesions is common, and intestinal bleeding is a frequent symptom. GISTs also may invade adjacent organs directly or spread via peritoneal seeding. Compared with gastric GISTs, small bowel GISTs tend to be more aggressive and have a worse prognosis. Metastases develop in nearly 50% of patients, primarily via the hematogenous route,

commonly involving the liver and peritoneum. GISTs smaller than 2 cm with a low mitotic index are generally considered benign with a very low risk of recurrence. About 5% of GIST cases are multiple, and an increased incidence is seen in patients with neurofibromatosis type 1. Gain-of-function mutations in exon 11 of the c-*kit* proto-oncogene are associated with most cases of GISTs [19].

Primary Lymphomas

Up to 40% of lymphomas develop in sites other than the lymph nodes, with the gut being the most common extralymphatic site [20]. Several patterns of small bowel lymphoma have been identified, including an infiltrating pattern which appears as wall thickening, an exophytic mass that sometimes simulates an adenocarcinoma or GIST, multifocal submucosal nodules within the small bowel, and single mass lesions which can lead to intussusceptions.

Four different histologic types of lymphomas may be found in the small bowel:

Celiac-Associated T-cell High-Grade Lymphoma

Enteropathy-associated T-cell lymphoma is a rare form of high-grade T-cell non-Hodgkin lymphoma (NHL) of the upper small intestine that is associated with celiac disease [21]. An abnormal clonal intraepithelial lymphocyte cell population is diffusely present throughout the gastrointestinal tract in approximately 80% of refractory celiac disease cases. These cells are characterized by a low ratio of CD_8^+/CD_3^+ and T-cell receptor (TCR)-γ gene rearrangement [22].

Burkitt-Type Lymphoma of the Small Intestine

Burkitt lymphoma is an aggressive type of B-cell lymphoma that has two major forms: endemic (African) and non-endemic (sporadic). The sporadic form usually involves abdominal organs, with the most common being the distal ileum, cecum, or mesentery. Burkitt lymphoma is a childhood tumor that can also be observed in adult patients. It is characterized by a high rate of malignant cell proliferation (indicated by ki-67 expression) and by morphologic features that are distinct from diffuse large B-cell lymphoma. Burkitt lymphoma can be seen in the setting of acquired immune deficiency syndrome (AIDS) or chronic immunosuppression [23].

Mucosa-Associated Lymphoid Tissue Lymphoma – Maltoma

Maltoma was first defined as a primary low-grade gastric B-cell lymphoma and immunoproliferative small intestinal disease. This definition was later extended to include several other extranodal low-grade B-cell NHLs. The gastric form is the most common and best characterized maltoma. These tumors tend to stay localized in the mucosal wall without involvement of regional lymph nodes. This type of malignancy has recently been linked with the response to bacterial infections [24].

Immunoproliferative Small Intestinal Disease (Mediterranean Lymphoma)

This is an unusual intestinal B-cell lymphoma that occurs mostly in children and young adults of Mediterranean ancestry, and is associated with a single protein abnormality. The mucosal IgA α-heavy chain has a deletion in its variable region [25]. Treatment with antibiotics can lead to remission, suggesting that the proliferative burst is due to an aberrant immunogenic response to bacterial infection. *Campylobacter jejuni* was shown to play a role in this disease, similar to the role of *Helicobacter pylori* in gastric MALT lymphoma [26].

Clinical Features (Table 34.1)

Small bowel tumors are usually asymptomatic in the early stages. The rarity of these tumors and the subtle and non-specific presenting symptoms may delay the diagnosis. The most frequent are abdominal pain, nausea, vomiting, and intestinal obstruction (50% of the patients undergo emergency surgery for intestinal obstruction) [27]. The nature of the symptoms depends mainly on the size and location of the tumor, with lesions distal to the ligament of Treitz tending to present with either obstruction or bleeding, while GISTs more commonly present with acute gastrointestinal bleeding. The most common laboratory abnormality is hypochromic microcytic anemia, and many of these patients have a positive test for fecal occult blood. Direct hyperbilirubinemia and increased alkaline phosphatase are usually found in cases of duodenal tumors as a consequence of extrahepatic biliary obstruction.

Table 34.1 Staging of small bowel carcinoma [according to the American Joint Committee on Cancer staging system. Greene FL, Page DL, Fleming ID, et al. AJCC Cancer Staging Manual, 6th edn, 2002. Springer; chapter 11].

Primary tumor stage (T)

TX	Primary tumor cannot be assessed
T0	No evidence of primary tumor is present
Tis	Carcinoma *in situ* is present
T1	Tumor invades the lamina propria or submucosa
T2	Tumor invades the muscularis propria
T3	Tumor invades through the muscularis propria into subserosa or into nonperitonealized perimuscular tissue (mesentery or retroperitoneum), with extension of < 2 cm
T4	Tumor penetrates the visceral peritoneum or directly invades other organs or structures

Regional lymph nodes (N)

NX	Regional lymph nodes cannot be assessed
N0	No regional lymph node metastasis is present
N1	Regional lymph node metastasis has occurred

Distant metastases (M)

MX	Presence of distant metastasis cannot be assessed
M0	No distant metastasis is present
M1	Distant metastasis has occurred

Stage grouping	T	N	M
Stage 0	Tis	N0	M0
Stage I	T1-2	N0	M0
Stage II	T3-4	N0	M0
Stage III	Any T	N1	M0
Stage IV	Any T	Any N	M1

Diagnosis

Early detection of a small bowel neoplasm is certainly desirable but a challenging prospect. The detection of small intestinal tumors by traditional imaging modalities is often compromised by overlapping bowel loops and suboptimal bowel distension. Newer techniques are expected to improve diagnostic capabilities.

Imaging Modalities

Small Bowel Follow-Through

This is the oldest barium study traditionally used for evaluation of the small bowel. The true value of this non-invasive test is open to question due to the reported wide range of sensitivity for tumor detection (30–90%) [28].

Enteroclysis

This is considered superior to small bowel follow-through due to the minute mucosal detail that can be demonstrated, its specificity and sensitivity. It is, however, a more difficult procedure for both the radiologist and the patient, requiring nasojejunal intubation and oral administration of large volumes of contrast material. The sensitivity of enteroclysis is as high as 95%, with 90% correct estimation of the actual size of the tumor.

Multidetector Computed Tomography Scans

Multidetector CT scans (MDCTs) produce high-resolution cross-sectional imaging of the abdomen and small bowel. The lumen of the small bowel must be distended with orally administered contrast material to demonstrate the wall thickening that characterizes small bowel tumors on CT. An MDCT allows multiplanar visualization of small bowel tumors, and demonstrates signs of small bowel obstruction as well as the mural and extramural extent of small bowel malignancies.

Multidetector Computed Tomography Enteroclysis

Multidetector CT enteroclysis (MDCT-E) shares the advantages of both conventional enteroclysis and cross-sectional imaging. This technique is more sensitive than conventional barium studies and less invasive than enteroscopy, and lesions as small as 5 mm can be identified. MDCT-E studies have shown 100% sensitivity and 85–95% concordance with enteroscopy [29]. The recent introduction of cellulose as the contrast material has significantly increased the sensitivity and specificity of CT enterography.

Magnetic Resonance Imaging and Magnetic Resonance Enteroclysis

The advantages of MRI over CT include excellent soft tissue contrast, absence of exposure to radiation and iodine contrast, and multiple contrast sources. MR enteroclysis includes small bowel intubation and the administration of a biphasic contrast agent. This protocol can provide anatomic demonstration of the normal intestinal wall, identification of wall thickening or timorous lesions, lesion characterization or evaluation of disease activity, and assessment of exoenteric/mesenteric disease extension [30].

FDG-Positron Emission Tomography

The role of positron emission tomography (PET) in the initial diagnosis of small bowel malignant tumors has not yet been established. It can serve to monitor response to treatment and is highly sensitive and specific for the evaluation of nodal and extranodal patients with malignant lymphomas [31].

Push Enteroscopy

Push enteroscopy permits evaluation of the proximal one-third of the small intestine to a distance that is approximately 50–100 cm beyond the ligament of Treitz. The diagnostic yield of this technique is reported to increase with a greater depth of scope insertion. Data on the diagnostic yield of small bowel tumors and polyps are limited to studies that have investigated push enteroscopy in the context of obscure gastrointestinal bleeding, with a reported yield in the range of 1–5% [32,33].

Video Capsule Endoscopy

Video capsule endoscopy (VCE) is safe, easy, minimally invasive, and patient-friendly, and has become a first-line tool in imaging and managing small bowel pathologies [34]. The utility of VCE has more than doubled the rate of detection of small bowel tumors from the precapsule endoscopy era of approximately 3% to today's 6–9% prevalence rate, when the procedure is done for obscure gastrointestinal bleeding. The detected small bowel tumors are malignant in more than 50% of cases [35]. VCE examinations reach the cecum about 80% of the time and luminal debris and bubbles interfere with viewing in some patients. Capsule retention is the major and, for all practical purposes, the only complication of VCE. The reported incidence of capsule retention ranges from 0% in healthy volunteers to 2% in obscure gastrointestinal hemorrhage, reaching up to 21% in individuals with suspected small bowel obstruction. The retention rate in patients with small bowel tumors may be around 10%.

Double Balloon Enteroscopy

Double balloon enteroscopy (DBE) is a novel endoscopic insertion technique that uses a high-resolution, dedicated video endoscope with a working length of 200 cm and two soft latex balloons, one attached to the tip of the endoscope and the other to the distal end of a soft, flexible overtube. The balloons can be inflated and deflated using an air pump that is controlled by the endoscopist while monitoring air pressure. DBE has been shown to be of both diagnostic and therapeutic value. DBE was found to be accurate in demonstrating the bleeding sites in 115 (75.7%) patients with obscure bleeding, of which 45 (39.1%) were due to small bowel tumors [36]. There are limitations associated with DBE, including concerns about the learning curve, the need for endoscopy on two separate days (transoral and then transanal approaches), limitations in visualization of the entire small bowel, miss rates for subepithelial lesions due to inadequate insufflation, its being a time-consuming procedure that requires a high level of ancillary staffing, the high level of sedation requirements, and patient tolerance and preferences. In addition, although uncommon, the reported incidence of severe complications associated with DBE ranges from 0% to 2.5% and these include pancreatitis, perforations, bleeding, abdominal pain, and fever.

Intraoperative Enteroscopy

This has been utilized since the 1980s and is an important diagnostic and potentially therapeutic endoscopic modality in suspected small bowel polyps and tumors [37]. It is considered to be the ultimate endoscopic evaluation of the small bowel. The reported complications include mucosal lacerations, perforations, prolonged ileus, abdominal abscess, and bowel ischemia.

Therapy

Benign Tumors

A simple endoscopic snare polypectomy is the treatment of choice for adenomatous polyps located within the reach of esophagogastroduodenoscopy. If this is not technically feasible, a local surgical excision is indicated, and close endoscopic follow-up is warranted. All patients with duodenal adenomas should undergo colonoscopy to rule out polyposis syndromes, especially FAP.

Lipomas should not be resected unless they are symptomatic.

Benign leiomyomas should be resected only if they are symptomatic, if they cannot be differentiated from GISTs, or if there is doubt about their being benign or malignant.

Neurofibromatas in patients with von Recklinghausen disease are considered to be benign and should not be resected unless they are symptomatic.

Hamartomatous polyps in PJS generally are not premalignant and they should only be resected if they become symptomatic (bleeding, intussusceptions,

obstruction), if their size exceeds 15 mm, or if they reveal macroscopic or microscopic features that are suspicious for malignant degeneration. Since polyps in PJS patients are abundant, and considering the high lifetime risk for having multiple interventions, appropriate surgical management consists of surgical enterectomy and polypectomy. If bowel resection is required, an absolute minimum length of bowel should be sacrificed in order to limit the risk for development of short bowel syndrome. Appropriate surveillance of the proband and his/her first-degree relatives is warranted.

Adenocarcinoma

Wide surgical resection of early lesions is the sole potentially curative treatment, but it is possible only in a minority of patients. The rarity of these tumors has resulted in a paucity of information on the benefits of adjuvant chemotherapy. There are reports of better overall survival for patients who receive combination treatment consisting of 5-fluorouracil (5-FU) alone or in combination with a variety of other agents [38]. In metastatic disease, a palliative surgical resection of the primary tumor and palliative chemotherapeutic treatment are frequently needed in order to prevent or treat complications, such as bowel obstruction or bleeding. Since there are no randomized clinical trials in the setting of small bowel tumors [38], the approach is similar to that of CRC.

Neuroendocrine Tumors

Surgery is the most effective treatment for the control of both local tumor effect and of endocrinopathy-related symptoms in the setting of unresectable or metastatic disease [39]. A thorough presurgical examination is essential to rule out synchronous or metachronous tumors (most likely adenocarcinomas), not only along the gastrointestinal tract, but also in the lung, prostate, cervix, and ovary. If liver metastases are present at diagnosis, the primary tumor should still be resected in order to avoid later complications, which may include obstruction, bleeding, and perforation.

In patients with moderate-to-severe symptoms, treatment with the somatostatin analogs, octreotide, and lanreotide is considered to be gold standard. The addition of interferon-α has shown to be effective in controlling carcinoid-related symptoms in patients resistant to somatostatin analogs [40]. Hepatic artery embolization or chemoembolization should be reserved for patients who have unresectable liver metastases without extrahepatic spread or for progressive disease and/or severe symptoms not responding to somatostatin analogs or interferon.

Lymphoma

The majority of primary intestinal low-grade lymphomas can be cured by surgery alone (resection of the affected segment of small bowel together with its adjacent mesentery). Aggressive chemotherapy is the mainstay of treatment in more advanced stages, while complete surgical resection is usually performed in order to alleviate symptoms of mass effect and to avoid complications during chemotherapy, even in advanced stages.

Remission can be induced by antibiotic treatment alone in Mediterranean lymphoma or in immunoproliferative small intestinal disease restricted to the mucosa and/or submucosa.

Gastrointestinal Stromal Tumors

The mainstay of resectable GIST treatment has been and continues to be surgery. The resectability of the tumor and the ability of the patient to tolerate a major resection must be carefully assessed. It is important to stress that although GISTs may present as a huge lesion, the "pushing" nature of tumor growth may allow adequate *en bloc* resection, leaving the pseudocapsule intact, thus avoiding intra-abdominal tumor spillage. Unlike adenocarcinoma or carcinoid tumor that spread thorough lymphatics, GISTs metastasize hematogenously, obviating the need for removal of lymphatic drainage in the mesentery. Dense adhesions often hamper resection. In the presence of metastatic disease, a local resection of the primary tumor may be considered for control of bleeding or relief of obstruction. Imatinib mesylate (Gleevec®), a selective tyrosine kinase inhibitor, has been shown to be effective in metastatic disease. It may also be used as a neoadjuvant drug in an attempt to downstage a borderline case to the point of making it resectable.

Take-home points

- Small bowel tumors are extremely rare and account for only 1–2% of all gastrointestinal malignancies. Two-thirds of these tumors are malignant.
- Adenocarcinoma is the most common malignancy (40%), followed by neuroendocrine tumors (carcinoid) (20–40%), lymphomas (14%), and gastrointestinal stromal tumors (11–13%).
- Small bowel tumors are usually asymptomatic in the early stages. The most frequent presenting symptoms are abdominal pain, nausea, vomiting, and intestinal obstruction.
- The diagnostic strategies include conventional non-invasive imaging (small bowel barium series, enteroclysis, computerized tomography, and magnetic resonance imaging), as well as the push, double balloon and video-capsule endoscopic modalities. The newer techniques have improved diagnostic accuracy.
- Since there are no data from clinical trials, therapy of small bowel adenocarcinoma is similar to that of colorectal cancer.

References

1 Jemal A, Siegel R, Ward E, Murray T, Xu J, Thun MJ. Cancer statistics, 2007. *CA Cancer J Clin* 2007; **57**: 43–66.

2 Hatzaras I, Palesty JA, Abir F, *et al*. Small-bowel tumors: epidemiologic and clinical characteristics of 1260 cases from the Connecticut tumor registy. *Arch Surg* 2007; **142**: 229–35.

3 Neugut AI, Jacobson JS, Suh S, Mukherjee R, Arber N. The epidemiology of cancer of the small bowel. *Cancer Epidemiol Biomarkers Prev* 1998; **7**: 243–51.

4 Ciresi DL, Scholten DJ. The continuing clinical dilemma of primary tumors of the small intestine. *Am Surg* 1995; **61**: 698–702; discussion 702–3.

5 Minardi AJ Jr, Zibari GB, Aultman DF, McMillan RW, McDonald JC. Small-bowel tumors. *J Am Coll Surg* 1998; **186**: 664–8.

6 Seifert E, Schulte F, Stolte M. Adenoma and carcinoma of the duodenum and papilla of Vater: a clinicopathologic study. *Am J Gastroenterol* 1992; **87**: 37–42.

7 Whiteman BJ, Janssens AR, Griffioen G, Lamers CB. Villous tumors of the duodenum. An analysis of the literature with emphasis on malignant transformation. *Neth J Med* 1993; **42**: 5–11.

8 Wirtzfeld DA, Petrelli NJ, Rodriguez-Bigas MA. Hamartomatous polyposis syndromes: molecular genetics, neoplastic risk, and surveillance recommendations. *Ann Surg Oncol* 2001; **8**: 319–27.

9 Dabaja BS, Suki D, Pro B, Bonnen M, Ajani J. Adenocarcinoma of the small bowel: presentation, prognostic factors, and outcome of 217 patients. *Cancer* 2004; **101**: 518–26.

10 Michelassi F, Testa G, Pomidor WJ, Lashner BJ, Block GE. Adenocarcinoma complicating Crohn's disease. *Dis Colon Rectum* 1993; **36**: 654–61.

11 Kaerlev L, Teglbjaerg PS, Sabroe S, *et al.* Medical risk factors for small-bowel adenocarcinoma with focus on Crohn disease: a European population-based case-control study. *Scand J Gastroenterol* 2001; **36**: 641–6.

12 Offerhaus GJ, Giardiello FM, Krush AJ, *et al.* The risk of upper gastrointestinal cancer in familial adenomatous polyposis. *Gastroenterology* 1992; **102**: 1980–2.

13 Wu AH, Yu MC, Mack TM. Smoking, alcohol use, dietary factors and risk of small intestinal adenocarcinoma. *Int J Cancer* 1997 **70**: 512–7.

14 Negri E, Bosetti C, La Vecchia C, Fioretti F, Conti E, Franceschi S. Risk factors for adenocarcinoma of the small intestine. *Int J Cancer* 1999; **82**: 171–4.

15 Polak JM. *Diagnostic Histopathology of Neuroendocrine Tumours.* Edinburgh: Churchill-Livingstone, 1993.

16 Rindi G, Capella C, Solcia E. Pathobiology and classification of digestive endocrine tumors. In: Mignon M, Colombel JF (eds). *Recent Advances in the Pathophysiology of Inflammatory Bowel Disease and Digestive Endocrine Tumors.* Montrouge: John Libbey Eurotext, 1999: 177–91.

17 Lebtahi R, Cadiot G, Sarda L, *et al.* Clinical impact of somatostatin receptor scintigraphy in the management of patients with neuroendocrine gastroenteropancreatic tumors. *J Nucl Med* 1997; **38**: 853–8.

18 Pidhorecky I, Cheney RT, Kraybill WG, Gibbs JF. Gastrointestinal stromal tumors: current diagnosis, biologic behavior, and management. *Ann Surg Oncol* 2000; **7**: 705–12.

19 Hirota S, Isozaki K, Moriyama Y, *et al.* Gain-of-function mutations of c-kit in human gastrointestinal stromal tumors. *Science* 1998; **279**: 577–80.

20 Crump M, Gospodarowicz M, Shepherd FA. Lymphoma of the gastrointestinal tract. *Semin Oncol* 1999; **26**: 324–37.

21 Catassi C, Bearzi I, Holmes GK. Association of celiac disease and intestinal lymphomas and other cancers. *Gastroenterology* 2005; **128** (4 Suppl 1): S79–86.

22 Verkarre V, Romana SP, Cellier C, *et al.* Recurrent partial trisomy 1q22-q44 in clonal intraepithelial lymphocytes in refractory celiac sprue. *Gastroenterology* 2003; **125**: 40–6.

23 Bishop PC, Rao VK, Wilson WH. Burkitt's lymphoma: molecular pathogenesis and treatment. *Cancer Invest* 2000; **18**: 574–583.

24 Isaacson P, Wright DH. Malignant lymphoma of mucosa-associated lymphoid tissue. A distinctive type of B-cell lymphoma. *Cancer* 1983; **52**: 1410–6.

25 Salem PA, Estephan FF. Immunoproliferative small intestinal disease: current concepts. *Cancer J* 2005; **11**: 374–82.

26 Lecuit M, Abachin E, Martin A, *et al.* Immunoproliferative small intestinal disease associated with *Campylobacter jejuni.* *N Engl J Med* 2004; **350**: 239–48.

27 Dabaja BS, Suki D, Pro B, Bonnen M, Ajani J. Adenocarcinoma of the small bowel: presentation, prognostic factors, and outcome of 217 patients. *Cancer* 2004; **101**: 518–26.

28 Korman MU. Radiologic evaluation and staging of small intestine neoplasms. *Eur J Radiol* 2002; **42**: 193–205.

29 Horton, KM; Fishman, EK Multidetector-row computed tomography and 3-dimensional computed tomography imaging of small bowel neoplasms: Current concept in diagnosis. *J Comput Assist Tomogr* 2004; **28**: 106–16

30 Semelka RC, John G, Kelekis NL, Burdeny DA, Ascher SM. Small bowel neoplastic disease: demonstration by MRI. *J Magn Reson Imaging* 1996; **6**: 855–60.

31 Kumar R, Xiu Y, Potenta S, *et al.* 18F-FDG PET for evaluation of the treatment response in patients with gastrointestinal tract lymphomas. *J Nucl Med* 2004; **45**: 1796–803.

32 Bessette, JR, Maglinte DD, Kelvin FM, Chernish SM. Primary malignant tumors in the small bowel: a comparison of the small-bowel enema and conventional follow-through examination. *AJR Am J Roentgenol* 1989; **153**: 741–4.

33 Chak A, Koehler MK, Sundaram SN, *et al.* Diagnostic and therapeutic impact of push enteroscopy: analysis of factors associated with positive findings. *Gastrointest Endosc* 1998; **47**: 18–22.

34 Triester SL, Leighton JA, Grigoris LI, *et al.* A meta-analysis of the yield of capsule endoscopy compared to other diagnostic modalities in patients with obscure gastrointestinal bleeding. *Am J Gastroenterol* 2005; **100**: 2407–18.

35 Pennazio M, Rondonotti E, de Franchis R. Capsule endoscopy in neoplastic diseases. *World J Gastroenterol* 2008; **14**: 5245–53.

36 Sun B, Rajan E, Cheng S, *et al.* Diagnostic yield and therapeutic impact of double-balloon enteroscopy in a large cohort of patients with obscure gastrointestinal bleeding. *Am J Gastroenterol* 2006; **101**: 2011–5.

37 Matsumoto T, Esaki M, Yanaru-Fujisawa R, *et al.* Small-intestinal involvement in familial adenomatous polyposis: evaluation by double-balloon endoscopy and intraoperative enteroscopy. *Gastrointestinal Endosc* 2008; **68**: 911–9.

38 Singhal N, Singhal D. Adjuvant chemotherapy for small intestine adenocarcinoma. *Cochrane Database Syst Rev* 2007: CD005202.

39 Kulke MH, Mayer RJ. Carcinoid tumors. *N Engl J Med* 1999; **340**: 858–68.

40 Modlin IM, Lye KD, Kidd M. A 5-decade analysis of 13,715 carcinoid tumors. *Cancer* 2003; **97**: 934–59.

CHAPTER 35

Small Intestinal Bacterial Overgrowth

Monthira Maneerattanaporn[1] and William D. Chey[2]

[1] Division of Gastroenterology, University of Michigan, Ann Arbor, MI, USA and Department of Medicine, Siriaj Hospital, Mahidol University, Bangkok, Thailand

[2] GI Physiology Laboratory, University of Michigan Health System, Ann Arbor, MI, USA

Summary

Small intestinal bacterial overgrowth (SIBO) is a condition that may cause a wide range of clinical and nutritional manifestations. Clinical suspicion must be high in patients with disorders that disrupt the small intestine's normal defenses against SIBO. There is a growing body of evidence to suggest that the prevalence of SIBO is higher in the elderly. Though an association between SIBO and IBS has been suggested, the available evidence is not conclusive. There is no currently available test that can be considered an adequate gold standard for the diagnosis of SIBO. Small bowel culture is highly specific but lacks sensitivity, particularly for distal SIBO. Carbohydrate breath tests are non-invasive and simple to perform but lack standardization and have not been adequately validated as a reliable surrogate means of identifying SIBO. Therapy of SIBO consists of antibiotics to decontaminate the small intestine, nutritional support to address the consequences of longstanding SIBO, and, when possible, correction of the underlying cause of SIBO.

Case

A 45-year-old woman was referred with complaints of bloating and chronic diarrhea.

Her bloating and diarrhea have been problematic for several months. She reports passing three to four loose bowel movements per day. She states that her stools occasionally float in the toilet bowl. She reports abdominal distension which can be severe enough to require loosening of the beltline of her pants. She also describes early satiety and malodorous flatus. Her symptoms worsen after eating a meal. She denies melena or hematochezia but does report progressive weight loss of 4.5 kg (10 pounds) over the past 6 months. She also reports the onset of difficulty driving at night and numbness and tingling of her lower extremities over the past few weeks. She has self-medicated with over-the-counter remedies, including simethicone, loperamide, and antacids, without benefit to her symptoms.

Her history of present illness began 5 years ago when she presented with Raynaud phenomenon. She was eventually diagnosed with systemic sclerosis after she had began to experience difficulty swallowing solids and liquids and noticed changes in the texture of her skin. Her current medications include methotrexate 25 mg/week, folate 1 mg/day, aspirin 81 mg/day, and verapamil 180 mg once daily.

She has no history of abdominal surgery or family history of gastrointestinal cancer.

Physical examination revealed a thin Caucasian female in non distress. Her body temperature is normal, blood pressure was 100/70 mmHg and pulse rate was 94 bpm. Her height was 152 cm (5 feet) and her weight was 47.6 kg (105 pounds). Positive findings included smooth, shiny skin with sclerodactyly consistent with her diagnosis of systemic sclerosis. There was an area of calcinosis cutis on her back. She also had crackles at both lung bases on deep inspiration and loud P_2 on precordial examination. Her abdomen was moderately distended with decreased bowel sounds but no succusion splash. Palpation revealed no masses or tenderness. Digital rectal examination revealed normal anal sphincter tone and hemeoccult-negative stool. Neurological examination revealed decreased sensation to pinprick but was otherwise non-focal.

Definition and Epidemiology

Small intestinal bacterial overgrowth (SIBO) has traditionally been defined by quantitative culture of aspirated juice from the proximal jejunum. The most widely accepted definition of SIBO is greater than 10^5 colony forming units of bacteria per milliliter of aspirate (CFU/mL). Some have argued that a lower threshold may be appropriate ($>10^3$ CFU/mL) if the bacteria species identified are absent from the saliva and gastric juice or are similar to those found in the colon [1,2]. SIBO is typically a byproduct of structural abnormalities involving the gastrointestinal tract or alterations in gut motor, secretory, or immunological function. There are few data addressing the prevalence of SIBO in healthy individuals. SIBO does appear to occur more commonly in the elderly. Recent work suggests that up to 15% of healthy elderly individuals will have an abnormal breath test result suggestive of SIBO [3,4]. Though still highly controversial, recent data also suggest an association between SIBO and the irritable bowel syndrome (IBS) [5].

Pathophysiology

The human gastrointestinal (GI) tract houses a diverse population of 300–500 bacterial species. The quantity and species of bacterial flora varies from the proximal to distal small intestine. Normal colony counts are 10^2 CFU/mL in proximal small intestine and increase to as high as 10^9 CFU/mL in the terminal ileum. In the proximal small intestine, Gram-positive, aerobic bacterial species are most common while Gram-negative, anaerobic bacteria are more common distally. In healthy individuals, the normal gut microflora is maintained by five major mechanisms [1,6,7]: gastric acid secretion, pancreatic enzyme secretion, small intestinal motility, structural integrity of the GI tract, and an intact gut immune system. The primary role of gastric acid is to reduce the bacterial content of food and to suppress bacterial growth within the proximal small intestine. Pancreatic enzymes also exert an antimicrobial effect within the proximal small intestine. Normal fasting small intestinal motility is critical to the prevention of bacterial overgrowth. Phase III of the migrating motor complex is composed of frequent peristaltic contractions which propel retained luminal debris and bacteria through the small intestine. Mechani-

cal obstruction predisposes to intestinal stasis. Further, the ileocecal valve provides a physical barrier to reflux of colonic contents into the terminal ileum. Disruption of any of these protective mechanisms can result in the development of SIBO (Figure 35.1).

Clinical Manifestation

SIBO can lead to both direct and indirect effects on the gut mucosa and luminal microenvironment. Bacterial adherence to the intestinal mucosa can result in direct injury, dysfunction, and alterations in gut immunology. Significant mucosal injury can lead to reduced brush border disaccharidase activity and altered small bowel permeability. In addition, bacterial metabolism and fermentation can compete with the host for nutritionally valuable substrates and lead to the production of byproducts which possess biologic activity or alter gut function (Figure 35.2).

The clinical consequences of SIBO span a spectrum ranging from asymptomatic to florid malabsorption. Most often, affected patients report non-specific symptoms including bloating, distension, abdominal cramping, and diarrhea. Diarrhea is usually multifactorial with contributions from malabsorption, maldigestion, bile acid deconjugation, protein losing enteropathy, and co-morbid disease processes. Numerous nutritional deficiencies have been reported, the most notable of which include vitamin B_{12} and fat-soluble vitamins. Specific clinical features can raise suspicion for such nutritional deficiencies; macrocytic anemia and peripheral neuropathy can be an indicator of B_{12} deficiency while night blindness and follicular hyperkeratosis can suggest vitamin A deficiency. Interestingly, as a consequence of bacterial synthesis, levels of folate and vitamin K are usually normal or elevated in the setting of SIBO.

Diagnosis

Aspiration of jejunal fluid for quantitative culture has been considered the gold standard for the diagnosis of SIBO. Though this technique is highly specific, small bowel aspiration for quantitative culture is far from a perfect gold standard for SIBO. Drawbacks of this technique include the invasive nature of sample collection,

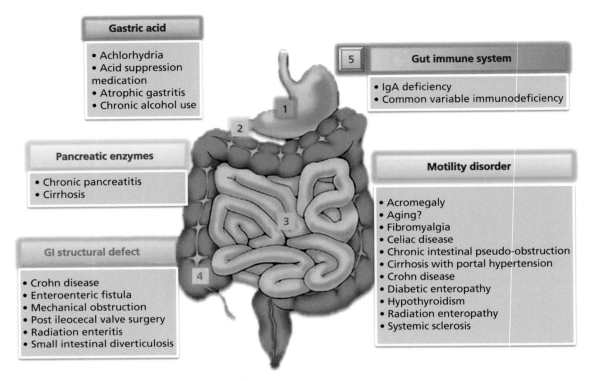

Gastric acid
- Achlorhydria
- Acid suppression medication
- Atrophic gastritis
- Chronic alcohol use

Gut immune system
- IgA deficiency
- Common variable immunodeficiency

Pancreatic enzymes
- Chronic pancreatitis
- Cirrhosis

Motility disorder
- Acromegaly
- Aging?
- Fibromyalgia
- Celiac disease
- Chronic intestinal pseudo-obstruction
- Cirrhosis with portal hypertension
- Crohn disease
- Diabetic enteropathy
- Hypothyroidism
- Radiation enteropathy
- Systemic sclerosis

GI structural defect
- Crohn disease
- Enteroenteric fistula
- Mechanical obstruction
- Post ileocecal valve surgery
- Radiation enteritis
- Small intestinal diverticulosis

Figure 35.1 Mechanisms to maintain normal gut microflora.

contamination of aspirated material by oral flora, the lack of sensitivity for detecting distal SIBO, expense, and the need for infrastructure and trained personnel to perform quantitative culture.

Many investigators and clinicians have utilized carbohydrate breath tests as a surrogate means of identifying SIBO. Breath tests rely upon the ability of intestinal bacteria to metabolize various carbohydrate substrates to hydrogen and/or methane gas which is rapidly absorbed across the intestinal epithelium and eventually excreted in the breath. After a carbohydrate load, a rapid rise in breath hydrogen or methane excretion may indicate the presence of SIBO (Figure 35.3) [8]. The most commonly used substrates for commercially available breath tests include lactulose and glucose. Each substrate offers unique advantages and disadvantages.

In the absence of SIBO, lactulose is not fermented or absorbed within the small intestine. When exposed to bacteria within the small intestine, lactulose is fermented to short-chain fatty acids and a number of gases including hydrogen and/or methane. Unfortunately, colonic bacteria will also ferment lactulose, making it difficult to interpret whether a positive breath test result truly represents SIBO or simply rapid orocecal transit. The optimal way in which to define a positive lactulose breath test remains controversial [8]. In one study which used quantitative small bowel culture as a gold standard, the sensitivity and specificity of the lactulose breath test was reported to be 68 and 44%, respectively [8,9].

The other substrate commonly used to test for SIBO is glucose. Glucose is avidly absorbed in the proximal small intestine. Because glucose typically does not reach the distal small bowel, the glucose breath test may be less sensitive than the lactulose breath test. On the other hand, the glucose breath test is likely more specific than the lactulose breath test [8,9]. Characteristics and performance of the commonly used tests for SIBO can be found in Table 35.1.

Other breath tests using D-xylose, ^{13}C-xylose, and cholyglycine have been described in the literature but

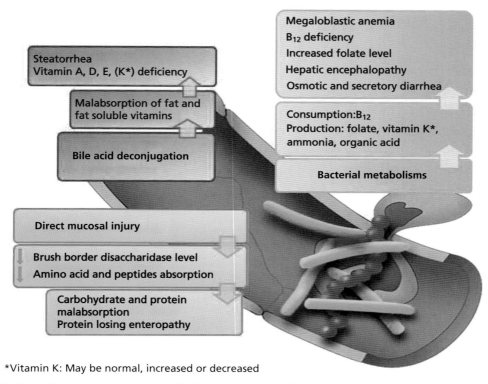

*Vitamin K: May be normal, increased or decreased

Figure 35.2 Effects of bacteria on gut mucosa and clinical consequences of small intestinal bacterial overgrowth.

have yielded conflicting results and are not widely available [8,10].

Treatment

The treatment of SIBO can be separated into several phases: acute antibiotic therapy to decontaminate the small intestine, repletion of vitamin deficiencies and correction of malnutrition, and management of any underlying disease process which might have been responsible for the development of SIBO.

Antibiotics are most commonly used to acutely decontaminate the small intestine. An ideal antibiotic for SIBO should possess activity against both aerobic and anaerobic enteric bacteria. A variety of antibiotics have been used to treat SIBO including amoxicillin–clavulanic acid, cefoxitin, ciprofloxacin, norfloxacin, metronidazole, neomycin, and doxycyclin. Most reports in the literature have recommended courses of 7 to 14 days. If a correct-

able underlying etiology for SIBO can be identified, a single course of antibiotics may result in a durable clinical response. In many cases, the underlying cause of SIBO cannot be identified or cannot be corrected. In these circumstances, repeated courses of antibiotics are often necessary. When SIBO is infrequent or only leads to mild clinical or nutritional consequences, it may be sufficient to wait for symptoms to recur before reinstituting a course of antibiotics. When patients have frequent or very severe bouts of SIBO, using rotating courses of antibiotics every 4–6 weeks can be very effective. Concerns with such a strategy include the development of *Clostridium difficile* colitis and multi-drug-resistant bacterial flora (Figure 35.4).

Rifaximin is a semisynthetic, non-absorbable oral antibiotic with a broad spectrum of action. This drug is concentrated in the GI tract and has recently been studied as a treatment for SIBO. Studies have utilized a variety of dosing schedules (400–550 mg two to three times per day for 7–14 days) [12,13]. In short-term studies utilizing

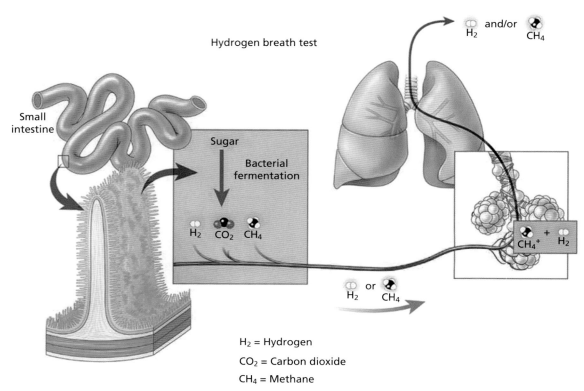

H₂ = Hydrogen

CO₂ = Carbon dioxide

CH₄ = Methane

Figure 35.3 Schematic for hydrogen breath testing. Reprinted from Saad RJ and Chey WD [8], © 2007, with permission from Elsevier.

Table 35.1 Comparison of the diagnostic tests for small intestinal bacterial overgrowth.

	Small intestinal aspiration for quantitative culture	Glucose breath test	Lactulose breath test
Advantages	Quantitative measurement Allows speciation of bacteria	Non-invasive Simple to perform Less costly than culture	
Disadvantages	Invasive High cost Technically difficult	Need specialized equipment, space, and technical support Abnormal thresholds not well validated	
False-positive results	Contamination from bacteria in upper GI tract	Rapid small bowel transit time	Rapid small bowel transit time
False-negative results	Inappropriate sample processing or culture techniques	Distal small intestinal bacterial overgrowth	Chronic lactose exposure? [10]
Sensitivity (%) [2,9,11]	56	62	16.7–68
Specificity (%) [2,9,11]	100	83	44–100

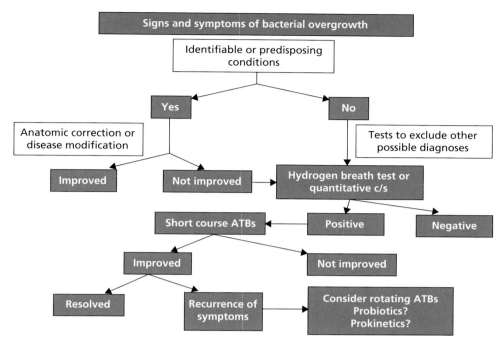

Figure 35.4 Treatment of small intestinal bacterial overgrowth. ATBs = antibiotics.

breath testing as a surrogate for SIBO, rifaximin has led to conversion of a positive to negative breath test result in up to 70% of patients [14,15]. In general, greater efficacy has been achieved by regimens utilizing higher doses of rifaximin. To date, little in the way of resistance to rifaximin has been reported.

There are scant data on the role of diet in the development, perpetuation, or recurrence of SIBO. Based on glucose breath test results, one study found SIBO to be more prevalent in subjects who consumed significantly less fiber, folic acid, and vitamins B_2 and B_6 than those without SIBO [14]. In another study, an elemental diet led to normalization of abnormal lactulose breath test results and improved symptoms in patients with IBS [15]. It is likely that diet does play a role in SIBO—for the worse and perhaps for the better. In fact, this concept underlies the notion that prebiotics might offer benefits for SIBO. Further work to understand the role of diet in patients with SIBO is eagerly awaited.

There are some data to suggest that prokinetic drugs, including motilin agonists and 5-HT$_4$ agonists, might offer a primary treatment option for SIBO in patients

with abnormal motility. It has also been suggested that prokinetic therapy might offer a means by which to prolong the duration of therapeutic benefit following intestinal decontamination with antibiotics. The available literature consists of small, methodologically flawed studies [1]. Further practical issues regarding the development of tolerance with chronic dosing (motilides) and lack of availability (5-HT$_4$ agonists) limit the role of prokinetic therapy in clinical practice.

Some investigators have suggested a potential role of probiotics for SIBO. To date, no methodologically rigorous studies have addressed this important issue.

Case continued

Her laboratory tests revealed mild anemia with hemoglobin of 9.6 g/dL (13–17.3 g/dL) and an elevated mean corpuscular volume of 111 fL (80–100 fL). A comprehensive metabolic profile revealed a low albumin level of 3.2 g/dL (3.5–4.9 g/dL). B_{12} level was decreased at 174 pg/mL (211–911 pg/mL). Other tests were within normal limits, including a thyroid stimulating hormone (TSH) level. She also underwent serological testing for celiac disease and inflammatory bowel disease, both of which were negative.

Stool studies for leukocytes, ova and parasite examination, Giardia antigen, and *Clostridium difficile* antigen were negative. A Sudan stain for qualitative fecal fat was positive.

A glucose hydrogen breath test was positive with a rise in breath hydrogen excretion of greater than 20 ppm within 30 min of ingesting 50 g of glucose.

She was diagnosed with small intestinal bacterial overgrowth, and started on a 10-day course of oral rifaximin 1.2 g/day, as well as selected vitamin and mineral supplements. Within a week, the patient experienced a dramatic improvement of her symptoms including bloating, flatus, and diarrhea.

Case summary

This patient was a 45-year-old woman with a well-established diagnosis of systemic sclerosis. She recently had developed new gastrointestinal symptoms, including diarrhea, abdominal distension, bloating, and malodorous flatus. She also had early satiety and impressive weight loss. Her physical examination and laboratory findings revealed a constellation of findings including anemia, hypoalbuminemia, and B_{12} deficiency. Her stool was positive for qualitative fecal fat suggesting the presence of steatorrhea.

Her glucose breath test was positive, which supported the diagnosis of small intestinal bacterial overgrowth. Subsequent small bowel follow through demonstrated areas of dilation with narrow separation between valvulae conniventes but wall thickening, findings consistent with her diagnosis of scleroderma. The patient responded very well to an acute course of oral antibiotics. Unfortunately, there is a high likelihood of recurrent bacterial overgrowth given her diagnosis of systemic sclerosis, which is associated with impaired motility and small bowel diverticulosis.

Long-term strategies that can be helpful in such patients include the use of prokinetic agents and/or rotating courses of oral antibiotics.

Take-home points

- In healthy individuals, the normal gut microflora is maintained by five major mechanisms: gastric acid secretion, pancreatic enzyme secretion, small intestinal motility, structural integrity of the GI tract, and an intact gut immune system. Abnormalities in any of these defensive mechanisms can lead to the development of SIBO.

- The clinical consequences of SIBO span a spectrum ranging from asymptomatic to florid malabsorption. Most commonly, patients present with non-specific symptoms such as bloating, cramping, and diarrhea.

- Aspiration of jejunal fluid for quantitative culture has been considered the gold standard for the diagnosis of SIBO. However, quantitative culture is invasive, complex to perform, expensive, and lacks sensitivity, particularly for distal SIBO.

- Breath tests utilizing glucose and lactulose are non-invasive and easy to perform but have not been adequately validated as an accurate means of identifying SIBO.

- Therapy of SIBO consists of antibiotics to decontaminate the small intestine, nutritional support to address the consequences of longstanding SIBO, and, when possible, correction of the underlying cause of SIBO.

References

1 Eamonn MM Quigley, Quera R. Small intestinal bacterial overgrowth: roles of antibiotics, prebiotics, and probiotics. *Gastroenterology* 2006; **130**: S78–S90.

2 Simre'n M, Stotzer P-O. Use and abuse of hydrogen breath tests. *Gut* 2005; **55**: 297–303.

3 Dukowicz AC, Lacy BE, Levine GM. Small intestinal bacterial overgrowth: A comprehensive review. *Gastroenterol Hepatol* 2007; **3**: 112–22.

4 Elphick DA, Chew TS, Higham SE, *et al.* Small bowel bacterial overgrowth in symptomatic older people: can it be diagnosed earlier? *Gerontology* 2005; **51**: 396–401.

5 Lupascu A, Gabrielli M, Lauritano EC, *et al.* Hydrogen glucose breath test to detect small intestinal bacterial overgrowth: a prevalence case–control study in irritable bowel syndrome. *Aliment Pharmacol Ther* 2005; **22**: 1157–60.

6 Pignata C, Budillon G, Monaco G, *et al.* Jejunal bacterial overgrowth and intestinal permeability in children with immunodeficiency syndromes. *Gut* 1990; **31**: 879–82.

7 Riordan SM, McIver CJ, Wakefield D, *et al.* Serum immunoglobulin and soluble IL-2 receptor levels in small intestinal overgrowth with indigenous gut flora. *Dig Dis Sci* 1999; **44**: 939–44.

8 Saad RJ, Chey WD. Breath test for gastrointestinal disease: The real deal or just a lot of hot air? *Gastroenterology* 2007; **133**: 1763–6.

9 Corazza GR, Menozzi MG, Strocchi A, *et al.* The diagnosis of small bowel bacterial overgrowth. Reliability of jejunal culture and inadequacy of breath hydrogen testing. *Gastroenterology* 1990; **98**: 302–9.

10 Romagnuolo J, Schiller D, Bailey RJ. Using breath tests wisely in a gastroenterology practice: an evidence-based review of indications and pitfalls in interpretation. *Am J Gastroenterol* 2002; **97**: 1113–26.

11 Riordan SM, McIver CJ, Walker BM, *et al.* The lactulose breath hydrogen test and small intestinal bacterial overgrowth. *Am J Gastroenterol* 1996; **91**: 1795–803.

12 Yang J, Lee HR, Low K, *et al.* Rifaximin versus other antibiotics in the primary treatment and retreatment of bacterial overgrowth in IBS. *Dig Dis Sci* 2008; **53**: 169–74.

13 Di Stefano M, Malservisi S, Veneto G, *et al.* Rifaximin versus chlortetracycline in the short-term treatment of small intestinal bacterial overgrowth. *Aliment Pharmacol Ther* 2000; **14**: 551–6.

14 Parlesak A, Klein B, Schecher K, *et al.* Prevalence of small bowel bacterial overgrowth and its association with nutrition intake in nonhospitalized older adults. *J Am Geriatr Soc* 2003; **51**: 768–73.

15 Pimentel M, Constantino T, Kong Y, *et al.* A 14-day elemental diet is highly effective in normalizing the lactulose breath test. *Dig Dis Sci* 2004; **49**: 73–7.

CHAPTER 36

Celiac Disease and Tropical Sprue

Alberto Rubio-Tapia and Joseph A. Murray

Division of Gastroenterology and Hepatology, Mayo Clinic, Rochester, MN, USA

Summary

Celiac disease and tropical sprue are the most frequent enteropathies that cause the malabsorption syndrome. While the pathophysiology of these disorders is quite different, some clinical manifestations, but especially the histologic findings, could be similar or even indistinguishable. This review summarizes recent advances in the diagnosis of celiac disease and tropical sprue with especial emphasis in the different clinical features and laboratory findings that may help in the differentiation of the sprue syndromes. Practical diagnostic and therapeutic algorithms are presented based on the most important clinical facts.

Case

A 50-year-old Caucasian man presented with involuntary loss of weight, diarrhea, and fatigue 3 months after a visit to southern Mexico, where his diarrhea began acutely. Macrocytic anemia and folic acid deficiency were detected. An EGD with mucosal biopsies of the small intestine was performed, revealing scalloping of the circular folds of the duodenum and partial villous atrophy in the microscopic evaluation, suggesting celiac disease or tropical sprue. Antibodies against endomysial and tissue transglutaminase were negative and the level of total immunoglobulin A was normal, making celiac disease unlikely. *Giardia* antigen and three stool samples were negative for the presence of cysts and trophozoites. The patient was successfully treated with folic acid and tetracycline.

Celiac Disease

Definition and Epidemiology

Celiac disease (CD) is an immune-mediated enteropathy induced by the ingestion of gluten (present in wheat, barley, and rye) in genetically susceptible individuals,

Practical Gastroenterology and Hepatology: Small and Large Intestine and Pancreas, 1st edition. Edited by Nicholas J. Talley, Sunanda V. Kane and Michael B. Wallace. © 2010 Blackwell Publishing Ltd.

which can affect any system or organ, and reverts to normal after the exclusion of gluten from the diet [1].

Epidemiological studies have shown that CD is common (prevalence around 0.5 to 1%) in many developed and developing countries, but most cases remain unrecognized [2]. The high prevalence (>5%) of CD among the African Saharawi population, and the recent evidence of a prevalence of CD comparable to Western countries in the Middle East are especially interesting [3]. CD is more frequent in females (by about 2 to 1) with onset of symptoms occurring at all ages. The prevalence of CD is higher in patients with type 1 diabetes mellitus, thyroiditis, autoimmune liver disorders, infertility, some chromosomal disorders, and family members than in the general population [1,4].

Clinical Features

CD has protean manifestations of variable severity that are summarized according the "celiac iceberg" model as classical, atypical, silent, or latent [5]. Classical CD refers to those patients with the florid malabsorption syndrome (this group of patients are at the top of the iceberg). Atypical CD is characterized by significant but generally mono-symptomatic extraintestinal manifestations. Silent CD refers to the presence of disease-specific autoimmunity with villous atrophy in the absence of any symptoms or apparent consequences. Latent disease refers to geneti-

Table 36.1 Serologic tests and their diagnostic accuracy in celiac disease.

Test (all IgA isotype antibodies)	Sensitivity (%)	Specificity (%)
Antigliadin [7]	<70	~90
Deamidated gliadin [7]	74	95
Endomysial [8]	91–98	99–100
Tissue transglutaminase [8]	95–98	94–98

Sensitivity and specificity varies between studies and according to the antigenic substrate used.

cally susceptible persons, without symptoms or histological evidence of CD, who will ultimately go on to develop the disease. In the iceberg model some atypical cases, but most especially silent and latent CD, are below the waterline [5]. Currently, non-classical symptoms are the clinical presentation in more than 50% of American patients with CD [1].

Diagnosis
Serologic Tests
CD is characterized by the development of antibodies directed against the components of the environmental factor (gliadin) or connective tissue. The sensitivity and specificity may vary among the antibodies (Table 36.1). It is important that the patient not reduce or exclude gluten in the diet before testing as all tests may become negative. Because the inferior accuracy of the standard antigliadin assays, the use of this test no longer is recommended [6]. The use of deamidated gliadin may increase specificity of the antigliadin test for celiac disease [7].

Tissue Transglutaminase Antibodies (tTGA)
The tTGA test by enzyme-linked immunosorbent assay is the screening test of choice for CD due to its technical simplicity and accuracy. The diagnostic performance is slightly better using human or human recombinant substrate (new generation kits) than when guinea pig is used. Overall, the tTGA sensitivity is in the range of 95–98% and the specificity greater than 94% [8].

Endomysial Antibodies (EMA)
EMA can be measured using an immunofluorescence technique. The overall sensitivity and specificity using monkey esophagus as substrate is 97% and 99%, respectively. The tests using human umbilical cord as substrate

have a lower sensitivity (90%) [8]. While the very high specificity makes EMA a very powerful serologic test, there are some disadvantages: the test is time-consuming, semiquantitative, and operator dependent [9].

Genetic Testing
CD is strongly associated with two human leukocyte antigens (HLA) haplotypes: DQ2 (encoded by DQA1*05 and DQB1*02) and/or DQ8 (encoded by DQA1*03 and DQB1*03) [1]. Patients with CD carry at least one of those two gene pairs (90–95% have DQ2). Typing of DNA from patients with CD can be easily performed from whole blood using sequence-specific primers or allele-specific oligonucleotide probes. Although approximately 30–35% of the general Caucasian population carries either the HLA-DQ2 or HLA-DQ8 haplotypes, only a small subset of these subjects have CD [4]. Thus, HLA genotyping in a clinical setting is useful to practically exclude the diagnosis of CD (high negative predictive value) when the at-risk gene pairs are absent, especially when the diagnosis is uncertain [1,5]. HLA genotyping may beneficial in symptomatic patients already on gluten-free diet (GFD) who also have a history of tropical travel and perhaps did not have celiac serology before the diet. In this usually difficult clinical situation the authors recommend carrying out both celiac serology and HLA typing because: (i) if doubly negative, treatment for tropical sprue is indicated and a GFD is not necessary; and (ii) if celiac serology is negative but patients are DQ2 or DQ8 positive, CD is not concluded, but after treatment for tropical sprue a gluten challenge maybe necessary to clarify whether the patient will require a life-long GFD.

Histopathology
Small bowel biopsy is the confirmatory test for CD. Multiple biopsies (ideally four to six biopsy specimens) of the duodenum are recommended as lesions can be patchy [5]. Correct orientation of the biopsy specimen is essential for accurate histological evaluation. Histologic findings include the combination of the following: increased number of intraepithelial lymphocytes (>25 for 100 epithelial cells), villous atrophy, and crypt hyperplasia. Biopsies are classified according the modified Marsh scale that recognizes four interrelated intestinal lesions in response to gluten: preinfiltrative (stage 0), infiltrative (stage I), hyperplastic (stage II), and destructive (stage

III-a to III-c) [10]. The original Marsh classification recognized a severe end-stage hypoplastic lesion (Stage IV), which is very rare [10].

Gluten Challenge

It is no longer necessary to re-challenge most patients with a well-established diagnosis of CD [1,6]. However, gluten challenge may be useful in patients started on a GFD without confirmatory histology (if the biopsy was taken elsewhere and is available for review, the challenge is unnecessary) or those with an equivocal diagnosis. The standard challenge includes four slices (~20 g of gluten) of whole wheat bread a day with serial clinical and serologic follow-up starting 4 weeks after reintroduction of gluten [5].

Suggested Diagnostic Approach

Celiac disease is most often detected with serologic tests [6]. However, serology alone does not suffice for diagnosis. The presumptive diagnosis of CD is usually made on the basis of an abnormal duodenal biopsy. Definitive diagnosis of CD is established after demonstration of response to the GFD [5,6]. Response to gluten withdrawal does not indicate CD in the patient with self-diagnosis or poorly investigated gastrointestinal symptoms [5] (Figure 36.1).

Treatment

The management of CD is a life-long, medically-supervised diet that is devoid of gluten [1]. Wheat (*Triticum* spp.), barley (*Hordeum vulgare*) and rye (*Secale cereale*) in all their forms are toxic to celiac patients [11]. Voluntary or accidental ingestion of gluten may occur as a result of lack of readily available gluten-free foods, eating outside of the home, cross-contamination (trace amounts of gluten in other non-gluten containing foods), and hidden sources of gluten [11]. Some vitamins or prescription and over-the-counter medications may contain gluten as inactive ingredient (hidden sources of gluten). Other important components of the initial management include the aggressive correction of dehydration and nutritional deficiencies when necessary [6]. All patients require assessment of the potential metabolic osteopathy by densitometry. Temporarily restricting lactose during a period of weeks may be beneficial in some cases [1].

Tropical Sprue

Definition and Epidemiology

Tropical sprue is an acquired disease of unknown etiology that affects residents and/or visitors in certain tropical areas (a zone centered on the equator and limited in latitude by the Tropic of Cancer in the northern hemisphere, and the Tropic of Capricorn in the southern hemisphere). As infectious agents are the most frequent cause of chronic diarrhea in a tropical environment, the diagnosis of tropical sprue requires the exclusion of active infection, especially by protozoa [12,13]. The prevalence of tropical sprue is unknown and maybe different among specific locations in tropical areas (e.g., high prevalence in South India and Philippines and a very low incidence in Africa) [14]. The incidence of tropical sprue appears to have decreased during the past decade, possibly because the widespread empiric use of antibiotics for the treatment of chronic diarrhea [13,14].

Pathophysiology

The etiology of tropical sprue is not known [15]. The favored hypothesis is that tropical sprue is either initiated or sustained by the complex interactions among as yet unidentified infectious agents, the enterocyte, and the immune system of the host [14,15]. The host risk factors (e.g., immunologic status or genetics) remain obscure, as well as the specific environmental trigger. Bacterial overgrowth, disturbed motility, and mucosal injury contribute to the manifestation of tropical sprue in a susceptible host [15]. The epidemiology of tropical sprue suggests an infectious etiology but extensive investigations have not yet identified or isolated any consistent causal agent [12]. Tropical enteropathy is the term used to describe nonspecific changes in the intestine (usually mild inflammation and partial villous atrophy) of asymptomatic subjects residing in tropical areas and should not be confused with tropical sprue.

Clinical Features

The onset of tropical sprue is usually insidious and is characterized by diarrhea, steatorrhea, abdominal pain, weight loss, fatigue, glossitis, multiple nutritional deficiencies, and loss of appetite [15].

Diagnosis

Tropical sprue should be considered in the differential diagnosis of chronic diarrhea in patients with a recent

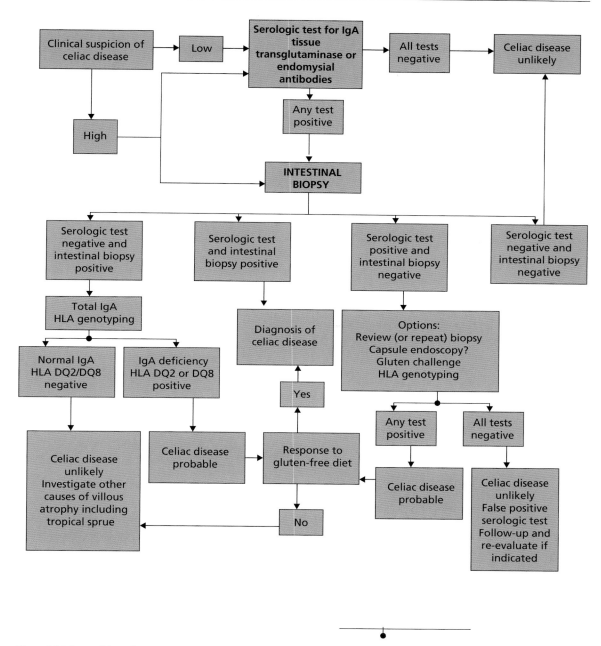

Figure 36.1 Proposal for a diagnostic algorithm for celiac disease.

Table 36.2 Diagnostic tests suggested for subjects with chronic diarrhea after a recent travel to tropical areas.

Test	Diagnosis suggested if test positive	Comment
Tissue transglutaminase antibody	Celiac disease	Requires intestinal biopsy as confirmatory test
Stool analysis for ova and trophozoites	Infectious diarrhea	Most common cause of persistent infectious diarrhea are protozoal infections
Giardia antigen in stool	Giardiasis	Stool analysis for cysts or trophozoites is not reliable
Endoscopy with intestinal biopsy and sampling of duodenal aspirate	Celiac disease Bacterial overgrowth Tropical sprue Giardiasis	Expensive and invasive test that requires case-by-case indication
Folic acid and β-carotene in serum –	Malabsorption syndrome All tests normal	Severe folic acid deficiency strongly suggests tropical sprue Normal tests suggest postinfective irritable bowel syndrome

Table 36.3 Differences between features of celiac disease and tropical sprue.

Feature	Celiac disease	Tropical sprue
Etiology	Immune-mediated disease	Unknown (possibly infectious)
Family history	Yes	No
Residence or travel to tropic areas	Not required	Yes
Gender difference	Yes (females)	No
Prevalence in the United States	1% of general population	Unknown
Endomysial or tissue transglutaminase antibodies	Yes	No
Iron-deficiency anemia	Common	Infrequent
Severe folic acid deficiency	Rare	Common
Intestinal involvement	Proximal	Proximal and distal
Treatment	Gluten-free diet	Oral tetracycline and folic acid

history of travel or residing in tropical areas [16] (Table 36.2). The histologic findings are non-specific and may be indistinguishable from that seen in celiac disease [1]. The D-xylose test and folic acid levels are usually abnormally low. Macrocytic anemia is a common finding [12]. Other indirect markers of malabsorption may be present, such as hypoalbuminemia, prolonged prothrombin time, and a low level of β-carotene. Indirect pancreatic test (e.g., pancreolauryl test) may be abnormal in as many as 64% of cases because of reversible exocrine pancreatic insufficiency related to a low pancreatic hormonal stimulation due to the loss of enterocytes [17]. While antigliadin antibodies could be positive (reflecting non-specific increased intestinal permeability), both tissue transglutaminase and endomysial antibodies are negative [5] (Table 36.3).

Treatment

Broad-spectrum antibiotics and folic acid are the treatment of choice [14]. The clinical response is usually rapid (within weeks) and complete. Recurrence is uncommon especially if the patient is not a resident or frequent traveler to tropical areas. Relapses are common in treated patients who return to, or remain in, tropical areas. Tetracycline is the antibiotic of choice and should be used for 3–6 months, usually in conjunction with folic acid [12,15]. Sulfonamide therapy may be an effective alternative in patients with allergy or other absolute contraindications for the use of tetracycline. Rifaximin, a non-absorbed antimicrobial drug with a broad spectrum of antimicrobial activity, which is effective for treatment of pathogen-negative traveler's diarrhea, is an attractive alternative therapy for tropical sprue but clinical trials are necessary to evaluate rifaximin safety and efficacy in tropical sprue. A gluten-free diet does not result in either clinical or histologic improvement in tropical sprue.

Take-home points

Diagnosis:
- The diagnosis of celiac disease is based on specific serology and an intestinal biopsy as a confirmatory test.
- History of either residing or recent travel to a tropical area may be a key to suspecting the diagnosis of tropical sprue.
- Marked folic acid deficiency is frequent in tropical sprue.
- Iron-deficiency anemia may be a the only sign or a clinical component of celiac disease.
- Clinical, serologic, and histologic response to a gluten free diet is characteristic of celiac disease.
- In those patients in whom tropical sprue is suspected and who lack specific serology for celiac disease, therapy for tropical sprue should be initiated.

Therapy:
- Correction of dehydration and nutritional deficiencies is an important part of the management of both celiac disease and tropical sprue.
- The gluten-free diet is the treatment of choice for celiac disease.
- Broad spectrum antibiotics and folic acid may result in a prompt clinical and histologic response in tropical sprue.

References

1 Green PH, Cellier C. Celiac disease. *N Engl J Med* 2007; **357**: 1731–43.

2 Fasano A, Berti I, Gerarduzzi T, *et al.* Prevalence of celiac disease in at-risk and not-at-risk groups in the United States: a large multicenter study. *Arch Intern Med* 2003; **163**: 286–92.

3 Catassi C. The world map of celiac disease. *Acta Gastroenterol Latinoam* 2005; **35**: 37–55.

4 Rubio-Tapia A, Van Dyke CT, Lahr BD, *et al.* Predictors of family risk for celiac disease: a population-based study. *Clin Gastroenterol Hepatol* 2008; **6**: 983–7.

5 Rostom A, Murray JA, Kagnoff MF. American Gastroenterological Association (AGA) Institute technical review on the diagnosis and management of celiac disease. *Gastroenterology* 2006; **131**: 1981–2002.

6 Schuppan D, Dennis MD, Kelly CP. Celiac disease: epidemiology, pathogenesis, diagnosis, and nutritional management. *Nutr Clin Care* 2005; **8**: 54–69.

7 Rashtak S, Ettore MW, Homburger HA, Murray JA. Comparative usefulness of deamidated gliadin antibodies in the diagnosis of celiac disease. *Clin Gastroenterol Hepatol* 2008; **6**: 426–32, quiz 370.

8 Lewis NR, Scott BB. Systematic review: the use of serology to exclude or diagnose coeliac disease (a comparison of the endomysial and tissue transglutaminase antibody tests). *Aliment Pharmacol Ther* 2006; **24**: 47–54.

9 Harewood GC, Murray JA. Diagnostic approach to a patient with suspected celiac disease: a cost analysis. *Dig Dis Sci* 2001; **46**: 2510–4.

10 Marsh MN. Gluten, major histocompatibility complex, and the small intestine. A molecular and immunobiologic approach to the spectrum of gluten sensitivity ("celiac sprue"). *Gastroenterology* 1992; **102**: 330–54.

11 See J, Murray JA. Gluten-free diet: the medical and nutrition management of celiac disease. *Nutr Clin Pract* 2006; **21**: 1–15.

12 Mathan VI. Diarrhoeal diseases. *Br Med Bull* 1998; **54**: 407–19.

13 Ramakrishna BS, Venkataraman S, Mukhopadhya A. Tropical malabsorption. *Postgrad Med J* 2006; **82**: 779–87.

14 Westergaard H. Tropical sprue. *Curr Treat Options Gastroenterol* 2004; **7**: 7–11.

15 Nath SK. Tropical sprue. *Curr Gastroenterol Rep* 2005; **7**: 343–9.

16 Farthing MJ. Tropical malabsorption. *Semin Gastrointest Dis* 2002; **13**: 221–31.

17 Morales M, Galvan E, Mery CM, *et al.* Exocrine pancreatic insufficiency in tropical sprue. *Digestion* 2001; **63**: 30–4.

CHAPTER 37
Whipple Disease

George T. Fantry

Division of Gastroenterology, University of Maryland School of Medicine, Baltimore, MD, USA

Summary

Whipple disease is a rare, chronic, systemic infection caused by *Tropheryma whipplei*. The symptoms and clinical findings are caused by chronic infection of the small intestine and other extraintestinal sites. Immune evasion and host interaction are important in the pathogenesis of infection. Clinical features include gastrointestinal and extraintestinal symptoms. Diarrhea is the most common presenting complaint. Arthritis is the most common extraintestinal symptom. Hyperpigmentation and peripheral lymphadenopathy are the most common physical findings. Small intestinal mucosal biopsy is the diagnostic test of choice. Infiltration of the lamina propria of the small intestine by large, foamy, PAS-positive macrophages containing Gram-positive, acid-fast-negative bacilli accompanied by lymphatic dilation is specific and diagnostic of Whipple disease. Antibiotic therapy usually results in dramatic improvement. The prognosis for patients with Whipple disease who receive effective antibiotic therapy is excellent.

Case

A 55-year-old Caucasian man presents with a longstanding history of seronegative arthritis, anemia, lethargy, weight loss, and recent intermittent fevers of uncertain etiology. He has visual disturbances and an unsteady gait. He has no gastrointestinal symptoms. Physical exam reveals severe cachexia, axillary adenopathy, and ataxia. Abdominal exam is benign. Laboratory evaluation reveals severe anemia, hypoalbuminemia, and an elevated erythrocyte sedimentation rate. Abdominal CT scan reveals thickening of jejunal folds and mesenteric adenopathy. Endoscopy reveals a normal duodenum. Duodenal biopsies reveal extensive infiltration of the lamina propria with PAS-positive, foamy macrophages. Electron microscopy reveals multiple bacilli with a characteristic cell wall and a pale central nucleoid. A diagnosis of Whipple disease is made. Treatment is instituted with parenteral penicillin G and streptomycin for 14 days followed by oral trimethoprim–sulfamethoxazole twice daily for 1 year. All symptoms rapidly improved over the course of a few weeks. Repeat endoscopy at 1 year revealed persistence of PAS-positive, foamy macrophages in the lamina propria; however, electron microscopy revealed no organisms consistent with treated Whipple disease.

Practical Gastroenterology and Hepatology: Small and Large Intestine and Pancreas, 1st edition. Edited by Nicholas J. Talley, Sunanda V. Kane and Michael B. Wallace. © 2010 Blackwell Publishing Ltd.

Definition and Epidemiology

Whipple disease [1,2] is a rare, chronic, systemic infection caused by *Tropheryma whipplei* [3–9]. The disease is most common between the fourth and sixth decades [10] with a male predominance. Whipple disease occurs predominantly in Caucasians and is more common in farmers and individuals involved in farm-related trades.

Pathophysiology

Immune Response

The symptoms and clinical findings in Whipple disease are caused by chronic infection of the small intestine and other extraintestinal sites with *T. whipplei*. Although *T. whipplei* may be a ubiquitous, commensal organism in the environment, its mode of transmission is uncertain. Immune evasion and host interaction are important in the pathogenesis of infection. There is evidence that abnormal host defense, specifically defects of monocyte/macrophage function, plays an important pathophysiologic role, leading to an inability of the host response to eliminate the bacteria.

Histopathology

The lamina propria of the small bowel mucosa is infiltrated by large, foamy macrophages distorting normal villous architecture, resulting in a blunted, club-like appearance. The cytoplasm of these macrophages is filled with large glycoprotein granules that stain with PAS. The lymphatic channels are dilated. Electron microscopy reveals rod-shaped bacillary bodies in the lamina propria. The bacilli have a characteristic cell wall and pale central nucleoid. The Whipple bacillus is acid-fast-negative. PAS-positive macrophages and the characteristic bacilli have been identified in many extraintestinal tissues, reflecting the systemic nature of the disease.

Clinical Features

Gastrointestinal Symptoms

Diarrhea or steatorrhea is the most common presenting complaint [10], however, it is not invariably present. Other intestinal symptoms include abdominal bloating, cramps, and anorexia. Weight loss is the second most common presenting complaint and is present before the initial evaluation in the majority of patients [10].

Extraintestinal Symptoms

Arthritis is the most common extraintestinal symptom and affects the majority of patients [10]. It often develops before the initial diagnosis of Whipple disease and is typically an intermittent, migratory arthritis of both the large and small joints. Fever, usually low grade and intermittent, is the second most common extraintestinal symptom [10]. Fatigue and generalized weakness are also common. Numerous other extraintestinal symptoms may develop, reflecting the systemic nature of the infection.

Neurological Symptoms

Central nervous system (CNS) involvement is common, however, symptoms related to CNS Whipple disease are present in a minority of patients. Neurological symptoms may occur with gastrointestinal symptoms or as isolated symptoms. The most common CNS symptoms are dementia, paralysis of gaze, and myoclonus.

Physical Findings

Hyperpigmentation and peripheral lymphadenopathy are the most common physical findings [10]. Emaciation, muscle wasting, peripheral edema, and peripheral neu-ropathy are often present. Abdominal findings may include mild distension, tenderness, or mass. Ascites, hepatomegaly, and splenomegaly are uncommon.

Additional physical findings may include fever, peripheral arthritis, heart murmurs, pleural or pericardial friction rubs, ocular abnormalities, and neurologic findings suggestive of CNS or cranial nerve involvement.

Radiologic and Endoscopic Findings

A small bowel series typically reveals marked thickening of the mucosal folds, most prominent in the proximal small bowel [10]. Abdominal computed tomography often reveals small bowel thickening, and massive para-aortic and retroperitoneal adenopathy [10]. On endoscopy, a characteristic finding of pale, shaggy, yellow mucosa in the postbulbar duodenum may be seen [11].

Laboratory Findings

Laboratory abnormalities, including low serum carotene levels, hypoalbuminemia, and electrolyte disturbances, are common [10]. Anemia is usually present secondary to chronic disease or iron deficiency [10]. The erythrocyte sedimentation rate is often elevated and the prothrombin time is frequently prolonged.

Diagnosis

Small intestinal mucosal biopsy is the diagnostic test of choice. Infiltration of the lamina propria of the small intestine by PAS-positive macrophages containing Gram-positive, acid-fast-negative bacilli accompanied by lymphatic dilation is specific and diagnostic of Whipple disease. Electron microscopy should be performed to verify the presence of the characteristic bacillus. Rarely, the diagnosis of Whipple disease is established in the absence of intestinal involvement by the identification of bacilli in involved tissues. Molecular diagnosis using PCR-based diagnostic tests may be useful in confirming the diagnosis of Whipple disease and in monitoring the response to antibiotic treatment [12–15].

Differential Diagnosis

Malabsorptive and Infiltrative Diseases of the Small Bowel

Other malabsorptive and infiltrative diseases of the small intestine, such as celiac disease and lymphoma, may present in a similar manner to Whipple disease. These diseases can be readily differentiated by small intestinal mucosal biopsy.

Small Bowel Infections

Mycobacterium avium complex (MAC) infection may mimic Whipple disease by causing infiltration of the lamina propria with PAS-positive macrophages [16], however, MAC bacilli are acid-fast. PAS-positive macrophages in the intestinal lamina propria can also be seen in systemic histoplasmosis, however, large, PAS-positive, rounded, encapsulated *Histoplasma* organisms are easily seen in macrophages.

Therapeutics

Antibiotic therapy usually results in dramatic improvement. Given concern for CNS involvement, treatment with an antibiotic that readily crosses the blood–brain barrier is appropriate [17,18]. One double-strength tablet of trimethoprim–sulfamethoxazole (TMP–SMX) given twice daily for 1 year is the best long-term option [10,17] (Table 37.1). Initial therapy with parenteral penicillin G and streptomycin for 10 to 14 days may be of additional benefit, resulting in a lower relapse rate [10,17]. In patients who are allergic to TMP–SMX, parenteral penicillin and streptomycin for 10 to 14 days followed by oral penicillin VK or ampicillin for 1 year is reasonable (Table 37.1).

Table 37.1 Treatment of Whipple disease.

Medication	Dose/frequency	Duration
Trimethoprim–sulfamethoxazole	160 mg/800 mg twice daily	1 year
	or	
Procaine penicillin G	1.2 million Units daily	2 weeks
+		
Streptomycin	1.0 g daily	2 weeks
+		
Trimethoprim–sulfamethoxazole	160 mg/800 mg twice daily	1 year

After 1 year of antibiotic therapy, a small intestinal mucosal biopsy should be repeated to document the absence of residual bacilli. Although PAS-positive macrophages may be present in the lamina propria for many years in patients treated for Whipple disease, the presence of bacilli on electron microscopy suggests inadequate treatment [19].

Prognosis

The prognosis for patients with Whipple disease who receive effective antibiotic therapy is excellent with rapid improvement in gastrointestinal and extraintestinal symptoms. Relapses are common [10,17]. Relapse of gastrointestinal symptoms and arthritis may occur early or late and respond favorably to further antibiotic treatment, whereas CNS relapses tend to occur late and respond poorly to additional antibiotic therapy. If relapse is suspected, small intestinal biopsy should be repeated to assess for the presence of free bacilli. The treatment of a relapse of Whipple disease is a repeat course of the initial antibiotic therapy.

Take-home points

Diagnosis:
- Consider Whipple disease in the setting of malabsorption, unexplained gastrointestinal symptoms, weight loss, seronegative arthritis, culture-negative endocarditis, and fever of unknown origin.
- Endoscopy with small bowel biopsy is indicated to diagnose Whipple disease.
- Characteristic, diagnostic, histopathologic, and electron microscopic features are present in the lamina propria of the duodenal mucosa.

Therapy:
- A 1-year course of antibiotics is highly effective in most patients.
- Relapse is common.

References

1 Whipple GH. A hitherto undescribed disease characterized anatomically by deposits of fat and fatty acids in the intestinal and mesenteric lymphatic tissues. *Bull Johns Hopkins Hosp* 1907; **18**: 382.

2 Dobbins WO III. Whipple's disease: a historical perspective. *QJM* 1985; **56**: 523–31.

3 Relman DA, Schmidt TM, MacDermott RP, Falkow S. Identification of the uncultured bacillus of Whipple's disease. *N Engl J Med* 1992; **327**: 293–301.

4 Wilson KH, Blitchington R, Frothingham R, Wilson JAP. Phylogeny of the Whipple's-disease-associated bacterium. *Lancet* 1991; **338**: 474–5.

5 Maiwald M, Ditton HJ, Von Herbay A, *et al*. Reassessment of the phylogenetic position of the bacterium associated with Whipple's disease and determination of the 16S-23S ribosomal intergenic spacer sequence. *Int J Syst Bacteriol* 1996; **46**: 1078–82.

6 Raoult D, Birg ML, La Scola B, *et al*. Cultivation of the bacillus of Whipple's disease. *N Engl J Med* 2000; **342**: 620–5.

7 Raoult D, La Scola B, Lecocq P, *et al*. Culture and immunological detection of Tropheryma whippelii from the duodenum of a patient with Whipple disease. *JAMA* 2001; **285**: 1039–43.

8 Fenollar F, Birg ML, Gauduchon V, Raoult D. Culture of *Tropheryma whipplei* from human samples: a 3-year experience (1999–2002). *J Clin Microbiol* 2003; **41**: 3816–22.

9 Bentley SD, Maiwald M, Murphy LD, *et al*. Sequencing and analysis of the genome of the Whipple's disease bacterium Tropheryma whipplei. *Lancet* 2003; **361**: 637–44.

10 Fleming JL, Wiesner RH, Shorter RG. Whipple's disease: clinical, biochemical, and histopathologic features and assessment of treatment in 29 patients. *Mayo Clin Proc* 1988; **63**: 539–51.

11 Geboes K, Ectors N, Heidbuchel H, *et al*. Whipple's disease. Endoscopic aspects before and after therapy. *Gastrointest Endosc* 1990; **36**: 247–52.

12 Von Herbay A, Ditton HJ, Maiwald M. Diagnostic application of a polymerase chain reaction assay for the Whipple's disease bacterium to intestinal biopsies. *Gastroenterology* 1996; **110**: 1735–43.

13 Ramzan NN, Loftus E, Burgart LJ. Diagnosis and monitoring of Whipple's disease by polymerase chain reaction. *Ann Intern Med* 1997; **126**: 520–7.

14 Muller C, Petermann D, Stain C, *et al*. Whipple's disease: comparison of histology with diagnosis based on polymerase chain reaction in four consecutive cases. *Gut* 1997; **40**: 425–7.

15 Pron B, Poyart C, Abachin C, *et al*. Diagnosis and follow-up of Whipple's disease by amplification of the 16S rRNA gene of *Tropheryma whippelii*. *World J Clin Microbiol Infect Dis* 1999; **18**: 62–5.

16 Gillin JS, Urmacher C, West R, Shike M. Disseminated *Mycobacterium avium-intracellulare* infection in acquired immunodeficiency syndrome mimicking Whipple's disease. *Gastroenterology* 1983; **85**: 1187–91.

17 Keinath RD, Merrell DE, Vlietstra R, Dobbins WO III. Antibiotic treatment and relapse in Whipple's disease. Long-term follow-up of 88 patients. *Gastroenterology* 1985; **88**: 1867–73.

18 Ryser RJ, Locksley RM, Eng SC, *et al*. Reversal of dementia associated with Whipple's disease by trimethoprim-sulfamethoxazole, drugs that penetrate the blood-brain barrier. *Gastroenterology* 1984; **86**: 745–52.

19 Von Herbay A, Maiwald M, Ditton HJ, Otto HF. Histology of intestinal Whipple's disease revisited. A study of 48 patients. *Virchows Arch* 1996; **429**: 335–43.

CHAPTER 38
Short Bowel Syndrome

David M. Shapiro and Alan L. Buchman

Division of Gastroenterology, Feinberg School of Medicine, Northwestern University, Chicago, IL, USA

Summary

Short bowel syndrome (SBS) is defined as malabsorption due to insufficient intestinal surface area, with an inability to sustain an adequate nutritional, electrolyte, or hydration status in the absence of specialized nutritional support. In adults, it is typically the consequence of extensive bowel resection, with loss of absorptive surface area. Over time, the intestine can adapt in order to ensure more efficient absorption. Overall, the most important aspects of the management of patients with SBS are to provide adequate nutrition, and to provide sufficient fluid and electrolytes to prevent dehydration. Anastomosis of the residual small bowel to the colon is the most important surgical procedure, enhancing the ability of the colon to become an energy-absorptive organ, and allowing for decreased dependence on total parenteral nutrition (TPN). The prognosis for patients with SBS depends on the patient's age, the type and extent of bowel resection, along with the underlying disease and health of residual intestine.

Case

A 57-year-old man with atrial fibrillation develops severe abdominal pain. He is diagnosed with an acute abdomen. He undergoes an emergent exploratory laparotomy, where an embolism is found in the superior mesenteric artery, and 200 cm of gangrenous small bowel is resected, and an ileostomy is created. Two days later, the patient undergoes a second-look surgery, and a jejunocolic anastomosis is created. TPN is initiated postoperatively, and, once bowel function returns, enteral nutrition is initiated with a goal of gradually decreasing the requirement for TPN.

Definition and Epidemiology

Intestinal failure is defined as an inability to sustain an adequate nutritional, electrolyte, or hydration status, in the absence of specialized nutritional support, and is often seen in patients with short bowel syndrome (SBS), which typically occurs in adults with less than 200 cm of functional intestine. However, the degree of intestinal

Practical Gastroenterology and Hepatology: Small and Large Intestine and Pancreas, 1st edition. Edited by Nicholas J. Talley, Sunanda V. Kane and Michael B. Wallace. © 2010 Blackwell Publishing Ltd.

function is better described in terms of energy absorption and loss, rather than the length of residual intestine, and some patients with SBS will not have sufficient loss of functional capacity so as to develop intestinal failure [1]. The patients at highest risk generally have a duodenostomy or a jejunoileal anastomosis with less than 35 cm of residual intestine, a jejunocolic or ileocolic anastomosis with less than 60 cm of residual intestine, or an end jejunostomy with less than 115 cm of residual intestine [2].

The incidence of SBS is difficult to assess given the lack of a national registry and prospective studies. However, based on multinational European data, the incidence and prevalence of severe SBS, necessitating long-term total parenteral nutrition (TPN), is estimated to be between 2 and 4 cases per 1 million persons per year [1]. These numbers, however, do not reflect patients who do not require TPN, and approximately 50–70% can successfully be weaned off TPN [3].

Pathophysiology

The major consequence of extensive bowel resection is loss of absorptive surface area, which results in malabsorption of nutrients, electrolytes, and water [4]. The degree of malabsorption is determined by the length and function of the remaining intestine, as well as the specific portions of small and large intestine resected, including whether the colon remains in continuity.

The length of the small intestine is estimated at 3 to 8 meters in the adult, and nutrient absorption is preserved until more than one half of the small intestine is removed [5]. Nutrient absorption may take place at any level of the small intestine; however, crypt morphology and microvillus enzyme and transporter activity predict a proximal to distal gradient in absorptive capacity and, as such, most macronutrients are absorbed in the proximal 100 cm of intestine [6,7].

Patients with a proximal jejunostomy have rapid gastric emptying of liquids, as well as rapid intestinal transit, both of which can severely limit nutrient digestive and absorptive processes. In addition, these patients are net secretors of salt and fluid, as jejunal fluid secretion is stimulated by oral intake and subsequent gastric emptying, so they excrete more fluid than they ingest. On unrestricted diets, these patients cannot absorb large volumes of water and electrolytes, and at least 100 cm of intact jejunum is required to maintain a positive water and electrolyte balance [8].

The intestine can adapt after bowel resection in order to ensure more efficient absorption. These changes are most pronounced in the ileum, which attains the morphologic characteristics of the jejunum, with increased villous density and height, as well as an increase in length. Conversely, the specialized cells of the terminal ileum, in which vitamin B_{12} and intrinsic factor receptors are located, and in which bile salts are absorbed, cannot be replaced by jejunal compensation. These adaptive changes may take up to 1 to 2 years to develop fully, and depend on the presence of food and biliary/pancreatic secretions. Because of this, patients with SBS are encouraged to start oral intake as soon as possible after surgery [9]. In addition, the colon becomes an important digestive organ in those with SBS. It has a large reserve absorptive capacity for sodium and water, and preservation of even part of the colon can significantly reduce fecal electrolyte and water losses [10].

Clinical Features

Ileal resection leads to interruption of the enterohepatic circulation of bile acids, resulting in decreased hepatic bile acid secretion and altered composition of bile. The bile becomes supersaturated with cholesterol, resulting in gall stone formation. Gall bladder hypomotility in the presence of TPN likely contributes to gall stone formation as well [10,11].

Fat malabsorption due to bile acid deficiency in patients with extensive ileal resection is associated with the development of oxalate kidney stones, as the unabsorbed long-chain fatty acids compete with oxalate for calcium, and a larger amount of free oxalate is lost to the colon, where it is absorbed and excreted by the kidney. Patients whose colon is in continuity generally should receive an oxalate-restricted diet [10].

Liver disease often develops in those requiring long-term TPN, with greater than 50% found to have severe liver disease after 5 years of TPN [12]. Liver failure will develop in approximately 15% of all TPN-dependent patients [13].

Other complications of SBS are catheter-related complications, including infection and occlusion, D-lactic acidosis, renal dysfunction, metabolic bone disease, memory deficits, and other neurologic abnormalities.

Differential Diagnosis

SBS may be a congenital or acquired condition. The causes of SBS in the pediatric population can be congenital or acquired, whereas in adults SBS typically results from surgical resection of bowel. In addition, functional SBS or intestinal failure may also occur in conditions of severe malabsorption, in which the bowel length is often intact (Table 38.1).

Therapeutics

Most available data on the treatment of SBS are based on retrospective analyses of case series, and are detailed below (Figure 38.1).

Medical Management

The most important aspects in the management of patients with SBS are to provide adequate nutrition, to provide sufficient fluid and electrolytes to prevent dehydration, and to correct and prevent acid–base disturbances. Furthermore, it is important to treat the

Table 38.1 Causes of short bowel syndrome and intestinal failure.

Adults

Catastrophic vascular accidents
    Superior mesenteric venous thrombosis
    Superior mesenteric arterial embolism
    Superior mesenteric arterial thrombosis
Chronic intestinal pseudo-obstruction*
Intestinal resection for tumor
Midgut volvulus
Multiple intestinal resections for Crohn disease
Radiation enteritis*
Refractory sprue*
Scleroderma and mixed connective tissue disease*
Trauma

Children

Congenital villous atrophy*
Extensive aganglionosis*
Gastroschisis
Jejunal or ileal atresia
Necrotizing enterocolitis
Microvillus inclusion disease*
Midgut volvulus

*Functional short bowel syndrome also may occur in conditions with severe malabsorption, in which bowel length remains intact.

Table 38.2 Therapeutic agents used to decrease intestinal transit and stool volume.

Agent	Dosage
Loperamide	4–6 mg four times daily
Diphenoxylate/atropine	2.5–5 mg four times daily
Codeine sulfate	15 mg two to four times daily
Ranitidine	300 mg twice daily
Omeprazole	40 mg twice daily
Octreotide	50–100 μg SC twice daily

underlying disorder, whenever possible, such as Crohn disease [5].

Medication absorption is often impaired in these patients, as absorption is a function of both intestinal surface area and contact time. The oral or enteral route for medications should be used whenever possible, in order to minimize TPN catheter manipulations. However, many medications are absorbed in the jejunum, and thus, in the absence of decreased intestinal transit time, absorption will be minimally impacted [5].

Massive enterectomy is associated with gastric hypersecretion for the initial 6 months [14,15], and these patients will benefit from acid reduction, which serves to reduce fluid losses [16–18]. High doses of oral H_2-receptor antagonists or proton pump inhibitors, or intravenous preparations, are typically necessary due to medication malabsorption.

In addition, excessive fluid losses typically require the use of antimotility agents, such as high doses of loperamide hydrochloride (4–16 mg/day) or diphenoxylate. If these agents are ineffective, codeine sulfate or tincture of opium are often necessary. Rarely, patients may require treatment with octreotide, which may be useful by

slowing intestinal transit and increasing water and sodium absorption [1] (Table 38.2).

Oral rehydration solutions (ORS) improve hydration and decrease TPN fluid requirements, especially in those patients with a proximal jejunostomy, or in those with less than 100 cm of jejunum remaining [17]. These solutions take advantage of the sodium–glucose cotransporter and the solvent drag that follows intracellular transport of sodium and water [19]. Optimal solutions have a sodium concentration of at least 90 mEq/L. The best and least expensive ORS is that recommended by the World Health Organization (WHO), with substantially more sodium than most commercially available solutions. Patients with SBS should be advised to avoid consumption of water and to drink ORS whenever thirsty [5].

Patients who have undergone massive enterectomy typically require TPN initially. Once the patient is hemodynamically stable, enteral nutrition should be started as soon as possible, and advanced gradually as tolerated. Once patients are able to eat, they should be encouraged to eat a regular diet, as modified below, and to eat substantially more than what was typical before the resection (hyperphagia), to compensate for the malabsorption. This may be accomplished by the use of multiple small meals, and is perhaps the single most important dietary intervention to reduce the need for TPN [5,20].

The absorption of nitrogenous macronutrients is least affected by the decreased intestinal absorptive surfaced area. It has been reasoned that if dietary protein were provided in a predigested form, it would be more readily absorbed. However, in seven patients with an end-jejunostomy, energy, carbohydrate, nitrogen, fat, electrolyte, fluid, and mineral absorption, as well as stool weight, were similar regardless of whether a peptide-based

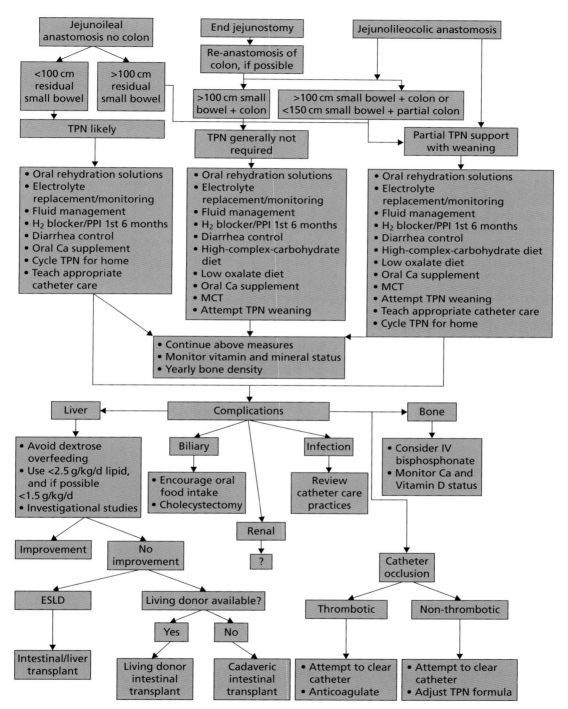

Figure 38.1 Management of short bowel syndrome. TPN, total parenteral nutrition; MCT, medium chain triglycerides; PPI, proton pump inhibitor, ESLD, end-stage liver disease. (Reprinted from Buchman AL, *et al.* [1], © 2003, with permission from Elsevier.)

enteral formula was provided. Based on this experience, the utility of peptide-based diets is largely without merit [21,22].

Most intestinal dissacharidases are present in highest concentration in the proximal small intestine, which often remains intact in patients who undergo massive enterectomy. In the absence of significant jejunal resection or documented lactase deficiency, lactose-containing foods should not be limited, as they are an important source of dietary calcium [23,24].

Patients with SBS whose colon is in continuity should consume a high-complex-carbohydrate diet, as starches, non-starch polysaccharides, and soluble fiber pass undigested into the colon, where bacteria ferment them into short-chain fatty acids (SCFAs), including butyrate, proprionate, and acetate. SCFAs provide fuel for the colonocyte and significantly reduce fecal energy losses. As such, the colon becomes an important digestive organ in patients with SBS [25,26]. Furthermore, sodium and water absorption are stimulated by SCFAs, although decreased fecal losses have not been documented clinically [27].

Lipid digestion may be impaired, as micelle formation is limited due to ileal bile salt malabsorption. Treatment with bile salt replacement, such as ox bile or the conjugated bile acid chylosarcosine, has been reported in a few patients, decreasing fecal fat in most, but leaving fecal volume unchanged or increased [28–32]. Cholestyramine may be useful in decreasing bile-salt-induced diarrhea in those with less than 100 cm of terminal ileum resected, but should not be used in patients with more than 100 cm of ileal resection, because it can worsen steatorrhea by binding dietary lipid [33].

In those patients with their colon in continuity, a high-fat diet can lead to more diarrhea. However, this must be balanced against the fact that fat is an important energy source, given its increased energy density when compared to carbohydrates. Overall, limited data are available to support the use of low-fat diets [34].

It is important to assess the vitamin and mineral status of these patients at regular intervals. It is unusual to develop water-soluble vitamin deficiencies, except in those with duodenostomies or proximal jejunostomies, because they are absorbed in the proximal jejunum. However, folate deficiency may develop in patients with proximal jejunal resection, and these patients should receive daily folate. In addition, vitamin B_{12} deficiency is

seen in patients who have greater than 60 cm of terminal ileum resected, and supplementation is necessary [5].

Fat soluble vitamin deficiencies are more common, and develop because of decreased bile salt reabsorption and associated fat maldigestion. Cholestyramine can cause fat-soluble vitamin deficiency as well, due to its effects of binding to bile salts, and should not be used if more than 100 cm of terminal ileum has been resected, as it will lead to enhanced malabsorption [33]. Vitamin A deficiency is characterized by night blindness and xerophthalmia. Vitamin D deficiency manifests as osteomalacia. Vitamin E deficiency manifests as hemolysis and various neurologic deficits. Vitamin K deficiency is uncommon in those patients with an intact colon, as 60% of vitamin K is synthesized by colonic bacteria; however, vitamin K deficiency can be seen in those without a residual colon or in those who have taken antibiotics [5].

Fecal losses of zinc and selenium can be significant, and deficiencies will develop. Zinc deficiency has been associated with growth abnormalities, delayed wound healing, and immune dysfunction. Selenium deficiency has been associated with various abnormalities, including cardiomyopathy, peripheral neuropathy, and proximal muscle weakness and pain [5].

The length of remaining bowel necessary to prevent dependence on TPN is approximately 100 cm in the absence of an intact colon, or 60 cm in the presence of a colon [2,6,35]. For those who require long-term TPN, gradual attempts should be made to wean the patients from parenteral nutrition, and approximately 50% can discontinue TPN and resume oral intake after 1–2 years [3]. Because TPN solutions are hypertonic, they are infused into a central vein. TPN is typically given in a continuous fashion in the initial postoperative phase, but over time the infusions are gradually compressed into to a cycled regimen (with adjustments to volume and nutritional support).

Growth factors have been studied in patients with SBS. A double-blinded, randomized, placebo controlled trial of growth hormone in 41 TPN-dependent patients, showed that TPN requirements in treated patients could be reduced by an additional 2 L/week over the reduction with standard therapies [36]. In addition, treatment with a synthetic analogue of glucagon-like peptide 2 (GLP 2), an intestinotrophic agent, has been shown to increase villous height, with increased fluid absorption, as well as modest improvements in energy absorption. However, these effects regressed once the medication was discontinued [37].

Surgical Management

Anastamosis of the small bowel to the colon is the most important surgical procedure, enhancing the ability of the colon to become an energy-absorptive organ, and allowing for decreased dependence on TPN. Other surgical procedures to taper dilated, non-functional intestine are available, but should be reserved for highly selected individuals with dilated, non-functional segments of intestine [1]. In the Bianchi procedure, the surgeon divides the dilated bowel and performs an end-to-end anastamosis, thereby doubling the bowel length [38]. In the serial transverse enteroplasty procedure (STEP), a linear staple is applied from alternating and opposite directions along the mesenteric border to incompletely divide the dilated intestine, which leads to tapering of the dilated intestine [39].

The main indication for intestinal transplantation is TPN-dependent SBS complicated by progressive liver disease, and as such, intestinal transplantation is often combined with liver transplantation. If patients are referred for evaluation for transplantation prior to the development of advanced fibrosis, isolated intestinal transplantation can be done. These patients have a better prognosis than those requiring a combined transplant. In addition, patients with significant fluid losses and refractory dehydration, despite appropriate medical management, are candidates for intestinal transplantation. Survival has improved considerably since intestinal transplantation was introduced, and patients who have undergone transplantation more recently have better survival, largely due to improved surgical techniques and improved immunosuppressive regimens [40,41]. And while the short-term survival in those receiving intestinal transplantation approaches 90%, the 5-year survival is closer to 50%, which is far worse than those requiring long-term home TPN. As such, intestinal transplantation is not a replacement for TPN. Along those lines, both premature intestinal transplantation, and late referral for transplantation, which often requires the addition of a liver graft, must be avoided. High-risk patients should be identified early and referred to a center where intestinal rehabilitation and transplantation are both practiced [42].

Prognosis

The prognosis for patients with SBS depends on the type and extent of bowel resection, along with the underlying disease and health of residual intestine. Patients with limited resections have an excellent prognosis, assuming careful management of their malabsorptive issues. As would be expected, patients with small bowel length less than 50 cm, including those with high jejunostomies and severe malabsorption, have a worse prognosis. In addition, mesenteric infarction as a cause for the bowel resection has a worse prognosis, as does radiation enteritis, when it leads to SBS. However, the overall prognosis, including survival and quality of life, are improving, largely because of increasing experience with long-term TPN and means of assessing nutritional needs [3].

Take-home points

- SBS is characterized by malabsorption due to insufficient intestinal surface area.
- SBS is usually the consequence of extensive bowel resection.
- Over time, the intestine can adapt to ensure more efficient absorption.
- Acid suppression and antimotility agents serve to decrease fluid losses.
- ORS improve dehydration and decrease TPN fluid requirements.
- Patients should generally be encouraged to eat a regular diet, and to eat substantially more than what was typical prior to the resection (hyperphagia).
- Approximately 50% of patients can discontinue TPN after 2 years.
- Anastamosis of the small bowel to the colon is the most important surgical procedure, allowing the colon to become an energy-absorptive organ.
- Prognosis depends on the type and extent of bowel resection, along with the underlying disease.

References

1 Buchman AL, Scolapio J, Fryer J. AGA technical review on short bowel syndrome and intestinal transplantation. *Gastroenterology* 2003; **124**: 1111–34.

2 Carbonnel F, Cosnes J, Chevret S, *et al*. The role of anatomic factors in nutritional autonomy after extensive small bowel resection. *J Parenter Enteral Nutr* 1996; **20**: 275–80.

3 Messing B, Crenn P, Beau P, *et al.* Long-term survival and parenteral nutrition dependence in adult patients with the short bowel syndrome. *Gastroenterology* 1999; **117**: 1043–50.

4 Andersson H, Bosaeus I, Brummer RJ, *et al.* Nutritional and metabolic consequences of extensive bowel resection. *Dig Dis* 1986; **4**: 193–202.

5 Buchman AL. Etiology and initial management of short bowel syndrome. *Gastroenterology* 2006; **130** (2 Suppl. 1): S5–S15.

6 Borgstrom B, Dahlqvist A, Lundh G, *et al.* Studies of intestinal digestion and absorption in the human. *J Clin Invest* 1957; **36**: 1521–36.

7 Clarke RM. Mucosal architecture and epithelial cell production rate in the small intestine of the albino rat. *J Anat* 1970; **107**: 519–29.

8 Nightingale JM, Lennard-Jones JE, Walker ER, *et al.* Jejunal efflux in short bowel syndrome. *Lancet* 1990; **336**: 765–8.

9 Cisler JJ, Buchman AL. Intestinal adaptation in short bowel syndrome. *J Invest Med* 2005; **53**: 402–13.

10 Nightingale JM, Lennard-Jones JE, Gertner, DJ, *et al.* Colonic preservation reduces need for parenteral therapy, increases incidence of renal stones, but does not change high prevalence of gall stones in patients with a short bowel. *Gut* 1992; **33**: 1493–7.

11 Roslyn JJ, Pitt HA, Mann LL, *et al.* Gallbladder disease in patients on long-term parenteral nutrition. *Gastroenterology* 1983; **84**: 148–54.

12 Cavicchi M, Beau P, Crenn P, *et al.* Prevalence of liver disease and contributing factors in patients receiving home parenteral nutrition for permanent intestinal failure. *Ann Intern Med* 2000; **132**: 525–32.

13 Chan S, McCowen KC, Bistrian BR, *et al.* Incidence, prognosis, and etiology of end-stage liver disease in patients receiving home total parenteral nutrition. *Surgery* 1999; **126**: 28–34.

14 Windsor CW, Fejfar J, Woodward DA. Gastric secretion after massive small bowel resection. *Gut* 1969; **10**: 779–86.

15 Williams NS, Evans P, King RF. Gastric acid secretion and gastrin production in the short bowel syndrome. *Gut* 1985; **26**: 914–9.

16 Jeppesen PB, Staun M, Tjellesen, L, *et al.* Effect of intravenous ranitidine and omeprazole on intestinal absorption of water, sodium, and macronutrients in patients with intestinal resection. *Gut* 1998; **43**: 763–9.

17 Jacobsen O, Ladefoged K, Stage JG, *et al.* Effects of cimetidine on jejunostomy effluents in patients with severe short-bowel syndrome. *Scand J Gastroenterol* 1986; **21**: 824–8.

18 Nightingale JM, Walker ER, Farthing MJ, *et al.* Effect of omeprazole on intestinal output in the short bowel syndrome. *Aliment Pharmacol Ther* 1991; **5**: 405–12.

19 Fordtran JS. Stimulation of active and passive sodium absorption by sugars in the human jejunum. *J Clin Invest* 1975; **55**: 728–37.

20 Cosnes J, Gendre JP, Evard D, *et al.* Compensatory enteral hyperalimentation for management of patients with severe short bowel syndrome. *Am J Clin Nutr* 1985; **41**: 1002–9.

21 McIntyre PB, Fitchew M, Lennard-Jones JE. Patients with a high jejunostomy do not need a special diet. *Gastroenterology* 1986; **91**: 25–33.

22 Levy E, Frileux P, Sandrucci, S, *et al.* Continuous enteral nutrition during the early adaptive stage of the short bowel syndrome. *Br J Surg* 1988; **75**: 549–53.

23 Marteau P, Messing B, Arrigoni E, *et al.* Do patients with short-bowel syndrome need a lactose-free diet? *Nutrition* 1997; **13**: 13–6.

24 Arrigoni E, Marteau P, Briet F, *et al.* Tolerance and absorption of lactose from milk and yogurt during short-bowel syndrome in humans. *Am J Clin Nutr* 1994; **60**: 926–9.

25 Bond JH, Currier BE, Buchwald H, *et al.* Colonic conservation of malabsorbed carbohydrate. *Gastroenterology* 1980; **78**: 444–7.

26 Cummings JH, Gibson GR, Macfarlane GT. Quantitative estimates of fermentation in the hind gut of man. *Acta Vet Scand* 1989; **86** (Suppl.): 76–82.

27 Nordgaard I, Hansen BS, Mortensen PB. Colon as a digestive organ in patients with short bowel. *Lancet* 1994; **343**: 373–6.

28 Little KH, Schiller LR, Bilhartz LE, *et al.* Treatment of severe steatorrhea with ox bile in an ileectomy patient with residual colon. *Dig Dis Sci* 1992; **37**: 929–33.

29 Fordtran JS, Bunch F, Davis GR. Ox bile treatment of severe steatorrhea in an ileectomy-ileostomy patient. *Gastroenterology* 1982; **82**: 564–8.

30 Djurdjevic D, Popvic O, Necic D, *et al.* Ox bile treatment of severe steatorrhea in a colectomy and ileectomy patient. *Gastroenterology* 1988; **95**: 1160.

31 Heydorn S, Jeppesen PB, Mortensen PB. Bile acid replacement therapy with cholylsarcosine for short-bowel syndrome. *Scand J Gastroenterol* 1999; **34**: 818–23.

32 Kapral C, Wewalka F, Praxmarer V, *et al.* Conjugated bile acid replacement therapy in short bowel syndrome patients with a residual colon. *Z Gastroenterol* 2004; **42**: 583–9.

33 Hofmann AF, Poley JR. Role of bile acid malabsorption in pathogenesis of diarrhea and steatorrhea in patients with ileal resection. I. Response to cholestyramine or replacement of dietary long chain triglyceride by medium chain triglyceride. *Gastroenterology* 1972; **62**: 918–34.

34 Woolf GM, Miller C, Kurian R, *et al.* Diet for patients with a short bowel: high fat or high carbohydrate? *Gastroenterology* 1983; **84**: 823–8.

35 Jeppesen PB, Mortensen PB. Intestinal failure defined by measurements of intestinal energy and wet weight absorption. *Gut* 2000; **46**: 701–6.

36 Byrne TA, Wilmore DW, Iyer K, *et al.* Growth hormone, glutamine, and an optimal diet reduces parenteral nutrition in patients with short bowel syndrome: a prospective, randomized, placebo-controlled, double-blind clinical trial. *Ann Surg* 2005; **242**: 655–61.

37 Palle B, Jeppesen PB, Consuelo M, *et al.* Treatment of short bowel patients with a glucagon-like peptide (GLP-2) analog, improves intestinal function in SBS patients. *Gastroenterology* 2002; **122**: A191.

38 Bianchi A. Intestinal loop lengthening—a technique for increasing small intestinal length. *J Pediatr Surg* 1980; **15**: 145–51.

39 Kim HB, Lee PW, Garza JW, *et al.* Serial transverse enteroplasty (STEP): a novel bowel lengthening procedure. *J Pediatr Surg* 2003; **38**: 425–9.

40 Fishbein TM, Kaufman SS, Florman SS, *et al.* Isolated intestinal transplantation: proof of clinical efficacy. *Transplantation* 2003; **76**: 636–40.

41 Lacaille F, Vass N, Sauvat, *et al.* Long-term outcome, growth and digestive function in children 2 to 18 years after intestinal transplantation. *Gut* 2008; **57**: 455–61.

42 Fryer JP. Intestinal transplantation: current status. *Gastroenterol Clin North Am* 2007; **36**: 145–59, vii.

CHAPTER 39
Protein-losing Gastroenteropathy

Lauren K. Schwartz[1] and Carol E. Semrad[2]

[1] Division of Gastroenterology, Mount Sinai Hospital, New York, NY, USA
[2] Gastroenterology Section, The University of Chicago, Chicago, IL, USA

Summary

Protein-losing gastroenteropathy (PLGE) is a condition characterized by excessive loss of serum proteins into the gastrointestinal tract that results in symptomatic hypoproteinemia. It can be due to a variety of diseases, intestinal or extraintestinal. Clinically, patients present with edema, ascites, and pericardial or pleural effusions. To make the diagnosis, excess fecal protein loss must be documented by measuring α-1-antitrypsin clearance or using nuclear scintigraphy. Further evaluation is then directed at establishing the underlying cause. Treatment goals include aggressive protein supplementation to improve nutritional status and stopping protein loss by treating the underlying disease when possible.

Case

A 72-year-old man is referred for chronic diarrhea, weight loss, and edema. He has a past history of diabetes and hypertension. Four years ago he began passing six to seven loose stools daily with associated gas/bloating and abdominal pain. He lost 36 kg (80 pounds) of weight. Four months ago he developed lower extremity edema. On physical examination he was well developed, heart and lungs were normal, and extremities with 4+ pitting edema. Outside evaluation showed low total protein and albumin levels, normal urinalysis, and negative stool studies. Esophagogastroduodenoscopy (EGD) and lower endoscopy with biopsies were unrevealing. Further evaluation shows increased fecal fat (70 g fat diet) of 15 g/day (normal <7 g/dL), increased α-1-antitrypsin level in the stool, and low vitamin B_{12} and zinc levels. Mesenteric Doppler study showed increased velocities of his celiac and superior mesenteric arteries. Video capsule endoscopy showed denuded areas predominantly in the jejunum (Figure 39.1). Upper double balloon enteroscopy confirmed denuded mucosa in the jejunum. Biopsies revealed active jejunitis with morphology typical of ischemia (Figure 39.2). Mesenteric angiography showed no vascular lesion amendable to by pass. The impression was chronic ischemic enteritis due to small

vessel disease causing malabsorption and protein-losing enteropathy. He was treated with prednisone with improvement in his diarrhea, serum protein levels, and edema.

Definition

The term protein-losing gastroenteropathy (PLGE) refers to the excessive loss of serum proteins into the gastrointestinal tract resulting in symptomatic hypoproteinemia. It is not a single condition but rather a manifestation of various disease states that compromise the gastrointestinal mucosal barrier and/or lymphatic flow.

Pathophysiology

Normally, a small amount of plasma proteins leak into the intestinal lumen where they are digested and reabsorbed for use in protein synthesis. In PLGE, up to 60% of plasma proteins are exuded into the intestinal lumen every day, overwhelming digestive and absorptive capacities and resulting in high fecal protein loss. Hypoproteinemia develops when the rate of protein loss exceeds the body's rate of protein synthesis [1,2]. Because the liver

Practical Gastroenterology and Hepatology: Small and Large Intestine and Pancreas, 1st edition. Edited by Nicholas J. Talley, Sunanda V. Kane and Michael B. Wallace. © 2010 Blackwell Publishing Ltd.

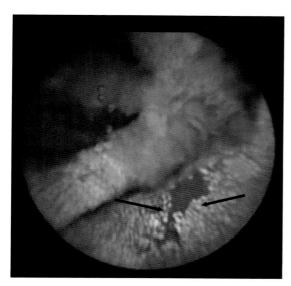

Figure 39.1 Denuded jejunal mucosa in protein-losing gastroenteropathy due to chronic intestinal ischemia.

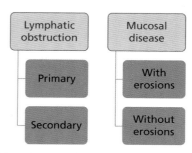

Figure 39.3 Mechanisms of protein-losing gastroenteropathy.

can only increase albumin synthesis by 25%, hypoalbuminemia quickly develops [3]. Reductions in other proteins with slow rates of synthesis (e.g., gamma globulins) are also common.

The two major mechanisms of PLGE are intestinal lymphatic obstruction and mucosal disease (Figure 39.3, Table 39.1). Lymphatic obstruction or impaired flow results in increased lymphatic pressure, rupture of lacteals, and protein leakage across the intestinal epithelium. Mucosal disease causes protein leakage due to an ulcerated epithelial barrier or increased permeability. The molecular basis of intestinal protein leakage due to the latter is unknown. Loss of heparin sulfate and syndecan-1 proteins on intestinal epithelial cells may be responsible [4].

Etiologies

• **Primary intestinal lymphangiectasia** is a rare disorder characterized by dilated intestinal lacteals that leak chylous fluid into the intestinal lumen. It classically presents in childhood or young adulthood with bilateral lower extremity edema. Most cases are sporadic although some occur as part of a syndrome (von Recklinghausen, Turner, Noonan, Klippel–Trenauny, Hennekam, yellow-nail syndromes) [5].

• **Secondary intestinal lymphangiectasia** refers to dilated intestinal lymphatics due to secondary causes of impaired lymphatic flow. These causes include cardiac conditions, lymphoma, tuberculosis, hepatic venous outflow obstruction, and chemotherapy. Cardiac and hepatic causes are believed to obstruct lymphatic flow due to venous congestion. The Fontan procedure, an operation for patients with a single ventricle, is also

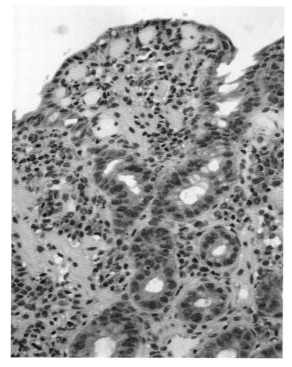

Figure 39.2 Jejunal biopsy with surface atrophy and regenerating crypts characteristic of ischemia. (Courtesy of Dr Jerrold Turner.)

Table 39.1 Causes of protein-losing gastroenteropathy.

Lymphatic obstruction		Mucosal disease	
Primary	**Secondary**	**Erosive**	**Non-erosive**
Intestinal lymphangiectasia Idiopathic Syndrome-associated	**Cardiac** Constrictive pericarditis Congestive heart failure Tricuspid regurgitation Congenital heart disease Fontan procedure	**Inflammatory** Crohn disease Ulcerative colitis Behçet disease Graft-versus-host disease	**Inflammatory** Celiac disease Allergic gastroenteropathy Eosinophilic gastroenteritis Collagenous colitis
Other congenital malformations Intestinal lymphatic hypoplasia Lymphangiomatosis	**Hepatobiliary** Hepatic vein outflow obstruction Portal hypertensive gastroenteropathy	**Esophageal and gastric** Erosive esophagitis and gastritis Esophageal and gastric ulcers	**Gastric** Ménétrier disease Lymphocytic gastritis Secretory hypertrophic gastropathy H. pylori infection
	Infectious Mesenteric tuberculosis Whipple disease	**Infectious** Clostridium difficile Invasive infectious enteritis	**Infectious** Bacterial overgrowth Tropical sprue Viral infection Parasitic infection Whipple disease
	Neoplastic Intestinal lymphoma Kaposi sarcoma	**Neoplastic** Lymphoma Gastric cancer Kaposi sarcoma Waldenstrom macroglobulinemia	**Collagen vascular** Systemic lupus erythematosus Sjögren disease Mixed connective tissue disease
	Toxic Chemotherapy Arsenic	**Toxic** NSAIDs Chemotherapy Radiation therapy	
	Other Mesenteric sarcoidosis Retroperitoneal fibrosis Mesenteric venous thrombosis	**Other** Intestina l ischemia Amyloidosis	

linked to venous congestion, but the underlying pathophysiology of protein loss appears more complex [6].

• **Mucosal disorders with erosions, ulcers, or denuded areas** have a clear breach in the epithelial barrier with concurrent inflammation which promotes protein loss. Examples include inflammatory bowel disease, intestinal ischemia (Figure 39.1), erosive gastritis, and non-steroidal anti-inflammatory drug (NSAID) enteropathy.

• **Mucosal disorders without erosions** are characterized by increased epithelial permeability in the absence of macroscopic injury. Classic examples include Ménétrier disease, celiac disease, eosinophilic gastroenteritis, and systemic lupus erythematosus.

Clinical Features

The most common presentation of PLGE is edema due to hypoproteinemia. Ascites and pleural and pericardial effusions may also occur. Low serum albumin levels are primarily responsible for loss of oncotic pressure and third-spacing of fluid. Decreased serum gamma globulin (IgM, IgA, IgG) levels are common, but generally do not lead to infectious complications. Other proteins with slow turn-over rates that are often reduced include transferrin, fibrinogen, α-1-antitrypsin, and ceruloplasmin.

In those with lymphatic obstruction, chylous fluid leaks across the intestinal epithelium into the lumen resulting in the loss of fat, fat-soluble vitamins (A, D, E, K), and lymphocytes as well as protein. Lymphopenia can result in impaired cellular immunity. Chylous effusions can also occur [5].

In patients with primary intestinal mucosal disease, abdominal bloating, diarrhea, malabsorption (fat and carbohydrate), and weight loss predominate and decreased protein absorption may contribute to low protein levels.

Diagnosis

The diagnosis of PLGE should be suspected when a patient presents with hypoproteinemia that is not explained by decreased protein intake or absorption. The first step to making a diagnosis is a history focused on diet intake and gastrointestinal symptoms. Hypoalbuminemia with a normal serum total protein level suggests impaired hepatic synthesis or renal losses (nephrotic syndrome), whereas hypoalbuminema with a low total protein suggests fecal loss (PLGE) or malnutrition.

Tests for Intestinal Protein Loss

The most sensitive test for fecal protein loss is α-1-antitrypsin clearance. α-1-antitrypsin is a glycoprotein that functions as a protease inhibitor. It is resistant to intestinal degradation and is excreted intact in the stool, making it an ideal endogenous marker of intestinal protein loss [7,8]. Plasma and stool concentrations of α-1-antitrypsin as well as stool volume must be measured. Stool is collected over 1–3 days as spot samples are unreliable. α-1-antitrypsin loss (mL/day) can be derived as follows:

$$\text{Clearance} = \frac{(\text{stool A1−AT concentration}) \times \left(\text{stool volume} \right)}{(\text{plasma A1−AT concentration})}$$

A1−AT = α-1-antitrypsin

concentration in mg/100 g dry stool weight

Normally, α-1-antitrypsin clearance is less than 13 mL/day. In patients with PLGE, clearance is greater than 24 mL/day and greater than 56 mL/day with diarrhea [9]. Diarrhea increases protein loss perhaps due to rapid transit or increased protein leakage. Gastrointestinal bleeding also elevates stool protein levels. In individuals with suspected esophageal or gastric protein loss (e.g., Ménétrier disease) the test may not be reliable because α-1-antitrypsin is degraded at a gastric pH less than 3. Acid suppressive therapy should be administered at the time of study to overcome this limitation [10,11].

Other methods to detect protein loss from the gastrointestinal tract involve:

1 Infusing radiolabeled macromolecules (e.g., chromium-51-albumin) into the blood stream and measuring fecal radioactivity to estimate clearance [12].

2 Nuclear scintigraphy to detect extravasation of tagged molecules (e.g., technetium-99 albumin) into the intestine [13].

The former technique is rarely used because it is costly and labor intensive. Nuclear scintigraphy is useful to both detect and localize the site of protein loss. It also allows documentation of response to therapy [14].

Tests to Determine Underlying Etiology

Once PLGE is established, efforts are directed to identify the underlying cause. Patient history is most valuable to guide tests. EGD, push enteroscopy, or colonoscopy with biopsies is indicated in those with suspected primary gastrointestinal disease. Video capsule endoscopy, computed tomography (CT) enterography, and small bowel series may be helpful in those with a patchy distribution of intestinal disease. In women with unexplained edema and PLGE, testing for systemic lupus erythematosus is warranted. In those with suspected cardiac disease, cardiac evaluation is indicated.

Therapy

The goals of therapy for a PLGE are twofold:
1 Reverse protein loss by treating the underlying disease
2 Dietary protein supplementation to improve nutritional status.

Treatment to reverse protein loss varies by disease and includes both medical and surgical therapies.

Medical Therapies

• **Corticosteroids** have been effective in collagen vascular diseases, inflammatory bowel disease, collagenous colitis, allergic eosinophilic gastroenteritis, amyloidosis, and after the Fontan operation. Use of other immunomodulators such as cyclosporine has also been reported [15].
• **Octreotide** has been effective in Ménétrier disease [16,17], amyloidosis [18], and intestinal lymphangiectasia [19].
• **Heparin** injections have been somewhat successful in post-Fontan PLGE [6]. Success in therapy may be related to an underlying loss of heparin sulfate on intestinal epithelial cells.
• **Antibiotics** are indicated for infectious causes of PLGE such as *Clostridium difficile*, tuberculosis, Whipple disease and *Helicobacter pylori*.
• **Chemotherapy** should be directed at underlying malignancies.
• **Biologics** such as antibodies to epidermal growth factor and TNF-α have been used for Ménétrier disease and inflammatory bowel disease, respectively.

Surgical Therapies

• **Cardiac surgery**: Definitive treatment of constrictive pericarditis entails removal of the pericardium. In post-Fontan patients, fenestration of the systemic venous pathway has been shown to reverse protein loss. Cardiac transplantation may be required for refractory PLGE in these patients.
• **Segmental intestinal resection**: Resection of diseased bowel segments reverses protein loss in Crohn disease [20] and localized intestinal lymphangiectasia [21].
• **Gastrectomy**: Subtotal or total gastrectomy is the definitive treatment for Ménétrier disease refractory to medical therapy.

Nutrition Support

Individuals with PLGE need to eat a high protein diet. They may require 2–3 g/kg dry weight of protein per day (an average adult requires 0.8–1.2 g/kg of protein per day). To estimate protein needs, fecal losses derived from α-1-antitrypsin clearance can be added to baseline daily requirements. Urine urea nitrogen balance can also be measured to ensure adequate protein intake. Dietary counseling by a registered dietician is recommended. High protein foods include meat, milk, cheese, and eggs. Modular protein concentrates and oral supplements can be used to increase protein intake. In patients who require tube feeding, high protein enteral feeds are available. Parenteral supplementation may be necessary if enteral intake fails.

In children with primary intestinal lymphangiectasia, a low-fat diet can reduce gastrointestinal symptoms, promote growth, and may improve hypoalbuminemia [22,23]. The efficacy of this approach is less well established in secondary lymphangiectasia. The dietary regimen restricts long chain triglycerides (LCT) which are absorbed into the lymphatic circulation and may increase lymphatic pressure and promote protein loss. In contrast, medium chain triglycerides (MCT) are absorbed into the portal system and do not aggravate lymphatic hypertension. Effective regimens limit LCT intake to 5–10 g/day (enough to meet essential fatty acid needs) and add MCTs oils to food and beverages for additional calories. A daily multivitamin plus individual supplements as needed are recommended.

Monitoring

Patients with PLGE should be monitored for protein levels and vitamin and mineral deficiencies. Fat-soluble vitamins (A, E, D, K) are of particular importance in those with lymphangiectasia because extravasated lymph fluid is rich in these vitamins. Monitor for essential fatty acid deficiency in those on a low-fat diet by measuring blood triene/tetrene ratio.

Take-home points

Diagnosis:

- Suspect protein-losing gastroenteropathy when both serum total protein and albumin levels are low (hypoproteinemia).

- α-1-antitrypsin clearance test quantifies fecal protein loss and establishes the diagnosis of protein-losing gastroenteropathy.

- Endoscopy with biopsy may help determine the cause of protein-losing gastroenteropathy in those with suspected mucosal disease.

Therapy:

- Treat the underlying disease to reverse intestinal protein loss.

- Provide a high-protein diet and protein-rich oral supplements or, if needed, parenteral protein to maintain nutritional status.

- Low-fat diets are effective in patients with intestinal lymphangiectasia.

References

1 Waldmann TA. Protein-losing enteropathy. *Gastroenterology* 1966; **50**: 422–43.

2 Laster L, Waldmann TA. Serum proteins and the gastrointestinal tract. *Med Ann Dist Columbia* 1965; **34**: 459–62.

3 Wochner RD, Weissman SM, Waldmann TA, *et al.* Direct measurement of the rates of synthesis of plasma proteins in control subjects and patients with gastrointestinal protein loss. *J Clin Invest* 1968; **47**: 971–82.

4 Bode L, Salvestrini C, Park PW, *et al.* Heparan sulfate and syndecan-1 are essential in maintaining murine and human intestinal epithelial barrier function. *J Clin Invest* 2008; **118**: 229–38.

5 Vignes S, Bellanger J. Primary intestinal lymphangiectasia (Waldmann's disease). *Orphanet J Rare Dis* 2008; **3**: 5.

6 Rychik J. Protein-losing enteropathy after Fontan operation. *Congenit Heart Dis* 2007; **2**: 288–300.

7 Bernier JJ, Florent C, Desmazures C, *et al.* Diagnosis of protein-losing enteropathy by gastrointestinal clearance of alpha1-antitrypsin. *Lancet* 1978; **2** (8093): 763–4.

8 Florent C, L'Hirondel C, Desmazures C, *et al.* Intestinal clearance of alpha 1-antitrypsin. A sensitive method for the detection of protein-losing enteropathy. *Gastroenterology* 1981; **81**: 777–80.

9 Strygler B, Nicar MJ, Santangelo WC, *et al.* Alpha 1-antitrypsin excretion in stool in normal subjects and in patients with gastrointestinal disorders. *Gastroenterology* 1990; **99**: 1380–7.

10 Florent C, Vidon N, Flourie B, *et al.* Gastric clearance of alpha-1-antitrypsin under cimetidine perfusion. New test to detect protein-losing gastropathy? *Dig Dis Sci* 1986; **31**: 12–15.

11 Reinhart WH, Weigand K, Kappeler M, *et al.* Comparison of gastrointestinal loss of alpha-1-antitrypsin and chromium-51-albumin in Menetrier's disease and the influence of ranitidine. *Digestion* 1983; **26**: 192–6.

12 Waldmann TA. Protein-losing enteropathy and kinetic studies of plasma protein metabolism. *Semin Nucl Med* 1972; **2**: 251–63.

13 Chiu NT, Lee BF, Hwang SJ, *et al.* Protein-losing enteropathy: diagnosis with (99m)Tc-labeled human serum albumin scintigraphy. *Radiology* 2001; **219**: 86–90.

14 Wang SJ, Tsai SC, Lan JL. Tc-99m albumin scintigraphy to monitor the effect of treatment in protein-losing gastroenteropathy. *Clin Nucl Med* 2000; **25**: 197–9.

15 Sunagawa T, Kinjo F, Gakiya I, *et al.* Successful long-term treatment with cyclosporin A in protein losing gastroenteropathy. *Intern Med* 2004; **43**: 397–9.

16 Yeaton P, Frierson HF Jr. Octreotide reduces enteral protein losses in Menetrier's disease. *Am J Gastroenterol* 1993; **88**: 95–8.

17 Green BT, Branch MS. Menetrier's disease treated with octreotide long-acting release. *Gastrointest Endosc* 2004; **60**: 1028–9.

18 Fushimi T, Takahashi Y, Kashima Y, *et al.* Severe protein losing enteropathy with intractable diarrhea due to systemic AA amyloidosis, successfully treated with corticosteroid and octreotide. *Amyloid* 2005; **12**: 48–53.

19 Filik L, Oguz P, Koksal A, *et al.* A case with intestinal lymphangiectasia successfully treated with slow-release octreotide. *Dig Liver Dis* 2004; **36**: 687–90.

20 Ferrante M, Penninckx F, De Hertogh G, *et al.* Protein-losing enteropathy in Crohn's disease. *Acta Gastroenterol Belg* 2006; **69**: 384–9.

21 Connor FL, Angelides S, Gibson M, *et al.* Successful resection of localized intestinal lymphangiectasia post-Fontan: role of (99m)technetium-dextran scintigraphy. *Pediatrics* 2003; **112**: e242–7.

22 Jeffries GH, Chapman A, Sleisenger MH. Low-fat diet in intestinal lymphangiectasia. it's effect on albumin metabolism. *N Engl J Med* 1964; **270**: 761–6.

23 Tift WL, Lloyd JK. Intestinal lymphangiectasia. Long-term results with MCT diet. *Arch Dis Child* 1975; **50**: 269–76.

CHAPTER 40

Acute Mesenteric Ischemia and Chronic Mesenteric Insufficiency

Timothy T. Nostrant

Department of Internal Medicine, University of Michigan, Ann Arbor, MI, USA

Summary

Acute mesenteric ischemia (AMI) is rare, but carries a high mortality if not diagnosed rapidly. Arterial obstruction second to embolus, thrombosis, or low blood flow states is most common. Mesenteric venous thrombosis should be suspected if the patient or family has a history for coagulation disorders, malignancy, intra-abdominal inflammation, or if the patient is taking thrombotic medications. Early diagnosis is mandatory. Surgery should be the first step if peritoneal signs are present and second-look surgery may be needed. Angiography is indicated if peritoneal signs are not found and angiographic treatment is anticipated. Intestinal vasoconstriction is the primary cause for bowel infarction and intra-arterial papaverine may be indicated in all forms of AMI, particularly those associated with low blood flow states. Mortality has decreased from 70 to 45% with the use of angiography/surgery early in suspected AMI. Chronic mesenteric insufficiency secondary to progressive atheromatous obstruction produces progressive weight loss with pain. Angiography is usually diagnostic. Surgical and angiographic treatments are available.

Case

A 62-year-old was hospitalized with an anterior wall myocardial infarction (MI) with ejection fraction of 20%. Two days after admission he develops severe central abdominal pain and hypotension. Physical exam of the abdomen was normal. The patient had a mild lactic acidosis and serum HCO_3 of 18 mmol/L. Plain film of the abdomen followed by CT angiography revealed ileus and lack of bowel enhancement in small bowel and right colon with a patent SMA and no mesenteric venous thrombosis. Angiography revealed a marked decrease in intestinal blood flow consistent with marked vasoconstriction. Intra-arterial papaverine resolved the vasoconstriction and the patient resolved his symptoms. Three months post this event the patient developed small bowel obstruction and surgery revealed a mid-small bowel stricture.

Acute/Chronic Mesenteric Ischemia

Acute mesenteric ischemia refers to the sudden onset of small intestinal hypoperfusion, which can be caused by non-obstructive, as well as obstructive, arterial, or venous flow reductions. The most common causes of arterial obstruction are emboli and thrombosis of atherosclerotic vessels. Venous outflow obstruction is usually secondary to thrombosis or intestinal strangulation. Non-occlusive arterial hypoperfusion is usually due to splanchnic vasoconstriction [1,2].

Chronic mesenteric ischemia/insufficiency is due to slow, progressive arterial narrowing of multiple atherosclerotic vessels associated with progressive pain and weight loss [3].

Vascular Anatomy/Function Mesenteric Circulation

The mesenteric vascular anatomy is shown in Figure 40.1 [4]. Extensive collateral circulation through the Arc of

Practical Gastroenterology and Hepatology: Small and Large Intestine and Pancreas, 1st edition. Edited by Nicholas J. Talley, Sunanda V. Kane and Michael B. Wallace. © 2010 Blackwell Publishing Ltd.

Riolan and marginal artery of Drummond (superior mesenteric artery [SMA], inferior mesenteric artery [IMA]) and pancreaticoduodenal arcade (celiac, SMA) allows for transient reductions in perfusion without consequence. Prolonged reductions will cause vasoconstriction, decreased collateral flow, and potentially intestinal ischemia.

The celiac axis is responsible for arterial flow to the upper gastrointestinal tract, pancreas, liver, and spleen.

The common hepatic artery usually gives rise to the gastroduodenal artery.

The superior mesenteric artery arises 1 cm below the celiac artery and terminates in the ileocolic artery. It supplies blood to the small intestines and colon proximal to the splenic flexure.

The inferior mesenteric artery arises 6–7 cm below the SMA and is responsible for the descending colon, sigmoid colon, and rectum.

Mesenteric Vascular Physiology

Arteriolar resistance is the major tool used to modulate splachnic blood flow, which varies from 10 to 35% of cardiac output. Direct arteriolar smooth muscle relaxation and indirect response to release of adenosine and other metabolites of mucosal ischemia are the major proposed mechanisms of autoregulation. Sympathetic nervous system and the renin–angiotensin axis may also contribute [5].

The intestine can compensate for a 75% acute reduction in flow for up to 12 h if collateral vessels are well developed. Longer periods of ischemia are associated with vasoconstriction to maintain peripheral arteriolar perfusion but reduces collateral flow [5,6].

Acute Mesenteric Ischemia

The major causes of intestinal ischemia are shown in Figure 40.2 [7,8]. The incidence of acute mesenteric ischemia is rising, likely secondary to an aging population

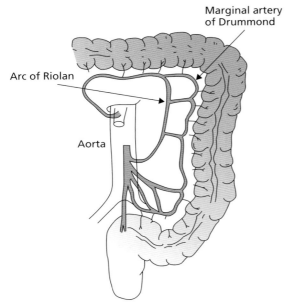

Figure 40.1 View of small bowel and colon mesenteric vasculature. Arc of Riolan and marginal artery of Drummond are mesenteric major collaterals. From Rosenblum GD, *et al.* [4], with permission from Elsevier.

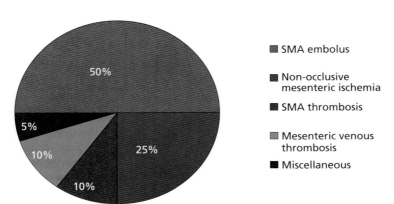

Figure 40.2 Etiologies of acute mesenteric ischemia. SMA, superior mesenteric artery.

and better cardiovascular care options for patients with severe cardiovascular disease. In younger patients, mesenteric venous insufficiency is the major cause [7].

Arterial emboli are secondary to clot dislodgement from the left atrium, left ventricle, and cardiac valves. The SMA is most vulnerable secondary to its narrow take off angle and large caliber. Emboli lodge at the orifice (15%) or just distal to the take off of the middle colic artery (85%). Emboli are multiple and the mid-jejunum is most vulnerable secondary to distance from collateral flow [8].

Acute thrombosis usually occurs in patients with chronic atherosclerotic mesenteric insufficiency or after abdominal trauma. Thrombosis usually occurs at the origin of multiple vessels, making revascularization difficult.

Mesenteric venous thrombosis is seen in patients with hypercoagulable states, portal hypertension, and inflammatory conditions such as infections, trauma, and pancreatitis. Malignancy, either through direct vascular compression or hypercoagulation, is another possibility. Mesenteric venous thrombosis leads to bowel wall edema, fluid loss, systemic hypotension, arterial vasoconstriction, and ultimate submucosal hemorrhage and bowel infarction.

Seventy-five percent of patients with mesenteric venous thrombosis have inherited thrombotic disorders with factor V Leiden causing resistance to activated protein C in 20 to 40% of patients [9]. Resistance to activated protein C not related to factor V Leiden mutation accounts for 10% of cases [9]. Prothrombin gene mutations are also seen in 8–10% of patients with venous thrombosis [9,10].

Non-occlusive Mesenteric Ischemia

Splanchnic hypoperfusion and vasoconstriction due to low flow cardiovascular states are the mechanisms proposed. Older patients with congestive heart with or without acute myocardial infarction on diuretics or digitalis are typical patients. Sepsis, cardiac arrhythmias, and α-adrenergic agonists have been described. Younger patients using cocaine may also develop mesenteric ischemia. Cardiac surgery with long aortic clamping times may also be a risk group. Prolonged vasoconstriction secondary to vasopressin and angiotensin is the major cause in cirrhosis and variceal bleeding. This form of intestinal ischemia accounts for 25% of patients now, but

had a much higher incidence before intensive care units and aggressive volume and vasodilatation support systems. Non-occlusive mesenteric ischemia still carries a high mortality (70%) due to diagnostic difficulties and limited treatment options in this critically ill group of patients [11].

Clinical Manifestations

Sudden-onset pain is predominant in most cases and out of proportion to physical exam. The pain is periumbilical or generalized and is associated with symptoms of sympathetic stimulation such as anxiety, tachycardia, or peripheral vasoconstriction. Nausea and vomiting occur in up to 50%. Bleeding is rare, but intense urgency with evacuation coupled with the above signs should raise suspicion in patients with risk factors such as congestive heart failure, recent myocardial infarction, heart arrhythmias, or coagulopathy. Hypotension and heart dysfunction may occur in patients with non-occlusive mesenteric ischemia. Severe pain lasting more than 2–3 h without discernible cause in a high-risk patient mandates immediate consideration for acute mesenteric ischemia and appropriate and rapid diagnostic testing. Acute mesenteric ischemia in moribund patients can present with sudden hypotension, sepsis, or coma without pain. High amylase or lipase levels without findings of pancreatitis should raise suspicion of AMI.

Diagnosis

Rapid diagnosis is essential because progression to infarction is associated with a high mortality. Intestinal viability approaches 100% if symptom duration before treatment is less than 12 h, 56% if it is between 12 and 24 h, and only 18% if diagnosis is more than 24 h after symptoms [12]. Diagnostic and treatment algorithms are outlined in Figures 40.3 and 40.4 [1].

Resuscitation for hypovolemia or cardiac rhythm disturbances is preeminent. Flat plate of the abdomen to look for visceral perforation, pneumatosis, or diffuse ileus followed by contrast computed tomography (CT) evaluation for proximal arterial occlusion or embolic disease and to exclude mesenteric venous thrombosis are the first steps if peritonitis is not present and suspicion is moderate. Since emboli can lodge distal to the orifice of the superior mesenteric artery, proximal occlusion on CT is most likely thrombosis with or without embolic disease. Embolic disease cannot be ruled out by a normal

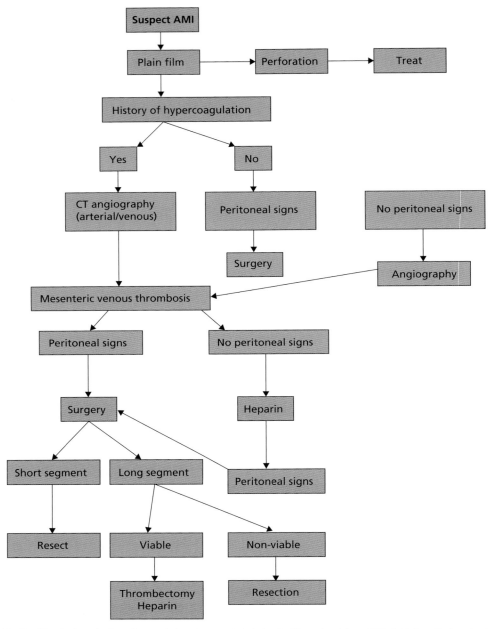

Figure 40.3 Algorithm for investigation of suspected acute mesenteric ischemia. (Reproduced from AGA Guideline. *Gastroenterology* 2000; 118: 951–3, with permission from Elsevier.)

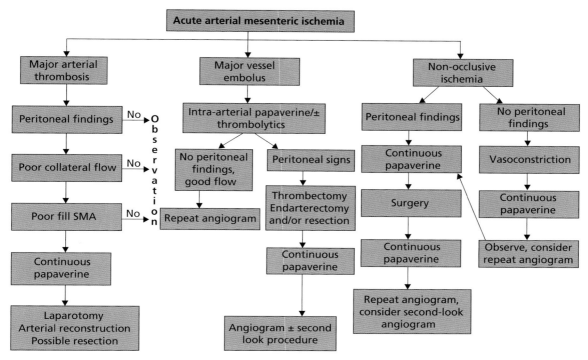

Figure 40.4 Algorithm for treatment of acute mesenteric ischemia (AMI). SMA, superior mesenteric artery. (Reproduced from AGA Guideline. *Gastroenterology* 2000; 118: 951–3, with permission from Elsevier.)

CT exam. The presence of intramural gas, portovenous gas, focal lack of bowel enhancement, or the presence of liver/spleen infarcts on CT had a sensitivity of 64% and 92%, respectively, but only portovenous gas sufficiently predicted transmural injury [13]. Laboratory tests, such as serum lactate, amylase, lipase, or the newer tests such as α-glutathione-S-transferase (α-GST) or intestinal fatty acid binding protein (I-FABP), take time and only in combination have high sensitivity and specificity for intestinal ischemia [14]. Strong clinical suspicion of mesenteric insufficiency warrants immediate angiography with vasodilators if applicable or immediate surgery if infarction is suspected.

Treatment Algorithms

The major cause of mortality in AMI is persistent vasoconstriction causing progressive necrosis leading to bowel infarction. This is seen in all conditions associated with AMI but is most predominate in non-occlusive intestinal ischemia. There have been no randomized controlled trials of any therapeutic intervention. Case–control trials are not comparable because of varying levels of ischemia and lack of matching of co-morbid conditions. Expert opinion is now, and also in the future, the likely basis for therapy utilization. Current guideline algorithms are shown in Figures 40.3 and 40.4. Mesenteric angiography for immediate diagnosis and intravenous vasodilators has been the major cause for mortality decline in the last 30 years (70 to 45%). (Figure 40.5) The major benefit is for arterial causes of AMI while multidetection row CT is best for mesenteric venous thrombosis (90%) [15]. The goal of treatment is to restore flow as quickly as possible. Vigorous rehydration, correction of arrhythmias, and systemic antibiotics to decrease intestinal bacterial translocation should be started (Evidence level C). All vasoconstrictors should be stopped. If vasopressors are required to maintain systemic blood pressure then dobutamine, low dose dopamine, or milrinone are preferred because of better mesenteric perfusion. Systemic anticoagulation should be administered to prevent thrombosis formation or propagation unless active intra-abdominal bleeding or large bowel infarction

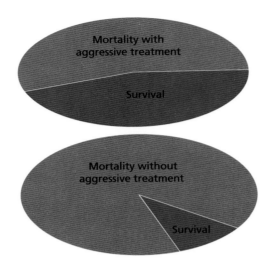

Figure 40.5 Outcome of acute mesenteric ischemia.

is suspected and immediate resection is anticipated. Anticoagulation is typically reinstated after surgery with or without resection to prevent further thrombosis.

Therapeutic options during angiography and surgery include intra-arterial vasodilators or antithrombotic agents, angioplasty with or without intra-arterial stenting, and embolectomy depending on the cause of AMI. Embolectomy during surgery using a balloon-tipped catheter has been the traditional treatment for mesenteric artery embolism with angiographic embolectomy or antithrombotics reserved for high-risk surgical patients without infarction. Postoperative arterial spasm can be attenuated by intra-arterial papaverine, which can be safely infused for up to 5 days. Persistent ischemic areas should be removed during initial surgery but a second-look surgery may need to be performed in the next 24–48 h to resect additional ischemic or gangrenous bowel.

Acute mesenteric arterial thrombosis is treated mainly with surgical vascular reconstruction and thrombectomy coupled with resection of non-viable segments. Survival post arterial reconstruction is associated with good patency rates and symptom-free survival (79% and 77%, respectively), but perioperative mortality can be as high as 52% [16]. Anticoagulation alone may be justified if chronic change is signaled by good collateral flow and peritoneal signs are not present.

Mesenteric venous thrombosis (MVT) treatment is predominately medical after necrotic bowel has been resected. Heparin should be given to all patients with MVT unless the risk for bleeding is considered to be too high. Long-term warfarin post the acute event is standard.

Non-occlusive mesenteric ischemia therapy is primarily intra-arterial papaverine to prevent vasoconstriction. Repeat angiography post discontinuation of papaverine can be performed in 24 h to verify continued resolution of vasoconstriction. Peritoneal signs warrant surgery but delay to reanatomosis may improve survival [17].

Chronic Mesenteric Insufficiency

Chronic mesenteric insufficiency CMI (intestinal angina) produces symptoms of predictable postprandial pain occurring 20–30 min postprandially. These symptoms usually progress over time to become continuous, associated with fear of eating and profound weight loss. Chronic mesenteric ischemia can present with recurrent gastric ulcers and gastroparesis and should be considered in the differential diagnosis of these disorders. Chronic atherosclerotic disease is usually the cause and involves at least two vessels in 91%, three vessels in 55%, and 7% including only the SMA and 2% involving the celiac axis [18].

Diagnosis can be suspected by non-invasive tests and confirmed with angiography. Non-invasive tests include provocative balloon tonometry to measure postprandial mural acidosis [19], MRI/CT angiography [20], duplex ultrasonography [21], and intestinal oxygen consumption [22]. Only balloon tonometry can show mural acidosis at the time of pain and return of normal pH after pain resolves showing mesenteric ischemia as the cause for pain [23]. Large studies have not been done but small studies have been promising. All other tests, including angiography, depend on exclusion of other diseases before CMI is likely.

Percutaneous mesenteric angioplasty (PTMA) with or without stent placement or surgical revascularization are the usual choices, but randomized control trials are absent. Retrospective reports of surgical revascularization have shown success rates from 59 to 100% and recurrent obstruction from 0 to 26.5% [24]. Mortality is low and the rates are best in the most recent studies. PTMA has only case reports but experience is increasing as the population ages and co-morbid illness increases

[25]. If rates close in on surgical rates, PTMA may become the treatment of choice.

Take-home points

- Decreased mesenteric arterial flow (thrombus, embolus) accounts for 60–70% of AMI and has a high mortality if diagnosis and treatment is delayed (70%).

- Risk factors for AMI include advanced age, atherosclerosis, low cardiac output, cardiac arrhythmias, cardiac valvular disease, recent myocardial ischemia or infarction, or mesenteric venous thrombosis (MVT). Hypercoagulation states or malignancy should be suspected in MVT.

- Mesenteric angiography with both diagnostic and treatment arms is still the gold standard although newer imaging modalities (CT, Doppler ultrasonography) are gaining in use. Rapid diagnosis is still paramount.

- Intestinal vasoconstriction is the major cause of bowel infarction in all forms of AMI and can be persistent. Vasodilator use should be frequent and may be prolonged.

- Long-term prognosis is good if the patient survives the acute event and the amount of bowel lost is small.

- Chronic mesenteric insufficiency is caused by progressive atherosclerosis leading to postprandial pain, weight loss, and fear of eating. Multiple vessel involvement is most common. Clinical history with mesenteric involvement of two or more vessels is required for intervention. Surgical vascular reconstruction or percutaneous transluminal mesenteric angioplasty with or without stenting is standard treatment.

References

1 American Gastroenterological Association Medical Position Statement: guidelines on intestinal ischemia. *Gastroenterology* 2000; **118**: 951–3.

2 Reinus JF, Brandt LJ, Boley SJ. Ischemic diseases of the bowel. *Gastroenterol Clin North Am* 1990; **19**: 319–43.

3 Moawad J, Gewertz BL. Chronic mesenteric ischemia. Clinical presentation and diagnosis. *Surg Clin North Am* 1997; **77**: 357–80.

4 Rosenblum GD, Boyle CM, Schwartz LB. The mesenteric circulation. Anatomy and physiology. *Surg Clin North Am* 1997; **77**: 289–306.

5 Boley SJ, Frieber W, Winslow PR, *et al*. Circulatory responses to acute reduction of superior mesenteric arterial flow. *Physiologist* 1969; **12**: 180.

6 Zimmerman BJ, Granger DN. Reperfusion injury. *Surg Clin North Am* 1992; **72**: 65–83.

7 Cappell MS. Intestinal (mesenteric) vasculopathy. I. Acute superior mesenteric arteriopathy and venopathy. *Gastroenterol Clin North Am* 1998; **27**: 783–825.

8 Batellier J, Kieny R. Superior mesenteric artery embolism: eighty-two cases. *Ann Vasc Surg* 1990; **4**: 112–16.

9 Amitrano L, Brancaccio V, Guardascione MA, *et al*. High prevalence of thrombophilic genotypes in patients with acute mesenteric vein thrombosis. *Am J Gastroenterol* 2001; **96**: 146–9.

10 de Visser MC, Rosendaal FR, Bertina RM. A reduced sensitivity for activated protein C in the absence of factor V Leiden increases the risk of venous thrombosis. *Blood* 1999; **93**: 1271–6.

11 Wilcox MG, Howard TJ, Plaskon LA. Current theories of pathogenesis and treatment of nonocclusive mesenteric ischemia. *Dig Dis Sci* 1995; **40**: 709–16.

12 LoboMartinez E, Carvajosa E, Sacco O, Martinez Molina E. Embolectomy in mesenterio ischemia. *Rev Esp Enferm Dig* 1993; **83**: 351–4.

13 Alpern MB, Glazer GM, Francis IR. Ischemic or infracted bowel: CT findings. *Radiology* 1988; **166**: 149–52.

14 Gearhart SL, Delaney CP, Senagore AJ, *et al*. Prospective assessment of the predictive value of alpha-glutathione S-transferase for intestinal ischemia. *Am Surg* 2003; **69**: 324–9.

15 Horton KM, Fishman EK. The current status of multidetector row CT and three-dimensional imaging of the small bowel. *Radiol Clin North Am* 2003; **41**: 199–212.

16 Rivitz SM, Geller SC, Hahn C, Waltman AC. Treatment of acute mesenteric venous thrombosis with transjugular intramesenteric urokinase infusion. *J Vasc Interv Radiol* 1995; **6**: 219–23.

17 Demirpolat G, Oran I, Tamsel S, *et al*. Acute mesenteric venous thrombosis. *N Engl J Med* 2001; **345**: 1683–8.

18 Tendler DA, LaMont JT. Chronic mesenteric ischemia. In: Rutgeerts P, ed. *UpToDate*, UpToDate, Waltham, MA, May 31st, 2008.

19 Kolkman JJ, Groeneveld AB. Occlusive and non-occlusive gastrointestinal ischaemia: A clinical review with special emphasis on the diagnostic value of tonometry. *Scan J Gastroenterol Suppl* 1998; **225**: 3–12.

20 Meaney JF, Prince MR, Nostrant TT, Stanley JC. Gadolinium-enhanced MR angiography of visceral arteries in patients with suspected chronic mesenteric ischemia. *J Magn Reson Imaging* 1997; **7**: 171–6.

21 Gentile AT, Moneta GL, Lee RW, *et al*. Usefulness of fasting and postprandial duplex ultrasound examinations for predicting high-grade superior mesenteric artery stenosis. *Am J Surg* 1995; **169**: 476–9.

22 Moneta GL. Screening for mesenteric vascular insufficiency and follow-up of mesenteric artery bypass procedures. *Semin Vasc Surg* 2001; **14**: 186–92.

23 Boley SJ, Brandt LJ, Veith FJ, *et al.* A new provocative test for chronic mesenteric ischemia. *Am J Gastroenterol* 1991; **86**: 888–91.

24 English WP, Pearce JD, Craven TE, *et al.* Chronic visceral ischemia: symptom-free survival after open surgical repair. *Vasc Endovascular Surg* 2004; **38**: 493–503.

25 Matsumoto AH, Tegtmeyer CJ, Fitzcharles EK, *et al.* Percutaneous transluminal angioplasty of visceral arterial stenoses: results and long-term clinical follow-up. *J Vasc Interv Radiol* 1995; **6**: 165–74.

CHAPTER 41
Small Intestinal Ulceration

Reza Y. Akhtar and Blair S. Lewis

Henry D. Janowitz Division of Gastroenterology, Mount Sinai School of Medicine, New York, NY, USA

Summary

The differential diagnoses of ulcers of the small bowel are well known. They include Crohn disease, non-steroidal anti-inflammatory drugs (NSAIDs), radiation, vasculitis, medication effects, some infections, and certain neoplasms. Yet when faced with the finding of ulceration in the small bowel, it can be difficult to come up with a final diagnosis. Crohn disease is most common but NSAID use is also very common. Then, how does a physician make the diagnosis of Crohn disease by the presence of ulcers seen only on endoscopy, capsule or otherwise? In the past, we were confident making the diagnosis in the clinical setting of pain and diarrhea in a young person in whom a small bowel series shows ileitis. We clearly should be able to do the same with endoscopic findings. That is to combine the clinical scenario with the endoscopic, instead of the radiographic, findings. There can be other evidence to support our diagnosis of Crohn disease including a family history of inflammatory bowel disease and abnormal serologies of antineutrophil cytoplasmic antibodies and anti-*Saccharomyces cerevisiae* antibodies, though this is not the intended use of these blood tests. Endoscopic biopsy typically cannot differentiate a Crohn ulcer from an NSAID ulcer. Other testing such as computed tomography scanning generally provides no additional information to endoscopy. Grading severity of inflammatory findings on capsule endoscopy can provide more certainty to making a final diagnosis.

Case

A 45-year-old female presented with a history of obscure gastrointestinal bleeding. Her first episode was at 20 years of age. Since then, multiple episodes ensued, occasionally requiring transfusion of packed red blood cells. Evaluations, including colonoscopy, esophagogastroduodenoscopy (EGD), and bleeding scan, were unrevealing. Additionally, computed tomography (CT) scan, Meckel scan, and small bowel series were normal. Her history was otherwise remarkable except for rare NSAID use and hypertension for which she takes diuretics.

Capsule endoscopy was performed and disclosed diffuse mucosal edema and erythema associated with scattered ulceration and luminal narrowing at the mid-ileum (Figure 41.1a,b). These findings correlated to an activity score of 1232. Serologies of ASCA (anti-*Saccharomyces cerevisiae* antibodies) and p-ANCA (perinuclear-staining antineutrophil cytoplasmic antibodies) were negative. Other laboratory values were unremarkable. Following the capsule exam, a double balloon enteroscopy from the transrectal approach was performed. Endoscopically, the area and affected regions of small bowel were identical to the capsule study. Biopsies were obtained and these revealed active inflammation. Clinical history, endoscopic appearance, and biopsies were consistent with Crohn disease.

Introduction

The differential diagnoses of ulcers of the small bowel are well known to clinicians. They include Crohn disease, non-steroidal anti-inflammatory drugs (NSAIDs) enteropathy, radiation enteropathy, as well as vasculitis, medication effects, some infections, and even certain neoplasms (Table 41.1). However, when faced with the finding of ulceration in the small bowel, it can be difficult to come up with a final diagnosis. Crohn disease is most common but we do not trust the patient who denies NSAID use since surreptitious use is common. In the patient reported in the Case, there is no history of radiation therapy and no history of medication use except the

Practical Gastroenterology and Hepatology: Small and Large Intestine and Pancreas, 1st edition. Edited by Nicholas J. Talley, Sunanda V. Kane and Michael B. Wallace. © 2010 Blackwell Publishing Ltd.

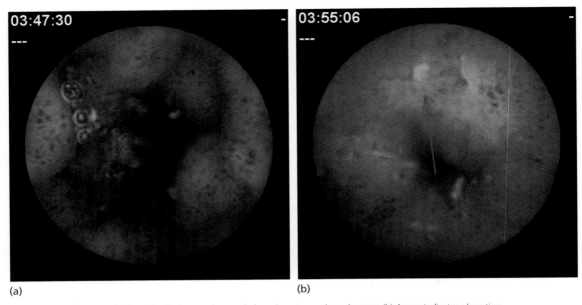

Figure 41.1 (a,b) Mucosal edema, luminal narrowing, and ulceration at capsule endoscopy. (b) Arrow indicates ulceration.

Table 41.1 Differential diagnoses of ulcerations in the small bowel.

Crohn disease
Ulcerative jejunoilietis
Zollinger–Ellison syndrome
Infections: mycobacterium, syphilis, typhoid, and histoplasmosis
Medications: potassium, non-steroidal anti-inflammatory drugs (NSAIDs)
Vasculitis: polyarteritis nodosa, Churg–Strauss disease, rheumatoid arthritis, systemic lupus erythematosis, Behçet disease, Wegener granulomatosis, cryoglobulinemia, Henoch–Schönlein purpura
Radiation enteritis
Meckel diverticulum
Duplication cyst
Graft-versus-host disease
Neoplasms: adenocarcinoma, carcinoid, lymphoma

limited NSAID use described. Infectious causes seem remote. Then how does a physician make the diagnosis of Crohn disease by the presence of ulcers seen only on capsule endoscopy? Of course we used to be confident in making this diagnosis in the proper clinical setting of pain and diarrhea in a young person in whom a small bowel series showed ileitis. We clearly should be able to do the same with capsule endoscopy. That is to combine

the clinical scenario with the endoscopic, instead of the radiographic, findings. This patient has no pain and no history of diarrhea, simply bleeding. This is known to occur in Crohn disease but it is an unusual presentation.

We look for other evidence to support our diagnosis of Crohn disease including a family history of inflammatory bowel disease (there was none), and sending serologies such as ANCA and ASCA (they were negative). These serologies help differentiate ulcerative colitis from Crohn disease but are now being used by physicians to confirm a diagnosis of suspected Crohn disease. Unfortunately, using these serologies for this purpose is not supported by the literature [1]. ASCA is detected in 39–70% of patients with Crohn disease and in only 0–5% of healthy subjects [1,2]. The sensitivity of ASCA in correctly identifying Crohn disease is 55%. ANCA are positive in 2–28% of Crohn patients and in 20–85% of ulcerative colitis patients. It also has a low sensitivity of diagnosing ulcerative colitis (56%).

Another way to diagnose Crohn disease is to have a tissue diagnosis. Double balloon enteroscopy is a method to deeply intubate the small bowel from either peroral or transrectal approaches [3]. Unfortunately, the hallmark finding of non-caseating granulomas are seen in a minority of cases [4]. Endoscopic biopsy cannot differentiate a Crohn ulcer from an NSAID ulcer, though, if suspected, neoplastic change can be excluded. Other methods, such as CT scanning, generally provides no additional information to capsule endoscopy [5]. Enlarged lymph nodes can be seen in chronic inflammatory changes and these finding may only fuel the thought that there is a neoplasm.

Capsule Endoscopy

Capsule endoscopy (CE) has provided us with the ability to detect mucosal inflammatory change of the small intestine often missed by other techniques. In a pooled data analysis, CE had a miss rate for ulcers of only 0.5% [6]. In this study, capsule was compared to ileocolonoscopy, push enteroscopy, and small bowel series. A meta-analysis of studies comparing CE to other imaging modalities of the small bowel for inflammatory bowel disease has established that CE has an incremental diagnostic yield of 25–40% over other modalities including CT enterography, small bowel series, and ileocolonoscopy [7]. A recent report described finding small bowel ulcers in 22 patients in whom no ulcers could be identified by any other means [8]. These included Crohn disease in nine, ulcerated neoplasms in three, and Behçet disease in two, among others. Yet despite the ability to detect ulcerations, turning this into a diagnosis has been difficult. The most common scenario clinically is oppo-

site to the case presented above. It typically involves applying capsule endoscopy in patients with symptoms of Crohn disease in an effort to find ulcerations. Suspicion of Crohn disease was previously defined at the discretion of the treating physician and usually was considered when a patient had either abdominal pain or persistent diarrhea. Yields of capsule endoscopy are low when performed in patients with abdominal pain alone [9] and in patients with abdominal pain and diarrhea alone [10]. The addition of a sign or symptom of inflammation increases the yield of capsule endoscopy. In the CEDAP-Plus study of 50 patients with suspected Crohn disease, signs of inflammation included elevated erythrocyte sedimentation rate, elevated C-reactive protein, thrombocytosis, and leukocytosis. The finding of one of these markers in addition to symptoms of pain and diarrhea increased the yield of capsule endoscopy with an odds ration of 3.2 [11]. The landmark study by Fireman enrolled patients with abdominal pain, diarrhea, anemia, and weight loss [12]. These patients had had symptoms for an average of 6.3 years and all had normal colonoscopies, EGD, and small bowel series. Crohn disease was diagnosed in 12 of the 17 by capsule endoscopy. In a consensus paper, the International Conference of Capsule Endoscopy defined which patients who should be suspected of having Crohn disease [13]. The algorithm presented in this paper includes individuals with symptoms plus either extraintestinal manifestations, inflammatory markers, or abnormal imaging studies (Figure 41.2). Unfortunately, these still do not help us with the patient

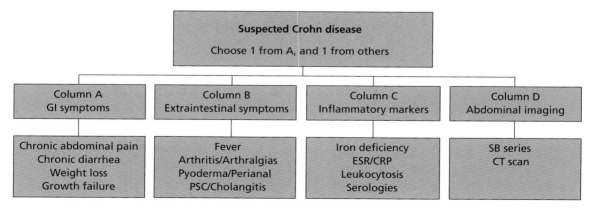

Figure 41.2 Criteria for suspected Crohn disease. PSC, primary sclerosing cholangitis; ESR, erythrocyte sedimentation rate; CRP, C-reactive protein; SB, small bowel; CT, computed tomography. (Adapted from Mergener K *et al. Endoscopy* 2007; 39: 895–909, with permission from Georg Thieme Verlag KG.)

described in the Case who has bleeding as the only symptom.

The presence of inflammatory changes in the small bowel cannot only be seen in a variety of disease states but can also be noted in normal individuals. Goldstein conducted a trial comparing the effects of naproxen, celecoxib, and placebo in the small bowel [14]. Prior to randomization, all volunteers were not allowed to take NSAIDs for a period of 2 weeks. He reported that 10.6% of the healthy volunteers had mucosal breaks after this run-in period. The study did not measure these ulcers and since these cases were excluded, we do not know their number or severity. Thus ulcers in the small bowel may be normal.

How does one make a diagnosis? These differing clinical scenarios point out the complexity of trying to make a diagnosis based on an endoscopic image alone. Are the ulcers seen on the capsule study in the Case at the start of this chapter a normal finding, secondary to her occasional NSAID use, or do they represent Crohn disease? Though a few small ulcers may be normal or may be secondary to NSAID use, most experts would agree that numerous, large ulcers could only mean Crohn disease. This is much like our feelings about ileitis seen on a small bowel series. These changes are quite pronounced and could never been felt to be normal or secondary to NSAID use. This necessity to grade the severity of inflammatory change noted on capsule exams raised the need for a scoring index. An index has been created and validated and is presently part of capsule software (Figure 41.3) [15]. This index evaluates three parameters: villous edema, ulceration, and stenosis. The severity of these changes is assessed by the number, size, and extent of the findings. Scores of below 135 designate normal or clinically insignificant mucosal inflammatory change, a score between 135 and 790 is considered mild, and a score of

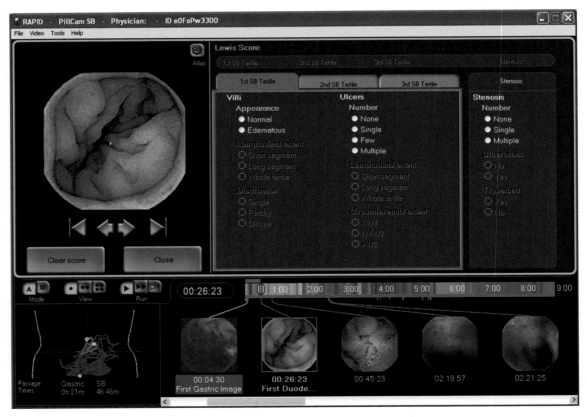

Figure 41.3 The screen view of the activity score. (Courtesy of Given Imaging, Stuttgart, Germany.)

790 or above is considered moderate to severe. It is recognized that the scoring index cannot at present differentiate the causes of inflammatory change in the small intestine. However, the score in the individual reported in the Case was 1232. This is well above the cutoff for moderate to severe inflammatory change of 790. This markedly elevated number strongly suggested that this patient has Crohn disease.

Take-home points

- A diagnosis of Crohn disease cannot be based solely on the appearance of ulcers. Circumferential ulcers and linear ulcers can be seen in both Crohn and NSAID enteropathy.
- The diagnosis of a small bowel ulcer seen on endoscopy has to be made with in conjunction with clinical factors.
- The mucosal activity index, part of small bowel capsule software, can be used to suggest a diagnosis.

References

1 Anand V, Russell A, Tyuyuki R, Fedorak R. Perinuclear cytoplasmic autoantibodies and anti-saccharomyces ceresvisiae antibodies as serological markers are not specific in the identification of Crohn's disease and ulcerative colitis. *Can J Gastroenterol* 2008; **22**: 33–6.

2 Peyrin-Biroulet L, Standaert-Vitse A, Branche J, Chamaillard M. IBD serological panels: facts and perspectives. *Inflamm Bowel Dis* 2007; **13**: 1561–6.

3 Semrad C. Role of double balloon enteroscopy in Crohn's disease. *Gastrointest Endosc* 2007; **66**: S94–5.

4 Pulimood A, Peter S, Rook G, Donoghue H. In situ PCR for Mycobacterium tuberculosis in endoscopic mucosal biopsy specimens of intestinal tuberculosis and Crohn disease. *Am J Clin Pathol* 2008; **129**: 846–51.

5 Solem C, Loftus E, Fletcher J, *et al*. Small-bowel imaging in Crohn's disease: a prospective, blinded, 4-way comparison trial. *Gastrointest Endosc* 2008; **68**: 255–66.

6 Lewis B, Eisen G, Friedman S. A pooled analysis to evaluate results of capsule endoscopy trials. *Endoscopy* 2005; **37**: 960–5.

7 Triester SL, Leighton JA, Leontiadis GI, *et al*. A meta-analysis of the yield of capsule endoscopy compared to other diagnostic modalities in patients with non-stricturing small bowel Crohn's disease. *Am J Gastroenterol* 2006; **101**: 954–64.

8 Ersoy O, Harmanci O, Aydinli, *et al*. Capability of capsule endoscopy in detecting small bowel ulcers. *Dig Dis Sci* 2009; **54**: 136–41.

9 Pada C, Pirozzi G, Riccioni M. Capsule endoscopy in patients with chronic abdominal pain. *Dig Liver Dis* 2006; **38**: 696–8.

10 Fry L, Carey E, Shiff A, *et al*. The yield of capsule endoscopy in patients with abdominal pain or diarrhea. *Endoscopy* 2006; **38**: 498–501.

11 May A, Manner H, Schneider M, *et al*. Prospective multicenter trial of capsule endoscopy in patients with chronic abdominal pain, diarrhea, and other signs and symptoms (CEDAP-Plus study). *Endoscopy* 2007; **39**: 606–12.

12 Fireman Z, Mahajna E, Broide E, *et al*. Diagnosing small bowel Crohn's disease with wireless capsule endoscopy. *Gut* 2003; **52**: 390–2.

13 Mergener K, Ponchon T, Gralnek I, *et al*. Literature review and recommendations for clinical application of small bowel capsule endoscopy based on a panel discussion by international experts. *Endoscopy* 2007; **39**: 895–909.

14 Goldstein JL, Eisen GM, Lewis B, *et al*. Video capsule endoscopy to prospectively assess small bowel injury with celecoxib, naproxen plus omeprazole, and placebo. *Clin Gastroenterol Hepatol* 2005; **3**: 133–41.

15 Gralnek I, DeFranchis R, Seidman E, *et al*. Development of a capsule endoscopy scoring index for small intestinal mucosal inflammatory change. *Aliment Pharmacol Ther* 2008; **27**: 146–54.

CHAPTER 42

Intestinal Obstruction and Pseudo-obstruction

Charlene M. Prather

Department of Medicine, Saint Louis University School of Medicine, St Louis, MO, USA

Summary

Identifying the etiology of abdominal pain, nausea, and vomiting often remains a challenge for clinicians. A laundry list of etiologies exists for these symptoms including acute gastroenteritis, peptic ulcer disease, metabolic etiologies, medication effects, gastroparesis, mechanical obstruction, and pseudo-obstruction. This review focuses on the diagnosis and management of intestinal mechanical obstruction, intestinal pseudo-obstruction, and differentiating the two. Early identification of complete mechanical obstruction and/or the presence of intestinal ischemia or peritonitis is paramount, as these patients benefit from early surgical intervention. Most patients with partial bowel obstruction may be managed medically. Clinical recognition of intestinal pseudo-obstruction avoids unnecessary surgery and directs treatment towards symptomatic management. The role of newer imaging techniques, CT and MR radiography and other, newer diagnostic techniques in intestinal pseudo-obstruction is also reviewed.

Case

A 65-year-old, long-time smoker presents to the Emergency Department with a 2-day history of worsening abdominal pain, distension, diarrhea, nausea, and vomiting. This is her third visit in the past several months, and she has been hospitalized each time for conservative treatment. She has responded each time to nasogastric suction and intravenous fluids. CT imaging reveals diffusely dilated loops of small bowel without evidence of a transition point or mass lesion. The dilation is noted to be worse than on previous films. She again responds symptomatically with decompression and bowel rest, but is noted to have a 4.5 kg (10 lb) weight loss since her last admission.

Introduction

Intestinal mechanical obstruction may be acute or chronic. Further, acute intestinal mechanical obstruction may be partial or complete. Almost by definition, chronic

Practical Gastroenterology and Hepatology: Small and Large Intestine and Pancreas, 1st edition. Edited by Nicholas J. Talley, Sunanda V. Kane and Michael B. Wallace. © 2010 Blackwell Publishing Ltd.

mechanical obstruction is partial (incomplete). Acute intestinal mechanical obstruction may be subdivided into three broad categories with the obstruction the result of: (i) abnormalities of the bowel wall; (ii) extrinsic compression; or (iii) intraluminal process. Abnormalities of the bowel wall include inflammatory or fibrotic strictures as in Crohn disease. The most common extrinsic etiology remains fibrous adhesions. Hernias would also fall in this category. Intraluminal causes of bowel obstruction include ingested foreign bodies, gall stones, parasites, and tumors. Adhesions, the most common cause of bowel obstruction, occur commonly following abdominal surgery. Adhesions develop in up to 93% of individuals with prior intra-abdominal surgery versus a prevalence of only 10% in patients without prior abdominal surgery [1]. Acute intestinal mechanical obstruction must further be subdivided into simple obstruction, without vascular compromise, versus obstruction complicated by vascular comprise and/or peritonitis, the latter requiring urgent surgical intervention.

The medical management of complete bowel obstruction remains relatively straight forward with management responsibilities most often falling to the surgeon.

Gastroenterologist expertise may be called upon when the presence of mechanical obstruction is in doubt to assist with the management of suspected ileus or pseudo-obstruction. The clinical presentation of intestinal pseudo-obstruction mimics mechanical obstruction with similar symptoms and dilated bowel loops, but no mechanical factor is present obstructing the intestine. Pseudo-obstruction may sometimes be referred to as a "functional" obstruction. Other descriptors of pseudo-obstruction include ileus or colonic pseudo-obstruction. These syndromes are acute and may occur in the postoperative period, result from medication effects, or metabolic abnormalities. Chronic intestinal pseudo-obstruction is a rare, severe intestinal motility disorder. It may be a primary digestive abnormality or result from underlying medical conditions such as systemic sclerosis, paraneoplastic phenomenon, or dysautonomia.

Intestinal Obstruction

The most common causes of acute mechanical intestinal obstruction are adhesive disease, hernias, and malignancy (Table 42.1). The level of obstruction may be at the small bowel or colon. Partial bowel obstruction indicates that some intestinal contents pass the level of block-age. In complete bowel obstruction no contents pass the level of obstruction. Complete bowel obstruction usually requires surgery. Partial obstruction is often managed conservatively. A recent review comprehensively outlines the pathophysiology of mechanical obstruction and its management [2]. Any abdominal surgery may result in the development of adhesions. The risk of symptomatic adhesive disease is reduced in laparoscopic surgery compared to laparotomy [3]. The presentation of intestinal obstruction varies depending upon the site of the obstruction and whether the obstruction is complete or partial. Most commonly, patients present with the acute onset of abdominal pain, nausea, and vomiting. Patients with more proximal bowel obstruction may describe the emesis of bilious materials. Patients with more distal obstructions may present with emesis of feculent material. The absence of passage of gas or stool suggests a complete bowel obstruction. Depending upon the duration of the bowel obstruction, signs of volume depletion may be present. In addition to determining if the obstruction is complete or partial, an early assessment for evidence of vascular compromise of the bowel or peritonitis remains critical. The presence of systemic toxicity or peritoneal signs suggests vascular compromise necessitating urgent surgical consultation for laparotomy.

Diagnosis

The diagnosis of mechanical bowel obstruction begins with a directed history and physical examination (Table 42.2). Initial laboratory testing to consider includes a complete blood count with differential, electrolytes, renal function, amylase, lipase, and lactate. All patients with

Table 42.1 Causes of mechanical bowel obstruction.

Common causes
  Adhesions
  Hernias
  Tumor
  Adenocarcinoma
  Lymphoma
  Metastatic tumor
  Crohn disease
  Foreign body
  Volvulus

Uncommon causes
  Intussusception
  Tumor
  Lipoma
  Meckel diverticulum
  Bezoars
  Gall stone
  Diverticular abscess
  Radiation strictures
  NSAID-induced strictures

Table 42.2 Making a diagnosis of mechanical bowel obstruction.

Directed history and physical examination
  Duration of symptoms
  Prior abdominal or pelvic surgery
  Prior abdominal radiation
  Character of pain
  Character of emesis
  Last bowel movement or passage of flatus
  Vital signs including checking for orthostasis
  Character of bowel sounds
  Presence of distension
  Presence of abdominal tenderness
  Presence of peritoneal signs

suspected bowel obstruction should first undergo an abdominal obstructive series (supine and upright images of the abdomen). In patients with atypical symptoms, history of inflammatory bowel disease, history of malignancy, or non-diagnostic obstructive series consideration should be given for early computed tomography (CT) radiography. In contrast to plain radiographs, CT radiography more reliably identifies the site and etiology of the bowel obstruction [4]. The absence of an obstructive bowel pattern does not exclude the presence of a complete bowel obstruction. False negatives may occur when the obstruction is very proximal and the patient is vomiting, closed loop syndromes, and in early complete or partial bowel obstruction. When the clinical picture does not fit with the initial radiographic findings, the early pursuit of CT radiography with IV contrast is recommended. CT radiography often identifies the presence of obstruction and/or strangulation and may identify the etiology [5]. When the diagnostic evaluation fails to identify presence of intestinal obstruction and the index of suspicion remains high, further evaluation may be necessary with small bowel radiography, including barium enteroclysis, CT, or magnetic resonance (MR) enterography (Table 42.3). CT or MR enterography may be particularly helpful in patients with suspected Crohn disease. The main advantage of MR enterography over CT enterography relates to the lack of radiation exposure. Although CT and MR radiography have similar sensitivity (~90%) for identifying inflammatory lesions of the bowel, the specificity of CT may be greater [6]. CT radi-

ography also appears better compared to MR for identifying masses as the cause of bowel obstruction.

Management (Figure 42.1)

The first step in the management of a patient with bowel obstruction remains fluid resuscitation with intravenous fluids and the correction of any underlying electrolyte abnormalities. Most patients should have a nasogastric tube placed to facilitate bowel decompression and prevent further bowel distension. A multidisciplinary approach is favored with early surgical consultation in patients with complete bowel obstruction or peritoneal signs. Patients with complete bowel obstruction, evidence of systemic toxicity, or peritoneal signs should undergo early surgical consultation. Partial obstruction related to adhesive disease may be managed conservatively with two-thirds to nearly 90% resolving spontaneously [7–9]. Careful observation is required with serial examinations of the abdomen to detect improvement or worsening and need for surgery.

Following initial management focused on fluid resuscitation and risk stratification, the focus moves toward identifying the location and underlying etiology of the obstruction. Reviewing the abdominal obstructive series and/or CT scan will provide a preliminary assessment of the obstruction location (Figures 42.2–42.8). The finding of a transition point on imaging with bowel dilated proximally and decompressed distally remains highly specific (though less sensitive) for bowel obstruction. The findings of small bowel loops larger than 3 cm diameter and

Table 42.3 Second-line diagnostic tests.

Test	Radiation exposure	IV contrast	Pros	Cons
Small bowel radiography	yes	no	More sensitive for identifying presence of obstruction Sensitivity for obstruction 93–98% (Dixon) Better at diagnosing closed loop syndromes	Less specific for identifying etiology Radiation exposure
CT radiography	yes	yes	Identifies etiology of obstruction Especially helpful in IBD Identifies presence of ischemia Shortest time to diagnosis	Radiation exposure IV contrast
MR radiography	no	yes	No radiation exposure High sensitivity for identifying obstruction Less able to identify masses Less able to identify inflammation	More limited availablity Lower specificity as to etiology

IBD, inflammatory bowel disease.

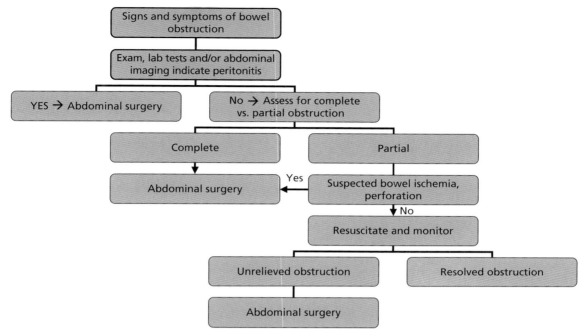

Figure 42.1 Algorithm outlining a management strategy in suspected bowel obstruction.

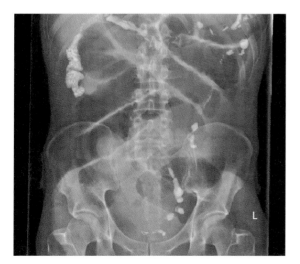

Figure 42.2 Plain, supine abdominal radiograph showing diffusely dilated small bowel. Note the presence of residual barium in a decompressed colon.

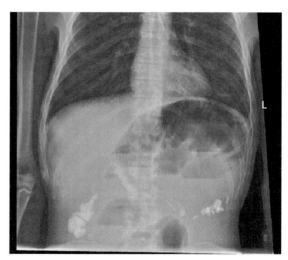

Figure 42.3 Upright abdominal radiograph showing dilated loops of small bowel and air–fluid levels in a patient with a partial small bowel obstruction.

colonic diameter greater the 6cm (10cm for cecum) indicate abnormally dilated bowel. In order to see this on plain films, some air must be present within the bowel. Thus, false negatives can be seen when the bowel is fluid filled, as in closed loop syndromes. Commonly used to differentiate mechanical obstruction from pseudo-

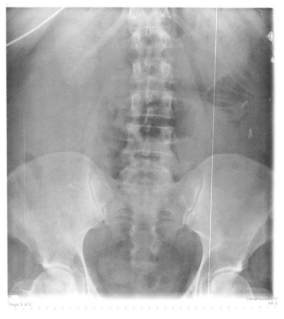

Figure 42.5 Patient presenting with recurrent episodes of abdominal pain, nausea, and vomiting. Note the presence of surgical clips and dilated loop of small bowel in the left upper quadrant.

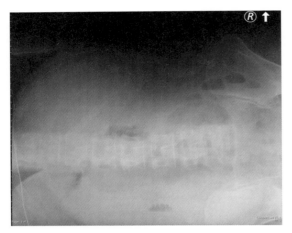

Figure 42.4 Lateral upright abdominal radiograph in a patient unable to stand. Note the presence of several air–fluid levels.

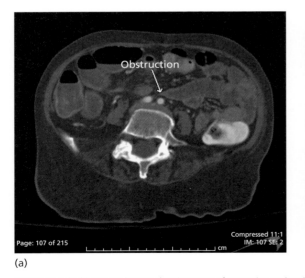

(a)

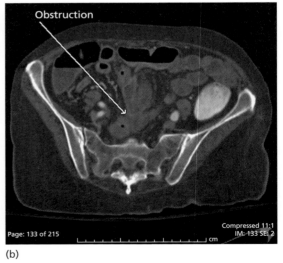

(b)

Figure 42.6 (a, b) Two CT images showing areas of narrowing and multiple loops of dilated bowel. Note the presence of contrast in a non-dilated colon. A laparotomy this patient was determined to have an internal hernia causing a partial obstruction.

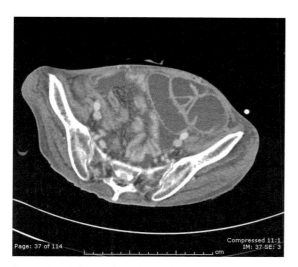

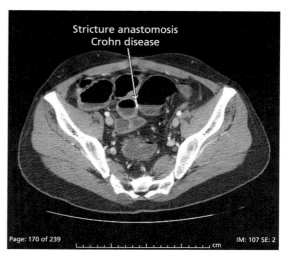

Figure 42.7 CT image of a patient with prior colonic resection for chronic ulcerative colitis presenting with nausea and vomiting. Note the dilated loops of bowel in the left pelvis compared to the decompressed loops of bowel in the right pelvis. At laparotomy an adhesive stricture was found.

Figure 42.8 CT enterography showed a narrowed anastomosis in a patient with Crohn disease and prior ileocolonic resection. Not the hypodense contrast in the bowel lumen compared to the higher density from IV contrast in the bowel wall. This patient was managed conservatively without surgery.

obstruction, the presence of air in the rectum on imaging makes complete small bowel obstruction or proximal colonic obstruction unlikely. Other abnormalities to look for when reviewing abdominal images include the presence of air under the diaphragm, air outside the bowel wall, air in the biliary tree or vasculature, abnormal bowel thickening, and the presence of stones or foreign bodies.

Further Diagnostic Imaging

The need for further diagnostic imaging results when there is difficulty in differentiating complete versus partial obstruction, and to assist in identifying the location and etiology of a partial bowel obstruction. CT with intravenous and oral contrast remains the most commonly used first step in this process. The advantage of CT remains its ability to detect vascular compromise and the specific cause of the obstruction. Non-visualization of oral contrast in the colon 12 h after ingestion on CT provides a reliable marker for complete bowel obstruction [10]. CT findings worrisome for strangulation include bowel wall thickening, pneumatosis intestinalis, mesenteric inflammatory changes, and poor contrast enhancement of the bowel. The sensitivity for identifying the location and cause of a partial bowel obstruction can be enhanced when using CT enterography. This technol-

ogy is increasingly available in community hospitals. Contrast is given orally or by enteric tube to distend the bowel lumen [11]. The luminal contrast used varies by institution, but usually includes the use of polyethylene glycol solutions (neutral contrast) or, less commonly, a dilute barium solution. Intravenous contrast is also used and images are obtained every 2–3 mm with reconstruction intervals of 1–1.5 mm. The goal is to create contrast differentiation between the intraluminal contents and the bowel wall (Figure 42.8). CT enterography plays a particularly important role in the evaluation of inflammatory bowel disease. It is also useful for detecting small bowel tumors and has an emerging diagnostic role in acute, obscure gastrointestinal bleeding. The role of CT or MR enterography in patients with bowel obstruction remains to be defined. One uncontrolled study assessing CT enterography in patients presenting to the emergency room with acute abdominal pain found it to be well tolerated and useful in identifying the source of abdominal pain in almost one-half of patients [12].

Complications and Recurrence

Intestinal strangulation and bowel necrosis result in significant morbidity and mortality. CT findings suggesting ischemia (e.g., reduced wall enhancement) have a sensi-

Table 42.4 Indications for operative intervention in bowel obstruction.

Complete bowel obstruction
Peritonitis
Evidence of ischemia
Closed loop syndrome
Failed conservative management (pSBO)
Obstructing neoplasms

tivity and specificity in the 90% range [10]. Additional clinical signs suggesting ischemia include leukocytosis and the presence of peritoneal signs on exam [13]. Early operative intervention is warranted in patients with signs and symptoms of complicated disease (Table 42.4).

Most patients undergoing open abdominal surgery develop adhesions (>90%). These are clinically symptomatic in a much smaller subset of patients, 10 to 15% [14]. In patients undergoing surgery for adhesion-induced bowel obstruction, the need for repeat adhesiolysis is common (10–30%) with risk factors including younger age, more frequent obstructive episodes, and prior non-operative management [15]. Laparascopic surgery is associated with a reduced incidence of bowel obstruction compared to open laparotomy. Although it is still not possible to prevent adhesive-related bowel obstruction, barrier substances and other materials reduce the development of adhesions with Seprafilm® (Genzyme Biosurgery) showing the most promise for preventing bowel obstruction [16,17].

Large Bowel Obstruction

Most cases of colonic obstruction result from neoplasms, most commonly colon cancer. Additional etiologies include colonic volvulus, inflammatory bowel disease, diverticular or ischemic strictures, and fecal impaction. Patients will typically describe abdominal pain and distension with an inability to pass stool or gas. Although nausea and vomiting may occur, they tend to occur later than with small bowel obstruction. Neoplasms and strictures tend to present with a gradual onset of symptoms, whereas volvulus presents acutely with a sudden onset of abdominal pain and distension. The initial evaluation of colonic obstruction is similar to that with small bowel obstruction. Plain abdominal radiographs (obstructive series) will frequently indicate the diagnosis. An important differentiation must be made between mechanical

obstruction and acute colonic pseudo-obstruction. Contrast enema radiography with water-soluble contrast will determine the presence or absence of an obstructing lesion more than 95% of the time [18].

Initial treatment of colonic obstruction begins with fluid resuscitation and correction of electrolyte abnormalities. Nasogastric tube suctioning may reduce nausea and vomiting, but have limited efficacy in reducing colonic distension. Likewise, rectal tubes may decompress the distal colon but do little to decompress the more proximal colon. As with small bowel obstruction, peritoneal findings and/or imaging results suggesting perforation or ischemia require urgent surgical intervention. The cause of the colonic obstruction will dictate the best therapeutic approach. For example, when obstruction is due to sigmoid volvulus and in the absence of peritoneal signs or ischemia, flexible sigmoidoscopy may be used to reduce the volvulus [19]. Cecal volvulus most commonly requires segmental resection. Fecal impaction as a cause of obstruction may be treated therapeutically by water-soluble contrast enema. Malignant obstruction typically requires surgical resection. In the setting of a distal (and possibly proximal), malignant partial colonic obstruction, endoscopic placement of a stent may facilitate bowel preparation, allowing a primary anastomosis rather than colostomy [20,21].

Intestinal Pseudo-obstruction

Chronic Intestinal Pseudo-obstruction

As the name implies, chronic intestinal pseudo-obstruction is characterized by chronic or recurrent episodes mimicking mechanical obstruction in the absence of any demonstrable obstructive lesion. Gastrointestinal motor function becomes uncoordinated with alterations in both fast and feed motor patterns. There may be a loss in the fasting period of phase III of the migrating motor complex (the "housekeeper" of the intestinal tract) resulting in retained debris in the stomach and bacterial overgrowth in the small intestine. Postprandially, normal mixing and propulsive motility are disrupted, resulting in nausea, vomiting, abdominal distension, and, most commonly, constipation. Diarrhea can result from overflow or small bowel bacterial overgrowth. In its most severe form, feeding difficulties result with malnutrition, weight loss, and death. Pseudo-obstruction results when

Table 42.5 Categories of intestinal pseudo-obstruction.

Chronic intestinal pseudo-obstruction
  Neuropathic
    Diabetes mellitus
    Postvagotomy
    Paraneoplastic
    Parkinson disease
    Dysautonomia
    Hirschsprung
    Chagas
    Inflammatory neuropathies (? autoimmune)
    Familial
  Myopathic
    Systemic sclerosis
    Ehlers–Danlos
    Familial (including mitochrondrial myopathies)
    Inflammatory myopathies (e.g., dermatomyositis)
  Mixed neuropathy/myopathy
    Amyloidosis
    Systemic sclerosis
    Radiation enteritis
  Iatrogenic
    Opiates
    Antipsychotics
    Antineoplastics

there has been significant disruption of the neural or muscular control of the gut. This may be primary (e.g., mitochondrial myopathy) or secondary (e.g., paraneoplastic). Pseudo-obstruction is most often categorized as neuropathic or myopathic (Table 42.5). The possibility of pseudo-obstruction should be considered in any patient presenting with recurrent "obstructive" episodes when no obstructing lesion can be found. This is particularly true in the setting of underlying diseases associated with pseudo-obstruction, including systemic sclerosis, diabetes mellitus, and neurologic disorders such as dysautonomia or Parkinson disease.

It remains imperative to exclude mechanical obstruction. Lesions that can be missed by routine imaging include retroperitoneal obstruction from masses (e.g., metastatic carcinoma) or fibrosis. Esophagogastroduodenoscopy (EGD) and CT radiography should be performed to exclude mechanical obstruction. Once mechanical obstruction has been definitively excluded, the evaluation moves towards identifying the cause of the pseudo-obstruction. While this differentiation can be initially suspected based on clinical findings and laboratory studies, small bowel manometry has traditionally provided the most definitive information, separating

myopathic from neuropathic and identifying unsuspected obstruction. Unfortunately, small bowel manometry is only available in highly specialized centers. A high index of suspicion is needed to identify paraneoplastic causes of pseudo-obstruction. This most commonly occurs with small cell lung cancer. Clues to this diagnosis include significant weight loss, older age, and history of smoking. The finding of positive antineoplastic antibodies (Anti-Hu, Anti-Ri N-type calcium channel antibody) indicates the need for further imaging to identifying occult malignancy.

Recent advances in motility testing include the use of a wireless device that measures intra-luminal pH, temperature, and pressure profiles as it travels through the digestive tract. The SmartPill® (Smartpill Corporation) provides a measure of gastric emptying, small bowel and colonic transit, and gastroduodenal motor patterns [22,23]. The use of the video capsule to assess small bowel motor patterns has also recently been described [24]. The availability of non-invasive techniques to facilitate the diagnosis of intestinal dysmotility is encouraging. However, the role of these newer, non-invasive techniques in the evaluation of intestinal motor dysfunctions remains to be defined. In particular, an ability to identify the underlying pathophysiology or direct treatment would be especially helpful.

The principles of managing pseudo-obstruction are the same regardless of the underlying cause. Initial attention addresses correcting fluid, electrolyte, and nutritional deficiencies. Metabolic disturbances affecting the gut should be considered and screened for in the appropriate setting (e.g., hypothyroidism, hyperparathyroidism, adrenal insufficiency). In the setting of dilated bowel and/or severe nausea and vomiting, nasogastric suction may be helpful in the acute setting. Pharmacotherapy with prokinetics would be ideal to restore the abnormal motor function, but there exists a paucity of available agents. Most pharmacotherapy addresses symptom treatment (Table 42.6). Metoclopramide remains the only FDA approved prokinetic agent. Its main efficacy in pseudo-obstruction may relate to its antiemetic properties. Careful monitoring for side effects is required, including dystonia, depression, exacerbation of Parkinson disease, galactorrhea, and tardive dyskinesia. Erythromycin at a dose of 3 mg/kg promptly empties the stomach. An effective prokinetic acutely, its efficacy long-term has been disappointing. In addition, it does not

Table 42.6 Management of intestinal pseudo-obstruction.

Fluid resuscitate

Correct electrolytes

Antiemetics
  Promethazine
  Prochlorperazine
  Ondansetron
  Granisetron
  Trimethobenzamide
  Metoclopramide

Look for and treat small bowel bacterial overgrowth
  Rifaximin
  Doxycycline
  Amoxicillin/clavulinic acid
  Ciprofloxacin
  Metronidazole

Analgesia
  Aim for non-narcotic control
  Tramadol
  Low-dose tricyclic antidepressants

Prokinetics
  Metoclopramide
  Erythromycin
  Domperidone
  Neostigmine

Table 42.7 Dietary suggestions in intestinal pseudo-obstruction.

Smaller volume, more frequent meals
Lower fat
Lower residue (avoiding difficult-to-process raw fruits and vegetables)
Pureed foods
Liquid nutrition supplements (preferably lower fat)

appear to improve symptoms and may exacerbate nausea and vomiting. Domperidone is not available in the United States, although it is widely available in other countries. A dopamine antagonist, it is an effective antiemetic with some prokinetic properties. It does not cause the central nervous system side effects seen with metoclopramide (except for elevation in prolactin and galactorrhea). Currently, no other prokinetics are approved in the United States. A 5-HT$_4$ antagonist prucalopride, a prokinetic, has been recently approved in Europe for irritable bowel syndrome and constipation. Its efficacy in pseudo-obstruction syndromes is unknown. Cisapride, a prokinetic agent previously shown to accelerate gastric emptying and improve symptoms in pseudo-obstruction, was removed from the market due to the induction of fatal cardiac dysrhythmias. Cisapride is available through an investigational limited access program through the FDA. Octreotide at a dose of 50 μg administered subcutaneously was shown to improve symptoms and reduce small bowel bacterial overgrowth in scleroderma [25]. In the absence of effective prokinetics, treat-

ment goals are to restore nutritional deficiencies and minimize symptoms.

For nutrition, enteral feeding should be attempted whenever possible. Although the underlying motor disturbance may be severe, in the absence of small bowel bacterial overgrowth, absorption often remains preserved. In patient with severe motor disturbances of the digestive tract (e.g., end-stage systemic sclerosis), parenteral nutrition may be needed. Oral nutrition, using a modified diet, may be successful in some patients (Table 42.7). When a patient is unable to ingest adequate nutrition orally, enteral tube feeding may be used (gastrostomy or jejunostomy). Patients with severe gastric emptying delay may require jejunal feeding tubes. Continuous, slow infusion of formula may be needed, as the gut may not tolerate bolus feedings or rapid infusion. Patients on modified diets should receive a general multivitamin and, when deficient, supplementation for other vitamin and mineral deficiencies. Patients with weight loss, unable to tolerate oral or enteral nutrition will require parenteral nutrition.

Symptom management includes the treatment of reflux disease, use of antiemetics, pain control, treatment of small bowel bacterial overgrowth, and diarrhea or constipation (when present). Providing alternatives to orally administered medications is essential. Consider orally dissolving, subcutaneous, and rectal administration of medications. Intravenous antiemetic administration is often required in the acute setting until oral intake can be resumed. When pain control with narcotics becomes necessary in the acute setting, a plan for discontinuation should be addressed early. Non-narcotic alternatives for treatment of pain include the use of acetaminophen, tramadol, low-dose tricyclic antidepressants (choosing one with the least anticholinergic effects), gabapentin, pregabalin, and lidocaine patches. Occasionally, non-steroidal anti-inflammatory drugs may be used, although risk for gastrointestinal toxicity must be considered. Treatment of bacterial overgrowth may be accomplished with intermittent or rotating antibiotics. Although antimicrobials limited to the gut are preferable (e.g., rifaximin), cost considerations dictate the more typical use of systemic antibiotics. Although autoimmune and inflammatory enteric neuropathies have been described, there exists minimal support for the use of prednisone or other immunosuppressants in the treatment of intestinal pseudo-obstruction.

Treatment of underlying medical conditions may improve the gastrointestinal disturbance. In patient with diabetes mellitus, proper glucose control remains important. Patients with active underlying rheumatologic conditions may also see improved GI symptoms with use of disease-modifying agents. Chronic intestinal pseudo-obstruction is a severe illness with up to 50% of individuals requiring supplemental nutrition and a mortality of 35% over 10 years [26]. Patients with refractory illness and those with complications from parenteral nutrition may benefit from abdominal visceral transplantation.

Enteric Dysmotility

The term "enteric dysmotility" has been coined to describe the subgroup of patients with severe gastrointestinal symptoms who do not have radiologic features of pseudo-obstruction. Required for the diagnosis is the presence of abnormal small bowel manometric findings, a specialized study not available at most centers [27]. Due the risk of subsequent adhesions and small bowel obstruction, the practice of full-thickness biopsy had been abandoned. Recent studies suggest another look at this strategy, especially now that laparoscopic biopsy can be obtained with minimal morbidity and no mortality. Investigators have identified the presence of an enteric inflammatory neuropathy in chronic intestinal pseudo-obstruction and in enteric dysmotility [28]. Interestingly, the manometric findings did not reliably predict the presence of neuropathy versus myopathy in this study, except in the most advanced stages of intestinal pseudo-obstruction. Importantly, early myopathic changes histologically were seen in individuals with neuropathic changes on manometry. The finding of enteric inflammatory neuropathy raises interesting questions about the treatment of these conditions. Consideration for full-thickness jejunal biopsy should be given in patients with intestinal pseudo-obstruction requiring abdominal surgery for other reasons. However, in order to recommend the routine performance of this invasive procedure, it will be necessary to demonstrate that we have treatments that can reverse or stabilize the underlying pathology and reduce symptoms with minimum morbidity.

Acute Colonic Pseudo-obstruction

Acute colonic pseudo-obstruction usually presents in hospitalized patients with other medical problems or recent surgical intervention. Risk factors include older age, surgery (including orthopedic surgery), narcotic pain control, and electrolyte abnormalities. A mortality of 30% highlights the medical seriousness of this condition. Patients present with progressive abdominal distension, pain, nausea, and vomiting. Abdominal radiography shows diffuse colonic dilatation. In the setting of peritoneal findings, fever, and/or leukocytosis, urgent surgical consultation is mandatory. As previously noted, mechanical obstruction should be excluded by CT scan or water-soluble contrast enema. Initial measures remove offending medications that slow motility and correct electrolyte abnormalities. Nasogastric tube suctioning, rectal tube placement and rotating the patient's position to facilitate gas passage are often employed with varying degrees of effectiveness. Neostigmine safely resolves colonic pseudo-obstruction in nearly 90% of cases. Cardiac monitoring is necessary and neostigmine should be avoided in the settings of significant bradycardia, active bronchospasm, or obstruction. Patients that fail to improve or have contraindications to neostigmine may be treated with endoscopic colon decompression, and, if evidence of toxicity, surgery.

Conclusion

Patients presenting with acute or recurring episodes of abdominal pain, nausea, vomiting, and abdominal distension with imaging suggesting obstruction must first undergo evaluation for mechanically obstructing lesions. When complete bowel obstruction is present or in the setting of peritonitis or suspected ischemia, early surgical intervention is warranted. Patients with partial bowel obstruction can usually be managed medically. Radiologic imaging helps to define the location and cause of most obstructions. Most cases of small bowel obstruction result from adhesive disease, whereas colonic obstruction is usually due to neoplasm. It remains essential to exclude mechanical obstruction in all patients with suspected intestinal pseudo-obstruction. A search for potentially treatable causes of secondary pseudo-obstruction must be undertaken, including evaluation for metabolic, rheumatologic, paraneoplastic, and medication-related adverse effects. In the absence of highly effective prokinetic agents, treatment is directed at correcting underlying nutritional deficiencies and control of symptoms. Newer imaging and diagnostic modalities for mechanical obstruction and pseudo-obstruction hold promise to more efficiently and non-invasively (or minimally invasively) identify the underlying problem. The development of novel treatments directed at reversing the effects of the underlying disease process may be possible with early diagnosis of intestinal pseudo-obstruction. Advances in operative techniques promise to reduce the development of adhesions and, hopefully, episodes of bowel obstruction.

Case continued

The patient undergoes a chest X-ray for a new cough and is found to have a mass. Her GI workup includes panendoscopy and is unremarkable. Serologic work up reveals positive paraneoplastic antibodies and she is diagnosed with small cell lung cancer and chronic pseudo-obstruction.

Take-home points

- Exclude mechanical obstruction first in patients with unexplained nausea, vomiting, and abdominal pain. Begin with an abdominal obstruction series during typical symptoms. If positive consider EGD, small bowel barium examination, and CT/MR enterography.

- Many patients with partial small bowel obstruction may be managed medically.

- Patients with complete bowel obstruction or signs of peritonitis typically require surgery.

- In the patient with older age, new-onset symptoms, profound weight loss, and/or a history of smoking, evaluate for malignancy.

- Address fluid, electrolyte, and nutritional status in all patients with obstruction or pseudo-obstruction.

- In patients with pseudo-obstruction, symptom management remains the cornerstone of therapy.

References

1 Menzies D, Ellis H. Intestinal obstruction from adhesions—how big is the problem? *Ann Roy Coll Surg Engl* 1990; **72**: 60–3.

2 Cappell MS, Batke M. Mechanical obstruction of the small bowel and colon. *Med Clin North Am* 2008; **92**: 575–97.

3 Gutt CN, Oniu T, Schemmer P, et al. Fewer adhesions induced by laparoscopic surgery? *Surg Endosc* 2004; **18**: 898–906.

4 Maglinte DD, Reyes BL, Harmon BH, et al. Reliability and role of plain film radiography and CT in the diagnosis of small-bowel obstruction. *AJR Am J Roentgenol* 1996; **167**: 1451–5.

5 Ha HK, Kim JS, Lee MS, et al. Differentiation of simple and strangulated small-bowel obstructions: usefulness of known CT criteria. *Radiology* 1997; **204**: 507–12.

6 Siddiki HA, Fidler JL, Fletcher JG, et al. Prospective comparison of state-of-the-art MR enterography and CT enterography in small-bowel Crohn's disease. *AJR Am J Roentgenol* 2009; **193**: 113–21.

7 Peetz DJ Jr, Gamelli RL, Pilcher DB. Intestinal intubation in acute, mechanical small-bowel obstruction. *Arch Surg* 1982; **117**: 334–6.

8 Brolin RE. Partial small bowel obstruction. *Surgery* 1984; **95**: 145–9.

9 Brolin RE, Krasna MJ, Mast BA. Use of tubes and radiographs in the management of small bowel obstruction. *Ann Surg* 1987; **206**: 126–33.

10 Mallo RD, Salem L, Lalani T, Flum DR. Computed tomography diagnosis of ischemia and complete obstruction in small bowel obstruction: a systematic review. *J Gastroint Surg* 2005; **9**: 690–4.

11 Fletcher JG. CT enterography technique: theme and variations. *Abdom Imag* 2009; **34**: 283–8.

12 Gourtsoyianni S, Zamboni GA, Romero JY, Raptopoulos VD. Routine use of modified CT Enterography in patients with acute abdominal pain. *Eur J Radiol* 2009; **69**: 388–92.

13 Jancelewicz T, Vu LT, Shawo AE, et al. Predicting strangulated small bowel obstruction: an old problem revisited. *J Gastroint Surg* 2009; **13**: 93–9.

14 Beck DE, Opelka FG, Bailey HR, et al. Incidence of small-bowel obstruction and adhesiolysis after open colorectal and general surgery. *Dis Colon Rectum* 1999; **42**: 241–8.

15 Barkan H, Webster S, Ozeran S. Factors predicting the recurrence of adhesive small-bowel obstruction. *Am J Surg* 1995; **170**: 361–5.

16 Fazio VW, Cohen Z, Fleshman JW, et al. Reduction in adhesive small-bowel obstruction by Seprafilm adhesion barrier after intestinal resection. *Dis Colon Rectum* 2006; **49**: 1–11.

17 Oncel M, Remzi FM, Senagore AJ, *et al*. Comparison of a novel liquid (Adcon-P) and a sodium hyaluronate and carboxymethylcellulose membrane (Seprafilm) in postsurgical adhesion formation in a murine model. *Dis Colon Rectum* 2003; **46**: 187–91.

18 Chapman AH, McNamara M, Porter G. The acute contrast enema in suspected large bowel obstruction: value and technique. *Clin Radiol* 1992; **46**: 273–8.

19 Oren D, Atamanalp SS, Aydinli B, *et al*. An algorithm for the management of sigmoid colon volvulus and the safety of primary resection: experience with 827 cases. *Dis Colon Rectum* 2007; **50**: 489–97.

20 Breitenstein S, Rickenbacher A, Berdajs D, *et al*. Systematic evaluation of surgical strategies for acute malignant left-sided colonic obstruction. *Br J Surg* 2007; **94**: 1451–60.

21 Dronamraju SS, Ramamurthy S, Kelly SB, Hayat M. Role of self-expanding metallic stents in the management of malignant obstruction of the proximal colon. *Dis Colon Rectum* 2009; **52**: 1657–61.

22 Cassilly D, Kantor S, Knight LC, *et al*. Gastric emptying of a non-digestible solid: assessment with simultaneous SmartPill pH and pressure capsule, antroduodenal manometry, gastric emptying scintigraphy. *Neurogastroenterol Motil* 2008; **20**: 311–9.

23 Kuo B, McCullum RW, Koch KZ, *et al*. Comparison of gastric emptying of a nondigestible capsule to a radio-labelled meal in healthy and gastroparetic subjects. *Aliment Pharmacol Therap* 2008; **27**: 186–96.

24 Malagelada C, De Iorio F, Azpiroz F, *et al*. New insight into intestinal motor function via noninvasive endoluminal image analysis. *Gastroenterology* 2008; **135**: 1155–62.

25 Soudah HC, Hasler WL, Owyang C. Effect of octreotide on intestinal motility and bacterial overgrowth in scleroderma. *N Engl J Med* 1991; **325**: 1461–7.

26 Lindberg G, Iwarzon M, Tornblom H. Clinical features and long-term survival in chronic intestinal pseudo-obstruction and enteric dysmotility. *Scand J Gastroenterol* 2009; **44**: 692–9.

27 Wingate D, Hongo M, Kellow J, *et al*. Disorders of gastrointestinal motility: towards a new classification. *J Gastroenterol Hepatol* 2002; **17**: S1–14.

28 Lindberg G, Törnblum H, Iwarzon M, *et al*. Full-thickness biopsy findings in chronic intestinal pseudo-obstruction and enteric dysmotility. *Gut* 2009; **58**: 1084–90.

PART 6

Diseases of the Colon and Rectum

CHAPTER 43
Ulcerative Colitis

Timothy L. Zisman[1] and Stephen B. Hanauer[2]

[1] Division of Gastroenterology, University of Washington Medical Center, Seattle, WA, USA
[2] Section of Gastroenterology, Hepatology and Nutrition, University of Chicago Medical Center, Chicago, IL, USA

Summary

Inflammatory bowel disease encompasses a spectrum between ulcerative colitis and Crohn disease. Ulcerative colitis is manifest by diffuse, continuous, and superficial inflammation that begins in the rectum and extends proximally to a variable extent in individual patients. In approximately 15% of patients with inflammatory bowel disease confined to the colon the pattern of inflammation is not distinguishable, necessitating the term indeterminate colitis or IBD-U (unclassified). Features that are helpful to discriminate between ulcerative colitis and Crohn disease include: family history, smoking history, presence of perianal manifestations, aphthous ulcerations, strictures, and fistulae. Therapeutic approaches are aimed at induction and maintenance of clinical remissions. Inductive agents include aminosalicylates, corticosteroids, cyclosporine, and monoclonal antibodies targeting tumor necrosis factor (TNF). Maintenance therapies include aminosalicylates, thiopurines, or anti-TNF agents. Colectomy is an option for refractory disease.

Case

A 20-year-old male with no past medical history presents with 2 months of rectal bleeding, increasingly loose stools associated with urgency, and nocturnal bowel movements. Additionally, he describes intermittent, subjective, low-grade fevers, a 4.5 kg (10 pound) weight loss and bilateral pain and swelling in his knees. He smokes a pack of cigarettes daily and his maternal uncle has ulcerative colitis. On physical exam his abdomen is soft and non-distended with mild, diffuse tenderness to palpation. Perianal exam reveals external skin tags with no fissure or fistula. Laboratory studies reveal mild leukocytosis with a left shift and microcytic anemia. Colonoscopy shows patchy inflammation of the entire colon with a normal terminal ileum.

Definition

Ulcerative colitis (UC) and Crohn disease (CD) encompass a spectrum of chronic idiopathic colitides [1]. The

Practical Gastroenterology and Hepatology: Small and Large Intestine and Pancreas, 1st edition. Edited by Nicholas J. Talley, Sunanda V. Kane and Michael B. Wallace. © 2010 Blackwell Publishing Ltd.

inflammation of UC is confined to the colon in a diffuse, continuous, and superficial (mucosal) pattern beginning at the anorectal junction and extending proximally to a distinct margin that differs amongst individuals. Approximately one-third of patients have disease limited to the rectum (ulcerative proctitis), one-third of patients have disease to the splenic flexure (proctosigmoiditis or left-sided colitis), and a third present with disease extending proximal to the splenic flexure up to the cecum (pancolitis). The term indeterminate colitis, or IBD-U (inflammatory bowel disease unclassified) has been used to describe patients with clinical and inflammatory features that are difficult to distinguish between classical UC and CD [2].

Epidemiology

The incidence of UC and CD in North America and Europe are similar, ranging from 2 to 14 cases per 100 000 population with a prevalence of 50–200 cases per 100 000 population [3]. While IBD colitis can occur from infancy to adulthood, there is a bimodal age distribution with the largest peak in the second–third decade of life and a smaller peak in the fifth–sixth decade of life. There is a roughly equal distribution between males and females.

Risk Factors

The primary risk factor for colitis is a family history of either UC or CD [3]. Appendectomy at a young age appears to be protective against the development of UC whereas cigarette smoking is the major environmental factor. Cigarette smoking is inversely ("protective") associated with UC but is positively associated with CD. Within families with a history of IBD, smokers tend to develop CD whereas non-smokers are more likely to develop UC [4].

Pathophysiology

Although the immunopathologic underpinnings of IBD remain elusive, a combination of genetic disposition and triggering environmental factors are hypothesized to lead to a chronic, dysregulated, acute inflammation [5]. Currently, up to 30 genes have been identified that are associated with IBD. The penetrance appears to be higher for CD where there is a higher concordance rate among monozygotic twins compared with dizygotic twins. While familial clustering of cases is well described, only 10–20% of patients with IBD have a positive family history.

Clinical Features

Ulcerative Colitis

Patients with UC typically experience rectal bleeding with urgency to evacuate, most commonly upon awakening or after meals. Many patients also describe increased stool frequency, nocturnal bowel movements, tenesmus, incontinence, and inability to pass gas without leakage of stool. Diarrhea is related to the extent of colonic involvement; patients with limited proctitis may describe constipation and difficulty evacuating with rectal bleeding. Patients with severe disease may present with fever, tachycardia, anorexia, and weight loss.

Indeterminate Colitis

Up to 15% of patients with IBD-colitis present with disease confined to the colon, but with features precluding distinct categorization as either UC or CD [2,6,7]. Clinical clues that signal suspicion for CD include a strong family history of CD, smoking at the time of diagnosis, perianal skin tags, nephrolithiasis, oral aphthae, and/or deep serpiginous ulcers at endoscopy. Patchy inflammation of the colon on endoscopy is indicative of CD; unless the colitis has been treated, in which case there may be some evidence of focal endoscopic findings.

Extra-intestinal Manifestations of IBD

UC is a systemic disease that can result in inflammation of organ systems aside from the gastrointestinal tract in 20–40% of patients [8]. Arthralgias and arthritis are the most common extraintestinal manifestation, affecting approximately one-quarter of patients with IBD. They are typically pauciarticular, involving larger joints, and parallel disease activity. Less commonly a polyarticular, symmetric arthritis or axial arthritis (ankylosing spondylitis, sacroiliitis) can present and progress independently of colitis [9].

Cutaneous lesions associated with colitis include erythema nodosum and pyoderma gangrenosum. Oral aphthous ulcers are fairly common but occur more often in patients with CD. Ocular manifestations can include uveitis (iritis), scleritis, or episcleritis.

Primary sclerosing cholangitis (PSC) is another disease of non-smokers that affects 3–4% of patients with UC or CD. The diagnosis is usually confirmed with magnetic resonance or endoscopic cholangiography showing a classic "beads on a string" in the small bile ducts, or a dominant stricture in the common hepatic or bile duct. Liver biopsy may be required in patients with involvement confined to the small intrahepatic ducts. Complications of PSC include acute cholangitis, choledocholithiasis, cholangiocarcinoma, and biliary cirrhosis.

Complications of IBD

Intestinal and systemic complications can occur in the setting of IBD-colitis [10]. Intestinal complications of UC include: hemorrhage, toxic megacolon, perforation, and neoplasia.

Extraintestinal complications are related to the pathophysiology or therapies associated with IBD-colitis.

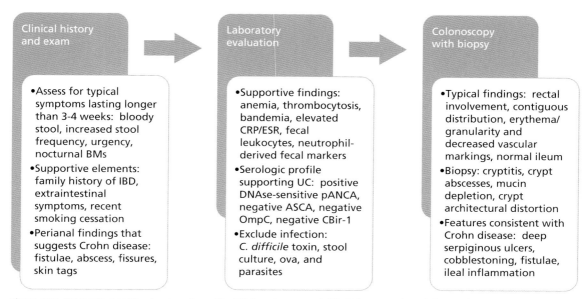

Figure 43.1 Diagnostic algorithm for ulcerative colitis. BM, bowel movement; IBD, inflammatory bowel disease; CRP, C-reactive protein; ESR, erythrocyte sedimentation rate; UC, ulcerative colitis; pANCA, perinuclear antineutrophil cytoplasmic antibody; ASCA, anti-*Saccharomyces cerevisiae* antibody; OmpC, antibody to *E. coli* outer membrane protein C; CBir1, antibody to CBir1 flagellin.

Osteopenia and osteoporosis can result from IBD itself or from chronic corticosteroid therapy such that patients with small bowel disease or those receiving chronic steroids should undergo bone mineral density testing and treatment for associated metabolic bone disease [11].

Anemia is common in IBD patients and is often multifactorial in etiology [12]. Iron deficiency is a common consequence of intestinal blood loss. IBD patients are at increased risk for thromboembolic events, likely attributable to chronic systemic inflammation [13].

Patients with IBD-colitis are at increased risk for colorectal carcinoma. Risk factors for neoplasia include younger age at diagnosis, long disease duration, and anatomic extent, family history of colorectal cancer, severity of inflammation, and coexisting PSC [14].

Diagnosis

Inflammatory bowel disease is a clinical diagnosis that involves comprehensive integration of history, physical findings, imaging, endoscopy, and histology. Serologic studies are evolving but are not yet definitive. No single test can conclusively establish the diagnosis, and exclu-

sion of other diseases that can mimic IBD is essential [1,15] (Figure 43.1).

Historical Factors

Although IBD can present at any age, the classic age of onset is during the second or third decade of life. A family history of IBD should increase suspicion of the diagnosis in a patient with typical symptoms. Smoking increases the risk of CD, whereas smoking cessation is associated with onset of UC. Use of aspirin or other non-steroidal anti-inflammatory drugs is a common precipitant of disease onset or exacerbation. Additionally, many patients present after an apparent episode of infectious diarrhea or recent exposure to antibiotics [3].

Physical Examination

The physical examination is frequently unrevealing in patients with mild to moderate colitis but those with severe or fulminant disease may demonstrate fever, tachycardia, abdominal distension, and tenderness.

Laboratory Evaluation

Laboratory studies are often normal in patients with mild disease. Anemia or electrolyte abnormalities may be present in a patient according to the chronicity and severity of symptoms. Erythrocyte sedimentation rate or C-reactive protein tend to parallel inflammatory activity but are not always reliable markers for individual patients [16]. In the setting of severe colitis patients may develop hypoalbuminemia, hypokalemia, or metabolic acidosis. Stool evaluation for ova and parasites, culture, and *Clostridium difficile* toxin are important to exclude infection at the time of initial diagnosis or disease relapse. Other stool markers of intestinal inflammation (calprotectin and lactoferrin) are being explored as diagnostic or prognostic tools [17]. Serologic evaluation for presence of antibodies to nuclear or gut luminal antigens is another exciting area of investigation. However, at this time, the role of these tests for diagnostic or prognostic purposes has not been solidly established [18].

Imaging

In the setting of colitis, colonoscopy has a primary role in diagnosis; however, advances in imaging continue to evolve beyond contrast barium studies. Computed tomography and magnetic resonance imaging provide additional information about bowel wall thickening and can better define the presence of extraintestinal complications such as abscesses or fistulae [19]. In the setting of severe colitis patients should have supine and upright abdominal radiographs performed to evaluate for megacolon, free air, or pneumatosis.

Endoscopy

Endoscopy is essential for establishing the diagnosis of colitis, determining the anatomical distribution of involvement, excluding complicating factors in patients not responding to therapy, assessing for disease recurrence in postoperative patients, and distinguishing CD from UC [20]. Although there are no endoscopic features that are pathognomonic for UC or for CD, certain findings are highly suggestive [1,6]. The classic endoscopic appearance of UC includes decreased vascular markings with diffuse erythema and granularity, extending proximally from the rectum in a continuous distribution. In patients receiving rectal therapy, the rectum may appear spared. Ulceration of the ileum or visualization of fistulae during colonoscopy are diagnostic features of CD while pseudopolyps may be present in either UC or CD. Wireless capsule endoscopy is not as helpful in the work up of UC as in CD [21].

Colonoscopy also serves as the cornerstone colorectal cancer prevention strategy in this high-risk population. Consensus guidelines recommend an initial screening colonoscopy in this high-risk patient group beginning 8–10 years after symptom onset, with subsequent surveillance colonoscopy every 1–2 years. Random biopsies as well as targeted biopsies of suspicious lesions should be obtained, and colectomy should be considered for patients in whom dysplasia or cancer is identified [14].

Pathology

Histologic features such as crypt architectural distortion suggest chronic injury and can aid in the distinction between acute self-limited colitis and chronic idiopathic IBD [15]. Typical histologic findings in early UC include acute cryptitis, crypt abscesses, mucin depletion, and plasma cell infiltration of the lamina propria.

Differential Diagnosis

The differential diagnosis of IBD is given in Table 43.1.

Case continued

The patient was initially started on oral mesalamine without improvement in his symptoms. Oral corticosteroids were then initiated and the patient achieved symptomatic remission, including resolution of his joint pains and low-grade fever. He was then transitioned to azathioprine for maintenance of remission and the steroids were withdrawn over the next few months.

Therapeutics

The goals of therapy in IBD patients are to induce and maintain symptomatic remission, and prevent complications of disease and therapies. The intensity of therapy used to induce remission generally dictates the effective maintenance strategies.

Current approaches to therapy include sequential induction to maintenance treatment according to the severity of symptoms at diagnosis [21–24] (Figure 43.2). Patients with mild UC (ambulatory patients with symptoms that do not have a major impact on quality of life and less than four to six bowel movements daily and without extraintestinal manifestations) can be treated

Table 43.1 Differential diagnosis of inflammatory bowel disease.

Bacterial colitis
    Salmonella
    Shigella
    Yersinia
    Campylobacter
    Enterohemorrhagic *E. coli*
    Enterotoxigenic *E. coli*
    Clostridium difficile
    Aeromonas
    Pleisiomonas

Viruses
    Cytomegalovirus
    Herpes simplex virus

Parasites
    Entamoeba histolytica

Microscopic colitis

Lymphocytic colitis

Collagenous colitis

Diverticular colitis

Ischemic colitis

Radiation enteritis/colitis

Celiac disease

Appendicitis

NSAID colitis

Neutropenic enterocolitis

Vasculitis

Sarcoidosis

Amyloidosis

with aminosalicylates. If symptoms completely resolve on aminosalicylates, maintenance therapy with an aminosalicylate should be continued. Patients with moderate to severe symptoms or those who fail to respond to aminosalicylates are induced with corticosteroids or an anti-TNF biologic. Steroid-induction more often requires maintenance therapy with a thiopurine, or anti-TNF biologic, in particular if the colitis is not controlled by high-dose (e.g., 4–5 g/day) mesalamine. Patients who fail steroid-induction or maintenance therapy with a thiopurine typically respond to anti-TNF induction and regularly scheduled maintenance therapy.

5-Aminosalicylates

Aminosalicylates (mesalamine, sulfasalazine, olsalazine, balsalazide) are first-line therapies for induction and remission of mild to moderate UC and, despite conflicting evidence, are often used early in the treatment algorithm for CD [22–25]. Several oral and rectally administered preparations are available, each employing unique mechanisms for delivering 5-ASA (mesalamine) to the colon. Specific delivery mechanisms include linking 5-ASA to a carrier molecule via an azo bond that is cleaved by colonic bacteria, use of moisture-dependent time-release granules that deliver 5-ASA throughout the bowel, or pH-dependent coatings that release 5-ASA in the terminal ileum and colon [26]. Mesalamine delivered topically, as an enema foam or suppository, is highly effective to treat distal colitis. Side effects are rare with this class of medications, but may include interstitial nephritis, pancreatitis, hepatitis, pneumonitis, or peri-

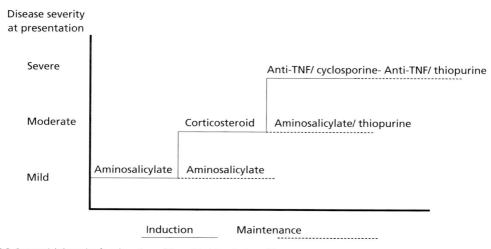

Figure 43.2 Sequential therapies for ulcerative colitis and indeterminate colitis.

carditis. Sulfasalazine is also associated with sulfa-related hypersensitivity.

Antibiotics

Antibiotics have no primary role in the treatment of UC.

Corticosteroids

Systemic corticosteroids are effective therapies to induce remission for moderate–severe colitis and can be delivered orally or intravenously [27]. However, the unacceptable adverse effect profile of steroids precludes their long-term use as maintenance therapies. Rectal steroids can be administered for patients with distal disease.

Thiopurine Immunosuppressants

Mercaptopurine (6-MP) and its prodrug azathioprine (AZA) are purine analogues that interfere with nucleic acid synthesis and exhibit anti-inflammatory properties through their cytotoxic effect on inflammatory cells [27]. They are effective therapies for maintenance of remission in UC and can facilitate withdrawal of steroids in patients who are otherwise steroid-dependent. Adverse effects include allergic reactions, infection, pancreatitis, bone marrow suppression, or hepatitis. Additionally, there is a slightly increased risk of lymphoma [28]. Bone marrow suppression and therapeutic efficacy are related to genetic polymorphisms of the thiopurine-*S*-methyltransferase (TPMT) enzyme which can be measured to allow customized dosing to enhance both safety and efficacy.

Cyclosporine

Intravenous cyclosporine can be used as salvage therapy to induce remission in severe UC refractory to intravenous steroids [23,24,27]. Although effective for short-term induction maintenance therapy with a thiopurine is required. Side effects include headache, tremor, paresthesias, seizures, hypertrichosis, hypertension, renal insufficiency, and opportunistic infections. The risk of pneumocystis pneumonia during cyclosporine therapy is substantial enough to warrant antimicrobial prophylaxis.

Tumor Necrosis Factor-α Inhibitors

Tumor necrosis factor (TNF) α is a pro-inflammatory cytokine that plays a key role in propagating the inflammatory cascade of IBD [27,29]. Monoclonal antibodies targeted against TNF include infliximab and adalim-

umab and an Fab′ fragment linked to polyethylene glycol (certolizumab pegol) which are highly effective at inducing and maintaining clinical, endoscopic, and histologic improvement in IBD patients refractory to conventional therapies and are effective for healing CD fistulae. Infliximab is approved for induction and maintenance in UC, whereas adalimumab and certolizumab are currently only approved for CD. The efficacy and safety profiles are comparable among the available anti-TNF agents. Opportunistic infections attributable to the immunosuppressive mechanism of these medications include fungal pneumonias and tuberculosis. Consequently, patients should be properly immunized (pneumonia, tetanus, influenza, HPV) and routinely tested for latent tuberculosis prior to initiation of an anti-TNF therapy. Other side effects include allergic reactions, infusion or injection site reactions, delayed hypersensitivity reactions, drug-induced lupus, heart failure, and demyelinating disease.

Surgical Therapy for UC

Indications for surgery in UC include medically refractory disease, inability to wean off steroids, toxic megacolon, perforation, or confirmed dysplasia or cancer. Surgical options include proctocolectomy with permanent ileostomy, or total colectomy with ileal pouch anal anastomosis. These surgeries are considered curative for UC, although half of patients can develop inflammation in the ileal pouch necessitating antibiotics, steroids, or anti-TNF agents [30].

Take-home points

- There are no pathognomonic markers for ulcerative colitis or Crohn disease.
- Diagnosis is based upon endoscopy, histology, and imaging.
- Therapeutic goals include induction and maintenance of clinical remissions.
- Aminosalicylates are inductive and maintenance therapies for mild–moderate disease.
- Corticosteroids are used to induce, but not maintain, remissions.
- Anti-TNF agents can induce and maintain remissions when conventional agents fail.
- Surgical removal of the colon is usually curative for UC.

References

1 Sands BE. From symptom to diagnosis: clinical distinctions among various forms of intestinal inflammation. *Gastroenterology* 2004; **126**: 1518–32.

2 Geboes K, Colombel JF, Greenstein A, *et al*. Indeterminate colitis: a review of the concept—what's in a name? *Inflamm Bowel Dis* 2008; **14**: 850–7.

3 Loftus EV Jr. Clinical epidemiology of inflammatory bowel disease: Incidence, prevalence, and environmental influences. *Gastroenterology* 2004; **126**: 1504–17.

4 Mahid SS, Minor KS, Soto RE, *et al*. Smoking and inflammatory bowel disease: a meta-analysis. *Mayo Clin Proc* 2006; **81**: 1462–71.

5 Xavier RJ, Podolsky DK. Unravelling the pathogenesis of inflammatory bowel disease. *Nature* 2007; **448**: 427–34.

6 Tremaine WJ. Review article: Indeterminate colitis— definition, diagnosis and management. *Aliment Pharmacol Therap* 2007; **25**: 13–7.

7 Martland GT, Shepherd NA. Indeterminate colitis: definition, diagnosis, implications and a plea for nosological sanity. *Histopathology* 2007; **50**: 83–96.

8 Ardizzone S, Puttini PS, Cassinotti A, *et al*. Extraintestinal manifestations of inflammatory bowel disease. *Dig Liver Dis* 2008; **40** (Suppl. 2): S253–9.

9 Williams H, Walker D, Orchard TR. Extraintestinal manifestations of inflammatory bowel disease. *Curr Gastroenterol Rep* 2008; **10**: 597–605.

10 Marrero F, Qadeer MA, Lashner BA. Severe complications of inflammatory bowel disease. *Med Clin North Am* 2008; **92**: 671.

11 Lichtenstein GR, Sands BE, Pazianas M. Prevention and treatment of osteoporosis in inflammatory bowel disease. *Inflammat Bowel Dis* 2006; **12**: 797–813.

12 Gasche C, Berstad A, Befrits R, *et al*. Guidelines on the diagnosis and management of iron deficiency and anemia in inflammatory bowel diseases. *Inflamm Bowel Dis* 2007; **13**: 1545–53.

13 Irving PM, Pasi KJ, Rampton DS. Thrombosis and inflammatory bowel disease. *Clin Gastroenterol Hepatol* 2005; **3**: 617–28.

14 Ullman T, Odze R, Farraye FA. Diagnosis and management of dysplasia in patients with ulcerative colitis and Crohn's disease of the colon. *Inflamm Bowel Dis* 2009; **15**: 630–8.

15 Yantiss RK, Odze RD. Diagnostic difficulties in inflammatory bowel disease pathology. *Histopathology* 2006; **48**: 116–32.

16 Jones J, Loftus EV, Panaccione R, *et al*. Relationships between disease activity and serum and fecal biomarkers in patients with Crohn's disease. *Clin Gastroenterol Hepatol* 2008; **6**: 1218–24.

17 Desai D, Faubion WA, Sandborn WJ. Review article: biological activity markers in inflammatory bowel disease. *Aliment Pharmacol Ther* 2007; **25**: 247–55.

18 Vermeire S, Vermeulen N, Van Assche G, *et al*. (Auto)Antibodies in inflammatory bowel diseases. *Gastroenterol Clin North Am* 2008; **37**: 429–38.

19 Bruining DH, Loftus EV. Evolving diagnostic strategies for inflammatory bowel disease. *Curr Gastroenterol Rep* 2006; **8**: 478–85.

20 Vanderheyden AD, Mitros FA. Pathologist surgeon interface in idiopathic inflammatory bowel disease. *Surg Clin North Am* 2007; **87**: 763–85.

21 Solem CA, Loftus EV, Fletcher JG, *et al*. Small-bowel imaging in Crohn's disease: a prospective, blinded, 4-way comparison trial. *Gastrointest Endosc* 2008; **68**: 255–66.

22 Lichtenstein GR, Hanauer SB, Sandborn WJ. Management of Crohn's disease in adults. *Am J Gastroenterol* 2009; **104**: 465–83.

23 Kornbluth A, Sachar DB. Ulcerative colitis practice guidelines in adults (update): American College of Gastroenterology, Practice Parameters Committee. *Am J Gastroenterol* 2004; **99**: 1371–85.

24 Travis SP, Stange EF, Lemann M, *et al*. European consensus on the diagnosis and management of ulcerative colitis: current management. *J Crohn's Colitis* 2008; **2**: 24–62.

25 Travis SP, *et al*. European evidence based consensus on the diagnosis and management of Crohn's disease: current management. *Gut* 2006; **55** (Suppl. 1): i16–35.

26 Sandborn WJ. Oral 5-ASA therapy in ulcerative colitis: what are the implications of the new formulations? *J Clin Gastroenterol* 2008; **42**: 338–44.

27 Lichtenstein GR, Abreu MT, Cohen R, *et al*. American Gastroenterological Association Institute technical review on corticosteroids, immunomodulators, and infliximab in inflammatory bowel disease. *Gastroenterology* 2006; **130**: 940–87.

28 Kandiel A, Fraser AG, Korelitz BI, *et al*. Increased risk of lymphoma among inflammatory bowel disease patients treated with azathioprine and 6-mercaptopurine. *Gut* 2005; **54**: 1121–5.

29 Clark M, Colombel JF, Feagan BC, *et al*. American Gastroenterological Association consensus development conference on the use of biologics in the treatment of inflammatory bowel disease, June 21–23, 2006. *Gastroenterology* 2007; **133**: 312–39.

30 Pardi DS, Sandborn WJ. Systematic review: the management of pouchitis. *Aliment Pharmacol Therap* 2006; **23**: 1087–96.

CHAPTER 44
Infectious Proctocolitis

Disaya Chavalitdhamrong, Gary C. Chen, and Rome Jutabha

Division of Digestive Diseases, David Geffen School of Medicine at UCLA, Los Angeles, CA, USA

Summary

Infectious diarrhea is a major cause of illness throughout the world. Acquisition of an enteric infection is the result of an interaction between the host factors that protect against infection and microbial virulence factors that function to overcome host defenses. The initial step in the diagnostic evaluation of a patient with acute diarrhea should be through complete history and physical examination. The nature of the illness and the appearance of the stool should be assessed. The goals of which are to identify those patients who may be at risk of severe illness or susceptible to complications and those who will benefit from specific therapy. Most cases are self-limiting and further evaluation is not needed. Diagnostic testing is indicated in severe diarrhea, bloody diarrhea, persistent diarrhea, recent use of antibiotics, and immunocompromised or elderly patients. Characteristics of diarrhea provide clues to the diagnosis. Stool tests, blood tests, radiologic studies, and endoscopic evaluation are useful tools for the diagnosis of the disease.

Case

A 58-year-old woman presented to the hospital with persistent left lower quadrant abdominal pain and diarrhea for 3 days. Two weeks before admission, the patient had left lower quadrant abdominal pain which was diagnosed as diverticulitis by CT scan showing sigmoid diverticulitis. A treatment with ciprofloxacin for 14 days was completed. Three days before her presentation, diarrhea developed, with crampy abdominal pain and no fever. Her diarrhea symptom did not improve after taking loperamide. There was no history of fever, chills, recent travel, or exposure to ill persons. Her temperature was 36.1°C, the pulse was 122, the respiratory rate was 16, and blood pressure was 145/90 mmHg. Physical examination was significant for moderate abdominal tenderness on palpation at left lower quadrant without rebound or guarding. She received IV hydration and her stool for *Clostridium difficile* toxins A and B were positive. She responded appropriately with oral metronidazole for 10 days with resolution of her abdominal pain and diarrhea within a few days.

Practical Gastroenterology and Hepatology: Small and Large Intestine and Pancreas, 1st edition. Edited by Nicholas J. Talley, Sunanda V. Kane and Michael B. Wallace. © 2010 Blackwell Publishing Ltd.

Introduction and Approach to the Patient

Infections of the lower gastrointestinal (GI) tract are a major cause of morbidity and mortality worldwide. The diagnostic approach includes a detailed history regarding the patient's demographics, travel history, epidemiological association, risk factors, medical history, and medication use, especially recent antibiotics use. The evidence of fever, peritoneal signs, mucous bloody diarrhea, or dysentery may be clues to infection with an invasive enteric pathogen, which will prompt further investigations (Figure 44.1).

The initial evaluation of patients should include the determination of the duration of symptoms, the frequency of diarrhea, and the characteristics of the stool. The degree of volume depletion should be determined and the initial therapy is rehydration. Then the patient should be categorized according to the setting into community acquired diarrhea, nosocomial diarrhea, or persistent diarrhea greater than 7 days. For community acquired diarrhea, culture or testing for *Salmonella*, *Shigella*, and *Campylobacter* is needed. Testing or culture for *E. coli* O125: H7 is warranted if there is a history of

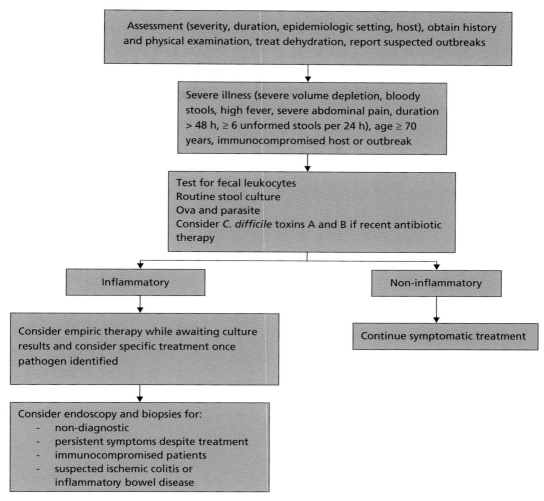

Figure 44.1 Approach to the patient with suspected infectious diarrhea.

bloody diarrhea or hemolytic–uremic syndrome. For nosocomial diarrhea, testing for *Clostridium difficile* toxins A and B is needed. For persistent diarrhea, consider protozoa, *Giardia*, *Cryptosporidium*, *Cyclospora*, and *Isospora belli*, and cytomegalovirus (also *Microsporidia* and *Mycobacterium avium* complex in HIV-positive patient). For orogenital/oroanal contact or rectal intercourse, tests for syphilis, herpes, *Chlamydia* and gonorrhea are needed.

Physical examination, stool studies, blood tests in selected cases, endoscopic examination, and serologic tests also play important roles in the workup process.

Antibiotics may prolong the duration of shedding of *Salmonella* and may increase the risk of life-threatening complications of Shiga toxin-producing *E. coli* infection. The benefit of antibiotics should be weighed against the cost, the risk of adverse reactions, and the risk of harmful eradication of normal flora or the induction of Shiga-toxin production.

The various forms of infectious proctocolitides have a wide spectrum of clinical, endoscopic, and histopathologic manifestations. Symptoms may range from mild to severe. Depending on the pathogen causing the proctocolitis, some require urgent medical treatment, whereas

Table 44.1 Infectious agents causing colitis, proctocolitis, and proctitis.

Colitis
　Salmonella species
　Yersinia species
　Vibrio parahaemolyticus
　Aeromonas hydrophila
　Plesiomonas shigelloides

Proctocolitis
　Clostridium difficile
　Campylobacter species
　Shigella species
　Enterohemorrhagic *Escherichia coli*
　Enteroinvasive *Escherichia coli*
　Entamoeba species
　Cytomegalovirus
　Chlamydia species
　Tuberculosis

Proctitis
　Herpesvirus
　Neisseria gonorrhoeae
　Treponema pallidum

others do not. The epidemiology, pathophysiology, clinical features, diagnosis, and management of each pathogen causing colitis, proctocolitis, and proctitis will be reviewed here (Table 44.1).

Colitis

Salmonella Colitis

Non-typhoidal *Salmonella* species are facultative anaerobic, Gram-negative bacilli that enter the body via the fecal–oral route. Outbreaks are associated with contaminated meats, eggs, and dairy products but can also occur in men who have sex with men (MSM). For the non-typhoidal species, *S. typhimurium* and *S. enteritidis* are the most common serotypes. The pathogenesis results from bacterial attachment to the M cells in the colon. The incubation period is 12–72 h. The ileum, appendix, and right colon are commonly involved. Patients usually present with nausea, vomiting, abdominal pain, and bloody diarrhea. Symptoms can last 2–3 weeks, and there is a high rate of mortality in the elderly. Colonoscopy findings include edema, hyperemia, friable mucosa, and apthous ulcerations [1]. Histological abnormalities range from edema of the lamina propria and inflammatory cell infiltration to disruption of the surface epithelium and microabscess formation [1]. An asymptomatic carrier state is possible, with the organisms harboring in the gall bladder. Diagnosis is made by stool or blood culture, rectal swab, or endoscopic biopsy. *Salmonella* colitis is usually self-limited, and does not require antibiotic treatment, which can prolong the intestinal carrier state and excretion of *Salmonella*. Quinolones and trimethoprim–sulfamethoxazole are effective and are recommended for patients at increased risk of complications (elderly, those with severe colitis, and immunocompromised patients).

Yersinia Colitis

Yersinia species are Gram-negative, facultative anaerobic coccobacilli. Two species produce GI illness: *Y. enterocolitica* (causes enterocolitis) and *Y. pseudotuberculosis* (causes mesenteric lymphadenitis). Contaminated food and water serve as the major routes of transmission. The incubation period is 1–11 days. Right lower quadrant abdominal pain, bloody diarrhea, nausea, vomiting, and fever are the most common symptoms [2]. Diarrhea can last 1–3 weeks. Erythema nodosum and reactive arthritis are the common infectious sequelae. Stool culture is the standard for diagnosis. Colonoscopy may show inflammation, friable mucosa, and ulcerations in the terminal ileum [2]. Histopathology shows lymphoid hyperplasia, epithelioid granulomas, and microabscesses [2]. The disease is usually self-limiting. However, treatment with tetracycline or ciprofloxacin should be considered in severe colitis, mesenteric adenitis, and erythema nodosum.

Vibrio parahemolyticus Colitis

Vibrio parahemolyticus is a Gram-negative rod that causes food poisoning, especially from raw seafood ingestion. The incubation period is 9–25 h. It causes watery or bloody diarrhea, abdominal pain, nausea, vomiting, and fever [3]. The median duration of illness is 2–3 days. Colonoscopy may show mucosal ulcerations. The diagnosis is confirmed by stool or rectal swab culture. The disease is usually self-limiting. The drug of choice is tetracycline, which can decrease the duration and severity of symptoms.

Aeromonas hydrophila Colitis

Aeromonas is a Gram-negative bacterium. *A. hydrophila* and *A. sobria* are the strains that cause GI illness in humans. Patients usually present with bloody diarrhea, abdominal cramps, vomiting, and fever [4]. Chronic colitis has been reported. Colonoscopy may show segmental colitis. Histopathology shows edema, friability, exudates, and loss of vascularity. Stool culture is the standard for diagnosis. Complications include hemolytic–uremic syndrome (HUS) and septicemia. Quinolones, trimethoprim–sulfamethoxazole, and tetracycline are effective.

Plesiomonas shigelloides Colitis

Plesiomonas is associated with the consumption of uncooked shellfish, particularly oysters, in the 48 h before the onset of GI illness [5]. Patients present with bloody diarrhea, vomiting, and fever [5]. The average duration of symptoms is 11 days [5]. Colonoscopy may show punctate lesions [5]. Asplenic patients are at increased risk of developing fulminant septic shock. Antibiotics reduce the duration of illness [6]. Most strains are susceptible to gentamicin, tetracycline, and trimethoprim–sulfamethoxazole.

Proctocolitis

Clostridium difficile Proctocolitis

Clostridium difficile is an anaerobic, spore-forming, Gram-positive rod. Toxin A, toxin B, and the binary toxin of *C. difficile* contribute to the disease. Alteration of the normal bacterial flora of the colon and the immune status of the host are important factors in the development of this disease. Although all antibiotics can predispose patients to the infection, clindamycin, ampicillin, amoxicillin, penicillin, cephalosporins, and fluoroquinolones are the most common culprits [7]. The risk factors for *C. difficile* infection (CDI) included antibiotic use, hospital admission, prolonged length of stay in a healthcare setting, serious underlying illness, immune-compromising conditions, aging, gastrointestinal surgery/manipulation, proton pump inhibitors, peripartum women, and heart transplant recipients [8]. The clinical presentation is variable, ranging from mild colitis, most pronounced in the rectosigmoid, to fulminant colitis, which could lead to toxic megacolon and perforation [9]. Symptoms can occur up to 6–10 weeks after antibiotic cessation and include systemic symptoms, lower abdominal cramping pain, profuse diarrhea, and lower GI

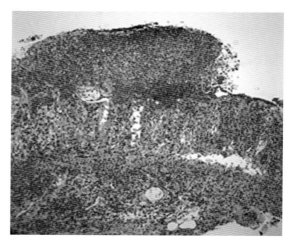

Figure 44.2 Histopathological picture of *Clostridium difficile* colitis. The histopathology of pseudomembranous colitis is demonstrative of a severe colitis. In mucosa pictured, there is an intense exudate compose of fibrin and necrotic cellular debris. This exudate is responsible for the gross impression of a pseudomembrane. Microscopically, the epithelium is largely destroyed. Only partial crypt lining and surface restitution can be found. The lamina propria is expanded by neutrophils. The overall picture gives the impression of an erupting necroinflammatory process. (Courtesy of Ananya Manuyakorn, MD.)

bleeding. The classical colonoscopy feature is pseudomembranous colitis. Histology shows neutrophilic inflammation of the colonic mucosa with patchy epithelial necrosis with overlying exudate that may erupt in a characteristic feature called "volcano" lesion (Figure 44.2). The stool cytotoxin assay is the gold standard for the diagnosis, but enzyme immunoassay to direct toxin for toxins A and B is widely used due to its same-day result and high concordance rate to the cytotoxin assay [10]. Treatment includes the discontinuation of the offending antibiotics and 10–14 days of oral or intravenous metronidazole 500 mg three times a day. Oral vancomycin (125–500 mg oral four times a day for 10–14 days) is recommended for patients who are critically ill, unable to tolerate metronidazole, pregnant, failed metronidazole therapy, or infection with metronidazole-resistant strains. Repeat testing to monitor response is not indicated. Contact isolation is essential in controlling the spread of the disease.

A new, hypervirulent strain of *C. difficile*, called NAP1/BI/027, has been implicated in *C. difficile* outbreaks associated with increased morbidity and mortality since

2000s [8]. The incidence of fulminant CDI is rising and the management is challenging. Oral vancomycin is the first-line treatment, intravenous metronidazole can be added, or vancomycin can be administered rectally (500 mg in 100 mL of normal saline every 6 h) [11]. Subtotal colectomy can be lifesaving in fulminant CDI. Intravenous immunoglobulin maybe a worthwhile intervention in fulminant CDI because a low concentration of *C. difficile* antitoxin is a risk factor for developing disease but its efficacy is uncertain.

Episodes of recurrent CDI are difficult to treat. Risk factors for recurrent CDI include the history of recurrence, continued use of antibiotics, concomitant receipt of antacid medications, elderly, and prolonged hospital stays [11,12]. For recurrent cases (20–25%), a repeat course of metronidazole should be given. After a second recurrence, oral vancomycin should be given [7]. Few studies have evaluated treatment options for recurrent *C. difficile* infection, but a prolonged, tapering, and pulse-dosed regimen of oral vancomycin is commonly used. Other potentially effective strategies for recurrent CDI include probiotics, rifaximin, toxin-binding resin (tolevamer), nitazoxanide, fecal transplantation, and intravenous immunoglobulin are promising but none have proven efficacy, therefore warranting further research [11].

Campylobacter Proctocolitis

Campylobacter organisms are Gram-negative rods, which cause a food-borne disease [13]. Species include *C. jejuni*, *C. fetus*, *C. coli*, *C. cinaedi*, *C. fennelliae*, *C. lari*, *C. upsaliensis*, and *C. hyointestinalis*. Colitis is typically caused by *C. jejuni* and *C. coli*. The incubation period is 2–5 days. Clinical presentations range from no symptoms to fulminant sepsis. Most patients have fever, abdominal pain, and diarrhea [13]. Infection starts in the jejunum and ileum and progresses distally and can cause mesenteric adenitis, toxic megacolon, and colonic perforation. Colonoscopy findings include mucosal edema, inflammation, and ulcerations. Biopsy shows acute colitis. *C. jejuni* also can trigger Guillain–Barré syndrome, reactive arthritis, and erythema nodosum, especially in HLA B27-positive patients [14]. However, symptoms usually resolve within 1 week without antimicrobial therapy in most patients. Antibiotics are given for prolonged symptoms, elderly patients, immunocompromised patients, and pregnant women. Macrolides are the treatment of choice because

Campylobacter has developed significant resistance against quinolones. Aminoglycosides or a carbapenem is indicated for bacteremia and should be given for 2–4 weeks to prevent relapse. *Campylobacter* can be identified by direct microscopic examination, routine stool, and blood cultures.

Shigella Proctocolitis

Shigella is a Gram-negative bacillus with four species: *S. dysenteriae*, *S. flexneri*, *S. boydii*, and *S. sonnei*. Outbreaks have been associated with food and water contaminations, but most transmission occurs via person-to-person contact. Shigella is highly virulent, as ingestion of only 10 organisms can cause disease [15]. The incubation period is 1–7 days. *S. dysenteriae* and *S. flexneri* commonly cause dysentery. Symptoms begin with fever, abdominal cramps, watery diarrhea, then dysentery. *S. dysenteriae* is the most virulent and causes toxic megacolon and perforation more frequently. Colonoscopy may show erythema, edema, and loss of vascularity, punctate hemorrhage, aphthoid erosions, mucosal friability, collar-button ulcers, and adherent grayish-white mucopurulent materials [16]. Histology findings may mimic inflammatory bowel disease. The diagnosis is made by stool culture, rectal swab, or by endoscopic biopsy. This disease is usually self-limiting. Antibiotics should be considered in the elderly, malnourished individuals, food handlers, health-care workers, and immunocompromised patients. Antibiotic therapy with trimethoprim–sulfamethoxazole or quinolones reduces illness duration, lowers mortality, and shortens the carrier state. Hygienic practices can reduce person-to-person transmission.

Enterohemorrhagic *Escherichia coli* (EHEC) Proctocolitis

EHEC strains are Shiga toxin-positive [17]. The most notable type is *E. coli* O157: H7. The fecal–oral route of transmission occurs due to ingestion of undercooked meat. The incubation period is 3–4 days, with the right colon as the most common affected site. Bloody diarrhea, vomiting, abdominal pain, and tenderness are common, often in the absence of fever [18]. The duration of illness is 7–10 days. Infection can trigger HUS and thrombotic thrombocytopenic purpura, particularly in the elderly [19]. Colonoscopy may show edema, hyperemia, hemorrhage, erosions, and ulcers. Histological findings include edema, submucosal hemorrhage, and fibrin exudation.

Diagnosis is made by stool culture. Treatment is mainly supportive. Treatment with antibiotics may increase the risk of HUS.

Enteroinvasive *Escherichia coli* (EIEC) Proctocolitis

The pathogenesis of EIEC is virtually identical to that of the *Shigella* species [20]. The incubation period is 2–3 days. The organisms invade the intestinal cells. Symptoms usually include fever, malaise, lower abdominal pain, and watery diarrhea, but dysentery can also be seen. Pathogens can be detected by DNA probe. Antibiotics treatment is often not needed.

Amebic Dysentery

Amebic colitis is caused by *Entamoeba histolytica* and *Entamoeba dispar*. Amebiasis is a common parasitic illness in the developing countries. In developed countries, it is seen in travelers to developing nations and in MSM. It exists in two forms in stool: the trophozoite and the cyst. Trophozoites adhere to colonic epithelial cells and cause colitis, especially in cecum and ascending colon, resulting in abdominal pain and bloody diarrhea. Rare complications, such as amoeboma, liver abscess, and rectovaginal fistulae, can also occur. Stool culture and serology are the mainstay of diagnosis. Colonoscopy may show the classic "flask-shaped" colonic ulcers (Figure 44.3) while histology shows cryptitis, crypt abscesses, ulcerations, and ingested red blood cells [21]. *E. dispar* infection needs no treatment. On the other hand, *E. histolytica* is treated with metronidazole 750 mg three times a day for 7–10 days and an amebicide such as iodoquinol 650 mg orally three times a day for 20 days. The latter is needed to eradicate the intestinal carrier state of amebiasis even in asymptomatic patients.

Cytomegalovirus (CMV) Proctocolitis

CMV is an enveloped, double-stranded DNA virus. The majority of active CMV disease is the result of reactivation of latent infection but primary infection can also occur, especially in an immunocompromised host (e.g., HIV positive or renal transplant patient). The symptoms are fever, weight loss, anorexia, malaise, abdominal pain, bloody diarrhea, and perforation. Endoscopic findings can vary from punctuate erosions to deep ulcerations and necrotizing colitis (Figure 44.4). Histopathology shows tissue destruction with the presence of cytomegalic cells. Diagnosis can be made by serology, culture, histology, or molecular assays [22]. Treatment is intravenous ganciclovir 5 mg/kg every 12 h intravenously for 14–21 days followed by 5 mg/kg every 24 h for 3–6 weeks. Maintenance therapy is with oral valganciclovir for 2–4 months to protect against relapse.

Chlamydial Proctocolitis

Chlamydia trachomatis is a Gram-negative, obligate, intracellular organism. *C. trachomatis* has lymphogranuloma venereum (LGV) and non-LGV strains, both of which can produce proctocolitis. The symptoms are

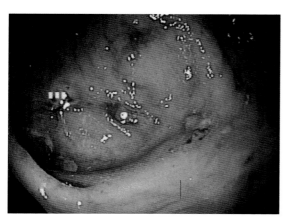

Figure 44.3 Amebic colitis: cecal ulcerations.

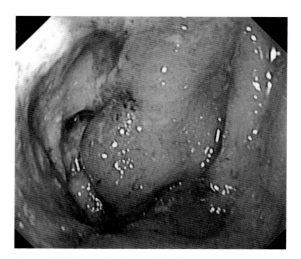

Figure 44.4 Cytomegalovirus proctitis: ulceration with luminal stenosis at rectum.

rectal pain, mucous bloody discharge, tenesmus, diarrhea, constipation, and left lower quadrant abdominal pain. The symptoms can be chronic, lasting from weeks to years, with complications of strictures, abscesses and fistulae, which can mimic Crohn disease [23]. Colonoscopy may show friable hemorrhagic mucosa, erosions, and ulcerations. Biopsy may show crypt abscesses and granulomas. Rectal swab specimen for Gram stain, culture, direct immunofluorescence, and enzyme-linked immunosorbent assay (ELISA) can help with the diagnosis. Doxycycline (100 mg orally twice a day for 7 days) or azithromycin (1 g orally once) is the treatment of choice.

Colorectal Tuberculosis

Mycobacterium tuberculosis and *Mycobacterium bovis* can involve the GI tract. The ileocecal area is affected in up to 90% of patients. The symptoms and signs include abdominal pain, diarrhea, weight loss, fever, abdominal tenderness, abdominal mass, and ascites. Colonic tuberculosis can cause deep transverse ulcers, colitis, and strictures (Figure 44.5). Rectal involvement is rare. Diagnosis can be made by biopsy showing caseating granulomas or acid-fast bacilli. Stool cultures can be done but diagnostic yield is low. About 90% of patients with GI tuberculosis respond to medical therapy if it is started early in the course [24].

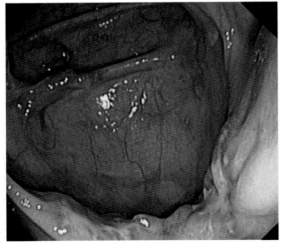

Figure 44.5 Tuberculosis: deep transverse ulcer at cecum.

Proctitis

Rectal infection is often a result of anal intercourse. The most common infections causing proctitis are herpes simplex virus, *Neisseria gonorrhoeae*, and syphilis.

Herpes Simplex Proctitis

Herpes simplex virus infection may present with systemic viral symptoms, perianal pain, discharge, constipation, and vesicles. The diagnosis can be made by viral culture, polymerase chain reaction (PCR), direct fluorescence antibody, Tzanck smear, and type-specific serologic tests. PCR is the most sensitive test. Symptomatic treatment for mild herpes simplex virus proctitis, but acyclovir (400 mg five times a day for 10 days) is recommended for severe disease [25].

Gonococcal Proctitis

Neisseria gonorrhea is a Gram-negative coccus. Gonococcal proctitis is associated with increase in the risk of acquiring HIV infection, probably due to diminished epithelial integrity. Typical symptoms are anal itching, irritation, painful defecation, sensation of rectal fullness, discharge, and constipation. Symptoms usually resolve rapidly, and patients can become asymptomatic carriers. The gold standard for diagnosis is rectal swab culture on Thayer–Martin agar. Multiple culture sites, such as urethral and pharyngeal cultures in men and endocervix in women, should be sampled if anorectal gonorrhea is suspected. The abnormalities noted on sigmoidoscopy usually are limited to the anal canal and rectum with the presence of pus, bleeding, erythema, friability, and superficial erosions. Histologically, patchy derangement of the columnar mucus-secreting cells, vascular engorgement and infiltration with neutrophils, lymphocytes, and plasma cells can be seen. Complications are rectal strictures, anal fistulae, fissures, perianal abscess, and rarely rectovaginal fistulae. Treatment with ceftriaxone (125 mg intramuscularly single dose) plus doxycycline is recommended due to the prevalence of concurrent chlamydial infection. Follow-up culture 7–10 days after therapy is essential to document cure [25].

Anorectal Syphilis

Anorectal syphilis due to *Treponema pallidum* infection is one of the most frequently misdiagnosed lesions in MSM. The incubation period is 2–8 weeks. The painless

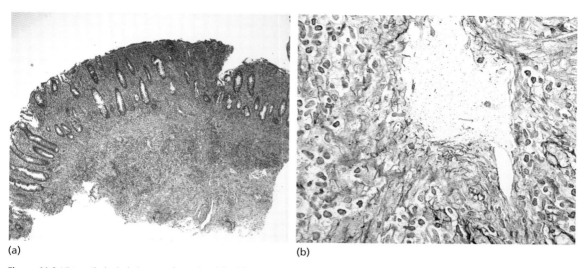

(a)   (b)

Figure 44.6 Histopathological pictures of rectal syphilis. (a) Rectal biopsy demonstrated dense predominantly plasma cell infiltrates within the mucosa and submucosa (H&E). (b) Steiner stain demonstrated numerous spirochete organisms, morphologically consistent with *Treponema pallidum*. The organisms concentrated particularly around blood vessels. (Courtesy of Galen Cortina, MD.)

chancre has well-demarcated indurated edges, a clean ulcer base, and usually heals spontaneously within 3–4 weeks. Symptoms are rectal pain, itching, bleeding, discharge, constipation, tenesmus, and tender inguinal nodes. Histologically, an intense plasma cell and lymphocyte infiltrate, necrotizing granuloma and *Treponema* can be present (Figure 44.6a,b). Secondary syphilis can be painful, and may include polyps, smooth lobulated masses, mucosal ulcerations, mucosal friability, and condyloma acuminatum. Diagnostic tests for syphilis include Venereal Disease Research Laboratory antigen test (VDRL), RPR, and FTA-ABS. Penicillin G (2.4 million units IM single dose or three doses for syphilis of more than 1 year's duration) is the treatment of choice [25].

for the majority of times when evaluating patients with infectious proctocolitis.

- Endoscopic evaluation usually is not necessary to establish the proper diagnosis and the endoscopic findings of infectious proctocolitis tend to be non-specific, often mimicking inflammatory bowel disease.
- Most cases of infectious proctocolitis are self-limiting and require supportive care only but antimicrobial therapy is necessary for certain pathogens and in certain patient populations, such as the elderly and immunocompromised patients.
- Proper hygiene, protected sex, and proper contact isolation can significantly decrease the transfer and spread of these pathogens.

Take-home points

- GI infections of the lower GI tract are a major cause of morbidity and mortality as well as utilization of health-care resources worldwide.
- Infectious proctocolitis can be caused by a variety of pathogens including bacteria, viruses, and parasites, which are most often transmitted by food and water as well as unprotected anal intercourse.
- A detailed, thorough history along with proper utilization of stool studies is keys to establish the proper diagnosis

References

1 Mandal BK, Mani V. Colonic involvement in salmonellosis. *Lancet* 1976; **1**: 887–8.
2 Vantrappen G, Ponette E, Geboes K, Bertrand P. Yersinia enteritis and enterocolitis: gastroenterological aspects. *Gastroenterology* 1977; **72**: 220–7.
3 Bolen JL, Zamiska SA, Greenough WB, 3rd. Clinical features in enteritis due to Vibrio parahemolyticus. *Am J Med* 1974; **57**: 638–41.

4 Holmberg SD, Schell WL, Fanning GR, *et al.* Aeromonas intestinal infections in the United States. *Ann Intern Med* 1986; **105**: 683–9.

5 Holmberg SD, Wachsmuth IK, Hickman-Brenner FW, *et al.* Plesiomonas enteric infections in the United States. *Ann Intern Med* 1986; **105**: 690–4.

6 Kain KC, Kelly MT. Clinical features, epidemiology, and treatment of Plesiomonas shigelloides diarrhea. *J Clin Microbiol* 1989; **27**: 998–1001.

7 Aslam S, Musher DM. An update on diagnosis, treatment, and prevention of Clostridium difficile-associated disease. *Gastroenterol Clin North Am* 2006; **35**: 315–35.

8 Hookman P, Barkin JS. Clostridium difficile associated infection, diarrhea and colitis. *World J Gastroenterol* 2009; **15**: 1554–80.

9 Adams SD, Mercer DW. Fulminant Clostridium difficile colitis. *Curr Opin Crit Care* 2007; **13**: 450–5.

10 Moyenuddin M, Williamson JC, Ohl CA. Clostridium difficile-associated diarrhea: current strategies for diagnosis and therapy. *Curr Gastroenterol Rep* 2002; **4**: 279–86.

11 Kelly CP. A 76-year-old man with recurrent Clostridium difficile-associated diarrhea: review of C. difficile infection. *JAMA* 2009; **301**: 954–62.

12 Garey KW, Sethi S, Yadav Y, DuPont HL. Meta-analysis to assess risk factors for recurrent Clostridium difficile infection. *J Hosp Infect* 2008; **70**: 298–304.

13 Allos BM, Blaser MJ. Campylobacter jejuni and the expanding spectrum of related infections. *Clin Infect Dis* 1995; **20**: 1092–9; quiz 100–1.

14 Allos BM. Campylobacter jejuni infections: update on emerging issues and trends. *Clin Infect Dis* 2001; **32**: 1201–6.

15 DuPont HL, Levine MM, Hornick RB, Formal SB. Inoculum size in shigellosis and implications for expected mode of transmission. *J Infect Dis* 1989; **159**: 1126–8.

16 Speelman P, Kabir I, Islam M. Distribution and spread of colonic lesions in shigellosis: a colonoscopic study. *J Infect Dis* 1984; **150**: 899–903.

17 Welinder-Olsson C, Kaijser B. Enterohemorrhagic Escherichia coli (EHEC). *Scand J Infect Dis* 2005; **37**: 405–16.

18 Ochoa TJ, Cleary TG. Epidemiology and spectrum of disease of Escherichia coli O157. *Curr Opin Infect Dis* 2003; **16**: 259–63.

19 Besser RE, Griffin PM, Slutsker L. Escherichia coli O157: H7 gastroenteritis and the hemolytic uremic syndrome: an emerging infectious disease. *Annu Rev Med* 1999; **50**: 355–67.

20 Tulloch EF, Jr., Ryan KJ, Formal SB, Franklin FA. Invasive enteropathic Escherichia coli dysentery. An outbreak in 28 adults. *Ann Intern Med* 1973; **79**: 13–7.

21 Lamps LW. Infective disorders of the gastrointestinal tract. *Histopathology* 2007; **50**: 55–63.

22 Bobak DA. Gastrointestinal infections caused by cytomegalovirus. *Curr Infect Dis Rep* 2003; **5**: 101–7.

23 Quinn TC, Goodell SE, Mkrtichian E, *et al.* Chlamydia trachomatis proctitis. *N Engl J Med* 1981; **305**: 195–200.

24 Marshall JB. Tuberculosis of the gastrointestinal tract and peritoneum. *Am J Gastroenterol* 1993; **88**: 989–99.

25 Fried R, Surawicz C. Proctitis and sexually transmissible diseases of the colon. *Curr Treat Options Gastroenterol* 2003; **6**: 263–70.

CHAPTER 45
Microscopic Colitis

Darrell S. Pardi

Inflammatory Bowel Disease Clinic, Division of Gastroenterology and Hepatology, Mayo Clinic, Rochester, MN, USA

Summary

Microscopic colitis is a common cause of chronic watery diarrhea, especially in the elderly. The incidence of this condition is increasing, perhaps due to an association with several commonly used medications. The two subtypes, lymphocytic and collagenous colitis, are only distinguishable histologically. The diagnosis relies on colon biopsies, which show an intraepithelial lymphocytosis and mixed lamina propria inflammation. In collagenous colitis, the subepithelial collagen band is thickened. The main differential diagnosis is irritable bowel syndrome, and histology is required to distinguish these entities. Several treatment options have been reported, but bismuth subsalicylate and budesonide seem to be the most effective. Many patients require maintenance therapy, but the prognosis is good, with most patients responding to treatment, and no known increased risk of colon cancer or death.

Case

A 68-year-old woman has a 10-month history of non-bloody diarrhea with abdominal pain. She has lost 4.5 kg (10 lb). She occasionally passes mucus per rectum but does not have steatorrhea. She has not had any travel or new medications. She has no medical history, and physical examination and laboratories, including stool studies, are normal. She has been diagnosed with irritable bowel syndrome, but has not responded to antidiarrheals or antispasmodics. She is referred for a second opinion.

Definition and Epidemiology

The term "microscopic colitis" was coined to describe patients with chronic watery diarrhea and normal sigmoidoscopy but inflammation on colon biopsies. Collagenous colitis has similar clinical and histologic features, with a thickened subepithelial collagen band. It is unclear if these conditions are distinct diseases or are variations of the same condition. Since the colon in collagenous colitis is grossly normal, it is also considered a form of "microscopic" colitis. Thus, microscopic colitis is an umbrella diagnosis, with two subtypes: collagenous colitis, with a thickened subepithelial collagen band, and lymphocytic colitis, without collagen thickening [1].

Microscopic colitis is found in 10–15% of patients with chronic diarrhea [2,3]. In Europe, the yearly incidence of collagenous and lymphocytic colitis is 0.6–5.2/100 000 each, with a prevalence of 10–15.7/100 000 [3–5]. In North America, the incidence appears to be slightly higher (4.6–9.8/100 000 each) [6,7], and increasing significantly [6] (Figure 45.1).

Microscopic colitis is more common in women and typically presents in the sixth to seventh decades [3–7], although a wide age range has been reported [8]. There are reports of families with microscopic colitis, but it is unclear whether these are chance associations or whether familial predisposition truly exists.

Pathophysiology

Pathophysiologic studies are typically small and often conflicting, such that a clear understanding of underlying mechanism(s) is not yet available. Several hypotheses

Practical Gastroenterology and Hepatology: Small and Large Intestine and Pancreas, 1st edition. Edited by Nicholas J. Talley, Sunanda V. Kane and Michael B. Wallace. © 2010 Blackwell Publishing Ltd.

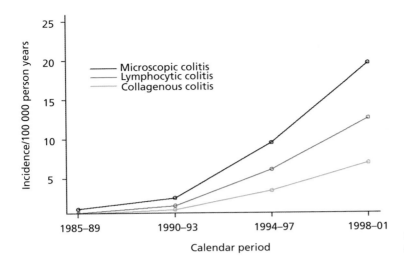

have been raised [8], and it is likely that "microscopic colitis" is a clinicopathologic syndrome that has several different mechanisms with similar histology. A detailed review of these data is beyond the scope of this chapter, but the entity of drug-induced microscopic colitis will be discussed further.

An association between microscopic colitis and non-steroidal anti-inflammatory drugs (NSAID) has been reported [9,10]. Some patients improve with discontinuation of NSAIDs, and recur after rechallenge. Finally, patients taking NSAIDs may be more likely to require steroids. Several other drugs have been implicated, including some of those most commonly prescribed: H_2 blockers, proton pump inhibitors, statins, serotonin reuptake inhibitors [8,9,11]. A comprehensive review of the literature on this issue [12] concluded that these and other medications had a high or intermediate likelihood of causing microscopic colitis based on the weight of evidence (Table 45.1). In patients with drug-induced microscopic colitis, remission is possible after discontinuation of the offending medication. Thus, this possibility should be considered in every patient before starting specific colitis therapy.

Clinical Features

The main symptom of microscopic colitis is chronic watery diarrhea, often with abdominal pain, mild weight

Table 45.1 Drugs with high or intermediate likelihood of causing microscopic colitis.

Drug (class)	Likelihood
Acarbose	High
Aspirin	High
Proton pump inhibitors	High
NSAIDs	High
H₂ receptor antagonists	High
SSRIs	High
Ticlopidine	High
Carbamazepine	Intermediate
Flutamide	Intermediate
Lisinopril	Intermediate
Levodopa/benserazide	Intermediate
Statins	Intermediate

Likelihood is based on strength of data, not on frequency with which the drug causes colitis. (Adapted from *Aliment Pharmacol Ther* 2005; **22**: 277–84 [12].)
NSAIDs, non-steroidal anti-inflammatory drugs; SSRIs, selective serotonin reuptake inhibitors.

loss, or fecal incontinence. Fecal leukocytes may be present, but dehydration is unusual. Arthralgias and various autoimmune conditions are common [8,11,13,14], including celiac disease, which is seen in 2–9% of patients [11,13,14]. This association should be considered in patients with sprue who do not respond to a gluten free diet and in those with microscopic colitis who have significant weight loss or any suggestion of

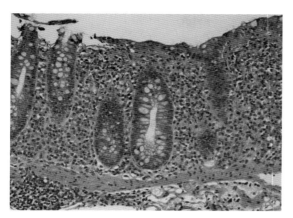

Figure 45.2 Lymphocytic colitis.

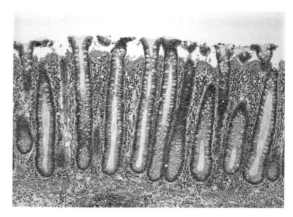

Figure 45.3 Collagenous colitis.

steatorrhea, and in those who do not respond to the usual treatments (see below).

Diagnosis

> **Case continued**
>
> The patient underwent colonoscopy, which was grossly normal. However, biopsies showed lymphocytic colitis.

Colonoscopy is typically normal or has mild changes such as erythema or edema. Colonic ulceration is uncommon, and when seen is likely related to use of NSAIDs. The most distinctive histologic feature is intraepithelial lymphocytosis (Figure 45.2), with more than 10–20 lymphocytes per 100 epithelial cells (normal <5). In addition, there is an acute and chronic inflammatory infiltrate in the lamina propria, often with surface epithelial damage. In collagenous colitis, the subepithelial collagen band is abnormally thickened (Figure 45.3).

Differential Diagnosis

The main differential diagnosis is diarrhea-predominant irritable bowel syndrome (IBS), which is approximately 100 times more common than microscopic colitis. There is no biologic or physiologic marker for IBS. The diagnosis is therefore symptom-based and the Manning and Rome criteria are widely used to identify IBS patients.

However, these criteria are not specific enough to establish the diagnosis of IBS without colon biopsies excluding microscopic colitis [15].

Therapeutics

> **Case continued**
>
> Trials of loperamide and bismuth subsalicylate were unhelpful. She was started on budesonide, 9 mg/day, with resolution of her diarrhea.

The use of NSAIDs or other medications that might be associated with microscopic colitis should be discontinued if possible. In addition, any other agent (e.g., dairy products) that may cause diarrhea should be avoided. Antidiarrheal therapy, such as loperamide or diphenoxylate, can be effective in mild cases [11,13,14]. If these agents are unsuccessful, bismuth subsalicylate may be beneficial [14,16].

If diarrhea does not respond to bismuth, the next therapeutic intervention considered often is mesalamine. However, large series have reported benefit in fewer than half of the patients treated with these drugs [11,13,14]. Cholestyramine may be more effective [8].

Patients refractory to these medications may respond to corticosteroids, which are the best therapies reported in the largest series (Table 45.2). Budesonide has been effective in controlled studies in collagenous and lymphocytic colitis [17], as well as in clinical experience [18].

Study [reference]	Pardi [14]	Olesen [11]	Bohr [13]
Type of colitis	Lymphocytic	Lymphocytic	Collagenous
Number of subjects	170	199	163
Antidiarrheals	73	70	71
Bismuth	73		
Mesalamine	45	50	50
Cholestyramine	65	57	59
Steroids	87	88	82
AZA/6-MP	20		

Table 45.2 Response to therapy in microscopic colitis.

Data are percentages and include complete and partial response. Response rates represent clinical experience and the results for different drugs are thus not directly comparable. Adapted from *Inflamm Bowel Dis* 2004; **10**: 860–70.)
AZA, azathioprine; 6-MP, 6-mercaptopurine.

Because of this efficacy, some physicians prescribe budesonide as first-line therapy in microscopic colitis. However, relapse after discontinuation is common [11,18], and many patients become steroid dependent. Thus, before starting corticosteroids, alternative diagnoses such as celiac disease, should be excluded. For steroid-refractory or dependent patients, immune modifiers such as azathioprine [14,19] can be considered. Alternatively, some clinicians use low-dose (3–6 mg/day) budesonide chronically [17].

Other treatments have been reported, but with limited experience [8]. Rarely, surgery is necessary. The response rates to various medications from three large uncontrolled series are listed in Table 45.2.

Most patients will respond to the treatment algorithm suggested above and outlined in Figure 45.4, but it is not clear how long to continue therapy, since many patients will have spontaneous or treatment-induced remissions and may not require long-term therapy. Treatment should be continued for 8–12 weeks, followed by tapering. For recurrent symptoms, maintenance therapy or episodic retreatment is used.

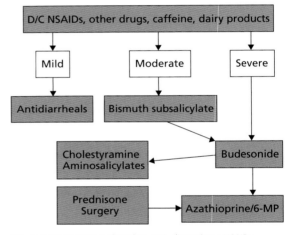

Figure 45.4 Treatment algorithm. D/C, discontinue; NSAIDs, non-steroidal anti-inflammatory drugs.

without full remission, some have intermittent symptoms and do not require maintenance therapy, but many (especially those requiring steroids) will [17]. There is no evidence of an increased risk of colon cancer or mortality.

Prognosis

Many patients have a waxing and waning course. Self-limited single attacks and spontaneous resolution have been reported [9,11]. The rate of spontaneous or treatment-induced complete remission with prolonged follow up ranges from 59 to 93% in lymphocytic colitis and from 2 to 92% in collagenous colitis [8,13,20]. Of those

Take-home points

- Microscopic colitis is a common cause of chronic watery diarrhea.
- It is more common in the elderly, and in females.
- Symptoms are similar to IBS; biopsies are required to distinguish these diagnoses.

- Some cases are associated with common medications.
- Celiac disease is more common in microscopic colitis.
- Bismuth subsalicylate appears to be an effective therapy.
- Budesonide is very effective, but recurrence is common after discontinuation.

References

1 Jessurun J, Yardley JH, Lee EL, *et al*. Microscopic and collagenous colitis: different names for the same condition? *Gastroenterology* 1986; **91**: 1583–4.

2 Fine KD, Seidel RH, Do K. The prevalence, anatomic distribution, and diagnosis of colonic causes of chronic diarrhea. *Gastrointest Endosc* 2000; **51**: 318–26.

3 Fernandez-Banares F, Salas A, Forne M, *et al*. Incidence of collagenous and lymphocytic colitis: a 5-year population-based study. *Am J Gastroenterol* 1999; **94**: 418–23.

4 Bohr J, Tysk C, Eriksson S, *et al*. Collagenous colitis in Orebro, Sweden, an epidemiological study 1984–1993. *Gut* 1995; **37**: 394–7.

5 Agnarsdottir M, Gunnlaugsson O, Orvar KB, *et al*. Collagenous and lymphocytic colitis in Iceland. *Dig Dis Sci* 2002; **47**: 1122–8.

6 Pardi DS, Loftus EV, Smyrk TC, *et al*. The epidemiology of microscopic colitis: a population-based study in Olmsted County, Minnesota. *Gut* 2007; **56**: 504–8.

7 Williams JJ, Kaplan GG, Makhija S, *et al*. Microscopic colitis-defining incidence rates and risk factors: a population-based study. *Clin Gastroenterol Hepatol* 2008; **6**: 35–40.

8 Pardi DS, Smyrk TC, Tremaine WJ, Sandborn WJ. Microscopic colitis: A review. *Am J Gastroenterol* 2002; **97**: 794–802.

9 Fernandez-Bavares F, Salos A, Estene M, *et al*. Collagenous and lymphocytic colitis: Evaluation of clinical and histological features, response to treatment and long-term follow-up. *Am J Gastroenterol* 2003; **98**: 340–7.

10 Riddell RH, Tanaka M, Mazzoleni G. Non-steroidal anti-inflammatory drugs as a possible cause of collagenous colitis: a case-control study. *Gut* 1992; **33**: 683–6.

11 Olesen M, Erickson S, Bohe J, *et al*. Lymphocytic colitis: A retrospective study of 199 Swedish patients. *Gut* 2004; **53**: 536–41.

12 Beaugerie L, Pardi DS. Drug-induced microscopic colitis: proposal for a scoring system and review of the literature. *Aliment Pharmacol Ther* 2005; **22**: 277–84.

13 Bohr J, Tysk C, Eriksson S, *et al*. Collagenous colitis: a retrospective study of clinical presentation and treatment in 163 patients. *Gut* 1996; **39**: 846–51.

14 Pardi DS, Ramnath VR, Loftus EV Jr, *et al*. Lymphocytic colitis: clinical features, treatment, and outcomes. *Am J Gastroenterol* 2002; **97**: 2829–33.

15 Limsui D, Pardi DS, Camilleri M, *et al*. Symptomatic overlap between irritable bowel syndrome and microscopic colitis. *Inflamm Bowel Dis* 2007; **13**: 175–81.

16 Fine K, Ogunji F, Lee E, *et al*. Randomized, double-blind, placebo-controlled trial of bismuth subsalicylate for microscopic colitis (abst). *Gastroenterology* 1999; **116**: A880.

17 Pardi DS. After budesonide, what next for collagenous colitis? *Gut* 2009; **58**: 3–4.

18 Abdalla AA, Faubion WA, Loftus EV, *et al*. The natural history of microscopic colitis treated with corticosteroids. *Gastroenterology* 2008; **134**: A121.

19 Pardi DS, Loftus EV, Tremaine WJ, *et al*. Treatment of refractory microscopic colitis with azathioprine and 6-mercaptopurine. *Gastroenterology* 2001; **120**: 1483–4.

20 Bonner GF, Petras RE, Cheong DMO, *et al*. Short- and long-term follow-up of treatment for lymphocytic and collagenous colitis. *Inflamm Bowel Dis* 2000; **6**: 85–91.

CHAPTER 46

Colonic Ischemia

Timothy T. Nostrant

Department of Internal Medicine, University of Michigan, Ann Arbor, MI, USA

Summary

Colonic ischemia is increasing in incidence. It accounts for 10% of all gastrointestinal events. Hypoperfusion and reperfusion injury are causative. The differential diagnosis is relatively small and usually clinical history is enough to make the diagnosis. CT examination followed by colonoscopy and biopsy if the patient is non-toxic confirms the diagnosis. Most resolve symptomatically in 1–2 days with radiographic and endoscopic resolution in 10–14 days. Progression to transmural necrosis occurs in 15% and manifests itself in the first few days by increasing pain, localized peritoneal findings, leukocytosis, and acidosis. Early surgery should be done if progression is evident. Aortic ilial reconstruction, renal transplant patients, and cardiac patients require close observation for progression. Newer theories for colonic ischemia are likely to come from the study of pharmacologic-induced ischemia.

Case

A 62-year-old man presents with 4 h of bilateral lower quadrant pain with recent passage of blood. He gives a history of two similar episodes that lasted 2 h each. Physical examination shows only mild lower left abdominal tenderness and grossly bloody stool. The patient takes diuretics for hypertension and digoxin for atrial fibrillation rate control. His laboratory tests show hemoglobin of 12.5 g%, hematocrit of 39, and white blood cell count of 12.0. CT of the abdomen reveals mild edema of the left colon and splenic flexure with no vascular or small bowel involvement. Unprepped colonoscopy shows multiple bluish black blebs in the left colon with ulcers at splenic flexure. Biopsies show acute mucosal necrosis, ghost crypt epithelial cells, and capillary hemorrhage. A diagnosis of ischemic colitis is made. The patient is treated with intravenous hydration. Diuretics and digoxin are stopped. The patient is well in 2 days.

Epidemiology

Colonic ischemia is the most common form of gastrointestinal ischemic injury (Figure 46.1). Its course is usually

mild with spontaneous resolution. Colonic ischemia is frequently misdiagnosed as inflammatory bowel disease or cancer. Estimates for colonic ischemia have the crude incidence of about 7.2 cases per 100 000 patient years. Some estimates have colonic ischemia accounting for one in 5000 colonoscopies, one in 700 office visits, and one in 2000 hospital admissions, with the incidence climbing. Most cases (90%) occur in patients over the age of 60 with no gender predilection [1,2].

Pathophysiology

Colonic ischemia is a result of hypoperfusion and reperfusion injury secondary to both anatomic and functional alterations in the mesenteric vasculature. Reperfusion accounts for most of the histologic and endoscopic damage, particularly when ischemia duration is short. During reperfusion, reactive oxygen species cause tissue damage, particularly in the mucosa since this is the most oxygen-deprived region during ischemia. Deeper layers can also be damaged if ischemia is more prolonged or more severe. These reactive oxygen species perioxidate lipid membranes, causing cell lysis, ghost epithelial cells, hemorrhagic mucosal necrosis, and subsequent fibrosis leading to radiologic and endoscopic thumbprinting,

Practical Gastroenterology and Hepatology: Small and Large Intestine and Pancreas, 1st edition. Edited by Nicholas J. Talley, Sunanda V. Kane and Michael B. Wallace. © 2010 Blackwell Publishing Ltd.

endoscopic ulcers, and deeper injury leading to pneumotosis, and finally perforation of the colonic wall. Although colonic ischemia has a full course from ischemic injury to a completely normal colon that is measured in days, 15% can progress to gangrene and perforation over the same period (Figure 46.2).

Major risk factors for colonic ischemia are listed in Table 46.1. Non-occlusive ischemia is the most common form of colonic ischemia and is the major reason why angiographic testing is rarely helpful. The "watershed areas" where blood flow is minimized between the superior mesenteric artery (SMA) and inferior mesenteric artery (IMA) vascular supplies are the most common areas of involvement. The vulnerable areas are the splenic flexure and rectosigmoid junction. Seventy-five percent of patients have left colon involvement with 25% limited to the splenic flexure. Rectal involvement is rare secondary to dual vascular supply through collateralization between the inferior mesenteric artery (mesenteric supply) and systemic circulation through hemorrhoidal

vessels (iliac arteries). Right colon involvement is seen in less than 10% of cases (Figure 46.3).

Specific forms of surgery are also complicated by colonic ischemia. Aortoiliac reconstruction has an incidence of colonic ischemia up to 7%. Many require surgical resection secondary to colonic gangrene. Multiple factors, such as sacrificed collaterals, vascular traction, and mesenteric hematoma, contribute to the injury. Renal transplantation with IMA vascular ligation is another contributor to colonic ischemia. Older-age patients, renal failure, fragile cardiopulmonary status, prior colonic resection with loss of collateral vessels, loss of perfusion secondary to cross clamping (particularly of both iliac vessels) are major contributors to hypoperfusion injury.

The superior mesenteric artery (right colon, transverse colon, splenic flexure) and inferior mesenteric arteries (left colon, sigmoid, rectum) are the major colonic vascular supply. Autoregulation of intestinal flow minimizes decreases in mesenteric blood flow during the postprandial state and systemic hypotension. The intestine can compensate for a 75% reduction in mesenteric blood flow for up to 12 h without apparent injury secondary to increased oxygen extraction. After several hours, vasoconstriction will occur with reduced collateral flow overcoming autoregulation attempts, producing increased ischemic injury. The colon is particularly vulnerable because the microvasculature plexus is less developed and is embedded in a thick muscular wall. Oxygen extraction is generally low for the entire intestine to maximize portal flow but relatively less blood is delivered to the colon (5–20%) versus 20–35% of cardiac output delivered to the small intestine [1,2].

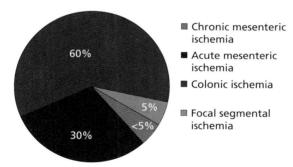

Figure 46.1 Intestinal ischemic syndromes.

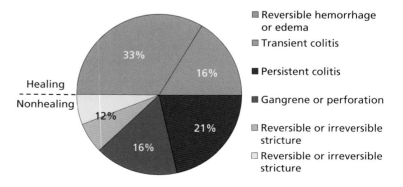

Figure 46.2 Various outcomes of colonic ischemia.

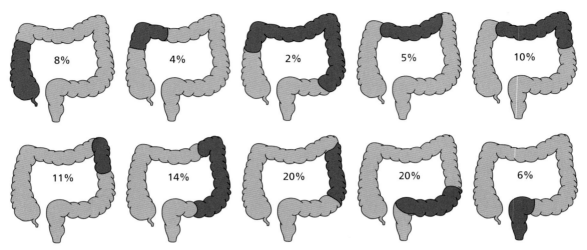

Figure 46.3 Mesenteric ischemia—colonic distribution (frequency).

Pharmacologic-induced Colon Injury

This causal mechanism has increased in incidence and potential importance since it may explain previously idiopathic cases [3]. Major classes of agents are listed in Table 46.1. Several classes offer insights into colonic ischemia.

Antibiotic-associated *C. difficile* and hemorrhagic colitis are important differentials. *C. difficile* is increasing secondary to widespread use of fluoroquinolone antibiotics. The organism producing the epidemic of *C. difficile* produces a high toxin burden and may be resistant to metronidazole. Acquisition is rapid in the hospital and mortality can be high, particularly in inflammatory bowel disease (IBD) patients. Older patients with co-morbidities are the population at highest risk for mortality. Endoscopic and biopsy findings can mimic colonic ischemia. Hemorrhagic colitis associated with penicillin use has a clinical course similar to colonic ischemia with predominate right-sided colitis. Direct toxin reaction to penicillin and overgrowth of *Klebsiella oxytoca* have been implicated. Prompt stoppage of penicillin usually results in complete resolution.

Constipation-inducing medications have a twofold increase in colonic ischemia. Calcium channel blockers, diuretics, digitalis, irritable bowel syndrome (IBS) medications, non-steroidal anti-inflammatory drugs (NSAIDs), and other inflammatory or chemotherapy

medications are most commonly implicated. Decreased colonic blood flow with colonic distension in areas with retained stool may be a common thread [3].

NSAIDs have been implicated in up to 10% of newly diagnosed colonic inflammation and may be a fivefold increased risk factor for colonic ischemia. Risk is also significant because of their over-the-counter status. Most patients are older and have been taking NSAIDs for a short time. Colonic symptoms mimic standard colonic ischemia and endoscopic findings include ulcers, strictures, perforation, and gangrene. Diaphragm-like strictures are likely pathognomonic, with pathology findings of fibrosis, hemorrhage, and coagulative necrosis. Increased leukotrienes producing mesenteric vasoconstriction with increased colonic permeability to toxins and luminal agents cause the colonic ischemia. Traditional NSAIDs are more commonly implicated but isolated reports of COX-2 specific agents producing colonic ischemia have been reported. Multiple risk factors, such as multiple NSAID use, co-morbid disease such as IBD, or atherosclerosis, will increase the risk of NSAID injury [3,4].

In serotonin modulator therapy, particularly in patients with IBS, but also in patients with migraines, both 5HT$_3$ antagonists (alosetron, cilansetron) and 5HT$_4$ agonists (tegaserod) may produce colonic ischemia, although the incidence is greater with 5HT$_3$ antagonists. The increased incidence of vasospastic disorders with

Table 46.1 Colonic ischemia—mechanisms.

Vascular occlusion—artery
Artery thrombosis
Cholesterol embolic
Aortic reconstruction
Renal transplantation (IMA occlusion/ligation)

Vascular occlusion—vein
Hypercoagulable state
Intra-abdominal enzyme release
Organ perforation
Pancreatitis
Antiphospholipid disease

Small vessel disease
Diabetes
Collagen vascular disease
Buerger disease (smoking)
Infiltrative vascular disease
Radiation
Amyloidosis

Non-occlusive colonic ischemia
Shock
Cardiac failure
Hemodialysis
Cardiopulmonary bypass
Colonoscopy (disinfectant colitis)

Pharmacologic agents
IBS drugs (alosetron, tageserod)
Digitalis
Cocaine
NSAIDs
Diuretics
Vasoactive substances (sympathominetics)

Infections
Pseudomembranous colitis (*C. difficile*)
Hemorrhagia colitis (antibiotics)
Shiga toxin colitis (*Shigella*, *E. coli* 0157: H7, other *E. coli*
  species)

Other conditions
Long distance running
Prolonged airline flights
Heat stroke
Lightening hits (neurogenic)

IBS, irritable bowel syndrome; IMA, inferior mesenteric artery;
NSAIDs, non-steroidal anti-inflammatory drugs.

increased intestinal ischemia has been reported in IBS patients without serotonin-modulating therapies. Alosetron has a reported incidence of 6.4 cases per 1000 patient years compared to 0.09 per 1000 patient years of placebo use. Adjudication of the entire postmarketing population yielded a rate of 1.0 case to 1000 patient years of use [5]. Most cases were reversible and less than 10% were associated with preischemic constipation. The mechanism is not fully understood but underlying atherosclerosis and cross talk between serotonin receptors producing vasoconstriction are implicated. Animal models have shown mesenteric vasoconstriction with $5HT_3$ antagonists but not $5HT_4$ agonists. $5HT_4$ agonists may increase colonic ischemia in patients who have other vasoconstrictive medications. Other comparative risk factor studies have shown an expected rate of 97 cases (tegaserod 20 cases) in an IBS population if the rate of colonic ischemia was 42/100000 patient years [1,5].

Intestinal ischemia is relatively common during extreme exercise. Common exercise scenarios producing ischemia are "Iron-Man Contests", marathon running, or continuous submarathon running with inadequate rehydration. Splanchnic mesenteric shunting, dehydration, hyponatremia, and skeletal muscle hyperperfusion are contributing factors. Bloody stools shortly after or during prolonged runs are common clinical presentations. Diagnosis is difficult and usually made clinically since testing will be normal unless done within 24h of the event [6].

Mesenteric venous thrombosis and acquired thrombotic conditions are relatively rare causes of colonic ischemia since the small bowel has the vast majority of the mesenteric venous flow. Thrombotic predilection may be a major contributor to colonic ischemia since one study comparing patients with colonic ischemia (36 patients), 18 patients with diverticulitis, and 52 healthy controls showed factor V Leiden mutations in 22.2 versus 0 and 3.8%, respectively, and 26 of the 36 patients with colonic ischemia (72%) had one or several prothrombotic effects [7].

Glutaraldehyde colitis secondary to poor clearing of endoscopes postdisinfection has become more frequent with increased volumes of endoscopy and strain on automated cleaners. The colitis occurs within 24h of a normal endoscopy and presents with urgency and bloody stools. The endoscopic findings look like ulcerative colitis but pathological findings are indistinguishable from ischemic colitis [8]. Resolution is usually rapid and should prompt evaluation of the endoscope cleaners and flushing procedures.

Clinical Manifestations

Most patients have a rapid onset of pain, commonly in the left side with mild to moderate tenderness. Bleeding will occur but can be delayed up to 24 h. A typical risk factor is usually not present, which is distinctly different than small bowel ischemia. Patients with colonic ischemia do not look severely ill and the pain is proportional to the findings on physical examination. Small bowel ischemia has severe pain typically with a normal physical exam and no gastrointestinal bleeding [9].

The natural history is usually short lived since ischemia is usually short in duration. The first findings are submucosal hemorrhages secondary to arterior/capillary injury and necrosis. Thumbprinting on radiological evaluation is the typical finding and is seen first on computed tomography (CT) scanning and as a latter finding on abdominal X-ray examination (only 30% of cases). The endoscopic correlate of this is the hemorrhagic phase (Figure 46.4). The next finding is longitudinal ulceration, which may involve only one wall or be circumferential. This is followed by mild mucosal scarring and then no abnormalities in many cases [10]. The natural history of ischemic colitis is usually less than 1 week with complete resolution the usual end point (Figure 46.4).

Progressive disease is seen in up to 20% of patients with severe colonic ischemia. Early thumbprinting with extensive colonic ulcerations may portend a worse course with increased mortality (29 versus 78% mortality). Symptoms lasting more than 24 h with signs of systemic toxicity (high white blood cell count, acidosis, fever, or segmental peritoneal findings) require aggressive diag-nostic testing to detect transmural injury or perforation and urgent surgical intervention. Risk factors for a poor prognosis include previous aortoilial reconstruction, renal transplant patients, previous colonic surgery, older age, co-morbid metabolic illness, colonic ischemia after myocardial infarction, and isolated right-sided colitis [2].

The common differential diagnoses include diverticulitis, infections, IBD, and complicated colon cancer or radiation colitis. Typically, patients with diverticulitis will have more fever and more leukocytosis with CT findings limited to the sigmoid colon. Splenic flexure thickening favors ischemia. Older patients have a lower incidence of IBD but differentiation from left side Crohn disease can be difficult. Rapid resolution with a normal colonoscopy or colonoscopy showing hemorrhagic necrosis predicts colonic ischemia. Infections with Shiga toxin-positive bacteria are particularly difficult since colonoscopy can show similar findings and biopsies can show mucosal necrosis with crypt epithelial loss (ghost crypts). Antibiotic use or recent dietary indiscretions are helpful but sporadic *Clostridium difficile* infection is increasing, and presumably safe but actually contaminated food use such as undercooked meats, contaminated vegetables, and even salad products have been implicated in colitis causation. Cultures for enterohemorrhagic *Escherichia coli* (EHEC) organisms, *Shigella*, *C. difficile*, and *Klebsiella oxytoca* (so-called antibiotic associated hemorrhagic colitis) should be done early [11,12]. Stopping offending drugs if clinically feasible should be done. Colonic cancer is usually in the differential of colonic strictures after resolved colonic ischemia and colonoscopy with biopsies will typically differentiate between them. Radiation colitis is a possibility in patients with prostate cancer radiation or female genitourinary radiation treatment. Microvascular damage with segmental ulcerations and fibrosis will be the endoscopic findings. Clinical history and endoscopic mucosal angiodysplasia, particularly in the rectum, will usually differentiate radiation-induced injury from uncomplicated colonic ischemia [13].

Diagnostic testing sequence depends on both time from presentation, the level of severity and systemic toxicity. CT examination to locate disease and look for potential complications is the first test. Free air or severe pneumatosis require urgent surgical evaluation. Segmental disease involving the left colon with splenic flexure or

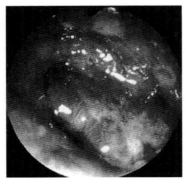

Figure 46.4 Colon ischemia—hemorrhagic phase.

isolated right colon without CT complications mandate urgent colonoscopic evaluation if the patient has no toxicity. Endoscopic findings are highly specific but biopsy confirmation should be done. Progressive symptoms or systemic toxicity require CT confirmation of progression or complications.

Therapy of Colonic Ischemia

In most cases, early recognition, supportive therapy, and stopping potential offending substances is all that is needed (Figure 46.5). Mortality with non-gangrenous colonic ischemia is 6%. Monitoring for progression is critical. If transmural injury is suspected, antibiotics are recommended based on animal studies showing increased bacterial translocation (Evidence Level C). Cardiac function and oxygenation should be maximized (Evidence Level C). If progression to transmural injury occurs, prompt colonic resection with appropriate margins is recommended.

Colonic infarction has a high mortality (50–75%) because of co-morbid disease. Most patients require an initial diverting colostomy with mucous fistula to assess for progressive interval damage requiring second look surgery with repeat resection if necessary (Evidence C). Aortoilial reconstruction has a high risk for transmural colonic ischemia requiring surgery.

Hypercoagulable states producing mesenteric venous thrombosis rarely cause colonic ischemia but, if present, anticoagulation may be required for at least 3–6 months but may be used lifelong (Evidence C).

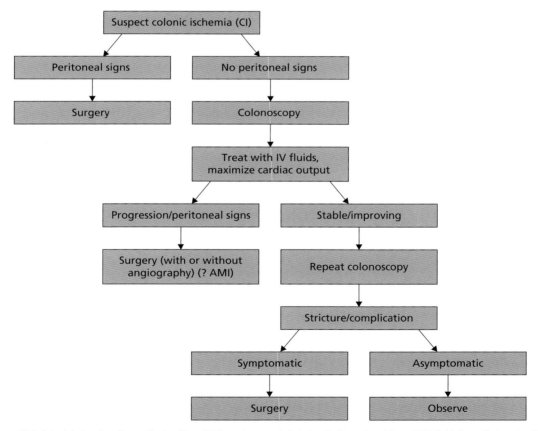

Figure 46.5 Colonic ischemia—diagnostic algorithm. (AMI, acute mesenteric ischemia. Reproduced from AGA Guidelines. *Gastroenterology* 2000; 118: 951–3, with permission from Elsevier.)

Take-home points

- Colonic ischemia is common and increasing in incidence.
- Multiple factors producing colonic ischemia are common including metabolic disease, atherosclerosis, advancing age of the population, surgery, and colonic ischemia-producing medications.
- Hypoperfusion with reperfusion injury is the cause of ischemic injury. Reperfusion is the usual cause for radiologic and endoscopic findings.
- Most cases are non-occlusive and spontaneously resolve without sequelae. Progression is associated with increasing pain, peritoneal findings, leukocytosis, and acidosis. Surgery should be done early if progression is evident.
- Colonic ischemia associated with surgery, cardiac failure, or renal transplantation requires prolonged observation because of high mortality.
- Look for infections, IBD, and pharmacologic agents as major treatable risk factors.
- CT examination followed by colonoscopy with biopsies will usually confirm the clinical diagnosis. Angiography is rarely helpful and barium enema is contraindicated in most cases.
- Colonic ischemia associated with pharmacologic agents is likely to shed light on pathophysiological mechanisms.

References

1 Higgins PD, Davis KL, Laine L. Systematic review: the epidemiology of ischemic colitis. *Aliment Pharmacol Ther* 2004; **19**: 729–38.

2 Brandt LJ, Boley SJ. AGA technical review on intestinal ischemia. American Gastrointestinal Association. *Gastroenterology* 2000; **118**: 954–68.

3 Hass DJ, Kozuch P, Brandt LJ. Pharmacologically mediated colonic ischemia. *Am J Gastroenterol* 2007; **102**: 1765–80.

4 Gibson GR, Whitacre EB, Ricotti CA. Colitis induced by NSAIDs. *Arch Intern Med* 1992; **152**: 625–32.

5 Chang L, Chey WD, Harris L, *et al.* Incidence of ischemic colitis and serious complications of constipation among patients using alosetron: systematic review of clinical trials and post marketing surveillance data. *Am J Gastroenterol* 2006; **101**: 1069–79.

6 Moses FM. Exercise-associated intestinal ischemia. *Curr Sports Med Rep* 2005; **4**: 91–5.

7 Koutroubakis IE, Sfiridaki A, Theodoropoulou A, Kouroumalis EA. Role of acquired and hereditary thrombotic risk factors in colonic ischemia of ambulatory patients. *Gastroenterology* 2001; **121**: 561–5.

8 West AB, Kuan S, Bennick M, Lagarde S. Glutaraldehyde colitis following endoscopy: clinical outbreak and pathological features and investigation of the outbreak. *Gastroenterology* 1995; **108**: 1250–5.

9 Greenwood DA, Brandt LJ, Reinus JF. Ischemic bowel disease in the elderly. *Gastroenterol Clin North Am* 2001; **30**: 445–73.

10 Zuckerman GR, Prakash E, Merriman RB, *et al.* The colon single-stripe sign and its relationship to ischemic colitis. *Am J Gastroenterol* 2003; **98**: 2018–22.

11 Beaugerie L, Metz M, Barbut F, *et al.* Klebsiella oxytoca as an agent of antibiotic associated hemorrhagic colitis. *Clin Gastroenterol Hepatol* 2003; **1**: 370–6.

12 Dignan CR, Greenson JK. Can ischemic colitis be differentiated from C. difficile colitis in biopsy specimens? *Am J Surg Pathol* 1997; **21**: 706–10.

13 Nostrant TT, Robertson JM, Lawrence TS. Radiation injury. In: Yamada T, ed. *Textbook of Gastroenterology*, 2nd edn. Philadelphia: JB Lippincott, 1995: 2524–36.

CHAPTER 47

Acute Diverticulitis

Chee-Chee H. Stucky[1] and Tonia M. Young-Fadok[2]

[1] Department of General Surgery, Mayo Clinic, Scottsdale, AZ, USA
[2] Division of Colorectal Surgery, Mayo Clinic, Scottsdale, AZ, USA

Summary

Diverticulitis occurs when diverticula present in the colonic wall become inflamed. This leads to micro- or macroscopic perforation of these sac-like protrusions. Diverticulitis can be divided into complicated and uncomplicated presentations, and the management differs based on the presentation. Surgical intervention is not always a necessity. This chapter summarizes the clinical manifestations and diagnosis of acute diverticulitis as well as current recommendations for medical and surgical management.

Case

A 70-year-old woman presented to the emergency room with a 3-day history of left lower quadrant pain, bloating, diarrhea, and nausea. Physical examination revealed a temperature of 38.0°C and laboratory evaluation showed leukocytosis. CT scan demonstrated diverticulosis of the sigmoid colon with associated bowel wall thickening and fat stranding but no pericolic fluid. The patient was admitted and made "nothing by mouth" (NPO) with IV fluid hydration. Metronidazole and ceftriaxone were started. After 2 days, the patient's abdominal pain and diarrhea had resolved. The patient was given clear liquids initially and diet was advanced as tolerated. Six weeks after discharge to home, the patient underwent colonoscopy and was found to have extensive diverticulosis involving the descending and sigmoid colon but no evidence of malignancy. This was her second hospitalization for diverticulitis, and at surgical consultation sigmoid resection was recommended.

Definition and Epidemiology

Diverticular disease of the colon refers to the presence of sac-like protrusions of the colonic wall. Diverticulitis is thought to occur by erosion of the diverticular wall by

Practical Gastroenterology and Hepatology: Small and Large Intestine and Pancreas, 1st edition. Edited by Nicholas J. Talley, Sunanda V. Kane and Michael B. Wallace. © 2010 Blackwell Publishing Ltd.

increased intraluminal pressure or inspissated food particles. This progresses to inflammation and focal necrosis, ultimately leading to micro- or macroscopic perforation of the diverticulum.

Recent epidemiologic studies have shown that the prevalence of diverticular disease increases with age, from less than 5% at age 40, to 30% by age 60, to 65% by age 85. There appears to be equal distribution between genders overall; however, certain age groups (elderly women, and obese young men) show gender specificity [1]. Geographic variation is a distinct feature of diverticulitis. Western countries have a higher prevalence rate (5 to 45%) than the corresponding age groups of the African and Asian countries (less than 0.2%). The location of disease also differs in that left-sided diverticulitis is more common in the Western countries while right-sided diverticulitis predominates otherwise. The incidence of diverticular disease appears to be related to lifestyle characteristics as seen by the increase in prevalence of diverticulosis in those countries which have adopted a more Western diet and sedentary daily routine [2].

Pathophysiology

The etiology of diverticular disease may be linked to lifestyle factors including, but likely not limited to, decreased

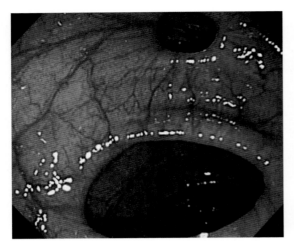

Figure 47.1 Diverticulum seen during colonoscopy with vasa recta vessels visible.

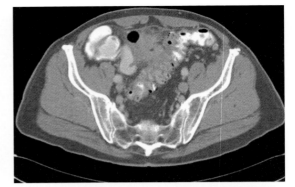

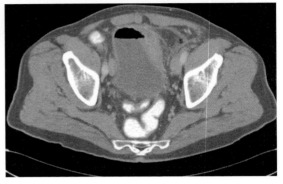

Figure 47.2 Colovesical fistula—the presence of air in the bladder is pathognomonic for this diagnosis.

dietary fiber intake, high intake of fat or red meat, lack of exercise, and obesity [3–5]. While historically patients have been advised to avoid seeds, corn, and nuts, this concept has yet to be proven clinically. This senior author has never seen a seed or a nut within even one of tens of thousands of diverticula!

Diverticula develop in areas of weakness, specifically the four points around the circumference of the colon where the vasa recta penetrate the circular muscle layer (Figure 47.1). Typically, these are "false" diverticula which do not contain all layers of the wall but just mucosa and submucosa herniated through the muscle layer. Ninety-five percent of diverticula are found in the sigmoid colon [6]. While there is no hypertrophy or hyperplasia of the bowel wall in these areas, there are structural changes including increased elastin deposition which may decrease the resistance of the wall to intra-luminal pressure [7].

Clinical Features

Acute diverticulitis can be divided into two presenta-tions: complicated and uncomplicated. Seventy-five percent of cases are uncomplicated and present with abdominal pain (usually in the left lower quadrant), changes in bowel habits, nausea, and vomiting. The pres-ence of pain for several days prior to seeking out medical

attention often aids in the differentiation of diverticulitis from other causes of acute abdominal symptoms. Also, up to one-half of patients have had one or more previous episodes of similar pain [8].

Low-grade fever and mild leukocytosis are fairly common signs of diverticulitis, but not always present. Other blood tests are typically normal or only mildly elevated and sterile pyuria may be seen on urinalysis.

Diverticular bleeding typically occurs in the absence of acute diverticulitis, but a history of painless melena or bright red blood per rectum is common in patients with diverticular disease [9].

Complicated diverticulitis with abscess, stricture, or fistula may present in similar fashion to uncomplicated diverticulitis. Some patients with fistula and stricture may even present with symptoms of pneumaturia (Figure 47.2) and obstruction, respectively, without a docu-mented prior episode of diverticulitis. Complicated diverticulitis in the form of free perforation, however,

Table 47.1 Differential diagnosis of left lower quadrant abdominal pain.

Colon cancer
Acute appendicitis
Crohn disease
Ischemic colitis
Pseudomembranous colitis
Viral gastroenteritis
Diverticular colitis
Ovarian cyst
Ovarian abscess
Ovarian torsion
Ectopic pregnancy

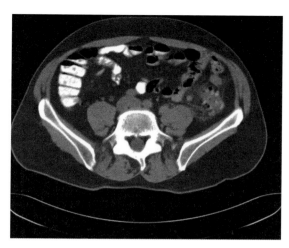

Figure 47.3 Uncomplicated diverticulitis: sigmoid wall thickening, fat stranding, and presence of diverticula.

presents as an acute abdomen with generalized peritonitis.

The rare occasion of right-sided diverticulitis may present with right lower quadrant pain and may be mistaken for acute appendicitis.

Diagnosis

The history and physical examination are essential in the diagnosis of acute diverticulitis, but further studies are necessary to confirm the diagnosis while ruling out other causes of the patient's signs and symptoms (Table 47.1). Routine abdominal and chest radiographs are commonly performed and aid in ruling out causes such as intestinal obstruction, but are otherwise no-contributory. Computed tomography (CT) of the abdomen and pelvis is the gold standard for diagnosis, assessment of severity, therapeutic intervention, and quantification of resolution of the disease. When performed with intravenous and oral contrast, features of acute diverticulitis include increased soft tissue density within pericolic fat, colonic diverticula, bowel wall thickening, and soft tissue masses representing phlegmon or pericolic fluid collections representing abscesses (Figure 47.2). CT evaluation has superior results when compared with barium enema or compression ultrasonography [10,11].

Once the acute episode has resolved, patients should undergo elective colonoscopy to rule out other lesions such as carcinoma (Figure 47.3). Barium enema plus flexible sigmoidoscopy is outdated; CT colography is only selectively available.

Treatment

Uncomplicated Diverticulitis

Therapy for acute diverticulitis depends on the presentation of the disease: complicated versus uncomplicated [12] (Figure 47.4). In the uncomplicated setting, there is a localized infection that requires bowel rest and antibiotics. In mild cases this may be safely achieved as an outpatient with oral antibiotics.

Those patients requiring intravenous fluid resuscitation, with high fever or leukocytosis, or significant comorbidities should be treated in the hospital setting. Elderly, immunosuppressed, and diabetic patients for example should undergo treatment as inpatients. Outpatients are restricted to clear liquids and started on an antibiotic regimen of ciprofloxacin and metronidazole. Amoxicillin–clavulanate and clindamycin may be used as alternatives. If signs and symptoms improve after 2 to 3 days, diet is advanced. These patients must receive explicit instruction to seek immediate medical attention if experiencing increase in fever or abdominal pain, if they are unable to consume adequate fluids, or if they fail to improve within 2 to 3 days. The possibility of abscess development should be explored in all patients who deteriorate or fail to improve. Intervention may include percutaneous drainage of abscesses or laparotomy under certain indications (Table 47.2).

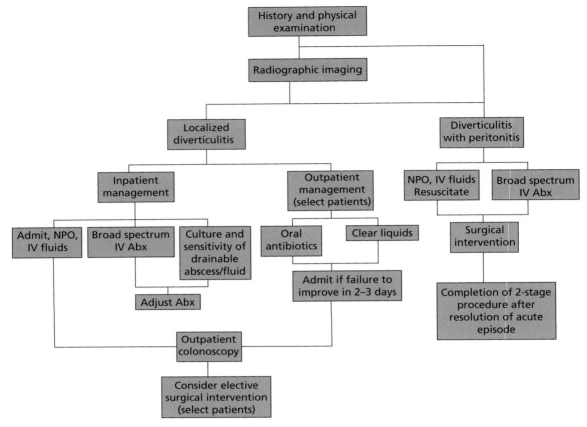

Figure 47.4 Flowchart for treatment of acute diverticulitis. NPO, nothing by mouth; IV, intravenous; Abx, antibiotics.

Table 47.2 Indications for surgery in at time of presentation in acute diverticulitis.

Peritonitis
Abscess (failed percutaneous drainage)
Obstruction, symptomatic
Clinical deterioration or failure to improve with medical therapy

Hospitalized patients are made NPO and given intravenous hydration. Empiric broad-spectrum intravenous antibiotics are directed at colonic anaerobic and Gram-negative flora. Metronidazole and third-generation cephalosporins, fluoroquinolones (ciprofloxacin or levofloxacin) or short courses of aminoglycosides may be used. Single agents with appropriate colonic flora coverage [13] include β-lactamase inhibitor combination antibiotics (ampicillin–sulbactam, piperacillin–tazobactam

or ticarcillin–clavulanate) or carbapenems (imipenem or meropenem). If drainage of any associated abscess is performed, antibiotic coverage is tailored once the causative organisms are identified.

As noted above, colonoscopy should be performed following successful conservative therapy for a first attack of diverticulitis. Thirty to 40% of patient will remain asymptomatic, 30 to 40% will have episodic abdominal cramps without frank diverticulitis, and 33% will proceed to a second attack of diverticulitis. It was generally believed that prognosis is worse with a second attack [1]. This is now not current belief. Most patients run "true-to-form", that is if they have attacks manageable as outpatients with oral antibiotics, subsequent attacks often will be of similar severity. In fact, 90% of patients who present with perforation have had no preceding attack, but have a factor that predisposes to this presentation.

Patients at increased risk of more severe attacks include young patients (less than 40 or 50 years of age) and the immunosuppressed [14].

Complicated Diverticulitis

Patients diagnosed with complicated diverticulitis undergo a more aggressive therapeutic regimen. In the case of peritonitis, immediate resuscitation, broad-spectrum antibiotics, and surgical exploration are performed in lieu of diagnostic studies. The mortality rate of perforated diverticulitis is 6% for purulent peritonitis and 35% for fecal peritonitis [15,16]. Examples of appropriate antibiotics include the combination of ampicillin or gentamicin plus metronidazole, imipenem/cilastin or piperacillin–tazobactam.

Diverticular obstruction must be differentiated from carcinoma. Whenever malignancy is suspected, resection is mandatory. Obstruction due to diverticulitis is rarely complete, and, therefore, patients may undergo appropriate bowel preparation prior to surgery.

With improvement in CT technology, small diverticular abscesses not amenable to drainage are found and may be treated with antibiotics. Whether these cases may be treated as uncomplicated diverticulitis is under further investigation. Abscesses larger than 3–4 cm require intervention, generally via percutaneous drainage and rarely surgery in cases of failed CT-guided drain placement. Macroperforation of diverticulitis leading to diffuse peritonitis is associated with a high mortality rate and surgical intervention is mandatory.

Surgery

Elective surgical intervention has typically been advised after a first attack of complicated diverticulitis (abscess, fistula, or stricture) or after two or more episodes of uncomplicated diverticulitis [17] (Table 47.3). More

Table 47.3 Indications for delayed operation after confirmed diverticulitis.

Abscess responding to percutaneous drainage
Symptomatic stricture
Fistula (colovesical, colovaginal, etc.)
Recurrent episodes
Inability to exclude carcinoma
Immunosuppression
Right-sided diverticulitis
? Young patient

recent data suggest that the limit of two episodes is not mandatory in uncomplicated diverticulitis, particularly if treated as an outpatient, and tailored advice is necessary, depending on the patient's age, preferences, and co-morbidities.

In the case of emergent surgical intervention in the patient with an acute abdomen, assessment of peritoneal contamination determines the advisability of a primary anastomosis versus a two-stage procedure. In the presence of fecal or purulent peritonitis, associated medical conditions, poor nutrition, immunosuppression, or emergency situations, two-stage procedures are indicated. The Hartmann procedure is a common approach which involves resection of the diseased colon, an end-colostomy, and creation of a rectal stump. The colostomy is closed 3 months later. Other two-stage procedures include primary anastomosis after resection, and a proximal diverting stoma with stoma closure at a later time. Single-stage procedures are less widely touted and include on-table washout of the proximal colon plus primary anastomosis; and laparoscopic evaluation, washout, and placement of drains *without* resection. The latter in particular requires additional data but is an attractive option. Currently, reported series have been highly selective [18,19].

Elective surgery after resolution of the acute episode of diverticulitis may be performed laparoscopically, and is the approach of choice for these authors. In this instance, resection and primary anastomosis are possible as long as adequate bowel preparation is achieved preoperatively and the bowel is well-vascularized, non-edematous and tension-free [20, 21].

Take-home points

Diagnosis:
- The diagnosis of diverticulitis is based on history and physical examination, with CT used for confirmation.

- History typically includes left lower quadrant abdominal pain, changes in bowel habits, and nausea or vomiting.

- Clinical signs may include fever and leukocytosis.

- Generalized abdominal tenderness suggests free perforation and peritonitis.

- The presence of abscess, obstruction, fistula, or perforation is classified as complicated diverticulitis.

- Colonoscopy should be performed after resolution of the acute episode to evaluate the extent of disease and rule out malignancy.

Therapy:
- Uncomplicated diverticulitis may be treated as an outpatient in selected circumstances in low-risk patients.
- Inpatient treatment includes NPO, intravenous fluids, and broad-spectrum antibiotics.
- Complicated diverticulitis with abscess requires intervention either by percutaneous drainage of associated abscesses or (rarely, with current interventional radiology techniques) surgery.
- Complicated diverticulitis with drained abscess, microperforation with phlegmon responsive to intravenous antibiotics, stricture, or fistula generally requires elective surgical intervention.
- Complicated diverticulitis with generalized peritonitis requires emergent laparoscopic or open exploration, with one- or two-stage procedure, or washout with drain placement.
- Surgical intervention commonly involves a two-stage procedure with stoma formation and delayed closure, but may be done laparoscopically or with primary anastomosis.

References

1 Parks TG. Natural history of diverticular disease of the colon. *Clin Gastroeneterol* 1975; **4**: 53–69.
2 Miura S, Kodaira S, Shatari T, *et al.* Recent trends in diverticulosis of the right colon in Japan: retrospective review in a regional hospital. *Dis Colon Rectum* 2000; **43**: 1383–9.
3 Aldoori WH, Giovannucci EL, Rimm EB, *et al.* A prospective study of diet and the risk of symptomatic diverticular disease in men. *Am J Clin Nutr* 1994; **60**: 757–64.
4 Aldoori WH, Giovannucci EL, Rimm EB, *et al.* A prospective study of alcohol, smoking, caffeine, and the risk of symptomatic diverticular disease in men. *Ann Epidemiol* 1995; **5**: 221–8.
5 Strate LL, Liu YL, Aldoori WH, *et al.* Obesity increases the risks of diverticulitis and diverticular bleeding. *Gastroenterology* 2009; **136**: 115–22.
6 Rodkey GV, Welch CE. Changing patterns in the surgical treatment of diverticular disease. *Ann Surg* 1984; **200**: 466–78.

7 Whiteway J, Morson BC. Elastosis in diverticular disease of the sigmoid colon. *Gut* 1985; **26**: 258–66.
8 Konvolink CW. Acute diverticulitis under age forty. *Am J Surg* 1994; **167**: 562–5.
9 Meyers MA, Alonso DR, Gray GF, *et al.* Pathogenesis of bleeding colonic diverticulosis. *Gastroenterology* 1976; **71**: 577–83.
10 Birnbaum BA, Balthazar EJ. CT of appendicitis and diverticulitis. *Radiol Clin North Am* 1994; **32**: 885–98.
11 Hulnick DH, Megibow AJ, Balthazar EJ, *et al.* Computed tomography in the evaluation of diverticulitis. *Radiology* 1984; **152**: 491–5.
12 Rafferty J, Shellito P, Hyman NH. Buie WD. Standards Committee of American Society of Colon and Rectal Surgeons. Practice parameters for sigmoid diverticulitis. *Dis Colon Rectum* 2006; **49**: 939–44.
13 Kellum JM, Sugerman HJ, Coppa GF, *et al.* Randomized, prospective comparison of cefoxitin and gentamicin-clindamycin in the treatment of acute colonic diverticulitis. *Clin Ther* 1992; **14**: 376–84.
14 Chautems RC, Ambrosetti P, Ludwig A, *et al.* Long-term follow-up after first acute episode of sigmoid diverticulitis: is surgery mandatory?: a prospective study of 118 patients. *Dis Colon Rectum* 2002; **45**: 962–6.
15 Nagorney DM, Adson MA, Pemberton JH. Sigmoid diverticulitis with perforation and generalized peritonitis. *Dis Colon Rectum* 1985; **28**: 71–5.
16 Morris CR, Harvey IM, Stebbings WS, Hart AR. Incidence of perforated diverticulitis and risk factors for death in a UK population. *Br J Surg* 2008: **95**: 876–81.
17 Stollman NH, Raskin JB. Diverticular disease of the colon. *J Clin Gastroenterol* 1999; **29**: 241–52.
18 Myers E, Hurley M, O'Sullivan GC, *et al.* Laparoscopic peritoneal lavage for generalized peritonitis due to perforated diverticulitis. *Br J Surg* 2008; **95**: 97–101
19 Franklin ME Jr, Portillo G, Trevino JM, *et al.* Long-term experience with the laparoscopic approach to perforated diverticulitis plus generalized peritonitis. *World J Surg* 2008; **32**: 1507–11.
20 Kohler L, Sauerland S, Neugebauer E. Diagnosis and treatment of diverticular disease: Results of a consensus development conference. The scientific Committee of the European Association for Endoscopic Surgery. *Surg Endosc* 1999; **13**: 430–6.
21 Scheidbach H, Schneider C, Rose J, *et al.* Laparoscopic approach to treatment of sigmoid diverticulitis: changes in the spectrum of indications and results of a prospective, multicenter study on 1,545 patients. *Dis Colon Rectum* 2004; **47**: 1883–8.

CHAPTER 48
Acute Colonic Pseudo-obstruction

Michael D. Saunders

Division of Gastroenterology, University of Washington Medical Center, Seattle, WA, USA

Summary

Acute colonic pseudo-obstruction (ACPO) is a syndrome of massive dilation of the colon without mechanical obstruction that develops in hospitalized patients with serious underlying medical and surgical conditions. ACPO is associated with significant morbidity and mortality, and, therefore, requires urgent gastroenterologic evaluation. Appropriate evaluation of the markedly distended colon involves excluding mechanical obstruction and other causes of toxic megacolon such as *Clostridium difficile* infection, and assessing for signs of ischemia and perforation. Increasing age, cecal diameter, delay in decompression, and status of the bowel significantly influence mortality, which is approximately 40% when ischemia or perforation is present. The risk of colonic perforation in ACPO increases when cecal diameter exceeds 12 cm and when the distension has been present for greater than 6 days. Appropriate management includes supportive therapy and selective use of neostigmine and colonoscopy for decompression. Early recognition and management are critical in minimizing complications.

Case

A 63-year-old man developed increasing abdominal distension 3 days after radical prostatectomy with bilateral lymph node dissection for prostate cancer. His postoperative course was complicated by atrial fibrillation with rapid ventricular response requiring intravenous rate control with calcium-channel antagonist medication in the ICU. The patient reported progressive cramping abdominal pain, bloating, and distension over a 3-day period. There was nausea but no vomiting. He was passing flatus but minimal stool. His past medical history was notable only for osteoarthritis and hypertension. His postoperative medications also included morphine administered by patient-controlled analgesia.

Abdominal radiographs revealed gaseous distension of large bowel with a cecal diameter of approximately 10 cm. There were no fevers and the leukocyte count was normal. Supportive therapy was instituted but the patient had progressive symptoms and distension despite these measures. Follow-up abdominal radiograph the next day showed persistent, marked cecal distension. Given the significant colonic dilation and non-response to over 24 h of supportive therapy, the patient was considered for

pharmacologic decompression with neostigmine. Although there had been atrial tachyarrythmias postoperatively, the rate had been adequately controlled and the rhythm had reverted to normal sinus spontaneously. Neostigmine, 2 mg intravenously, was administered with prompt evacuation of flatus and stool, and resolution of colonic distension by subsequent radiograph. No adverse reactions to the infusion were noted. He made a full recovery and was discharged home a week later.

Definition and Epidemiology

Intestinal pseudo-obstruction is a term used to characterize a clinical syndrome with symptoms, signs, and radiographic appearance of bowel obstruction without a mechanical cause [1]. According to presentation, pseudo-obstruction syndromes can be subdivided into acute and chronic forms. Acute colonic pseudo-obstruction (ACPO) is characterized by massive colonic dilation with symptoms and signs of colonic obstruction without mechanical blockage [1]. Chronic colonic pseudo-obstruction represents an entirely different disorder in pathogenesis, presentation, and management, and will be briefly discussed at the end of this review.

Practical Gastroenterology and Hepatology: Small and Large Intestine and Pancreas, 1st edition. Edited by Nicholas J. Talley, Sunanda V. Kane and Michael B. Wallace. © 2010 Blackwell Publishing Ltd.

ACPO is an important cause of morbidity and mortality, which can be substantial because of serious concomitant illness. Ischemia and perforation are the feared complications of ACPO. Spontaneous perforation has been reported in 3 to 15% of cases with a mortality rate estimated at 50% or higher when this occurs [2]. The clinical presentation of ACPO has been extensively documented in the literature. However, despite the accurate description of this condition, its diagnosis remains difficult and is often delayed. Early recognition and prompt appropriate management are critical to minimizing poor outcomes. Thus, ACPO represents a true gastroenterologic emergency.

The main issues for the clinician to consider are:

1 What is the correct diagnosis?

2 Is ischemia or perforation present?

3 What is the appropriate evaluation and management?

The exact incidence of ACPO is unknown. In the retrospective series of patients undergoing orthopedic procedures reported by Norwood *et al.* [3], the incidence of ACPO was 1.3, 1.19, and 0.65% following hip replacement, spinal operations, and knee replacement, respectively. ACPO most often affects those in late middle age (mean of 60 years of age), with a slight male predominance (60%) [4]. ACPO occurs almost exclusively in hospitalized or institutionalized patients with serious underlying medical and surgical conditions. Abdominal distension usually develops over 3 to 7 days but can occur as rapidly as 24 to 48 hours. In surgical patients, symptoms and signs develop at a mean of 5 days postoperatively.

Pathophysiology

The pathogenesis of ACPO is not completely understood although it likely results from an alteration in the autonomic regulation of colonic motor function. Colonic pseudo-obstruction was first described in 1948 by Sir Heneage Ogilive, who reported two patients with chronic colonic dilation associated with malignant infiltration of the celiac plexus. Ogilvie attributed the syndrome to sympathetic deprivation. A better understanding of the autonomic nervous system in the gut has modified this hypothesis. The parasympathetic nerves to the right colon are supplied by the vagus nerve. The distal colon receives its parasympathetic nerve innervation from the

sacral cord (S2–4). The sympathetic innervation to the colon is via the celiac and mesenteric ganglia. The parasympathetic nervous system increases contractility, whereas the sympathetic nerves decrease motility [5]. An imbalance in autonomic innervation, produced by a variety of factors, leads to excessive parasympathetic suppression or sympathetic stimulation. Because the vagal supply to the large bowel terminates at the splenic flexure and the parasympathetic innervation of the left colon originates from the sacral plexus, it has been proposed that transient parasympathetic impairment at the sacral plexus may cause atony of the distal large bowel and functional obstruction [6]. Alternatively, hyperactivity of inhibitory neurons to the large bowel, due to increased sympathetic drive, may play an important role in the pathophysiology of ACPO [5]. Mechanoreceptors located within the wall of the large intestine, when stimulated by distension, activate a reflex pathway whose final effect, via efferent sympathetic nerves targeting the myenteric plexus or smooth muscle layers, is the inhibition of colonic motility (colocolonic reflex) [5]. However, despite improved knowledge on the pathophysiology of colonic motility, the precise mechanisms underlying ACPO remain poorly understood.

Clinical Features

The clinical features of ACPO include abdominal distension, abdominal pain (80%), and nausea and/or vomiting (60%) [4]. Passage of flatus or stool is reported in up to 40% of patients. No significant differences were noted in symptoms of patients with ischemic or perforated bowel, except for a higher incidence of fever [4]. On examination, the abdomen is tympanitic and bowel sounds are typically present. Fever, marked abdominal tenderness, and leukocytosis are more common in patients with ischemia or perforation but also occur in those who have not developed these complications [4].

The vast majority of patients (>95%) with ACPO have the syndrome in association with a predisposing factor or clinical condition (Table 48.1). In a large retrospective series of 400 patients, the most common predisposing conditions were non-operative trauma (11%), infections (10%), and cardiac disease (10%) [4]. Cesarean section and hip surgery were the most common surgical procedures. In a retrospective series of orthopedic surgical

Table 48.1 Predisposing conditions associated with acute colonic pseudo-obstruction: an analysis of 400 cases.*

Condition	Number	Percent rate
Trauma (non-operative)	45	11.3
Infection (pneumonia, sepsis most common)	40	10.0
Cardiac (myocardial infarction, heart failure)	40	10.0
Obstetrics/gynecology	39	9.8
Abdominal/pelvic surgery	37	9.3
Neurologic (Parkinson disease, spinal cord injury, multiple sclerosis, Alzheimer disease)	37	9.3
Orthopedic surgery	29	7.3
Miscellaneous medical conditions (metabolic, cancer, respiratory failure, renal failure)	128	32
Miscellaneous surgical conditions (urologic, thoracic, neurosurgery)	47	11.8

*Associated conditions of approximately 400 patients, reported by Vanek *et al.* [4]. Some patients had more than one associated condition.

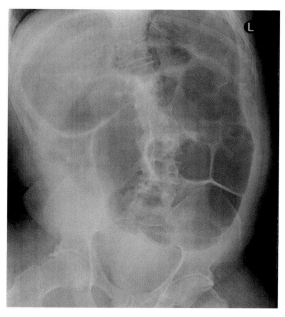

Figure 48.1 Plain abdominal radiographs of a patient with acute colonic pseudo-obstruction demonstrating marked colonic dilation mimicking mechanical obstruction. Varying degrees of small intestinal dilation are evident.

patients, ACPO patients were evaluated for potential exacerbating or contributing factors compared to age-matched controls [3]. In comparison to control patients, patients who developed ACPO had significantly lower postoperative serum sodium, a higher serum urea, and remained in hospital longer. In another retrospective analysis of 48 patients, the spine or retroperitoneum had been traumatized or manipulated in 52% [7]. Over half the patients were receiving narcotics, and electrolyte abnormalities were present in approximately two-thirds. Thus, multiple metabolic, pharmacologic, or traumatic factors appear to alter the autonomic regulation of colonic function resulting in pseudo-obstruction. The mechanisms through which these different conditions temporarily suppress colonic motility and induce dilation are unknown.

Diagnosis

The diagnosis of ACPO is suggested by the clinical presentation and confirmed by plain abdominal radio-

graphs, which show varying degrees of colonic dilation (Figure 48.1). The right colon and cecum show the most marked distension, and "cutoffs" at the splenic flexure and descending colon are common. This distribution of colonic dilation may be caused by the different origins of the proximal and distal parasympathetic nerve supply to the colon. Air fluid levels and dilatation can also be seen in the small bowel.

The differential diagnosis of acute colonic distension in hospitalized or institutionalized patients includes:
- Mechanical obstruction
- Toxic megacolon due to severe *Clostridium difficile* infection
- ACPO.

The appropriate urgent evaluation of a patient with suspected ACPO, therefore, includes excluding mechanical obstruction and other causes of a toxic megacolon such as *Clostridium difficile*, and assessment for signs of peritonitis or perforation which would warrant urgent surgical intervention. Estimation should be made on the degree and duration of colonic distension. If on plain abdominal radiographs air is not seen throughout all colonic segments including the rectosigmoid, then a computed tomography scan or a water-soluble contrast enema should be performed to exclude distal obstruction. Stool should be submitted for *Clostridium difficile* toxin assay. In addition, empiric treatment for *Clostridium difficile* while awaiting stool results or a limited sigmoidoscopic examination assessing for the presence of pseudomembranes is reasonable if one needs an immediate diagnosis based on the severity of the patient's condition.

The assessment for ischemia or perforation includes both clinical examination and imaging studies. Fever, abdominal tenderness, and leukocytosis are more common in patients with ischemia but also occur in those who have not developed these complications. Plain abdominal radiographs and computed tomography should be assessed for evidence of free peritoneal air and pneumatosis of the bowel wall.

Therapeutics

An evidenced-based guideline for the treatment of ACPO has been published by the American Society of Gastrointestinal Endoscopy [8]. A proposed algorithm for the management of ACPO is detailed in Figure 48.2. The

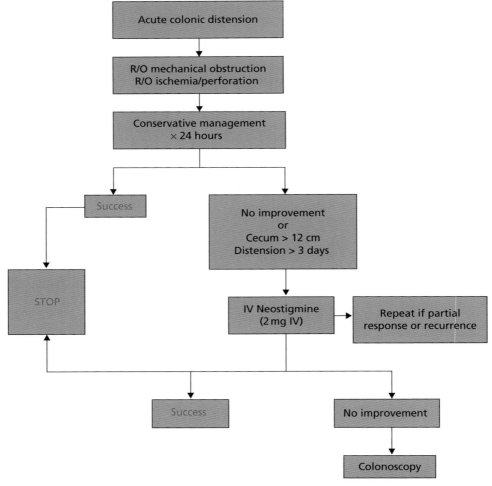

Figure 48.2 Management algorithm for acute colonic pseudo-obstruction. R/O, rule out.

clinical dilemma facing the clinician caring for a patient with ACPO is whether to treat the patient with conservative measures and close observation versus proceeding with medical or endoscopic decompression of the dilated colon.

Treatment options for ACPO include appropriate supportive measures, pharmacologic therapy, colonoscopic decompression, and surgery. Despite extensive literature documenting the clinical features of ACPO, there are few controlled clinical trials on the treatment of this condition, and most evidence for efficacy of treatments comes from anecdotal reports, retrospective reviews, or uncontrolled studies.

Supportive Therapy

Supportive therapy (Table 48.2) is the preferred initial management of ACPO and should be instituted in all patients [8]. Patients are given nothing by mouth. Intravenous fluids and electrolytes imbalances are corrected. Nasogastric suction is provided to limit swallowed air from contributing further to colonic distension. Laxatives are avoided, particularly lactulose, which provides substrate for colonic bacterial fermentation, resulting in further gas production. A rectal tube should be inserted and attached to gravity drainage. Medications that can adversely affect colonic motility, such as opiates, anticholinergics, and calcium-channel antagonists are discontinued if possible. Mobilization and ambulation of patients are encouraged, and the patients' position in bed should be changed frequently. The knee–hand position has been advocated by some to stimulate motility and promote colonic emptying [8]. Serial physical examinations and daily abdominal radiographs help closely monitor the progress of the patient. The benefits of any particular component of these supportive measures are unknown as these measures have not been studied individually.

Table 48.2 Supportive therapy for acute colonic pseudo-obstruction.

Nothing by mouth
Correct fluid and electrolyte imbalances
Nasogastric suction
Rectal tube decompression
Limit offending medications
Frequent position changes, ambulate if possible

Conservative management is successful as the primary treatment in the majority of patients. Sloyer *et al.* reported 25 cancer patients with ACPO (mostly non-gastrointestinal malignancies) [9]. The mean cecal diameter was 11.7 cm (range 9–18 cm). Of the 24 patients treated conservatively, 23 (96%) improved by clinical and radiologic criteria with the median time to improvement of 1.6 days (mean 3 days). There were no perforations or ACPO-related deaths. In another retrospective series of 151 patients, 117 (77%) had spontaneous resolution of ACPO with conservative treatment [10]. These studies demonstrate that the initial management of ACPO should be directed towards eliminating or reducing factors known to contribute to the problem.

The decision to intervene with medical therapy, colonoscopy, or surgery is dictated by the patient's clinical status. Knowing that the risk of colonic perforation is greatest with cecal diameter greater than 12 cm [4] and when distension has been present for more than 6 days [11], patients with marked cecal distension (>10 cm) of significant duration (>3–4 days) and those not improving after 24–48 h of supportive therapy are candidates for further intervention. In the absence of signs of overt peritonitis or perforation, medical therapy with neostigmine should be considered the initial therapy of choice.

Medical Therapy

Neostigmine

The only randomized, controlled therapeutic trial for ACPO involves intravenous neostigmine [12]. Neostigmine, a reversible acetylcholinesterase inhibitor, indirectly stimulates muscarinic receptors, thereby enhancing colonic motor activity, inducing colonic propulsion, and accelerating transit. The rationale for using neostigmine stems from the imbalance in autonomic regulation of colonic function that is proposed to occur in ACPO. Neostigmine, administered intravenously, has a rapid onset of action (1–20 min) and short duration (1–2 h) [13]. The elimination half-life averages 80 min, which is prolonged in patients with renal insufficiency.

A randomized, double-blind, placebo-controlled trial evaluated neostigmine in patients with ACPO with a cecal diameter of greater than 10 cm and no response to 24 h of conservative therapy [12]. Exclusion criteria were suspected ischemia or perforation, pregnancy, severe active bronchospasm, cardiac arrhythmias, and renal failure. Patients were randomized to receive neostigmine,

2 mg, or saline by intravenous infusion over 3–5 min. A clinical response was observed in 10 of 11 patients (91%) randomized to receive neostigmine compared to 0 of 10 receiving placebo. The median time to response was 4 min. Eight patients not responding to initial infusion (seven placebo, one neostigmine) were administered open-label neostigmine, and all had prompt decompression. Of the 18 patients who received neostigmine, either initially or during open-label treatment, 17 (94%) had a clinical response. The recurrence of colonic distension after neostigmine decompression was low (11%). The most common side effects observed with neostigmine were mild abdominal cramping and excessive salivation. Symptomatic bradycardia requiring atropine occurred in two of 19 patients.

Neostigmine was also evaluated in a double-blinded, placebo-controlled trial involving 24 critically ill, ventilated patients with ileus (defined as absence of stools for 3 days) [14]. No details of the extent and duration of colonic distension were provided. Neostigmine was administered as a continuous infusion (0.4 mg/h for 24 h). Of the 13 patients receiving neostigmine, 11 passed stools, whereas none of the placebo-treated patients passed stools (p < 0.001). No acute serious adverse events occurred but three patients had ischemic colonic complications 7–10 days after treatment.

There are also several non-controlled, open-label and retrospective series supporting the use of neostigmine in this condition [10,15–21]. Collectively, rapid decompression of colonic distension was observed in 87% of patients with a recurrence rate of approximately 10% (Table 48.3). In the prospective series reported by Mehta *et al.* [21], a response to neostigmine was more likely in the postoperative setting (11 of 15 (73%) vs. 1 of 4 (25%), P = 0.07), and less likely in those with electrolyte imbalance or receiving antimotility agents (3 of 15 (20%) vs. 4 of 4, P = 0.003). This study highlights the importance of correcting electrolyte abnormalities and limiting exacerbating medications.

Repeated infusions or more prolonged treatment with neostigmine have not been fully evaluated. There have been reports of patients with ACPO receiving repeated

Table 48.3 Neostigmine for colonic decompression in patients with acute colonic pseudo-obstruction.

Study	Number	Design	Dose	Decompression	Recurrence
Ponec (1999) [12]	21 (neostigmine 11, placebo 10)	RCT (OL in non-responders)	2.0 mg IV over 3–5 min	10/11 in RCT 17/18 total	2
Huthcinson (1992) [15]	11	OL	2.5 mg IV in 1 min.	8/11	0
Stephenson (1995) [16]	12	OL	2.5 mg IV over 1–3 min	12/12 (2 patients required 2 doses)	1
Turegano-Fuentes (1997) [17]	16	OL	2.5 mg IV over 60 min	12/16	0
Trevisani (2000) [18]	28	OL	2.5 mg IV over 3 min	26/28	0
Paran (2000) [19]	11	OL	2.5 mg IV over 60 min	10/11 (2 patients required 2 doses)	0
Abeyta (2001) [20]	8	Retrospective	2.0 mg IV	6/8 (2 patients required 2 doses)	0
Loftus (2002) [10]	18	Retrospective	2.0 mg IV	16/18	5
Mehta (2006) [21]	19	Prospective	2.0 mg IV	16/19	6
Total	141			123 (87%)	14 (10%)

RCT, randomized controlled trial; OL, open-label trial.

Table 48.4 Suggested protocol for administration of neostigmine in acute colonic pseudo-obstruction.

Neostigmine, 2 mg, intravenous infusion over 3–5 min

Atropine available at bedside

Patient kept supine, on bedpan

Continuous electrocardiographic monitoring with vital signs for 30 min

Continuous physician assessment for 15–30 min

---

infusions and prolonged treatment with resolution [22]. This experience suggest that cautious repeated infusions can be successful and merits further study in patients with persistent or recurrent pseudo-obstruction.

Although neostigmine was associated with a favorable safety profile in the reported clinical trials, caution should be used when administering the medication. Neostigmine should be given with the patient kept supine in bed with continuous electrocardiographic monitoring, physician assessment, and vital signs for 15–30 min following administration (Table 48.4). Contraindications to its use include mechanical obstruction, presence of ischemia or perforation, pregnancy, uncontrolled cardiac arrhythmias, severe active bronchospasm, and renal insufficiency (serum creatinine >3 mg/dL).

The cost of neostigmine for a 2 mg ampule for parenteral use is approximately $3 [12]. The cost to the patient after storage and handling fees are included is approximately $15.

Thus, neostigmine appears to be an effective, safe, and inexpensive method of colonic decompression in ACPO. The published data support its use as the initial therapy of choice for patients not responding to conservative therapy if there are no contraindications to its use. In patients with only a partial response or recurrence after an initial infusion, a second dose is reasonable and often successful. If the patient fails to respond after two doses, proceeding with colonoscopic decompression is advised.

Other Pharmacologic Therapy

Administration of polyethylene glycol electrolyte solution (PEG) in patients with ACPO after initial resolution may decrease the recurrence rate of colonic dilation. Sgouros *et al.* [23] evaluated PEG in a randomized, controlled trial in ACPO patients who had initial resolution of colonic dilation. The study enrolled 30 patients with cecal diameter 10 cm or greater that had resolution of the

colonic dilation with either neostigmine (22 patients) or endoscopic decompression (eight patients). Patients were then randomized to receive daily PEG 29.5 g or placebo. Recurrence was defined as a cecal diameter of 8 cm or greater with a concomitant 10% increase after the initial successful decompression. Five (33%) patients in the placebo group had recurrent cecal dilation compared with none in the PEG group (P = 0.04). Therapy with PEG resulted in a significant increase in stool and flatus output, decrease in colonic distension on radiographic measurements, and improvement in abdominal girth [23].

There are few data on strategies to prevent the development of ACPO. A recent randomized controlled clinical study evaluated whether lactulose or PEG were effective in promoting defecation in critically ill patients, whether either of the two is superior, and whether the use of enteral laxatives is related to clinical outcome [24]. Three hundred and eight consecutive patients with multiple organ failure were included. ACPO occurred in 4.1% of patients in the placebo group, 5.5% of patients in the lactulose group, and 1.0% of patients in the polyethylene glycol group. Thus, it appears that the use of PEG in critically ill patients to promote defecation may prevent the development of ACPO, and that its use following a pseudo-obstruction episode decreases the recurrence rate.

There are only anecdotal case reports using other prokinetic agents, such as erythromycin, in ACPO.

There are no data in ACPO on the use of other newly-developed prokinetic agents such as the selective chloride channel activator, lubiprostone, or opioid antagonist, alvimopan.

Endoscopic Decompression

Procedural Aspects

Non-surgical approaches to mechanical decompression have included radiologic placement of decompression tubes, colonoscopy with or without placement of a decompression tube, and percutaneous cecostomy performed through a either an endoscopic or radiologic approach. Colonoscopic decompression is preferred among these invasive, non-surgical options given the reported experience in the literature, now totaling many hundreds of patients [8].

Colonic decompression is the initial invasive procedure of choice for patients with marked cecal distension

(>10 cm) of significant duration (>3–4 days), not improving after 24–48 h of supportive therapy, and who have contraindications to or fail neostigmine. Colonoscopy is performed to prevent bowel ischemia and perforation. It should not be performed if overt peritonitis or perforation are present.

There is no well-defined standard of care regarding the use of colonoscopy in ACPO [8]. Colonoscopic decompression can be helpful in ACPO, but it is associated with a greater risk of complications, is not completely effective, and can be followed by recurrence. Oral laxatives and bowel preparations should not be administered prior to colonoscopy. Enemas can be given but the stool is usually already liquefied and whether their use facilitates colonoscopy in this setting is uncertain. Patients are often debilitated and bed-bound, thus making the administration of enemas impractical. Conscious sedation is achieved using primarily benzodiazepines, titrated to patient comfort. One should limit or use only low doses of narcotic analgesics given their deleterious effects on colonic motility.

The necessary materials needed for colonoscopic decompression are detailed in Table 48.5. Colonoscopes with large-diameter accessory channels (3.8 mm) or the dual channel colonoscope (Olympus® CF-2T160C), are preferable for optimal suctioning of stool and gas. The dual-channel scope with its 3.7 mm and 3.2 mm accessory channels has the advantage of not only superior suctioning capability but also in allowing continued suctioning during placement of the decompression tube. The colonoscope should be advanced as far as possible. Prolonged attempts at cecal intubation are not necessary because reaching the hepatic flexure usually suffices. Air insufflation should be minimized and the entire colon need not be examined. Gas should be aspirated and the viability of the mucosa assessed during slow withdrawal of the endoscope.

A tube for decompression should be placed in the right colon with the aid of a guidewire and fluoroscopic guidance. Commercially available, disposable, over-the-wire colon decompression tubes are available (Wilson-Cook® 14 French Colon Decompression Set). This disposable kit includes a guiding catheter (6 French, 181 cm length), guidewire (0.035 inch, 480 cm length), and decompression catheter (14 French, 175 cm length). The cost for this kit is $129 (USD). The drainage catheter consists of 10 elongated side ports for faster drainage (Figure 48.3). Alternatively, one can use a "home-made" model consisting of an 18 French Levine tube with the tip cut off and passed over a Savary or American guidewire (210 cm). The cost of this home-made model is approximately $160 (Levine tube $20; guidewire $140). The length of the Levine tube (80 cm) is shorter than the commercially-available catheters but placement into the right colon is usually feasible. The larger size of the Levine tube (18 versus 14 French) is advantageous.

The guidewire is advanced through the accessory channel of the colonoscope into the cecal pole or ascending colon. The endoscope is then removed from the patient as the guidewire is inserted, using fluoroscopy to make sure the wire tip remains in place. Following endoscope removal, the decompression tube is passed over the guidewire, using fluoroscopy to prevent loop formation and ensure tube placement into the right colon (Figure

Table 48.5 Recommended materials for colonoscopic decompression in acute colonic pseudo-obstruction.

Equipment	Comment
Colonoscope	
Olympus® CF-Q160AL	Large therapeutic channel (3.8 mm)
Olympus® CF-2T160C	Dual-channel (3.7 mm, 3.2 mm); insertion tube outer diameter 13.7 mm
Guidewire	
Wilson-Cook®	0.035 inch, 480 cm length; included in decompression kit
Savary or American guidewire	Length 210 cm
Decompression tube	
Wilson-Cook® Colon Decompression kit	14 French; length 175 cm
Levin tube	18 French; length 80 cm

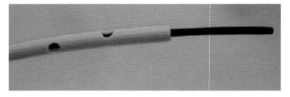

Figure 48.3 Colonic decompression tube with guidewire and side holes.

48.4). The guidewire is removed and the tube connected to gravity drainage.

The decompression tube should be flushed every 6 h with saline to prevent clogging. The tube generally passes spontaneously over 3 days as peristalsis improves. If it has not passed spontaneously after 72 h, the tube is removed.

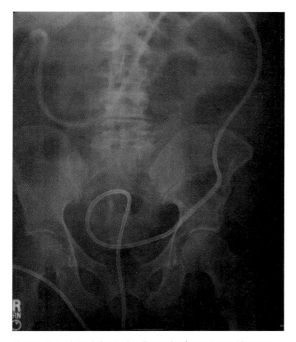

Figure 48.4 Plain abdominal radiograph of a patient with acute colonic pseudo-obstruction with colonic decompression tube placed into the right colon.

Efficacy
The efficacy of colonoscopic decompression has not been established in randomized clinical trials. However, successful colonoscopic decompression has been reported in many retrospective series (Table 48.6), now totaling many hundreds of patients [7,25–28]. Rex reviewed the available literature of patients with ACPO treated with colonoscopy [29]. Among 292 reported patients, 69% were estimated to have a successful initial decompression, determined by a reduction in radiographically measured cecal diameter. Forty percent of patients treated without decompression tube placement had at least one recurrence, requiring an additional colonoscopy. Thus, an initial decompression colonoscopy without tube placement can be considered to be definitive therapy in less than 50% of patients [29]. To improve the therapeutic benefit, decompression tube placement at the time of colonoscopy is strongly recommended. The value of decompression tubes has not been evaluated in controlled trials, but anecdotal evidence suggests that it may lower the recurrence rate. In the series reported by Geller *et al.* [28], the overall clinical success of colonoscopic decompression was 88%. However, in procedures where a decompression tube was not placed the clinical success was poor (25%).

Safety
The complication rate of decompression colonoscopy in ACPO ranges from approximately 1 to 5% (Table 48.6) [7,25–28], with perforation being the most feared adverse event, occurring in approximately 3% [28].

Table 48.6 Colonoscopic decompression in acute colonic pseudo-obstruction.

Study (author/year)	Number of patients	Successful initial decompression (%)	Overall colonoscopic success (%)	Complications (%)
Nivatvongs (1982) [25]	22	68	73	<1 (no perforations)
Strodel (1983) [26]	44	61	73	2 (1 perforation)
Bode (1984) [27]	22	68	77	4.5 (1 perforation)
Jetmore (1992) [7]	45	84	36	<1 (no perforations)
Geller (1996) [28]	41	95	88	5 (2 perforations)

Percutaneous Cecostomy

Percutaneous cecostomy, performed either radiologically or endoscopically, can be considered in high surgical risk patients [30]. A small case series described five patients with ACPO in which percutaneous endoscopic cecostomy was the definitive treatment [30]. This approach is modeled after the percutaneous endoscopic gastrostomy pull technique. There were no complications reported with tube placement in ACPO patients in these small series. It is uncertain when percutaneous endoscopic cecostomy should be considered over other forms of mechanical decompression, such as colonoscopy with decompression tube placement or surgical cecostomy. At the present time, percutaneous endoscopic cecostomy should be reserved for patients failing neostigmine and colonoscopic decompression who have no evidence of ischemia or perforation and who are felt to be at high risk for surgery.

Surgical Therapy

Surgical management is reserved for patients with signs of colonic ischemia or perforation or who fail endoscopic and pharmacologic efforts. Surgical intervention is associated with significant morbidity and mortality, likely related to the severity of the patients' underlying medical condition. In a large retrospective series, 179 patients underwent surgery for ACPO with resulting morbidity and mortality rates of 6 and 30%, respectively [4]. The type of surgery performed depends on the status of the bowel. Without perforated or ischemic bowel, cecostomy is the procedure of choice because the success rate is high, morbidity is relatively low, and the procedure can be performed under local anesthesia [4]. In cases of ischemic or perforated bowel, segmental or subtotal resection is indicated, with either exteriorization or primary anastomosis.

Prognosis

The outcome of patients with ACPO is determined by multiple factors. The severity of the underlying illness has the greatest influence on patient outcome. ACPO often afflicts debilitated patients, which explains the significant morbidity and mortality even with successful treatment of the colonic dilation. Other factors that influence outcome are increasing age, maximal cecal diameter,

delay in decompression, and status of the bowel [4]. The risk of spontaneous colon perforation in ACPO is low but clearly exists. Rex summed all available reports in the literature and determined the risk of spontaneous perforation to be approximately 3% [29]. The mortality rate in ACPO is approximately 40% when ischemia or perforation are present compared to 15% in patients with viable bowel [4]. Retrospective analyses of patients with ACPO [4,11] have attempted to identify clinical factors that predict which patients are more likely to have complications such as ischemia or perforation. Based on LaPlace's law, increasing diameters accelerate the rise in tension experienced by the colon wall. The risk of colonic perforation has been reported to increase with cecal diameter greater than 12 cm [4] and when distension has been present for more than 6 days [11]. In the large retrospective series, no cases of perforation were seen with a cecal diameter less than 12 cm [4]. However, at diameters greater than 12 cm, there was no clear relationship between risk of ischemia or perforation and the size of the cecum. The duration and progression of colonic distension may be more important. Johnson and Rice reported a mean duration of distension in patients who perforated of 6 days compared to 2 days in those who did not [11]. A twofold increase in mortality occurs when cecal diameter is greater than 14 cm and a fivefold increase when delay in decompression is greater than 7 days [4]. Thus, the decision to intervene with medical therapy, colonoscopy, or surgery is dictated by the patient's clinical status.

Chronic Colonic Pseudo-obstruction

Chronic colonic pseudo-obstruction (CCPO) is a rare and highly morbid syndrome characterized by impaired gastrointestinal propulsion together with symptoms and signs of bowel obstruction in the absence of any lesions occluding the gut lumen. It can be classified as either "secondary" to a wide array of recognized pathological conditions or idiopathic. A detailed review of this condition is beyond the scope of this chapter.

CCPO represents an entirely different disorder in pathogenesis, presentation, and management when compared to ACPO (Table 48.7). CCPO is usually an indolent and progressive condition rather than occurring in acutely ill, hospitalized patients as in ACPO. Emerging

Table 48.7 Differences between acute and chronic colonic pseudo-obstruction.

	Acute	Chronic
Setting	Hospitalized; acutely ill	Outpatient; indolent
Pathogenesis	Imbalance between sympathetic and parasympathetic nervous system	Reduced interstitial cells of Cajal*
Risk of perforation	High	Low
Involvement of other bowel segments	Rare	Frequent
Management	Neostigmine, colonoscopic decompression	Nutritional support, antibiotics, prokinetics

*He CL, Burgart L, Wang L, et al. Gastroenterology 2000; **118**: 14–21.

evidence suggests that the density of the interstitial cells of Cajal (ICC) is reduced in the colon of patients with chronic pseudo-obstruction and in patients with slow-transit constipation. Other segments of bowel such as the small bowel and stomach are often involved concurrently in CCPO. Management is primarily directed at providing appropriate nutritional support, prokinetics, and antibiotics for bacterial overgrowth.

Take-home points

- Conservative therapy is recommended as the initial preferred management.
- Potentially contributory metabolic, infectious, and pharmacologic factors should be identified and corrected.
- Active intervention is indicated for patients at risk of perforation and/or failing conservative therapy.
- Neostigmine is effective in the majority of patients as compared to placebo in a randomized clinical trial.
- Colonic decompression is the initial invasive procedure of choice for patients failing or who have contraindications to neostigmine.
- Surgical decompression should be reserved for patients with peritonitis or perforation and for those failing endoscopic and medical therapy.

References

1 Saunders MD. Acute colonic pseudo-obstruction. *Gastrointest Endoscopy Clin N Am* 2007; **17**: 341–60.

2 Rex DK. Colonoscopy and acute colonic pseudo-obstruction. *Gastrointest Endosc Clin N Am* 1997; **7**: 499–508.

3 Norwood MG, Lykostratis H, Garcea G, et al. Acute colonic pseudo-obstruction following major orthopedic surgery. *Colorect Dis* 2005; **7**: 496–9.

4 Vanek VW, Al-Salti M. Acute pseudo-obstruction of the colon (Ogilivie's syndrome). An analysis of 400 cases. *Dis Colon Rectum* 1986; **29**: 203–10.

5 De Giorgio R, Barbara G, Stanghellini V, et al. The pharmacologic treatment of acute colonic pseudo-obstruction. *Aliment Pharmacol Ther* 2001; **15**: 1717–27.

6 Spira IA, Rodrigues R, Wolff WI. Pseudo-obstruction of the colon. *Am J Gastroenterol* 1976; **65**: 397–408.

7 Jetmore AB, Timmcke AE, Gathright Jr BJ, et al. Ogilvie's syndrome: Colonoscopic decompression and analysis of predisposing factors. *Dis Colon Rectum* 1992; **35**: 1135–42.

8 Eisen GM, Baron TH, Dominitz JA, et al. Acute colonic pseudo-obstruction. *Gastrointest Endosc* 2002; **56**: 789–92.

9 Sloyer AF, Panella VS, Demas BE, et al. Ogilvie's syndrome. Successful management without colonoscopy. *Dig Dis Sci* 1988; **33**: 1391–6.

10 Loftus CG, Harewood GC, Baron TH. Assessment of predictors of response to neostigmine for acute colonic pseudo-obstruction. *Am J Gastroenterol* 2002; **97**: 3118–22.

11 Johnson CD, Rice RP. The radiographic evaluation of gross cecal distention. *Am J Radiol* 1985; **145**: 1211–7.

12 Ponec RJ, Saunders MD, Kimmey MB. Neostigmine for the treatment of acute colonic pseudo-obstruction. *N Engl J Med* 1999; **341**: 137–41.

13 Aquilonius SM, Hartvig P. Clinical pharmacokinetics of cholinesterase inhibitors. *Clin Pharmacokinet* 1986; **11**: 236–49.

14 van der Spoel JI, Oudemans-van Straaten HM, Stoutenbecek CP, et al. Neostigmine resolves critical illness-related colonic ileus in intensive care patients with multiple organ failure—a prospective, double-blind, placebo-controlled trial. *Intensive Care Med* 2001; **27**: 822–7.

15 Hutchinson R, Griffiths C. Acute colonic pseudo-obstruction: A pharmacologic approach. *Ann R Coll Surg Engl* 1992; **74**: 364–7.

16 Stephenson BM, Morgan AR, Salaman JR, *et al.* Ogilvie's syndrome: A new approach to an old problem. *Dis Colon Rectum* 1995; **38**: 424–7.

17 Turegano-Fuentes F, Munoz-Jimenez F, Del Valle-Hernandez E, *et al.* Early resolution of Ogilvie's syndrome with intravenous neostigmine. A simple, effective treatment. *Dis Colon Rectum* 1997; **40**: 1353–7.

18 Trevisani GT, Hyman NH, Church JM. Neostigmine: safe and effective treatment for acute colonic pseudo-obstruction. *Dis Colon Rectum* 2000; **43**: 599–603.

19 Paran H, Silverberg D, Mayo A, *et al.* Treatment of acute colonic pseudo-obstruction with neostigmine. *J Am Coll Surg* 2000; **190**: 315–18.

20 Abeyta BJ, Albrecht RM, Schermer CR. Retrospective study of neostigmine for the treatment of acute colonic pseudo-obstruction. *Am Surg* 2001; **67**: 265–8.

21 Mehta R, John A, Nair P, *et al.* Factors predicting successful outcome following neostigmine therapy in acute colonic pseudo-obstruction: a prospective study. *J Gastroenterol Hepatol* 2006; **21**: 459–61.

22 Cherta I, Forne M, Quintana S, *et al.* Prolonged treatment with neostigmine for resolution of acute colonic pseudo-obstruction. *Aliment Pharmacol Ther* 2006; **23**: 1678–9.

23 Sgouros SN, Vlachogiannakos J, Vassilliadis K, *et al.* Effect of polyethylene glycol electrolyte balanced solution on patients with acute colonic-pseudo-obstruction after resolution of colonic dilation: a prospective, randomized, placebo controlled trial. *Gut* 2006; **55**: 638–42.

24 van der Spoel JI, Oudemans-van Straaten HM, Kuiper MA, *et al.* Laxation of critically ill patients with lactulose or polyethylene glycol: A two-center randomized, double-blind, placebo-controlled trial. *Crit Care Med* 2007; **35**: 2726–31.

25 Nivatvongs S, Vermeulen FD, Fang DT. Colonoscopic decompression of acute pseudo-obstruction of the colon. *Ann Surg* 1982; **196**: 598–600.

26 Strodel WE, Nostrant TT, Eckhauser FE, *et al.* Therapeutic and diagnostic colonoscopy in non-obstructive colonic dilatation. *Ann Surg* 1983; **19**: 416–21.

27 Bode WE, Beart RW, Spencer RJ, *et al.* Colonoscopic decompression for acute pseudo-obstruction of the colon (Ogilvie's syndrome): report of 22 cases and review of the literature. *Am J Surg* 1984; **147**: 243–5.

28 Geller A, Petersen BT, Gostout CJ. Endoscopic decompression for acute colonic pseudo-obstruction. *Gastrointest Endosc* 1996; **44**: 144–50.

29 Rex DK. Acute colonic pseudo-obstruction (Ogilvie's syndrome). *Gastroenterologist* 1994; **2**: 223–38.

30 Ramage JI, Baron TH. Percutaneous endoscopic cecostomy: a case series. *Gastrointest Endosc* 2003; **57**: 752–5.

CHAPTER 49
Colonic Polyps and Colon Cancer

John B. Kisiel and Paul J. Limburg

Division of Gastroenterology and Hepatology, Mayo Clinic, Rochester, MN, USA

Summary

Globally, more than 1 million new cases of colorectal cancer (CRC) are diagnosed each year and CRC accounts for 10% of all cancer deaths. Symptoms (i.e., hematochezia, melena, change in bowel habits, etc.) and signs (i.e., anemia, positive fecal occult blood test, etc.) of CRC can be subtle and non-specific, but often indicate relatively advanced-stage disease. Since prognosis is inversely associated with CRC stage, early detection of premalignant adenomas or locally-invasive cancers is a clinical priority. Therapy for invasive malignancy is multimodal and can involve surgery, chemotherapy, and radiation therapy. Although not universally applied, guidelines have been developed for post-therapeutic CRC surveillance to detect recurrent and metachronous lesions.

Case

A 42-year-old man presents to his primary care physician with a chief complaint of rectal bleeding. He is generally healthy and takes no medications. Review of his family history is significant for uterine cancer, diagnosed in his mother at the age of 32 years, and colon cancer, diagnosed in his maternal uncle at the age of 54 years.

Definition and Epidemiology

In 2009, approximately 146 970 incident and 49 920 fatal colorectal cancer (CRC) cases are expected in the United States [1]. By gender, CRC incidence rates are 59.0 and 43.6 cases per 100 000 person-years for men and women, respectively [2]. Overall, CRC accounts for approximately 10% of all US cancer deaths. At the histologic level, CRC represents a variety of heterogeneous subtypes [3]. However, because adenocarcinoma represents the large majority of malignant colorectal tumors, CRC is used to refer to colorectal adenocarcinoma throughout the remainder of this chapter. Adenomatous polyps, also

Practical Gastroenterology and Hepatology: Small and Large Intestine and Pancreas, 1st edition. Edited by Nicholas J. Talley, Sunanda V. Kane and Michael B. Wallace. © 2010 Blackwell Publishing Ltd.

known as adenomas, are regarded as non-obligate precursor lesions for most CRCs and typically exhibit a raised, polypoid appearance at the macroscopic level. Adenoma morphology may resemble branched tubules ("tubular"), show villi arranged in a frond-like pattern ("villous"), or contain mixed features ("tubulovillous"). Large size (>1 cm), high dysplasia grade, and/or villous morphology typically comprise "advanced" adenomas, which are more closely related to CRC [4]. Macroscopically flat or depressed lesions, which account for approximately 10% of all adenomas, also appear to have higher malignant potential [5]. Adenoma prevalence rates are difficult to discern for average-risk adults. Available data suggest that 29-45% of asymptomatic persons in screening cohort studies may have one or more colorectal adenomas [6,7].

Hyperplastic polyps (HPPs) are characterized by increased glandular cells with relatively reduced cytoplasm, but nuclear atypia, stratification, and hyperchromatism are absent. Small, distally located HPPs do not appear to be associated with increased CRC risk, while HPPS of 1 cm or more in diameter, 30 or more in total number, and/or with mixed adenomatous features are thought to confer at least some risk elevation, particularly when coupled with a strong family history of CRC [4]. Serrated adenomas have been more recently recognized and are characterized by hyperplastic architecture with accompanying dysplastic features, such as abnormal crypt epithelium and nuclear atypia, supporting a premalignant phenotype. The magnitude of CRC risk associated with these serrated adenomas represents an area of active investigation [4,8].

Pathophysiology

Multiple molecular events have been linked to the sequential progression from normal mucosa to adenomatous polyp to adenocarcinoma (Figure 49.1) [9]. At the genetic level, mutations in the *APC* gene (chromosome 5q) are thought to lead to disrupted cell cycle regulation [10] and subsequent colorectal tumorigenesis. Similar *APC* mutations have been documented in familial and non-familial CRC cases [11]. Genetic alterations in *DCC*, *K-ras*, *p53* and other growth regulating genes

have been identified in a substantial proportion of CRC cases as well [12,13]. COX-2 protein expression appears to be inducible in colorectal neoplasia, with absent or low-level concentrations in normal colorectal mucosa. Loss of DNA mismatch repair (MMR) protein expression is associated with microsatellite instability. Deficient MMR protein status can be caused by germline mutation in or epigenetic silencing of *MLH1*, *MSH2*, *PMS1*, *PMS2*, and/or *MSH6*. Among older women, approximately 20–30% of CRC cases appear to arise from methylation-induced suppression of *MLH1*. Hypermethylation of other genes, including *p14* and *p16*, has been shown in 25 and 35% of non-familial CRC cases, respectively [14,15].

Host Factors

CRC risk increases with advancing age, with cumulative incidence rates of 1:20 and 1:18 after age 90 years for women and men, respectively (Table 49.1). Subsite-spe-

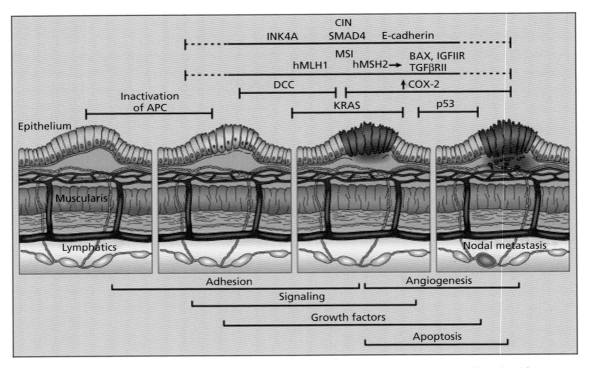

Figure 49.1 Adenoma-to-carcinoma sequence and associated molecular alterations in colon cancer development. (Reproduced from Compton C, *et al*. Colon cancer. In: Abeloff MD, ed. *Abeloff's Clinical Oncology*, 4th edn. Philadelphia: Churchill Livingstone Elsevier, 2008, with permission from Elsevier.)

Table 49.1 Cumulative risk of developing colorectal cancer across 10-year age categories, by gender.

Age (years)	Cumulative risk			
	Women		Men	
	%	1 in	%	1 in
20	0.002	50000	0.002	50000
30	0.018	5556	0.016	6250
40	0.077	1299	0.079	1266
50	0.273	366	0.300	333
60	0.775	129	0.942	106
70	1.740	57	2.197	46
80	3.207	31	3.909	26
90	4.585	22	5.093	20

Data obtained using Fast Stats: An interactive tool for access to SEER cancer statistics. Surveillance Research Program, National Cancer Institute. http://seer.cancer.gov/faststats (Accessed on 4-1-2010)

cific CRC incidence rates also differ by gender, with the female:male rate ratio higher in the proximal (cecum, ascending and transverse, including both flexures) versus distal (descending, sigmoid, rectum) colorectum. Race/ethnicity may also contribute to CRC risk, since incidence and mortality rates are consistently higher among African-Americans relative to Caucasians [16]. However, the primary reasons for these rate differences remain incompletely defined.

Past Medical History

Prior history of colorectal adenoma(s) corresponds with a three- to sixfold increase in risk for subsequent, metachronous neoplasia [4]. Advanced adenomas (i.e., ≥1 cm diameter, high-grade dyplasia, villous morphology) and three or more adenomas in total are associated with higher recurrence risks. Patients who have undergone prior CRC resection are prone to developing recurrent primary and second primary tumors, typically within 3 years.

Chronic ulcerative colitis (CUC) is associated with progressively increasing CRC risk over time, with cumulative incidence rates ranging from 2 to 18% after 10–30 years of disease. In addition to CUC duration, colitis extent (pancolitis > distal colitis > proctitis), concomi-

tant primary sclerosing cholangitis, and family history of CRC appear to be risk modifiers. Data regarding CRC risks for patients with Crohn disease are more limited, but the magnitude of the association appears to be similar to CUC. Interestingly, recent data from Olmsted County, MN showed comparable CRC incidence rates between patients with inflammatory bowel disease and a regional reference population, which the authors speculated was due to increasingly widespread use of maintenance therapy and surveillance colonoscopy [17].

Type 2 diabetes mellitus has been positively associated with CRC risk in multiple observational studies, presumably because insulin and/or insulin-like growth factors have growth promoting effects in the colorectal mucosa [18]. Excess body weight, particularly when centrally distributed (visceral adiposity) may also increase CRC risk through an insulin-mediated mechanism. Of note, recent long-term follow-up data suggest that overall cancer mortality is reduced among morbidly obese patients who undergo bariatric surgery [19,20].

Family History

In the US, approximately 15–25% of all CRC cases exhibit familial clustering. Several heritable syndromes are well recognized, as discussed below. In the absence of a defined heritable syndrome, family history of CRC in one or more first-degree relatives increases CRC risk by about two to fourfold [21].

Familial adenomatous polyposis (FAP) results from a mutated *APC* gene and is characterized by hundreds to thousands of colorectal adenomas that usually develop sometime during adolescence. As many as one in five FAP patients have new-onset mutations (i.e., no known family history of polyposis). Extracolonic features of FAP include duodenal adenomas, gastric (fundic) gland hyperplasia, mandibular osteomas, and supernumerary teeth. Unless total proctocolectomy is performed, CRC is essentially universal with a mean age at diagnosis of approximately 40 years. Attenuated FAP is associated with relatively fewer colorectal adenomas (<100) and later onset of CRC (mean age approximately 55 years).

Hereditary non-polyposis colorectal cancer (HNPCC) syndrome is distinguished by germline mutations in *MLH1, MSH2, PMS1, PMS2,* or *MSH6.* The median age for CRC diagnosis is 46 years. Other cancer risks are also increased, including uterine, ovarian, gastric, genitourinary tract, small bowel, and hepatobiliary. Clinical and

Table 49.2 Proposed clinical criteria for the diagnosis of hereditary non-polyposis colon cancer.

Revised International Collaborative Group–HNPCC Criteria (Amsterdam criteria II)	Revised Bethesda Guidelines for testing colorectal tumors for microsatellite instability (MSI)
There should be at least 3 relatives with an HNPCC-associated cancer (CRC, cancer of the endometrium, small bowel, ureter, or renal pelvis)	Tumors from individuals should be tested for MSI in the following situations:
One should be a first-degree relative of the other 2	Colorectal cancer diagnosed in a patient who is less than 50 years of age
At least 1 should be diagnosed before age 50	Presence of synchronous, metachronous colorectal, or other HNPCC-associated tumors* regardless of age
At least 2 successive generations should be affected	Colorectal cancer with the MSI-H† histology‡ diagnosed in a patient who is less than 60 years of age
Familial adenomatous polyposis should be excluded in the CRC case(s) if any	Colorectal cancer diagnosed in one or more first-degree relatives with an HNPCC-related tumor, with one of the cancers being diagnosed under age 50 years
Tumors should be verified by pathological examination	Colorectal cancer diagnosed in two or more first- or second-degree relatives with HNPCC-related tumors, regardless of age

CRC, colorectal cancer.
*Hereditary non-polyposis colorectal cancer (HNPCC)-related tumors include colorectal, endometrial, stomach, ovarian, pancreas, ureter and renal pelvis, biliary tract, and brain (usually glioblastoma as seen in Turcot syndrome) tumors, sebaceous gland adenomas and keratoacanthomas in Muir–Torre syndrome, and carcinoma of the small bowel.
†MSI-H = microsatellite instability-high in tumors refers to changes in two or more of the five National Cancer Institute-recommended panels of microsatellite markers.
‡Presence of tumor infiltrating lymphocytes, Crohn-like lymphocytic reaction, mucinous/signet-ring differentiation, or medullary growth pattern.

laboratory data can be used to recognize high-risk patients and/or families (Table 49.2) [22,23]. Muir–Torre syndrome is an HNPCC variant wherein affected individuals (women : men = 1 : 2) may present with sebaceous neoplasms in addition to the cancer types noted above.

MYH-associated polyposis (MAP) is a recently described, autosomal recessive syndrome with a colorectal adenoma burden similar to attenuated FAP, although patients with more than 100 adenomas have been described. Upper gastrointestinal adenomas can be found in MAP patients, although the true incidence of these extracolonic lesions is not yet known. Biallelic mutation carriers have an 80% cumulative risk of CRC by age 70 years [24], while the CRC risk for monoallelic carriers remains incompletely defined. Turcot syndrome refers to a familial predisposition for both colonic polyposis and central nervous system tumors and likely represents a constellation of molecular features that can be variants of either FAP or HNPCC.

Peutz–Jeghers syndrome (PJS) is characterized by multiple hamartomatous polyps scattered throughout the upper and lower gastrointestinal tract. Up to 60% of PJS patients are found to have germline mutations in the *LKB1* (*STK11*) gene. Other clinical features include melanin deposition around the lips, buccal mucosa, face, genitalia, hands, and feet. CRC risk is thought to be increased by foci of adenomatous epithelium within PJS polyps. Cancers of the small bowel, pancreas, biliary tree, gall bladder, ovaries, and testes are also relatively more common among PJS patients. In juvenile polyposis syndrome, mucous retention polyps can arise in the colon, stomach, and/or other parts of the gastrointestinal tract, which may cause bleeding or obstruction during childhood. Both *PTEN* and *SMAD4* mutations have been identified in JPS patients.

Environmental Exposures

Differences in CRC incidence, prevalence, and mortality rates by global region [25] support the hypothesis that colorectal carcinogenesis is influenced by environmental factors. Although numerous exposure agents have been associated with increased CRC risk, risk factor modification is not generally incorporated into CRC prevention guidelines. A "westernized" diet (high fat, low fiber, low fruit and vegetable intake) can stimulate tumor formation in animal models. Tobacco smoke contains a number of potential carcinogens, including polycyclic aromatic hydrocarbons (PAHs), nitrosamines, and aromatic amines. Cigarette smoking has been linked to a two to threefold increase in CRC risk, most noticeably after a prolonged latency period of at least three decades. Emerging data suggest that cigarette smoking may be differentially associated with CRCs that exhibit microsatellite instability [26]. Colonic microflora can generate procarcinogenic metabolites [27,28]. While no specific bacterial organisms have been convincingly established as CRC risk factors, further investigation in this area will likely be informative.

Prevention

Early detection remains the cornerstone of CRC risk reduction. Average-risk screening should begin at age 50 years, although recent national guidelines differ slightly with respect to specifically endorsed test options and the age at which to consider discontinuing CRC screening [29,30]. For high-risk patients, earlier, more frequent screening and surveillance is typically recommended, as discussed in greater detail in Chapter 31. Chemoprevention, which refers to the use of chemical compounds to interrupt carcinogenesis, may serve as a complementary CRC prevention strategy. Non-steroidal anti-inflammatory drugs, selective cyclo-oxygenase-2 (COX-2) inhibitors, di-fluoromethylornithine (DFMO), calcium, and other compounds have been investigated as candidate CRC chemoprevention agents, but their clinical application has been limited by unacceptable toxicity [31] and/or insufficient efficacy in trials reported to date.

Clinical Features

CRC signs and symptoms are rather non-specific and are further influenced by tumor size, stage, anatomic subsite, and distribution of distant metastases, when present.

Patients with late-stage CRCs tend to exhibit more obvious signs and symptoms than patients with early-stage tumors. General clinical features of CRC include hematochezia, melena, anemia, abdominal pain, change in bowel habits, involuntary weight loss, nausea, vomiting, and fatigue. CRCs arising from the proximal colon tend to be associated with occult bleeding and iron-deficiency, whereas cancers originating in the distal colon or rectum may produce narrow-caliber stools, fecal urgency, and overt bleeding. About one in five CRC patients present with distant metastases, manifested by hepatosplenomegaly, palpable lymphadenopathy (i.e., left supraclavicular nodes), or other signs and symptoms referable to the affected organ site(s).

Diagnosis

Case continued

The patient undergoes diagnostic colonoscopy with findings of a 2.5 cm sessile mass in the ascending colon and a 1.5 cm pedunculated polyp in the rectum. Biopsy samples were interpreted as showing invasive adenocarcinoma (with tumor infiltrating lymphocytes and a Crohn-like lymphocytic reaction) and tubulovillous adenoma, low-grade dysplasia from the proximal and distal lesions, respectively.

Colonoscopy is the test of choice for diagnostic evaluation of the lower gastrointestinal tract, since macroscopic assessment, mucosal sampling, and, when needed, therapeutic intervention (i.e., polypectomy) can be performed during a single procedure. Computed tomography (CT) colonography can serve as a useful adjunct to colonoscopy when technical challenges, obstructing lesions, concomitant medications (such as anticoagulants), or other factors do not permit complete diagnostic evaluation. Since synchronous cancers may be found in approximately 5% of all CRC cases [32], full structural assessment is required. Once the CRC diagnosis is established, preoperative staging with abdominopelvic CT and chest X-ray is typically performed to exclude distant metastases. For rectal cancers, endorectal ultrasound is helpful for determining the depth of mural invasion and extent of regional lymph node involvement. Measurement of carcinoembryonic antigen (CEA) may provide additional prognostic information [33], although this test is not universally recommended. Definitive CRC stage is deter-

Table 49.3 Standard treatment recommendations for colorectal cancer, by presenting stage.

Presenting stage	TNM classification	Colon cancer		Rectal cancer	
		Standard treatment	5-Year survival (%)	Standard treatment	5-Year survival (%)
Stage I	T1 N0 M0 T2 N0 M0	Surgical resection	93	Surgical resection	72
Stage II	T3 N0 M0 T4 N0 M0	Surgical resection; consider adjuvant chemotherapy if pathologic features suggest high recurrence risk	72–85	Neoadjuvant chemo/radiation therapy + surgical resection + adjuvant chemo/radiation therapy	52
Stage III	Any T N1 M0 Any T N2 M0	Surgical resection with adjuvant chemotherapy	44–83	Neoadjuvant chemo/radiation therapy + surgical resection + adjuvant chemo/radiation therapy	37
Stage IV	Any T Any N M1	Chemotherapy and/or symptomatic care; consider potentially curative treatment for isolated liver or lung metastases	8	Chemotherapy and/or symptomatic care; consider potentially curative treatment for isolated liver or lung metastases	4

Data obtained from O'Connell *et al*. [34] and Jessup *et al*. [35].

Primary tumor (T)	Regional lymph nodes (N)	Distant metastases (M)
T0 No evidence of primary tumor	N0 no regional lymph node metastases	M0 no distant metastases
T1 tumor invades submucosa	N1 metastases in 1–3 regional lymph nodes	M1 distant metastases
T2 tumor invades muscularis propria	N2 metastases in ≥4 regional lymph nodes	
T3 tumor invades through muscularis propria		
T4 tumor invades surrounding organs or structures		

mined from the surgical resection specimen, using the TNM classification system (Table 49.3).

Differential Diagnosis

Due to the non-specific nature of CRC-related signs and symptoms, formulation of an efficient differential diagnosis can be challenging. Given the relatively high CRC incidence rate among the general population, colonoscopy should be incorporated into the diagnostic algorithm for any of the common clinical features cited above. Atypical colorectal cancer subtypes are discussed elsewhere (see Chapter 6). Malignant tumors that can metastasize to the colorectum include breast, ovary, prostate, lung, or stomach cancers. Lymphomas and malignant melanomas may originate from or spread to the colorectum. Benign lesions such as endometriosis,

Crohn disease, or solitary rectal ulcer syndrome can also mimic CRC, but these diagnoses are readily distinguishable by histology.

Therapeutics

Case continued

The patient underwent a colon cancer staging evaluation, including CT scan of the abdomen and pelvis that showed no signs of distant metastases. Based on the patient's age, family history, and cancer histology, HNPCC was strongly suspected. Further testing of the tumor specimen revealed that the ascending colon cancer exhibited the microsatellite instability-high phenotype. The patient was referred for genetic counseling and a germline mutation was detected in *MLH1*.

CRC treatment is determined largely by TMN stage and may include surgical intervention, chemotherapy, and/or radiation therapy (Table 49.3). Surgical resection is generally the mainstay of CRC therapy, unless contraindicated by tumor stage, patient co-morbidities, or other factors. At least 12 regional lymph nodes should be removed along with the primary tumor for definitive pathologic staging. Anastomotic site recurrence rates for all CRC are 2–4% but may be as much as 10 times higher for rectal cancers, due to differences in surgical technique and/or tumor biology [36]. Resection of isolated liver and lung metastases appears to improve the survival rate for some patients [37,38].

Postoperative (also known as "adjuvant") chemotherapy is routinely recommended for stage III CRCs and may be considered for select stage II CRCs [39], using one of several combination regimens including 5-fluorouracil (5-FU), leucovorin, and oxaliplatin (collectively referred to as FOLFOX). In a large, randomized, controlled trial of subjects with stage II or III CRC, adjuvant FOLFOX therapy improved the 3-year disease free survival rate from 72.9 to 78.2% [40]. On average, treating 19 patients with FOLFOX instead of 5-FU and leucovorin would prevent one additional CRC recurrence at 3 years. However, the added benefit of oxaliplatin is counter-balanced by possible drug-induced toxicities, such as peripheral neuropathy.

An array of chemotherapy options exists for patients with metastatic CRC (Table 49.4) [39]. First-line combi-

Table 49.4 Colorectal cancer chemotherapeutic agents.

Agent	Mechanism of action	Indications	Common toxicities
5- Fluorouracil (5-FU)	Blocks the enzyme thymidylate synthase, which is essential for DNA synthesis	Multiple uses in combination with other agents in the adjuvant (postoperative) and palliative settings	Nausea, diarrhea Myelosuppression Fatigue
Capecitabine	Blocks thymidylate synthase (orally administered prodrug converted to 5-FU)	Multiple uses in combination with other agents in the adjuvant (postoperative) and metastatic setting	Nausea, diarrhea Myelosuppression Fatigue Palmar–plantar syndrome (hand–foot syndrome)
Oxaliplatin	Inhibits DNA replication and transcription by forming inter- and intra-strand DNA adducts/cross-links	Used in combination with 5-FU, LV (FOLFOX) in the adjuvant (postoperative) and metastatic setting	Peripheral neuropathy Nausea, diarrhea Fatigue Myelosuppression Hypersensitivity
Irinotecan	Inhibits topoisomerase I, an enzyme that facilitates the uncoiling and recoiling of DNA during replication	Used alone or in combination with 5FU, LV (FOLFIRI) in the metastatic setting	Cholinergic (acute diarrhea) Nausea, late diarrhea Fatigue Myelosuppression Alopecia
Bevacizumab	Monoclonal antibody that binds to VEGF ligand	Used in combination with either FOLFOX or FOLFIRI in the metastatic setting	Hypertension Arterial thrombotic events Impaired wound healing Gastrointestinal perforation
Cetuximab	Monoclonal antibody to EGFR (chimeric) that blocks the ligand-binding site	Used with irinotecan or as a single agent in the metastatic setting	Acneform rash Hypersensitivity Hypomagnesemia Fatigue
Panitumumab	Monoclonal antibody to EGFR (fully humanized) that blocks the ligand-binding site	Used as a single agent in the metastatic setting	Acneform rash Hypomagnesemia Fatigue

EGFR, epidermal growth factor receptor; VEGF, vascular endothelial growth factor; LV, leucovorin.
From Asmis TR and Saltz L [39].

nation therapy with either FOLFOX or FOLFIRI (substituting irinotectan for oxaliplatin) appears to provide a response rate (defined as a composite of either complete disappearance of all detectable disease or as a decrease in tumor size by RECIST criteria) of 31–56%, with a median progression-free survival of 7–8 months. [41,42]. Further benefits might be achieved by adding a biologic agent such as bevacizumab.

External beam radiation therapy combined with systemic chemotherapy is used to treat locally advanced (T3, T4, and/or node-positive) rectal cancers. In a landmark study from 1985, the Gastrointestinal Tumor Study Group found a 33% recurrence rate among patients with locally advanced, surgically treated rectal cancer who received postoperative combination chemotherapy and radiation therapy, compared to a 55% recurrence rate for patients treated with surgery alone, after 80 months of follow-up [43]. The number needed treat (NNT) with adjuvant combination therapy to prevent one additional recurrence was five in this cohort. Subsequent, large trials have further defined the benefits of radiation therapy for treating locally advanced rectal cancer [44–47], with preoperative (also known as "neoadjuvant") chemoradiotherapy to down-size the tumor, now considered standard of care [48]. Most patients who receive neoadjuvant chemoradiation therapy are also candidates for adjuvant chemotherapy. For recurrent rectal cancers, long-term survival can be achieved for some patients using surgical resection, intraoperative radiation therapy, and adjuvant chemoradiation therapy [49].

Patients who develop bowel obstruction or other complications of locally advanced or metastatic disease may benefit from palliative chemotherapy or radiation therapy. Palliation through mechanical stenting and decompression techniques is also feasible, as discussed in Chapter 32.

Prognosis

CRC stage at diagnosis is a strong predictor of survival (Table 49.3) [50,51]. After definitive treatment, the presence of residual tumor, lymphovascular invasion, and elevated CEA level are robust predictors of worsened prognosis. Additional important prognostic factors include tumor grade and residual tumor after neoadjuvant therapy. Newer methods for histologic and molecular prognostication are under active research. Although prognosis for limited-stage disease is excellent, patients with a history of CRC are at increased risk for recurrent primary and/or second primary tumors. Guidelines for post-CRC treatment surveillance [36] are discussed in Chapter 31.

Take-home points

- CRC is the fourth most common incident and second most common fatal cancer in the United States.

- Most, if not all, CRCs are preceded by macroscopically identifiable dysplastic lesions (adenomas) that can be detected and removed through effective screening.

- Personal history (colorectal adenomas, inflammatory bowel disease, diabetes mellitus) and family history (with or without a defined heritable syndrome) can affect CRC risk.

- Environmental factors such as diet, obesity, and smoking also appear to adversely affect colorectal carcinogenesis.

- CRC signs and symptoms are non-specific, influenced by tumor site and typically signify more advanced-stage disease. Colonoscopy is the diagnostic test of choice.

- Preoperative staging evaluation is performed to define local invasion, regional lymph node involvement and distant metastases. Common tests include chest X-ray, CT scan of the abdomen and pelvis, and endoscopic ultrasound (rectal cancers).

- Surgical resection is the primary treatment modality. Adjuvant chemotherapy should be recommended for patients with stage III, and some stage II, colon cancers. Neoadjuvant and adjuvant chemoradiation therapy are typically recommended for stage II and III rectal cancer patients.

- CRC prognosis is inversely associated with pathologic stage.

References

1 Jemal A, Siegel R, Ward E, *et al.* Cancer statistics, 2009. *CA Cancer J Clin* 2009; **59**: 225–49.

2 Edwards BK, Ward E, Kohler BA, *et al.* Annual report to the nation on the status of cancer, 1975–2006, featuring colorectal cancer trends and impact of interventions (risk factors, screening, and treatment) to reduce future rates. *Cancer* 2010; **116**: 544–73.

3 Jass JR, Sobin LH, Watanabe H. The World Health Organization's histologic classification of gastrointestinal tumors. A commentary on the second edition. *Cancer* 1990; **66**: 2162–7.

4 Winawer SJ, Zauber AG, Fletcher RH, *et al.* Guidelines for colonoscopy surveillance after polypectomy: a consensus update by the US Multi-Society Task Force on Colorectal Cancer and the American Cancer Society. *Gastroenterology* 2006; **130**: 1872–85.

5 Soetikno RM, Kaltenbach T, Rouse RV, *et al.* Prevalence of nonpolypoid (flat and depressed) colorectal neoplasms in asymptomatic and symptomatic adults. *JAMA* 2008; **299**: 1027–35.

6 Winawer SJ, Zauber AG, O'Brien MJ, *et al.* Randomized comparison of surveillance intervals after colonoscopic removal of newly diagnosed adenomatous polyps. The National Polyp Study Workgroup. *N Engl J Med* 1993; **328**: 901–6.

7 Pickhardt PJ, Choi JR, Hwang I, *et al.* Computed tomographic virtual colonoscopy to screen for colorectal neoplasia in asymptomatic adults. *N Engl J Med* 2003; **349**: 2191–200.

8 Cappell MS. Pathophysiology, clinical presentation, and management of colon cancer. *Gastroenterol Clin North Am* 2008; **37**: 1–24, v.

9 Abeloff MD. *Abeloff's Clinical Oncology*, 4th edn. Philadelphia: Churchill Livingstone/Elsevier 2008.

10 Bodmer WF, Bailey CJ, Bodmer J, *et al.* Localization of the gene for familial adenomatous polyposis on chromosome 5. *Nature* 1987; **328**: 614–6.

11 Suraweera N, Duval A, Reperant M, *et al.* Evaluation of tumor microsatellite instability using five quasimonomorphic mononucleotide repeats and pentaplex PCR. *Gastroenterology* 2002; **123**: 1804–11.

12 Vogelstein B, Fearon ER, Hamilton SR, *et al.* Genetic alterations during colorectal-tumor development. *N Engl J Med* 1988; **319**: 525–32.

13 Robbins DH, Itzkowitz SH. The molecular and genetic basis of colon cancer. *Med Clin North Am* 2002; **86**: 1467–95.

14 Burri N, Shaw P, Bouzourene H, *et al.* Methylation silencing and mutations of the p14ARF and p16INK4a genes in colon cancer. *Lab Invest* 2001; **81**: 217–29.

15 Shannon BA, Iacopetta BJ. Methylation of the hMLH1, p16, and MDR1 genes in colorectal carcinoma: associations with clinicopathological features. *Cancer Lett* 2001; **167**: 91–7.

16 Cheng X, Chen VW, Steele B, *et al.* Subsite-specific incidence rate and stage of disease in colorectal cancer by race, gender, and age group in the United States, 1992–1997. *Cancer* 2001; **92**: 2547–54.

17 Jess T, Loftus EV, Jr., Velayos FS, *et al.* Risk of intestinal cancer in inflammatory bowel disease: a population-based study from olmsted county, Minnesota. *Gastroenterology* 2006; **130**: 1039–46.

18 Giovannucci E. Modifiable risk factors for colon cancer. *Gastroenterol Clin North Am* 2002; **31**: 925–43.

19 Sjostrom L, Narbro K, Sjostrom CD, *et al.* Effects of bariatric surgery on mortality in Swedish obese subjects. *N Engl J Med* 2007; **357**: 741–52.

20 Adams TD, Gress RE, Smith SC, *et al.* Long-term mortality after gastric bypass surgery. *N Engl J Med* 2007; **357**: 753–61.

21 Butterworth AS, Higgins JP, Pharoah P. Relative and absolute risk of colorectal cancer for individuals with a family history: a meta-analysis. *Eur J Cancer* 2006; **42**: 216–27.

22 Vasen HF, Watson P, Mecklin JP, Lynch HT. New clinical criteria for hereditary nonpolyposis colorectal cancer (HNPCC, Lynch syndrome) proposed by the International Collaborative group on HNPCC. *Gastroenterology* 1999; **116**: 1453–6.

23 Umar A, Boland CR, Terdiman JP, *et al.* Revised Bethesda Guidelines for hereditary nonpolyposis colorectal cancer (Lynch syndrome) and microsatellite instability. *J Nat Cancer Instit* 2004; **96**: 261–8.

24 Jenkins MA, Croitoru ME, Monga N, *et al.* Risk of colorectal cancer in monoallelic and biallelic carriers of MYH mutations: a population-based case-family study. *Cancer Epidemiol Biomar* 2006; **15**: 312–4.

25 Kamangar F, Dores GM, Anderson WF. Patterns of cancer incidence, mortality, and prevalence across five continents: defining priorities to reduce cancer disparities in different geographic regions of the world. *J Clin Oncol* 2006; **24**: 2137–50.

26 Neugut AI, Terry MB. Cigarette smoking and microsatellite instability: causal pathway or marker-defined subset of colon tumors? *J Nat Cancer Instit* 2000; **92**: 1791–3.

27 Hope ME, Hold GL, Kain R, El-Omar EM. Sporadic colorectal cancer—role of the commensal microbiota. *FEMS Microbiol Lett* 2005; **244**: 1–7.

28 Wang X, Huycke MM. Extracellular superoxide production by Enterococcus faecalis promotes chromosomal instability in mammalian cells. *Gastroenterology* 2007; **132**: 551–61.

29 Levin B, Lieberman DA, McFarland B, *et al.* Screening and surveillance for the early detection of colorectal cancer and adenomatous polyps, 2008: a joint guideline from the American Cancer Society, the US Multi-Society Task Force on Colorectal Cancer, and the American College of Radiology. *Gastroenterology* 2008; **134**: 1570–95.

30 U.S. Preventative Services Task Force. Screening for Colorectal Cancer: U.S. Preventive Services Task Force Recommendation. *Ann Intern Med* 2008; **149**: 627–37.

31 Psaty BM, Potter JD. Risks and benefits of celecoxib to prevent recurrent adenomas. *N Engl J Med* 2006; **355**: 950–2.

32 Langevin JM, Nivatvongs S. The true incidence of synchronous cancer of the large bowel. A prospective study. *Am J Surg* 1984; **147**: 330–3.

33 Locker GY, Hamilton S, Harris J, *et al.* ASCO 2006 update of recommendations for the use of tumor markers in gastro-intestinal cancer. *J Clin Oncol* 2006; **24**: 5313–27.

34 O'Connell JB, Maggard MA, Ko CY. Colon cancer survival rates with the new American Joint Committee on Cancer sixth edition staging. *J Natl Cancer Inst* 2004; **96**: 1420–5.

35 Jessup JM, Stewart AK, Menck HR. The National Cancer Data Base report on patterns of care for adenocarcinoma of the rectum, 1985–95. *Cancer* 1998; **83**: 2408–18.

36 Rex DK, Kahi CJ, Levin B, *et al.* Guidelines for colonoscopy surveillance after cancer resection: a consensus update by the American Cancer Society and the US Multi-Society Task Force on Colorectal Cancer. *Gastroenterology* 2006; **130**: 1865–71.

37 Simmonds PC, Primrose JN, Colquitt JL, *et al.* Surgical resection of hepatic metastases from colorectal cancer: a sys-tematic review of published studies. *Br J Cancer* 2006; **94**: 982–99.

38 Yedibela S, Klein P, Feuchter K, *et al.* Surgical management of pulmonary metastases from colorectal cancer in 153 patients. *Ann Surg Oncol* 2006; **13**: 1538–44.

39 Asmis TR, Saltz L. Systemic therapy for colon cancer. *Gastroenterol Clin North Am* 2008; **37**: 287–95, ix.

40 Andre T, Boni C, Mounedji-Boudiaf L, *et al.* Oxaliplatin, fluorouracil, and leucovorin as adjuvant treatment for colon cancer. *N Engl J Med* 2004; **350**: 2343–51.

41 Tournigand C, Andre T, Achille E, *et al.* FOLFIRI followed by FOLFOX6 or the reverse sequence in advanced colorectal cancer: a randomized GERCOR study. *J Clin Oncol* 2004; **22**: 229–37.

42 Colucci G, Gebbia V, Paoletti G, *et al.* Phase III randomized trial of FOLFIRI versus FOLFOX4 in the treatment of advanced colorectal cancer: a multicenter study of the Gruppo Oncologico Dell'Italia Meridionale. *J Clin Oncol* 2005; **23**: 4866–75.

43 Gastrointestinal Tumor Study Group. Prolongation of the disease-free interval in surgically treated rectal carcinoma.. *N Engl J Med* 1985; **312**: 1465–72.

44 Fisher B, Wolmark N, Rockette H, *et al.* Postoperative adju-vant chemotherapy or radiation therapy for rectal cancer: results from NSABP protocol R-01. *J Nat Cancer Instit* 1988; **80**: 21–9.

45 Krook JE, Moertel CG, Gunderson LL, *et al.* Effective surgi-cal adjuvant therapy for high-risk rectal carcinoma. *N Engl J Med* 1991; **324**: 709–15.

46 Kapiteijn E, Marijnen CA, Nagtegaal ID, *et al.* Preoperative radiotherapy combined with total mesorectal excision for resectable rectal cancer. *N Engl J Med* 2001; **345**: 638–46.

47 Robertson JM. The role of radiation therapy for colorectal cancer. *Gastroenterol Clin North Am* 2008; **37**: 269–85, ix.

48 Van Cutsem EJ, Oliveira J. Colon cancer: ESMO clinical recommendations for diagnosis, adjuvant treatment and follow-up. *Ann Oncol* 2008; **19** (Suppl. 2): ii29–30.

49 Hahnloser D, Haddock MG, Nelson H. Intraoperative radio-therapy in the multimodality approach to colorectal cancer. *Surg Oncol Clin North Am* 2003; **12**: 993–1013, ix.

50 Jessup JM, Stewart AK, Menck HR. The National Cancer Data Base report on patterns of care for adenocarcinoma of the rectum, 1985–95. *Cancer* 1998; **83**: 2408–18.

51 O'Connell JB, Maggard MA, Ko CY. Colon cancer survival rates with the new American Joint Committee on Cancer sixth edition staging. *J Nat Cancer Instit* 2004; **96**: 1420–5.

CHAPTER 50

Clostridium difficile Infection and Pseudomembranous Colitis

Alan C. Moss and John Thomas LaMont

Beth Israel Deaconess Medical Center, Boston, MA, USA

Summary

Colonization of the colon with *Clostridium difficile* bacteria can lead to a range of outcomes from asymptomatic carriage, to pseudomembranous colitis, to fulminant colitis. The incidence and severity of this infection have increased in the last 5 years, probably related to the emergence of a highly toxigenic strain associated with hospital outbreaks.

Standard treatment for *C. difficile*-associated diarrhea (CDAD) includes stopping the implicated antibiotics, commencing oral metronidazole therapy, and correction of secondary dehydration. *C. difficile* has not developed resistance to metronidazole or vancomycin, hence initial response to these agents exceeds 90% in clinical trials. Recurrent infection usually responds to re-treatment with metronidazole or vancomycin, or pulse-tapered therapy. Control measures to minimize the risk of hospital-acquired infections remain an important preventative strategy.

Case

A 68-year-old woman complained of a 2-week history of loose stool and abdominal cramps. One month ago she was treated by her primary care physician for a sinus infection with amoxicillin. In addition to diarrhea, she noticed some blood mixed with her stool. She is a diabetic and takes metformin. Her last colonoscopy 2 years ago showed diverticula only.

Definition and Epidemiology

Clostridium difficile infection (CDI) and *Clostridium difficile*-associated diarrhea (CDAD) describe the development of diarrhea that occurs in patients infected with toxin-producing *Clostridium difficile* bacteria [1]. "Pseudomembranous colitis" refers to the endoscopic appearance of scattered white mucosal plaques that can appear in the colon in patients with CDI (Figure 50.1). The pres-

Practical Gastroenterology and Hepatology: Small and Large Intestine and Pancreas, 1st edition. Edited by Nicholas J. Talley, Sunanda V. Kane and Michael B. Wallace. © 2010 Blackwell Publishing Ltd.

ence of *C. difficile* in the colon does not always infer active infection, as asymptomatic carriage has been reported in up to 14% of hospitalized adults receiving antibiotics, and up to 70% of healthy infants [2].

The incidence of CDI rose steadily from the 1970s but remained stable throughout the 1990s at 30–40 cases per 100 000. Since 2000, however, there has been a steep rise in the incidence of this disease (84 per 100 000 in 2005), and the severity of disease has also increased, particularly in elderly patients. Sporadic outbreaks associated with severe morbidity and mortality in Canada and the US have been linked to the virulent NAP-1/027 strain that produces large quantities of toxins (A, B, and binary toxin), and is relatively resistant to fluoroquinolones [3].

Risk factors traditionally associated with the development of CDI include current or recent antibiotic use, advanced age, hospitalization, and co-morbid illnesses [4]. Inflammatory bowel disease (IBD) has recently been recognized as an additional factor, being present in 16% of CDI cases in one series [5]. The Center for Disease Control has recently documented infection in previously healthy young adults with no hospital or antibiotic exposure [6].

Pathophysiology

Oral ingestion of *C. difficile* spores leads to the colonization of the large bowel in some patients following antibiotic exposure, which reduces the ability of the normal flora to resist colonization. These spores are resistant to heat and antibiotics, and widely contaminate the hospital environment. Colitis in *C. difficile* infection is related to its two exotoxins (A and B), which bind to and enter colonic epithelial cells, and disrupt the cellular cytoskeleton [7]. These alterations lead to apoptosis and disintegration of the epithelial barrier function. In addition, *C. difficile* toxins can activate neutrophils, stimulate monocytes and epithelial cells to release interleukin-8 (IL-8), and induce tumor necrosis factor-α (TNF-α) release by macrophages. These result in colonic mucosal inflammation, microulceration and, in some patients, pseudomembrane formation. Toxin B appears to be more potent in inducing colitis than toxin A. The NAP-1/027 strain also produces a non-A/non-B binary toxin, but the role of this toxin in colitis is unclear.

Since not every colonized individual develops CDI, differences in certain host factors probably influence the outcome of infection including:

- The binding of toxin to epithelial receptors
- Production of IgG and IgA antitoxin antibodies
- IL-8 production by colonic inflammatory cells

Although 50–70% of healthy infants up to age 12 months are transiently colonized with toxigenic strains, they are protected from diarrhea, possibly due to absent receptors or ineffective toxin-receptor binding in the presence of breast milk [8]. Hospitalized patients with asymptomatic *C. difficile* colonization have higher serum IgG antitoxin antibodies directed at toxin A than those with CDI, and high levels of these antitoxins appear to protect against recurrence in patients following initial infection [2,9]. Since IL-8-mediated neutrophil recruitment to the colon is central to CDI, patients with polymorphisms in the gene for this chemokine have increased susceptibility to this disease [10].

Clinical Features of *C. difficile* Infection

Patients with CDI typically develop frequent, semiformed or watery diarrhea, in association with crampy abdominal pain [11]. The loose stool is usually non-bloody, but urgency and incontinence may develop in elderly patients. Patients with severe or fulminant disease may develop ileus, peritoneal signs, or shock. Peripheral edema or ascites has been observed due to a secondary protein-losing enteropathy and hypoalbuminemia [12]. *C. difficile* is rarely invasive, but there are rare case reports of reactive arthritis after CDI, or incidental *C. difficile* infection of skin, blood, or bone as part of a polymicrobial infection [13,14]. In patients with an ileostomy or ileal pouch, CDI can cause profuse stoma output or diarrhea.

Clinical signs of CDI are non-specific, and include low-grade fever, diffuse abdominal tenderness, and dehydration. The development of fulminant colitis or megacolon will manifest as ileus and abdominal distension, accompanied by hypotension, diffuse guarding, and rebound tenderness or rigidity if perforation occurs. Associated features include dehydration, hypokalemia, colonic hemorrhage, perforation, and sepsis [15]. Leukocytosis greater than 15000 cells/mm^3 is common, and CDI should always be considered in elderly patients with clinical deterioration and an elevated white count, even in the absence of severe diarrhea.

There are no validated clinical scores for determining disease severity or risk of adverse outcomes in patients with CDI. A recent clinical trial used a novel score (Table 50.1) to classify disease severity with the following parameters: age, temperature, albumin, white blood cell (WBC) count, endoscopic findings, and intensive care unit requirement [15]. This has not been matched with risk of adverse outcomes. A retrospective study of 1600 cases from Canada identified a number of factors associated with a higher risk of complicated CDI, which they

Table 50.1 Criteria to classify *Clostridium difficile* infection severity; score ≥2 within 48h classified as "severe CDAD".

Factor	Points
Age >60 years	1
Temperature >38.3°C	1
Albumin level <2.5 mg/dL	1
WBC count >15000 cells/mm^3	1
Pseudomembranous colitis on endoscopy	2
Treatment in intensive care unit	2

Adapted from [15].

Table 50.2 Risk factors for severe/complicated *Clostridium difficile* infection (SC-CDI) in those not infected with the hypervirulent NAP1/027 strain.

Risk factor	Odds ratio of SC-CDI
Age >65 years	2.1
Tube feeding within 2 months	2.0
Immunosuppression	2.7
WBC >20 × 10⁹/L	3.65
Creatinine	
>100 μmol/L	2.65
>200 μmol/L	4.21

Modified from [16].

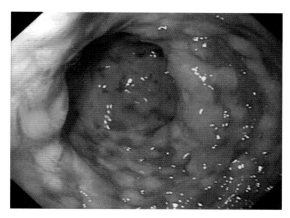

Figure 50.1 Endoscopic image of pseudomembranous colitis in patient with *Clostridium difficile* infection.

defined as death, sepsis, megacolon, perforation, or emergency colectomy (Table 50.2) [16].

Diagnosis

The standard test is an enzyme immunoassay (EIA) for toxins A and B in stool. Testing for either toxin alone may lead to false negative results, as some strains produce only A or B toxin. Toxin EIA has a specificity close to 100%, but sensitivity is limited by the fact that the EIA does not detect small concentrations of toxins. The authors routinely recommend repeat testing in three separate stool samples in patients suspected to have CDI in whom the initial EIA is negative, which has been shown to increase the diagnostic yield [11]. The advantage of the EIA is that results are available within 24 h, unlike toxin bioassays, which may take 2–3 days to develop and read. Once the patient starts treatment, stools may remain toxin-positive for up to 7 days or longer. We do not recommend repeat toxin assays to confirm elimination of toxin at the end of successful therapy.

Endoscopy (sigmoidoscopy or colonoscopy) is not required to diagnose CDI, but may be helpful in atypical presentations, or when there is a high suspicion for CDI despite negative toxin assays. Endoscopic findings can range from simple erythema and friability, to patchy or confluent ulcers with pseudomembranes (Figure 50.1) [17]. It is important to note that the maximally-affected areas may occasionally be proximal to the sigmoid. The

risk of perforation is increased in patients with extensive ulceration or a dilated colon. In this situation a simple examination of the rectum without air insufflation is advisable.

Case continued

A stool sample was sent for enteric pathogen culture and *C. difficile* toxin immunoassay. The toxin test is negative and stool cultures are pending. Labs drawn at the time show a white cell count of 15 × 10⁹.

Differential Diagnosis

The differential diagnosis for patients presenting with diarrhea is long and covered elsewhere in this volume (see Chapter 19). In hospitalized patients with diarrhea, especially those treated with antibiotics, the following specific causes of diarrhea should also be considered:

• Antibiotic-associated osmotic diarrhea: this occurs when antibiotics disrupt the normal bacterial metabolism of dietary carbohydrates in the colonic lumen. The subsequent accumulation of non-absorbed carbohydrates causes an osmotic diarrhea. This is usually mild and disappears with fasting or cessation of the antibiotics.

• Infectious diarrhea: other organisms that cause colitis during or after antibiotic use are *Staphylococcus aureus, Salmonella*, and *Clostridium perfringens. Klebsiella oxytoca* was recently reported to cause an antibiotic-associated hemorrhagic colitis [18]. Rotavirus and cytomegalovirus infection may also cause diarrhea in hospitalized patients.

- Inflammatory bowel disease: patients with established or undiagnosed IBD sometimes experience a flare of disease activity during, or after, antibiotic use, presumably due to alterations in colonic flora that trigger active inflammation.

Treatment

Treatment of CDI has four main tenets, which apply to all cases of confirmed CDI:
- Discontinue the causative antibiotics (if possible)
- Initiate anti-*C. difficile* antibiotic therapy
- Monitor for, and manage, complications
- Initiate infection control measures.

The choice of antibiotic regimen to treat confirmed CDI depends on whether it is an initial infection or relapse, and the severity of the infection itself. As noted in Table 50.1, patients aged over 65 years, those with a high white cell count, and those with an elevated creatinine are at higher risk of severe disease.

Initial CDI

For initial treatment of uncomplicated CDI, oral metronidazole, 250 mg four times daily for 10–14 days, is the treatment of choice. As it is excreted in the bile, intravenous (IV) administration of metronidazole is also effective. The advantages of metronidazole are its low cost, and its comparable efficacy to vancomycin for non-severe CDI in randomized controlled trials [15]. The disadvantages are its side-effects, including nausea and metallic taste during therapy. It is worth noting that a recent outbreak in Canada was associated with an unusually high rate (26%) of patients who failed to respond to metronidazole, but this may reflect a higher proportion of patients with severe disease due to the hypervirulent NAP-1/027 strain [19]. Vancomycin 125 mg orally four times daily is an alternative choice, but is not effective if given IV as it is excreted primarily by the kidney. The disadvantages to using vancomycin are its higher costs, and concerns about the proliferation of vancomycin-resistant enterococci. Importantly, metronidazole or

vancomycin resistance has not been documented in *C. difficile*.

In severe CDI (Tables 50.1 and 50.2) oral vancomycin 125 mg four times a day is significantly more effective than metronidazole [15], and is the drug of choice. In the presence of ileus, or in patients unable to take oral medications, vancomycin may be given via nasogastric tube or as a retention enema (500 mg four times per day) [20]. Patients with fulminant colitis require IV metronidazole (500 mg three times per day), in addition to vancomycin (500 mg four times per day) and review by a surgeon to consider urgent colectomy.

Recurrent CDI

Recurrence occurs in about 20% of patients of successfully treated patients, regardless of initial therapy, and may result either from environmental re-infection with a different strain of *C. difficile* or persistence, via spores in the colon, of the same strain responsible for the initial episode. Positive stool toxin tests in patients with recurrence of diarrhea are not always helpful, as colonized patients can produce toxin which is neutralized by antitoxin antibodies, thus preventing colitis. Other causes of diarrhea such as other infections, IBD flares, or postinfectious irritable bowel syndrome may mimic relapse of *C. difficile* (see Differential Diagnosis).

The first recurrence is usually treated with a repeat 14-day course of metronidazole or vancomycin, in the same dosage used for the initial episode, with recovery expected in about 80–90%. After the first recurrence patients are at high risk of developing further recurrences, up to 50% in one study [21]. Some patients require treatment for multiple symptomatic recurrences. The following treatment strategies are used in patients with multiple relapse (Figure 50.2):
- Vancomycin taper and pulse regimen, to eradicate remnant spores as they convert to the vegetative state in the colon [21]
- Vancomycin taper and pulse regimen followed by a 4-week course of probiotics, such as *Saccharomyces boulardii* to prevent re-growth of *C. difficile* [22]
- Vancomycin for 14 days followed by rifaximin for 14 days [23].

Other options such as intravenous immunoglobulin (IVIG), bacterotherapy with fecal transplantation, or toxin binders such as cholestyramine are resorted to in some patients with multiple relapses.

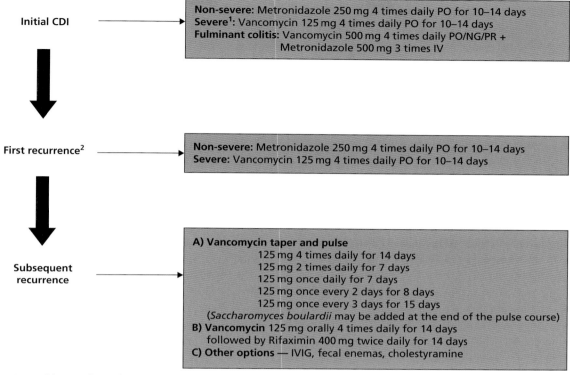

Figure 50.2 Flow chart of suggested management of *Clostridium difficile* infection (CDI).

Case continued

The patient started oral metronidazole 250 mg four times per day for presumed acute CDI. Her diarrhea resolved within 4 days. A second stool sample prior to initiation of therapy was positive for *C. difficile* toxin.

A few days after she finished the course of metronidazole the patient was admitted to hospital with profuse watery diarrhea. She has no features of severe disease, but her initial *C. difficile* toxin test was positive..

Prognosis

As discussed above, most patients (>90%) treated for an initial episode of uncomplicated CDI are symptom-free after 7 days treatment with metronidazole or vancomycin. The proportion of patients who developed severe or complicated disease in 800 non-epidemic patients was 11%, and the 30-day mortality was 8% in this cohort [16]. However, during the recent NAP-1/027 epidemic the 30-day mortality attributable to CDI rose to 23% [24]. After initial treatment for non-severe disease, approximately 20% of patients develop at least one episode of recurrence, and at least half of these will proceed to further relapses of CDI.

Take-home points

- *Clostridium difficile* infection (CDI) is increasing in incidence and severity worldwide, partially due to the emergence of hypervirulent strains.

- Although associated with antibiotic use in most case, infection should be also considered in otherwise healthy individuals with no known antibiotic exposure, and in patients with IBD flares.

- Immunoassay for toxin A and B is the diagnostic test of choice, but should be repeated in those with likely infection and a negative initial result.
- Oral metronidazole or vancomycin are very effective initial therapies, and should be repeated in those with a first recurrence.
- Recurrent disease occurs in about 20% of cases, but a number of regimens have been used with success.

References

1 Kelly CP, LaMont JT. Clostridium difficile: more difficult than ever. *N Engl J Med* 2008; 1932–40.

2 Kyne L, Warny M, Qamar A, Kelly CP. Asymptomatic carriage of Clostridium difficile and serum levels of IgG antibody against toxin A. *N Engl J Med* 2000; **342**: 390–7.

3 McDonald LC, Killgore GE, Thompson A, *et al.* An epidemic, toxin gene-variant strain of Clostridium difficile. *N Engl J Med* 2005; **353**: 2433–41.

4 Barbut F, Petit JC. Epidemiology of Clostridium difficile-associated infections. *Clin Microbiol Infect* 2001; **7**: 405–10.

5 Issa M, Vijayapal A, Graham MB, *et al.* Impact of Clostridium difficile on inflammatory bowel disease. *Clin Gastroenterol Hepatol* 2007; **5**: 345–51.

6 Severe Clostridium difficile-associated disease in populations previously at low risk—four states, 2005. *Morb Mortal Wkly Rep* 2005; **54**: 1201–5.

7 Just I, Selzer J, Wilm M, *et al.* Glucosylation of Rho proteins by Clostridium difficile toxin B. *Nature* 1995; **375**: 500–3.

8 Rolfe RD, Song W. Immunoglobulin and non-immunoglobulin components of human milk inhibit Clostridium difficile toxin A-receptor binding. *J Med Microbiol* 1995; **42**: 10–9.

9 Kyne L, Warny M, Qamar A, Kelly CP. Association between antibody response to toxin A and protection against recurrent Clostridium difficile diarrhoea. *Lancet* 2001; **357**: 189–93.

10 Jiang ZD, DuPont HL, Garey K, *et al.* A common polymorphism in the interleukin 8 gene promoter is associated with Clostridium difficile diarrhea. *Am J Gastroenterol* 2006; **101**: 1112–6.

11 Manabe YC, Vinetz JM, Moore RD, *et al.* Clostridium difficile colitis: an efficient clinical approach to diagnosis. *Ann Intern Med* 1995; **123**: 835–40.

12 Dansinger ML, Johnson S, Jansen PC, *et al.* Protein-losing enteropathy is associated with Clostridium difficile diarrhea but not with asymptomatic colonization: a prospective, case-control study. *Clin Infect Dis* 1996; **22**: 932–7.

13 Birnbaum J, Bartlett JG, Gelber AC. Clostridium difficile: an under-recognized cause of reactive arthritis? *Clin Rheumatol* 2008; **27**: 253–5.

14 Garcia-Lechuz JM, Hernangomez S, Juan RS, *et al.* Extra-intestinal infections caused by Clostridium difficile. *Clin Microbiol Infect* 2001; **7**: 453–7.

15 Zar FA, Bakkanagari SR, Moorthi KM, Davis MB. A comparison of vancomycin and metronidazole for the treatment of Clostridium difficile-associated diarrhea, stratified by disease severity. *Clin Infect Dis* 2007; **45**: 302–7.

16 Pepin J, Valiquette L, Gagnon S, *et al.* Outcomes of Clostridium difficile-associated disease treated with metronidazole or vancomycin before and after the emergence of NAP1/027. *Am J Gastroenterol* 2007; **102**: 2781–8.

17 Seppala K, Hjelt L, Sipponen P. Colonoscopy in the diagnosis of antibiotic-associated colitis. A prospective study. *Scand J Gastroenterol* 1981; **16**: 465–8.

18 Hogenauer C, Langner C, Beubler E, *et al.* Klebsiella oxytoca as a causative organism of antibiotic-associated hemorrhagic colitis. *N Engl J Med* 2006; **355**: 2418–26.

19 Pepin J, Alary ME, Valiquette L, *et al.* Increasing risk of relapse after treatment of Clostridium difficile colitis in Quebec, Canada. *Clin Infect Dis* 2005; **40**: 1591–7.

20 Apisarnthanarak A, Razavi B, Mundy LM. Adjunctive intracolonic vancomycin for severe Clostridium difficile colitis: case series and review of the literature. *Clin Infect Dis* 2002; **35**: 690–6.

21 McFarland LV, Elmer GW, Surawicz CM. Breaking the cycle: treatment strategies for 163 cases of recurrent Clostridium difficile disease. *Am J Gastroenterol* 2002; **97**: 1769–75.

22 McFarland LV, Surawicz CM, Greenberg RN, *et al.* A randomized placebo-controlled trial of *Saccharomyces boulardii* in combination with standard antibiotics for Clostridium difficile disease. *JAMA* 1994; **271**: 1913–8.

23 Johnson S, Schriever C, Galang M, *et al.* Interruption of recurrent Clostridium difficile-associated diarrhea episodes by serial therapy with vancomycin and rifaximin. *Clin Infect Dis* 2007; **44**: 846–8.

24 Pepin J, Valiquette L, Cossette B. Mortality attributable to nosocomial Clostridium difficile-associated disease during an epidemic caused by a hypervirulent strain in Quebec. *Can Med Assoc J* 2005; **173**: 1037–42.

CHAPTER 51
Anorectal Testing

Karthik Ravi and Adil E. Bharucha

Clinical Enteric Neuroscience Translational and Epidemiological Research Program, Division of
Gastroenterology and Hepatology, Mayo Clinic, Rochester, MN, USA

Summary

Anal manometry and a rectal balloon expulsion test, occasionally supplemented by defecography, are necessary
for diagnosing functional defecatory disorders. Diagnostic testing is also useful for evaluating the
pathophysiology and guiding management in fecal incontinence. Anal resting and squeeze pressures measured
by manometry reflect predominantly internal and external anal sphincter function, respectively. Disordered
defecation is diagnosed by assessing rectal balloon expulsion and the rectoanal pressure gradient during
simulated evacuation. Endoanal ultrasound and magnetic resonance imaging (MRI) visualize anal sphincter
defects, scars, and atrophy. Both tests are comparable for the internal sphincter but only MRI identifies external
sphincter atrophy. Barium defecography can characterize rectal evacuation and pelvic floor function and thereby
reveal evacuation disorders, excessive perineal descent, and rectoceles. Dynamic MRI provides similar information
and also images the bladder and genital organs. Since the measurement of pudendal nerve latencies suffers
from several limitations, anal sphincter electromyography is recommended when neurogenic sphincter weakness
is suspected.

Case

A 40-year-old woman was referred with chronic constipation
for 10 years. On her current regimen of polyethylene glycol
(Miralax 17 g) daily, she had one bowel movement every 5
days. Her stools were small hard pellets, that is Bristol stool
form score was 1. Defecation required considerable straining
and she felt unsatisfied thereafter. However, she denied anal
digitation or a sense of anorectal blockage. Her dietary fiber
content was adequate. The past medical history was
non-contributory; she had two uncomplicated vaginal
deliveries. While the abdominal examination was
unremarkable, digital rectal examination revealed external
hemorrhoids, normal anal resting tone, a normal
puborectalis lift to voluntary command, and reduced (<1 cm)
perineal descent during simulated evacuation.

Anal manometry identified increased average anal resting
and normal anal squeeze pressures of 100 (normal is
<90 mmHg) and 180 mmHg (normal is <220 mmHg),
respectively. The rectoanal inhibitory reflex was present.
Rectal sensory thresholds for first sensation, desire to

defecate, and urgency were normal. The rectal balloon
expulsion test was abnormal.

A diagnosis of pelvic floor dysfunction was made. The
patient completed 18 sessions of pelvic floor retraining by
biofeedback therapy over a 2-week period. Three months
later, the patient reported taking a fiber supplement
(psyllium 15 g daily) and passing one bowel movement every
other day. She did not strain and felt satisfied thereafter.

In summary, an integrated assessment of the clinical
features, rectal examination, and anorectal manometry are
useful for identifying defecatory disorders, which should be
treated with pelvic floor retraining by biofeedback therapy.

Tests of Function

Anorectal Manometry

Measurement

Anorectal manometry measures anal resting and squeeze
pressures, the rectoanal inhibitory reflex, and rectoanal
pressure changes during straining [1]. The manometric
catheter assembly includes a rectal balloon and either
solid state or water perfused pressure transducers located

Practical Gastroenterology and Hepatology: Small and Large
Intestine and Pancreas, 1st edition. Edited by Nicholas J. Talley,
Sunanda V. Kane and Michael B. Wallace. © 2010 Blackwell
Publishing Ltd.

in the anal canal. However, catheter design is not standardized. The sensors may be radially staggered at 1-cm intervals or located around the circumferential axis at one or two levels along the longitudinal axis. Because the sphincter is not symmetric, anal pressures should preferably be simultaneously measured. The catheter is gradually withdrawn in 0.5- or 1-cm steps from the rectum to the anal verge (i.e., station pull-through procedure). Squeeze pressure should be measured by asking patients to squeeze (i.e., contract) the anal sphincter for 20 s, and then averaging pressures over this duration. The rectoanal inhibitory reflex is assessed by measuring anal pressures during rapid, intermittent, rectal balloon inflation with incremental 10- or 15-mL aliquots. The rectoanal pressure gradient is measured during simulated evacuation of an inflated rectal balloon, typically by 50 mL. Defecation is normally accompanied by increased intrarectal pressure and anal relaxation (Figure 51.1).

To account for anal sphincter asymmetry, anal resting and squeeze pressures should be summarized by averaging pressures in all four quadrants. Resting pressures are probably less susceptible to artifact than are squeeze pressures. Because pressures are lower in women and in older people, anal pressures should be compared against normal values obtained in age- and gender-matched subjects by the same technique [2].

Clinical Utility

Anal resting and squeeze pressures are frequently reduced in fecal incontinence (FI) [3,4]. The pattern of disturbances may provide clues to underlying pathophysiology (Table 51.1). However, even patients with anal weakness may have other disturbances, for example, diarrhea, disturbances of rectal compliance, and/or sensation [11]. Anorectal testing is necessary for discriminating functional defecatory disorders from other causes of chronic constipation (e.g., slow transit constipation, irritable bowel syndrome) [12]. Features of an evacuation disorder on anal manometry include increased anal resting pressure, impaired relaxation or paradoxical contraction of the anal sphincter during simulated evacuation (i.e., dyssynergia), or inadequate augmentation of rectal pressure during simulated evacuation (Figure 51.1).

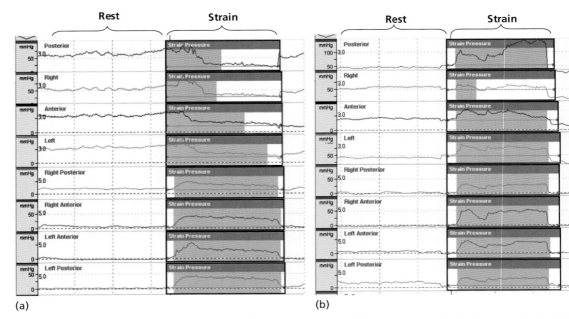

(a)   (b)

Figure 51.1 Rectoanal pressure changes during straining. In both tracings, the upper four sensors were located in the anal canal 3 cm from the verge, while the lower four sensors were located in the rectum, 5 cm from the anal verge. (a) The normal tracing shows anal relaxation coordinated with increased intrarectal pressure. (b) The dyssynergic pattern is characterized by increased intrarectal and intra-anal pressure. (From Bharucha AE. Bharucha AE. Update of tests of colon and rectal structure and function. *J Clin Gastroenterol* 2006; **40**(2): 96–103. (Review), with permission from Wolters Kluwer Health.)

Table 51.1 Anorectal sensorimotor disturbances in fecal incontinence (from Bharucha AE. Fecal incontinence. *Gastroenterology* **124**(6): 1672–1685, 2003, with permission from Elsevier).

Etiologic factor	Anal sphincter pressure	Threshold for internal sphincter relaxation	Threshold for external sphincter contraction	Rectal sensation*	Rectal compliance	Pelvic floor function
"Idiopathic"	↓	↓	↓	↓ or ↑	↓	↓
Diabetes mellitus[5]	R ↓ S ↓	↔	↑	↓↓	↔	
Multiple sclerosis[5]	R ↔ S ↓↓	↓	↑	↓↓	↔	
Elderly patients with fecal impaction and incontinence[6]	R ↔; S ↔	↓	↑	↓		↓
Acute radiation proctitis[7]	R ↓ S ↓	NA	NA	↔	↓	NA
Chronic radiation injury[8]	NA	NA	NA	↑	↓	NA
Ulcerative colitis[9]	S ↓ incontinent patients	↓ (active colitis only)	NA	↑ (active colitis only)	↓ (active colitis only)	NA
Spinal cord injury—high spinal lesion, i.e. T12 or higher[10]	R ↔ S ↓	↓	↔	↓	↓	NA
Low spinal lesion, i.e. below T12	R ↓ S ↓	↔	↓	↓	↔	NA

Information pertains to patients with underlying disease and fecal incontinence.

↑, increased; ↓, decreased; ↔, no change; R, resting; S. squeeze sphincter pressure; NA, not available

*Rectal sensation expressed as volume thresholds for perception; ↑ sensation indicates volume threshold for perception was lower compared to normals

Anorectal manometry is conducted in the horizontal position and expulsion efforts do not mimic the colorectal coordination or stool delivery involved in normal defecation. Manometry may over diagnose dyssynergia [13]. Anal "resting" pressures may also be increased in patients who cannot relax completely or have anal fissures. Although a rectoanal pressure gradient (i.e., the ratio of the highest rectal to the lowest anal pressure) during straining of less than 1.5 is considered abnormal (i.e., suggestive of disordered defecation), additional studies in healthy subjects are necessary [14].

Rectal Balloon Expulsion

Measurement

Patients are asked to expel a water-filled balloon while seated on a commode in a private setting. The balloon is inflated either by a fixed volume, typically 50 mL [15], or alternatively by a variable volume until patients experience the desire to defecate [16]. Healthy people require less than 60 s to expel the balloon. Alternatively, the amount of external traction required to facilitate expulsion of a rectal balloon filled with water can be assessed [17]. Patients with pelvic floor dysfunction require more external assistance (i.e., traction) to expel a balloon

Clinical Utility

In one study, the balloon expulsion test was 87.5% sensitive and 89% specific for diagnosing functional defecation disorders [16]. Thus, the rectal balloon expulsion test is a very useful screening test for a rectal evacuation disorder. However, this test does not define the mechanisms of disordered defecation. For example, even patients with reduced rectal sensation may not perceive the desire to defecate when a rectal balloon is distended, causing an abnormal rectal balloon expulsion test. Conversely, patients with pelvic floor dysfunction may have a false-negative test, that is they may expel a balloon by straining excessively. Therefore, a normal balloon expulsion study does not always exclude a functional defecation disorder.

Rectal Sensation

Measurement

Rectal sensation is assessed by progressively distending a balloon, generally with a syringe. A barostat, which is used in research studies and some clinical laboratories, provides a more refined assessment since the balloon can be inflated in a controlled manner. Thresholds for first perception, desire to defecate, and severe urgency are measured during distension and results are influenced by techniques [18]. An alternative approach is to measure the intensity of perception by visual analog scales during distension of varying magnitude [18].

Clinical Utility

Thresholds for rectal sensation may be normal, reduced or increased in FI [3,4]. Rectal hyposensitivity is also observed and may explain a diminished desire to defecate in chronic constipation [19]. However, whether reduced rectal sensation reflects afferent nerve dysfunction, and/or is secondary to habituation to the presence of stool, is unclear. Sensory retraining by biofeedback therapy can improve rectal sensation.

Rectal Compliance

Measurement

Rectal compliance is measured by assessing the pressure–volume relationships, either by manually inflating a balloon or by distending a highly compliant polyethylene balloon with a barostat [18]. The barostat technique is preferable because the rate of distension is controlled and because a polyethylene balloon, in contrast to a latex balloon, is infinitely compliant. Patients are examined in a semiprone position to reduce pelvic hydrostatic pressure. Rectal pressure–volume relationships and sensation can be measured simultaneously during distension.

Clinical Utility

Reduced rectal compliance may cause symptoms of rectal urgency and frequent defecation in ulcerative and radiation proctitis. The rectal capacity (i.e., the balloon volume at the maximum imposed pressure), is reduced in a subset of women with idiopathic FI [4]. Moreover, reduced rectal capacity is associated with the symptom of urgency and with rectal hypersensitivity in FI. Further studies are necessary to ascertain if rectal capacity can be increased by pharmacologic approaches.

Pudendal Nerve Terminal Motor Latency

The clinical utility of pudendal nerve terminal motor latency (PNTML) is limited by several methodologic issues [20]. Contrary to earlier studies, more recent studies suggest that prolonged latency does not predict success, or lack thereof, after anal sphincteroplasty. A position statement issued by the American Gastroenterological Association (AGA) recommended that PNTML should not be used in the evaluation of FI [20].

Needle Electromyography of the External Sphincter

Measurement

Electromyography (EMG) provides a sensitive measure of denervation and can identify myopathic damage, neurogenic damage, or mixed injury [4]. Each side of the external anal sphincter (EAS) is examined with one or two concentric needle insertions. The puborectalis muscle is examined by inserting a needle in the midline between the anus and tip of the coccyx, passing it through the EAS and into the deeper puborectalis. Insertional activity at rest, motor unit potential amplitude and duration, percent polyphasia, and recruitment following mild-to-moderate voluntary muscle contraction are assessed.

Clinical Utility

Anal EMG should be considered in patients with clinically suspected neurogenic sphincter weakness. Neurogenic changes isolated to the external anal sphincter may be caused by injury at any level along the lower motor neuron. Therefore, pudendal neuropathy can be diagnosed with certainty only when neurogenic changes affect not only anterior but also posterior quadrants of the sphincter or when the anal sphincter and ischiocavernosus muscle are both involved. Needle EMG of the puborectalis can be used to distinguish disorders that affect this muscle and the external sphincter muscle selectively or in combination.

Tests of Structure

Endoanal Ultrasound

Measurement

Endoanal ultrasound (EUS) is conducted with patients in the lateral or prone position. Endoscopic visualization is not necessary for ultrasound examination in most patients with FI. Two-dimensional (2D) EUS takes 10–

15 min and provides a 360° view. Three-dimensional (3D) imaging continuously captures 3D images as the probe is withdrawn through the anal canal. Only 3D images can characterize sphincter length and volume [21].

The sphincter appearance is characterized as normal, mild focal thinning, marked focal thinning, defect, or atrophy [4]. The location of these abnormalities is described in the cross-sectional plane and in the longitudinal axis of the anal canal. A focal, full thickness, hypoechoic defect in the external sphincter is considered to be a scar, generally secondary to a prior tear, while diffuse reduction in muscle bulk reflects atrophy. The internal sphincter is distinctly visualized by EUS and becomes thinner with age [22]. Internal sphincter atrophy is identified by diffuse thinning of the sphincter (measured diameter ≤1 mm). However, it can be challenging to visualize the external sphincter and to discriminate between an external anal sphincter tear and a scar by EUS.

Clinical Utility
Occult sphincter defects, which are recognized by imaging only, occur in up to 35% of primiparous women [23]. Overt anal sphincter tears occur in up to 18% of all vaginal deliveries. Postpartum FI is more common in women with than without sphincter tears after vaginal delivery. Sphincter defects related to obstetric trauma, which more frequently affects the external than the internal sphincter, can be recognized by 2D and 3D US. However, 3D US is better than 2D US for distinguishing external sphincter defects from defects in surrounding structures (i.e., transverse perinei and puboanalis muscle) [24]. Two-dimensional US may overestimate the prevalence of anal sphincter defects, perhaps explaining why only a small proportion of women with anal sphincter defects visualized by 2D US have FI.

Internal sphincter defects probably reflect more severe injury than isolated external sphincter defects. Among women with a delivery complicated by an anal sphincter tear, internal sphincter tears were more likely in women who had a fourth-degree than a third-degree sphincter tear [25]. Among women with postpartum sphincter tears, the severity of FI was greater in those with, than those without, internal sphincter defects [23].

Tests of Structure and Function

Dynamic Proctography (Defecography)
Measurement
Anorectal anatomy and pelvic floor motion are visualized by fluoroscopy. Images are obtained at rest, while patients squeeze the anal sphincter and pelvic floor muscles, and during simulated defecation [18]. Enemas may be required for patients with stool in the rectum. The rectum is filled with a paste which has a consistency of stool and is less likely to leak than liquid barium. Enteroceles can be visualized by opacifying the small intestine with oral barium given 60 min prior to examination. The vagina can be opacified with barium paste, permitting identification of vaginal prolapse.

In addition to rectal evacuation, anorectal motion is quantified by measuring changes in the anorectal angle and the location of the anorectal junction during these maneuvers. The anorectal angle is measured between axes drawn through the anal canal and the rectum. Since the bony landmarks may not be visualized in the same image as the anorectum, anorectal descent is generally measured with reference to the commode [26].

Clinical Utility
Barium proctography is useful when the results of anorectal manometry and rectal balloon expulsion do not concur, are inconsistent with the clinical impression, and/or to identify anatomic abnormalities [12]. Features of disordered defecation include inadequate perineal descent (i.e., <2 cm), inadequate change in the anorectal angle from rest to defecation, impaired and delayed rectal evacuation, and reduced puborectalis relaxation or paradoxical puborectalis contraction during evacuation [27]. The commonest findings in incontinent patients include spontaneous leakage of contrast through a patulous anal canal, a more obtuse resting anorectal angle, and a smaller reduction in the anorectal angle during voluntary contraction of the pelvic floor. A more obtuse anorectal angle at rest may reflect pelvic floor muscle weakness and is very useful for discriminating between controls and FI [27].

Since asymptomatic subjects may also have findings suggestive of disordered defecation, the diagnosis should be based on an integrated assessment of clinical features and test results. For anorectal angle measurements, the intraobserver reproducibility is excellent but interob-

Rest   Evacuation   Rest   Squeeze

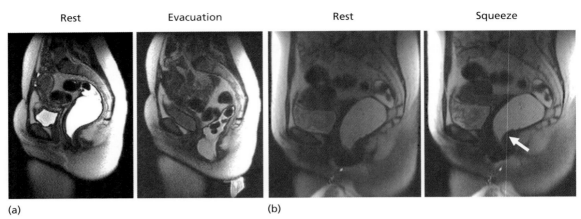

(a)   (b)

Figure 51.2 (a) Dynamic MRI images of normal puborectalis relaxation, perineal descent (2.6 cm), and opening of the anal canal during rectal evacuation in an asymptomatic subject. (b) During squeeze, the anal canal was elevated upward and anteriorly by pelvic floor contraction. Observe the increased indentation (white arrow), reflecting contraction of the puborectalis muscle on the posterior rectal wall during squeeze (i.e., contraction of pelvic floor muscles). (From Bharucha AE, Fletcher JG, Seide B, Riederer SJ, Zinsmeister AR. Phenotypic variation in functional disorders of defecation. *Gastroenterology* 2005; **128**(5): 1199–210, with permission from Elsevier.)

server reproducibility is variable. Indeed, discrepancies between features of disordered defecation and completeness of rectal evacuation, and between anal manometry and defecography occur even in healthy subjects. Despite these limitations, barium proctography may be useful in selected patients.

Pelvic Magnetic Resonance Imaging

Measurement

No preparation is necessary prior to MRI. Before imaging, patients are instructed in the maneuvers (i.e., anal squeeze and simulated defecation) to be performed during the examination. A combined examination (i.e., static and dynamic MRI) can be performed in approximately 45–60 min. Endoluminal imaging is generally performed prior to dynamic imaging because residual rectal or vaginal contrast, used to assess rectal evacuation, can cause near-field artifacts [4].

After endoanal imaging, approximately 180 mL of ultrasound gel is added to the rectum. Dynamic images are acquired during squeeze and rectal evacuation. Thereafter, patients are asked to empty their bladder and rectum in the toilet and dynamic images are acquired during a Valsalva maneuver [4,28–30]. Real-time image reconstruction allows patients to be coached during maneuvers.

Normally, the anorectal junction moves anterior–superiorly, indicating contraction of the puborectalis

muscle during the squeeze maneuver (Figure 51.2). During evacuation, the perineum should descend and the puborectalis indentation should become less pronounced, indicating puborectalis relaxation. When the bladder or rectum is full, the levator plate may limit small bowel and uterine descent. Consequently, enteroceles and uterine prolapse may not be adequately appreciated. Therefore, evacuation should be reimaged as the sagittal plane after patients are allowed to use a toilet. Finally, contiguous coronal images are acquired at rest and during a Valsalva maneuver to better visualize rectal prolapse and to detect eventration or hernias of the levator muscle and lateral rectoceles.

Anorectal motion and rectal evacuation are evaluated as described for evacuation proctography. Normal values for anorectal motion in asymptomatic subjects are summarized elsewhere [30]. Interobserver correlations for anorectal angle measurements by MR proctography are excellent; however, it is important to recognize that the normal ranges (i.e., 10th–90th percentile values) for these parameters in asymptomatic subjects are fairly wide and are also affected by age [4,31].

Clinical Utility

The anorectal angle change during defecation is reduced, reflecting impaired puborectalis relaxation in defecatory disorders [30]. Similar to barium proctography, the diagnosis of disordered defecation should not be based only

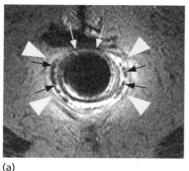
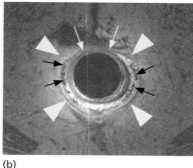
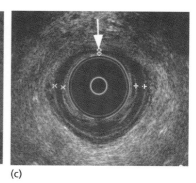

(a) (b) (c)

Figure 51.3 Endoanal (a) fast spin-echo T2-weighted and (b) spin-echo T1-weighted MR images demonstrate marked atrophy of the external anal sphincter (arrowheads) in a 75-year-old incontinent patient, making the internal anal longitudinal muscle prominent (black arrows). (c) Corresponding endoanal ultrasound images identified patchy thinning of the internal sphincter also seen on the MR images (white arrows), but not external sphincter atrophy. (From Bharucha AE, Fletcher JG, Harper CM, Hough D, Daube JR, Stevens C, Seide B, Riederer SJ, Zinsmeister AR. Relationship between symptoms and disordered continence mechanisms in women with idiopathic fecal incontinence. *Gut* **54**: 546–55, 2005. Reproduced with permission from the BMJ Publishing Group.)

on changes in the anorectal angle or puborectalis indentation during evacuation because these features may not conform to the anticipated "normal" pattern even in some asymptomatic subjects. Conversely, these parameters may be normal in some patients with clinical and manometric features of an evacuation disorder [30,32].

In addition to impaired evacuation, patients with defecatory disorders also have impaired anorectal motion when they squeeze or contract the anal sphincter and pelvic floor [30]. Perineal descent may be normal, reduced, or increased, suggesting perhaps that the natural history of pelvic floor disorders is characterized by a transition from reduced perineal descent to increasing perineal descent as the pelvic floor becomes weaker. Over time, the descending perineum syndrome may cause a pudendal neuropathy and lead to incontinence [33].

It is easier to measure anorectal and pelvic motion by MRI than barium proctography because the bladder, vagina, small bowel, peritoneum, and bony landmarks are visualized more distinctly with MRI. Dynamic MRI may be more sensitive than fluoroscopic defecography for detecting enteroceles. Since subtle or transitory intussusception or prolapse may not be evident on MRI, fluoroscopic defecography should be performed if these conditions are suspected but are not evident during MRI.

Although imaging generally reveals distinct patterns in patients with FI and defecatory disorders, there is some overlap because these conditions may coexist. Anal sphincter and puborectalis injury, which may be partly attributable to obstetric trauma, are more frequently observed in FI than in defecatory disorders [30]. While endoanal US and MRI are comparable for identifying internal sphincter abnormalities, MRI is superior to US for identifying external sphincter atrophy, which may be severe in up to one-fifth of incontinent patients, but is uncommon in asymptomatic controls [30,34] (Figure 51.3). Reduced anal resting pressure may manifest as a patulous anal canal filled with rectal contrast. Anorectal motion from rest to squeeze may be reduced, which suggests impaired voluntary contraction, either due to a limited effort or to weakness of the puborectalis muscle.

Conclusions

The multifaceted mechanisms responsible for fecal continence and defecation can be assessed by a variety of tests. These tests should be conducted by rigorous techniques and interpreted in the context of the clinical features. There is consensus that anal manometry and rectal balloon expulsion tests are necessary for diagnosing defecatory disorders in constipated patients. In FI, the need for and extent of diagnostic testing is guided by the patient's age, symptom severity, bowel habits, and response to conservative measures. One or more anorectal sensorimotor dysfunctions occur in patients with anorectal symptoms; the pattern of anorectal sensorimotor dysfunctions may explain symptoms, facilitate an understanding of the underlying pathophysiology, and guide therapy. Anal manometry provides a useful starting point in FI. Additional testing is guided by clinical features and the results of manometry. The impact of diagnostic testing on management is currently limited but will continue to evolve with development of newer therapeutic approaches.

Acknowledgments

This work was supported in part by Grant R01 DK 78924 from the National Institutes of Health, US Public Health Service.

Take-home points

- Anorectal manometry and rectal balloon expulsion tests generally suffice for confirming a clinically suspected defecatory disorder.
- Anal manometry and imaging can characterize sphincter weakness and damage, respectively in fecal incontinence.
- Endoanal ultrasound and MRI are probably equivalent for visualizing the internal sphincter. Pelvic MRI is better than ultrasound for identifying external sphincter abnormalities, particularly atrophy.
- The methods for anal manometry are not standardized. Age, gender, and clinical features should be considered when interpreting anorectal tests.

References

1 Bharucha AE, Seide B, Fox JC, Zinsmeister AR. Day-to-day reproducibility of anorectal sensorimotor assessments in healthy subjects. *Neurogastroenterol Motility* 2004; **16**: 241–50.

2 Fox JC, Fletcher JG, Zinsmeister AR, Seide B, Riederer SJ, Bharucha AE. Effect of aging on anorectal and pelvic floor functions in females. *Dis Colon Rectum* 2006; **49**: 1726–35 [erratum in *Dis Colon Rectum* 2007; **50**: 404].

3 Sun WM, Donnelly TC, Read NW. Utility of a combined test of anorectal manometry, electromyography, and sensation in determining the mechanism of "idiopathic" faecal incontinence. *Gut* 1992; **33**: 807–13.

4 Bharucha AE, Fletcher JG, Harper CM, *et al.* Relationship between symptoms and disordered continence mechanisms in women with idiopathic fecal incontinence. *Gut* 2005; **54**: 546–55.

5 Caruana BJ, Wald A, Hinds JP, Eidelman BH. Anorectal sensory and motor function in neurogenic fecal inconti-

nence. Comparison between multiple sclerosis and diabetes mellitus. *Gastroenterology* 1991; **100**: 465–70.

6 Read NW, Abouzekry L. Why do patients with faecal impaction have faecal incontinence. *Gut* 1986; **27**: 283–7.

7 Yeoh EK, Russo A, Botten R, *et al.* Acute effects of therapeutic irradiation for prostatic carcinoma on anorectal function. *Gut* 1998; **43**: 123–7.

8 Varma JS, Smith AN, Busuttil A. Correlation of clinical and manometric abnormalities of rectal function following chronic radiation injury. *Br J Surg* 1985; **72**: 875–8.

9 Rao SS, Read NW, Davison PA, Bannister JJ, Holdsworth CD. Anorectal sensitivity and responses to rectal distention in patients with ulcerative colitis. *Gastroenterology* 1987; **93**: 1270–5.

10 Sun WM, Read NW, Donnelly TC. Anorectal function in incontinent patients with cerebrospinal disease. *Gastroenterology* 1990; **99**: 1372–9.

11 Bharucha A. Fecal incontinence. *Gastroenterology* 2003; **124**: 1672–85.

12 Bharucha AE, Wald A, Enck P, Rao S. Functional anorectal disorders. *Gastroenterology* 2006; **130**: 1510–8.

13 Voderholzer WA, Neuhaus DA, Klauser AG, Tzavella K, Muller-Lissner SA, Schindlbeck NE. Paradoxical sphincter contraction is rarely indicative of anismus. *Gut* 1997; **41**: 258–62.

14 Rao SS, Welcher KD, Leistikow JS. Obstructive defecation: a failure of rectoanal coordination. *Am J Gastroenterol* 1998; **93**: 1042–50.

15 Rao SS, Azpiroz F, Diamant N, Enck P, Tougas G, Wald A. Minimum standards of anorectal manometry. *Neurogastroenterol Motility* 2002; **14**: 553–9.

16 Minguez M, Herreros B, Sanchiz V, *et al.* Predictive value of the balloon expulsion test for excluding the diagnosis of pelvic floor dyssynergia in constipation. *Gastroenterology* 2004; **126**: 57–62.

17 Pezim ME, Pemberton JH, Levin KE, Litchy WJ, Phillips SF. Parameters of anorectal and colonic motility in health and in severe constipation. *Dis Colon Rectum* 1993; **36**: 484–91.

18 Bharucha AE. Update of tests of colon and rectal structure and function. *J Clin Gastroenterol* 2006; **40**: 96–103.

19 Gladman MA, Lunniss PJ, Scott SM, Swash M. Rectal hyposensitivity. *Am J Gastroenterol* 2006; **101**: 1140–51.

20 Diamant NE, Kamm MA, Wald A, Whitehead WE. American Gastroenterological Association Medical Position Statement on Anorectal Testing Techniques. *Gastroenterology* 1999; **116**: 732–60.

21 Santoro GA, Fortling B. The advantages of volume rendering in three-dimensional endosonography of the anorectum. *Dis Colon Rectum* 2007; **50**: 359–68.

22 Huebner M, Margulies RU, Fenner DE, Ashton-Miller JA, Bitar KN, DeLancey JOL. Age effects on internal anal sphinc-

ter thickness and diameter in nulliparous females. *Dis Colon Rectum* 2007; **50**: 1405–11.

23 Wheeler TL, 2nd, Richter HE. Delivery method, anal sphincter tears and fecal incontinence: new information on a persistent problem. *Curr Opin Obstet Gynecol* 2007; **19**: 474–9.

24 Williams AB, Bartram CI, Halligan S, Spencer JA, Nicholls RJ, Kmiot WA. Anal sphincter damage after vaginal delivery using three-dimensional endosonography. *Obstet Gynecol* 2001; **97**: 770–5.

25 Bradley CS, Richter HE, Gutman RE, *et al.* Risk factors for sonographic internal anal sphincter gaps 6–12 months after delivery complicated by anal sphincter tear. *Am J Obstet Gynecol* 2007; **197**: 310.e1–5.

26 Bartram CI, Turnbull GK, Lennard-Jones JE. Evacuation proctography: an investigation of rectal expulsion in 20 subjects without defecatory disturbance. *Gastrointest Radiol* 1988; **13**: 72–80.

27 Agachan F, Pfeifer J, Wexner SD. Defecography and proctography. Results of 744 patients. *Dis Colon Rectum* 1996; **39**: 899–905.

28 Kelvin FM, Maglinte DD, Hale DS, Benson JT. Female pelvic organ prolapse: a comparison of triphasic dynamic MR imaging and triphasic fluoroscopic cystocolpoproctography. *AJR Am J Roentgenol* 2000; **174**: 81–8.

29 Pannu HK, Kaufman HS, Cundiff GW, Genadry R, Bluemke DA, Fishman EK. Dynamic MR imaging of pelvic organ prolapse: spectrum of abnormalities. *Radiographics* 2000; **20**: 1567–82.

30 Bharucha AE, Fletcher JG, Seide B, Riederer SJ, Zinsmeister AR. Phenotypic Variation in functional disorders of defecation. *Gastroenterology* 2005; **128**: 1199–210.

31 Fox JC, Fletcher JG, Zinsmeister AR, Seide B, Riederer SJ, Bharucha AE. Effect of aging on anorectal and pelvic floor functions in females. *Dis Colon Rectum* 2006; **49**: 1726–35.

32 Halligan S, Bartram CI, Park HJ, Kamm MA. Proctographic features of anismus. *Radiology* 1995; **197**: 679–82.

33 Bartolo DC, Jarratt JA, Read MG, Donnelly TC, Read NW. The role of partial denervation of the puborectalis in idiopathic faecal incontinence. *Br J Surg* 1983; **70**: 664–7.

34 Terra MP, Beets-Tan RG, van der Hulst VP, *et al.* MRI in evaluating atrophy of the external anal sphincter in patients with fecal incontinence. *AJR Am J Roentgenol* 2006; **187**: 991–9.

CHAPTER 52

Abdominal Abscesses and Gastrointestinal Fistula

Faten N. Aberra and Gary R. Lichtenstein

Division of Gastroenterology, Hospital of the University of Pennsylvania, Philadelphia, PA, USA

Summary

Abdominal abscesses and gastrointestinal fistula are complications or manifestations of several diseases. In this review, the pathophysiology, clinical presentation, diagnostic testing, and therapeutics of abdominal abscesses and gastrointestinal fistula are provided as a guide for the clinician.

Case

A 60–year-old male presents with a 2-day history of crampy left–lower abdominal pain. The day of presentation he has a fever to 102°F. He has no change in his bowel habits and currently has two to three bowel movements per day. He denies hematochezia, melena, nausea, and vomiting. He is otherwise healthy, takes no medications, and has no medication allergies. He denies tobacco, drinks alcohol occasionally, and denies illicit drug use. He has no family history of gastrointestinal diseases. His physical exam was remarkable for mild tenderness to palpation in the left lower quadrant of the abdomen, and mild voluntary guarding in the left lower quadrant without rebound tenderness.

Definition and Epidemiology

Abdominal abscesses are usually a result of perforation of hollow viscera and may occur in the setting of a fistula. A gastrointestinal fistula is an abnormal connection from the luminal gastrointestinal tract to another epithelium-lined organ or vessel. Fistulae may occur anywhere in the gastrointestinal tract, esophagus to anus, and usually in the setting of active luminal mucosal disease. Gastroin-

Practical Gastroenterology and Hepatology: Small and Large Intestine and Pancreas, 1st edition. Edited by Nicholas J. Talley, Sunanda V. Kane and Michael B. Wallace. © 2010 Blackwell Publishing Ltd.

testinal fistulae are classified anatomically as internal and external (Table 52.1). Examples of internal fistula are intestinal-to-intestinal fistula such as enteroenteric, enterocolonic, and gastrocolic. Fistulae may also form from between the gastrointestinal tract and another internal organ such as rectovaginal and enterovesicular fistulae. Examples of external fistula include enterocutaneous and perianal fistula. From the most common to the least common type of gastrointestinal fistulae are perianal, enteroenteric, rectovaginal, enterocutaneous, enterovesicular, and enteroabdominal. Fistulae may also be classified by level of fluid output (low, moderate, high).

Pathophysiology

The development of fistulae and abdominal abscesses are both usually related to perforation of a hollow gastrointestinal organ either leading to a walled off connection to another site or resulting in abscess formation without frank peritonitis. Mechanisms of perforation that may predispose to either abdominal abscess or fistula include foreign body perforation (ingested, blunt, or iatrogenic), extrinsic bowel obstruction, intrinsic bowel obstruction, loss of gastrointestinal wall integrity, gastrointestinal ischemia, and infection [1]. The most common causes for abdominal abscesses are appendicitis, diverticulitis,

Table 52.1 Types of gastrointestinal fistulae.

Internal fistulae
   Esophageal (cervical, thoracic)
   Enteroenteric
   Enterovesical
   Colovesical
   Ileocolonic
   Colocolic
   Cholecystoduodenal

External fistulae
   Enterocutaneous
   Colocutaneous
   Rectovaginal
   Perianal

Table 52.2 Causes of gastrointestinal fistulae.

Crohn disease
Infections (HIV related, tuberculosis, actinomycoses)
Malignancy
Diverticulitis
Radiation
Ischemia
Postoperative-anastomotic
Foreign body
Trauma
Hidradenitis
Peptic ulcer disease
Appendicitis
Lye ingestion

Crohn disease, cholecystectomy, complication of acute pancreatitis, peptic ulcer, tumor, blunt trauma, and ischemic colitis [2]. Bacteria such *Bacteroides fragilis* and *Escherichia coli* are commonly isolated from abscesses from secondary bacterial peritonitis, whereas *Candida*, *Enterococcus, Enterobacter,* and *Staphylococcus epidermis* may be cultured from nosocomial-related abscesses.

Gastrointestinal fistulae may form due to Crohn disease, a foreign body, radiation enteritis, infection (such as tuberculosis), tumor, diverticulitis, peptic ulcer disease, appendicitis, and postoperative at a surgical anastomosis (Table 52.2). Fifteen to twenty-five percent of gastrointestinal fistulae occur spontaneously and the majority, 75–85%, are iatrogenic, postoperative [3]. The most common cause of spontaneous gastrointestinal fistula in the developed world is Crohn disease.

Clinical Features

In the setting of an abdominal abscess the clinical presentation may vary; patients may present with localized abdominal pain, back pain, fever, localized mass on exam, and/or frank sepsis. The location of abdominal pain and physical exam findings are dependent on the site of an abscess. Patients may also present with sciatica-type pain, flank pain, and psoas sign in the setting of iliopsoas involvement. In patients with aggressive disease, there may be peritoneal signs due to abdominal spread of infection.

Most internal fistulae may not present with clinical symptoms or signs and may go unrecognized until found incidentally on radiologic examination. Internal fistulae that may eventually cause symptoms include enterovesical, rectovaginal, and enterocolonic. Enterovesical fistulae cause recurrent urinary tract infections with urinary cultures often revealing several bacteria species. Patients may notice pneumaturia and fecaluria. Rectovaginal fistula may present with increased vaginal discharge. Enterocolonic fistula may cause increased stool output that may be difficult to differentiate from a typical flare caused by exacerbation of mucosal ulceration. External fistula, such has enterocutaneous and perianal, present with discharge from the cutaneous opening.

Diagnosis

In the setting of a possible intra-abdominal abscess, cross-sectional imaging is recommended to help determine the site and cause. Computed tomography (CT) with intravenous and oral contrast is the diagnostic test of choice due to the ability to detect abscesses in many locations in the abdomen [2].

For gastrointestinal fistula, the initial diagnostic test is based on the site suspected. For an abdominal site of involvement, CT scan may be sufficient. Other modalities that may be needed to confirm the presence of a fistula include barium studies (upper gastrointestinal series, small bowel follow through, or barium enema), and injection of dye into the fistula cutaneous opening with contrast flowing to the fistula site of origin ("fistulogram") [4]. In the setting of suspected fistula in the pelvic or perianal locations, magnetic resonance imaging

(MRI) has better sensitivity than CT scan, 76–100% for pelvic MRI versus 24–60% for pelvic CT scan [5]. Additional tests that may aid in diagnosing pelvic or perianal fistula include endoscopic ultrasound (EUS), with a diagnostic accuracy of 56–100%, and digital rectal exam under anesthesia by an experienced surgeon with diagnostic accuracy as high as 91%. In cases of an unknown cause of a pelvic or perianal fistula, endoscopic evaluation of the intestinal mucosa may be necessary to determine the etiology. In cases of suspected external fistula from a postoperative wound, at the bedside patients may be given oral methylene blue or charcoal with wound drainage assessed for a change in color due to the presence of these compounds.

Case continued

Blood work revealed a white blood cell count of 16 000/mm³. A CT scan of the abdomen and pelvis with oral and intravenous contrast revealed multiple pericolonic abscesses adjacent to the distal sigmoid colon, the largest 11.5 cm in length × 4.1 cm in width, and two smaller abscesses (5.8 × 4.5 cm and 1.8 × 3.7 cm) (Figure 52.1).

Therapeutics

Abdominal Abscess

Management of an abdominal abscess depends on the location and cause. Initial treatment requires removal of

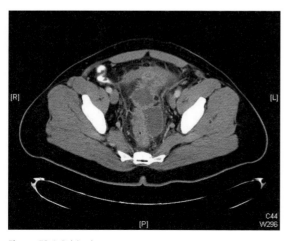

Figure 52.1 Pelvic abscess.

the abscess by percutaneous and/or surgical drainage and adjunctive antimicrobial therapy [4]. Feasibility of percutaneous drainage needs to be assessed based on the clinic scenario and location of the abscess. In the setting of multiple, complex, multiloculated abscesses, percutaneous drainage may not be beneficial. If possible, a catheter is placed to aspirate an abscess, fluid sent for Gram stain and culture, and the catheter is left in place, followed for daily output and clinical response. If clinical response (continued fever and/or leukocytosis) is poor, repeat cross-sectional imaging may be needed to monitor the abscess site. Once there is minimal drainage, less than 15–20 mL/day, and appropriate clinical response, the catheter may be removed.

Peridiverticular Abscesses
For abscesses less than 4 cm, patients may be treated conservatively with antibiotics and bowel rest [6]. Larger abscesses require drainage and CT-guided percutaneous drainage is an option, based on the location of the abscess and the clinical condition of the patient. Drainage may prevent urgent surgery that may require a two-stage operation (temporary stoma) and allow for elective surgery leading to a one-stage operation. Treatment also entails antimicrobial therapy, with aerobic and anaerobic coverage.

Periappendical Abscesses
When a periappendiceal abscess is detected preoperatively, patients have better long-term outcome if managed initially by percutaneous drainage and antimicrobial therapy followed by elective surgery [7].

Gastrointestinal Fistulae

Spontaneous closure of a fistula is more likely to occur if drainage output is low (<500 mL/day), located in the proximal small bowel, secondary to anastomotic breakdown, a long fistulous tract, a new fistula, and in a young (<40 years of age) patient that is well nourished [8] (Table 52.3). Otherwise, surgical closure and/or therapy is directed at the underlying cause.

Initial management of gastrointestinal fistula involves volume repletion and electrolyte and acid/base correction. If patients are malnourished, total parenteral nutrition (TPN) is needed. For high-output proximal fistulae, nasogastric tube suction, gastric acid suppression, TPN, and bowel rest including avoidance of enteral feeds prox-

Table 52.3 Factors influencing spontaneous closure of fistulae.

	Positive factors	Negative factors
Anatomic characteristics	Long fistulae (>2 cm)	Short fistulae (<2 cm) Distal obstruction Diseased adjacent bowel Abdominal wall defect
Origin	Esophageal, duodenum, jejunum	Gastric, lateral duodenum, ileum
Etiology	Anastomosis breakdown	Malignancy Infection Radiation enteritis Crohn disease Anastomosis dehiscence
Fistula output	<500 mL/day	>500 mL/day
Duration	<6 weeks	>6 weeks
Malnutrition	None	Present

imal to the fistula is warranted [9]. Octreotide, a somatostatin analogue, may also help in decreasing fistula output but controlled studies have failed to verify this. In the setting of sepsis, therapy is directed at assuring adequate drainage of the fistula (surgical or percutaneous) and treating with antimicrobials. Endoscopic or percutaneous fibrin glue injection into a fistulous track may also be attempted in patients that fail conservative management. Short tracts tend to have poor outcomes. Fistulae that persist for more than 4–6 weeks, sepsis or abscess formation, distal intestinal obstruction, or bleeding are indications for surgery.

Surgical Emergencies

Esophageal fistulae tend to require urgent evaluation due to the surrounding organs, such as the respiratory system and aorta. Malignant esophagorespiratory fistulae (ERF) can often be palliated with self-expanding metallic stents. Benign ERF, including postoperative, anastomotic leaks, can often be treated with temporary placement of a self-expanding, removable, plastic stent. Chest tube drainage is often needed as these are frequently associated with infected pleural effusions or empyema.

Additionally, aortoenteric fistula may occur in the setting of aortic vascular grafts that erode into the gastrointestinal tract. The most frequent location in the gastrointestinal tract affected is the duodenum. Suspected aortoenteric fistula is a surgical emergency. Any fistula in the setting of sepsis and/or abscess requires urgent antimicrobial therapy and drainage.

Fistulizing Crohn disease

Fistulae occur in a third of Crohn disease patients with the most common location in the perianal region. Treatment of fistulae include medical therapy with antibiotics, immunomodulators (azathioprine, methotrexate, or cyclosporine), and/or antitumor necrosis factor alpha (anti-TNF-α) therapy (infliximab, adalimumab, or certolizumab).

A concomitant abscess needs to be excluded prior to initiating immunosuppressants. Surgery may also be needed based on the type and severity of disease. Asymptomatic internal fistulae rarely require therapy.

Enterocutaneous Fistulae

High-output fistulae occur in the setting of proximal small bowel involvement (>500 mL/day) and cause severe volume depletion [10]. Initial management of these patients involves volume repletion. In the postoperative setting, a fistulous opening is usually in the area of a wound and it is imperative to protect the healing skin from infection due to the drainage either by an ostomy bag or a catheter for high-output fistula. High-output fistulae will rarely close spontaneously and will require surgical closure.

Fistulae that are low output and arising from Crohn disease may be treated initially medically with azathioprine (or 6-mercaptopurine), methotrexate, or anti-TNF-α therapy (infliximab, adalimumab, or certolizumab).

Perianal Fistulae

Treatment of perianal fistula is based on several factors. The first factor is the understanding of the anatomy of the fistulous track in relation to the anal sphincter. Anal fistula anatomic location, based on the Parks classification, is divided into superficial (or submucosal), intersphincteric, trans-sphincteric, suprasphincteric, and extrasphincteric [11,12].

For Crohn disease-related perianal fistulae, classification is divided into simple and complex fistula. Simple fistulae are located below most of the anal sphincter (superficial or intersphincteric (low track) location) and have one track. Complex fistulae go through the intersphincteric (high track), trans-sphincteric, and suprasphincteric region and may have multiple tracks.

Simple fistulae respond well to therapy. Initial therapy is an antibiotic, metronidazole with or without ciprofloxacin for the fistula, and treating mucosal Crohn disease if present. Patients without rectal mucosal Crohn disease may respond well to fistulotomy, whereas patients with mucosal involvement may benefit from seton placement rather than fistulotomy due to poor wound healing. Treatment with immunomodulators (azathioprine or methotrexate) or anti-TNF-α therapy may also be considered.

Treatment of complex fistulae usually entails a combination of surgical and medical therapy. Complex fistulae may be associated with concomitant perianal abscess. In the setting of intractable disease, colonic or ileal diversion may allow for rectal/perianal healing and in severe cases proctocolectomy may be necessary.

Rectovaginal Fistulae

The decision for surgical or medical therapy depends on the clinical scenario. Surgical therapy such as fistulotomy and mucosal flap may be considered. For Crohn disease-related fistula, medical therapy may be considered prior to surgery.

Enterovesical and Colovesical Fistula

Initial Crohn disease-related fistulae may be treated with medical therapy, but recurrent urinary tract infection is an indication for surgery. Surgery usually involves resection of bowel involved and closure of the bladder defect. Colovesicular fistulae are more commonly a consequence of diverticular disease and require surgical intervention.

Internal Fistula

Asymptomatic internal fistulae, such as enteroenteric fistulae, do not require surgical intervention and may be observed as long as the cause has been identified. If the fistula is a consequence of Crohn disease, then treatment with an immunomodulator may be considered. Internal fistulae, such as cologastric and coloduodenal, may cause significant symptoms due to bypass of intestine. These fistulae may be treated medically if a consequence of Crohn disease. If medical management fails, surgery is recommended. Internal fistulae that are associated with sepsis and abscess should be surgically treated.

Case continued

Intravenous ampicillin/sulbactam and bowel rest was initiated. Interventional radiology was consulted and ultrasound-guided perirectal drainage with catheter placement was completed. Antibiotics and TPN were continued and 2 weeks later fluoroscopic assessment and CT scan of the abdomen and pelvis revealed resolution of the complex abscess. A colonoscopy 6 weeks later revealed sigmoid diverticula and diverticulitis as the likely cause for the abscess.

Take-home points

- Most gastrointestinal fistulae are iatrogenic, postoperative.
- Crohn disease is the most common cause for spontaneous gastrointestinal fistulae in the developed world.
- If an abdominal abscess is suspected, then cross-sectional imaging, preferably CT, scan should be completed for diagnosis.
- The cornerstone of treatment of an abdominal abscess is drainage, surgical or percutaneous, along with antimicrobial therapy.
- The cause, location, and duration of fistulae are predictors of healing.

References

1 Langell JT, Mulvihill SJ. Gastrointestinal perforation and the acute abdomen. *Med Clin North Am* 2008; **92**: 599–625, viii–ix.

2 Minei JP, Champine JG. Abdominal abscesses and gastrointestinal fistulas. In: Feldman M, Friedman L, Sleisenger M, eds. *Sleisenger and Fordtran's Gastrointestinal and Liver Disease, Pathophysiology/ Diagnosis/ Management*, 7th edn. Philadelphia: Saunders, 2002: 431–45.

3 Berry SM, Fischer JE. Classification and pathophysiology of enterocutaneous fistulas. *Surg Clin North Am* 1996; **76**: 1009–18.

4 Thomas HA. Radiologic investigation and treatment of gastrointestinal fistulas. *Surg Clin North Am* 1996; **76**: 1081–94.

5 Osterman MT, Lichtenstein GR. Infliximab in fistulizing Crohn's disease. *Gastroenterol Clin North Am* 2006; **35**: 795–820.

6 Jacobs DO. Clinical practice. Diverticulitis. *N Engl J Med* 2007; **357**: 2057–66.

7 Dominguez EP, Sweeney JF, Choi YU. Diagnosis and management of diverticulitis and appendicitis. *Gastroenterol Clin North Am* 2006; **35**: 367–91.

8 Campos AC, Meguid MM, Coelho JC. Factors influencing outcome in patients with gastrointestinal fistula. *Surg Clin North Am* 1996; **76**: 1191–8.

9 Foster CE, 3rd, Lefor AT. General management of gastrointestinal fistulas. Recognition, stabilization, and correction of fluid and electrolyte imbalances. *Surg Clin North Am* 1996; **76**: 1019–33.

10 Tassiopoulos AK, Baum G, Halverson JD. Small bowel fistulas. *Surg Clin North Am* 1996; **76**: 1175–81.

11 Williams JG, Farrands PA, Williams AB, *et al.* The treatment of anal fistula: ACPGBI position statement. *Colorectal Dis* 2007; **9** (Suppl. 4): 18–50.

12 American Gastroenterological Association Clinical Practice Committee. American Gastroenterological Association medical position statement: perianal Crohn's disease. *Gastroenterology* 2003; **125**: 1503–7.

CHAPTER 53

Acute Appendicitis

Patricia Sylla and Richard Hodin

Department of Surgery, Harvard Medical School, Massachusetts General Hospital, Boston, MA, USA

Summary

Acute appendicitis is the most common abdominal surgical emergency. Careful history taking and focused physical examination are essential for accurate diagnosis. CT scan has become a routine adjunct in the work-up and is particularly helpful in female patients and in patients with atypical presentation. Prompt operative management with perioperative antibiotic prophylaxis is the mainstay of treatment. Open and laparoscopic appendectomy are associated with low morbidity and mortality. The laparoscopic approach is associated with lower wound infection rate and shorter hospital stays despite longer operative time and higher costs. Delay in presentation, diagnosis, or treatment of acute appendicitis is associated with increased risk of perforation resulting in higher infectious complications. Patients presenting with perforated appendicitis with a phlegmon or abscess can be managed with immediate appendectomy or non-operatively with antibiotics, bowel rest, and percutaneous drainage, followed by either expectant management or interval appendectomy. Although immediate appendectomy is feasible, it can be technically challenging and is associated with a higher incidence of complications than conservative management.

Case

A 27-year-old male presents to the emergency department (ED) complaining of abdominal pain for the past 13 h. He describes the pain as gradual in onset and initially centered around the umbilicus that progressively intensified to become constant, severe, and predominantly right-sided. He also reports nausea and anorexia and had one normal bowel movement prior to coming to the ED which did not alleviate the pain. He denies fevers, urinary symptoms, diarrhea, bloody stools, or previous similar episodes. Upon evaluation, his temperature is 100.2°F and the rest of the vital signs are within normal limits. Abdominal evaluation is remarkable for tap tenderness over McBurney point with localized right lower quadrant tenderness on light palpation associated with guarding and rebound tenderness. The pain is reproduced upon flexion at the right hip. The remainder of his physical examination is unremarkable. Blood chemistry, liver function test, and urinalysis are within normal limits. His white blood cell count is elevated to 18.8 10³/mm³ with 85% polymorphonuclear cells. Abdominal CT scan with intravenous and rectal contrast was performed which

demonstrates a dilated and non-filling appendix measuring 1.2 cm in diameter with wall thickening and surrounding fat stranding (Figure 53.1a,b). Broad-spectrum antibiotics were administered intravenously and the patient was brought to the operating room for planned laparoscopic appendectomy (Figure 53.2; Video 16).

Definition and Epidemiology

Acute appendicitis is the most common acute abdominal surgical emergency. Approximately 250 000 appendectomies are performed each year in the United States [1]. The highest incidence of appendicitis is found in the 10 to 19-year-old age group with male predominance across all age groups (1.4 : 1) [1]. There is significant heterogeneity in the clinical course of acute appendicitis. There is evidence that early appendicitis may resolve spontaneously or if treated with antibiotics alone [2], particularly in children with symptoms for less than 24 h [3]. On the other hand, progression to perforated appendicitis is well documented and associated with substantial morbidity. The goal of treatment remains early diagnosis and prompt operative intervention.

Practical Gastroenterology and Hepatology: Small and Large Intestine and Pancreas, 1st edition. Edited by Nicholas J. Talley, Sunanda V. Kane and Michael B. Wallace. © 2010 Blackwell Publishing Ltd.

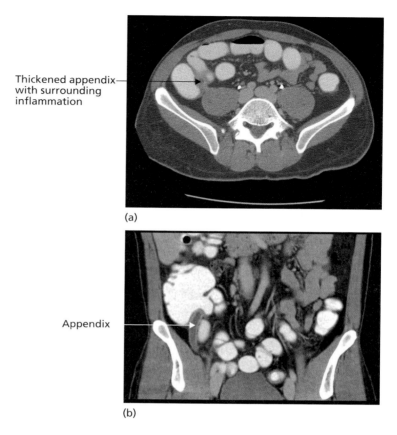

Thickened appendix with surrounding inflammation

(a)

Appendix

(b)

Figure 53.1 Computed tomography of the abdomen and pelvis with oral and rectal contrast. Axial (a) and coronal (b) views were obtained following administration of oral and intravenous contrast which demonstrates a fluid-filled and dilated appendix with a thickened wall extending from the base of the cecum. There are inflammatory changes in the adjacent fat tissue.

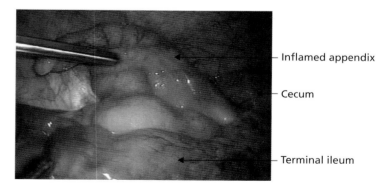

Inflamed appendix

Cecum

Terminal ileum

Figure 53.2 Intraoperative picture during laparoscopic appendectomy in the patient described in the Case. The appendix is acutely inflamed with wall thickening and a purulent exudate. Note the adjacent terminal ileum.

Anatomy and Pathophysiology

Anatomy

The appendix is a tubular structure measuring 2 to 10 cm in length, originating as an antimesenteric outpouching from the cecum during the sixth to eighth week of gestation. It can be traced from the point of confluence of the three taeniae coli of the cecum. The mesoappendix contains the appendicular artery which originates from the ileocolic artery. During embryologic development, the appendix becomes displaced with rotation of the colon, resulting in variations in its final anatomic location. The appendix is found in a retrocecal position in two-thirds and in the pelvis in one-third of patients with resultant differences in the clinical presentation of acute appendicitis.

Pathophysiology

The etiology of appendicitis is most commonly attributed to acute obstruction of the appendiceal lumen. In children, common causes of obstruction include lymphoid hyperplasia from bacterial infection (*Escherichia coli*, *Yersinia*, *Salmonella*, *Shigella*), parasitic infestation (*Entamoeba histolitica*), and viral infection (measles, chicken pox, and cytomegalovirus). In adults, etiologies of luminal obstruction include fecaliths (inspissated fecal material), fibrosis, neoplasia (carcinoid, adenocarcinoma), parasites, or foreign bodies. Obstruction of the appendiceal lumen in the setting of ongoing mucous secretion causes a rise in luminal pressure, promoting bacterial overgrowth with progressive obstruction of venous and lymphatic outflow and wall edema. This leads to obstruction of arterial inflow, leading to wall ischemia, progression to necrosis, and translocation of enteric bacteria leading to full-thickness gangrene. Perforation of the appendix is found in 4–14% of patients [4] and results in either a localized periappendiceal inflammatory mass or phlegmon, a well-circumscribed periappendiceal abscess, or diffuse peritonitis.

Clinical Features

The appendix is lined by visceral peritoneum which is supplied by the autonomic nervous system. The inflammatory process, mediated by local and systemic inflammatory markers, leads to inflammation of the visceral peritoneum which is perceived as a dull and aching, poorly localized discomfort. Subsequent irritation of the parietal peritoneum lining the abdominal cavity is mediated by somatic nerves and is perceived as sharp, localized, and severe. This distinction between visceral and parietal peritoneum is crucial in understanding the evolution in symptoms and physical findings associated with acute appendicitis. The classic history of pain starting in the periumbilical region and migrating to the right lower quadrant, however, is only elicited in about 50% of

patients [5] and, therefore, a high degree of clinical suspicion is often required.

The majority of patients with acute appendicitis present for medical evaluation within 12 to 48 h of symptom onset. Early symptoms include dull epigastric or periumbilical pain associated with nausea, anorexia, and generalized malaise. As inflammation progresses, the pain migrates to the right lower quadrant with localized peritonitis characterized by focal tenderness and rigidity of the overlying muscles. As the pain localizes to the right lower quadrant, it typically becomes constant and more intense and is aggravated by movement. Most patients presenting within 24 h of onset of symptoms have non-perforated appendiceal inflammation with or without gangrene.

Delayed presentation (symptoms for 48 h or longer) is associated with a higher incidence of perforation, ranging from 37 to 65% [6,7]. Delays in diagnosis are due to either late presentation or atypical clinical presentation, which is common at extremes of age (less than 3 and older than 60) [8]. Atypical symptoms can also be related to variations in the location of the appendix. Location in the pelvis often leads to presentation with right flank pain, dysuria, or tenesmus due to proximity of the inflamed appendix to the ureter and rectum.

Diagnosis

History and physical examination findings are the mainstay of diagnosis of acute appendicitis.

Physical Examination

In acute non-perforated appendicitis, the patient may have a normal or low-grade temperature. High temperature and tachycardia on presentation correlate with perforated appendicitis. Examination of the abdomen very early in the course of appendicitis may be non-specific. Later findings include focal tenderness on palpation at McBurney point, the intersection of the middle and lateral thirds of a line drawn from the umbilicus to the anterior superior iliac spine. There may be differences in the location of the point of maximal tenderness from the variable location of the appendix. The presence of muscle rigidity is manifested by involuntary guarding. As muscle spasm in the right lower quadrant increases, rebound tenderness can be elicited. Various maneuvers can elicit pain that indicates peritoneal irritation from appendiceal inflammation [9]. The obturator sign refers to right lower quadrant pain elicited upon passive internal rotation of the flexed right hip as a result of the inflammatory process. The iliopsoas sign is elicited by passive extension of the right thigh with the patient positioned in the left lateral decubitus position, and suggests a retrocecal inflamed appendix overlying the right psoas muscle. In addition, pain can be elicited through Rovsing sign, where pressure applied in the left lower quadrant triggers pain in the right lower quadrant. As inflammation progresses, pain is exacerbated with coughing or other strenuous movements (Dunphy sign). Rectal examination may demonstrate tenderness when the appendix is located adjacent to the rectum. However, the above physical findings are non-specific and can be associated with other abdominal and pelvic pathology. Advanced appendiceal pathology is often associated with tenderness on palpation beyond the right lower quadrant, guarding, and rebound tenderness [10]. When perforation occurs, it may progress to localized or generalized peritonitis. Physical examination should include a pelvic exam in all females presenting with abdominal pain to rule out a gynecologic etiology.

Diagnostic Tests

Laboratory

Mild leukocytosis is common, although it is a non-specific finding associated with other abdominal pathology and may be within normal limits if obtained early in the inflammatory process. A left shift or predominance of neutrophils or bandemia on peripheral blood smear, with or without leukocytosis, supports the diagnosis of appendicitis, particularly in combination with other signs and symptoms. Urinalysis may show mild microscopic hematuria or pyuria due to the proximity of the ureter to the inflamed appendix. Gross hematuria combined with right flank pain helps differentiate acute appendicitis from nephrolithiasis. A pregnancy test should be performed in all female patients of child-bearing age to exclude intrauterine or ectopic pregnancy.

Radiologic Tests

1 Abdominal radiographs are of little use in patients with suspected acute appendicitis. Appendiceal fecaliths are very rarely visualized. Plain radiographs are helpful to rule out other abdominal pathology such as bowel perforation or obstruction in patients presenting with non-specific symptoms and physical findings.

2 Abdominal ultrasound: abdominal sonography is most helpful in pediatric patients. Demonstration of a non-compressible, blind-ending, tubular structure 6 mm or greater in anteroposterior diameter with associated focal tenderness and periappendiceal fluid suggests a diagnosis of acute appendicitis with 75–90 % sensitivity, 86–100% specificity, positive predictive value 89–93%, and overall accuracy 90–94% [11]. Transvaginal ultrasound in patients with abdominal pain and equivocal physical findings can help differentiate acute appendicitis from gynecologic pathology. Both abdominal and transvaginal sonography rely on the experience of the operator for accurate interpretation.

3 Abdominal computed tomography: CT scanning of the abdomen and pelvis has become a routine part of the work-up of patients with suspected acute appendicitis in some centers. Multislice spiral dual-contrast-enhanced CT scan is performed with oral and intravenous contrast and has 90–100% sensitivity, 91–99% specificity, positive predictive value 95–97%, and accuracy 94–100 % for acute appendicitis [11]. CT scan images can be reformatted to provide 1 mm-thin slices through the right iliac fossa with axial and coronal views, thereby improving diagnostic accuracy. Comparable accuracy can be obtained with single-contrast CT or "appendiceal" scan where only rectal contrast is used. CT findings suggestive of acute appendicitis include a distended appendix with a thickened wall (>2 mm) and periappendiceal inflammation (Figure 53.1a,b). Additional findings may include an appendicolith and a "target sign" with concentric thickening of the inflamed appendiceal wall. The degree of periappendiceal inflammation ranges from fat stranding to phlegmon and abscess formation. Advantages of CT scanning include that it is not operator-dependent and allows evaluation of the entire abdomen and pelvis for other pathology.

There is ongoing controversy as to whether a CT scan should be offered routinely to all patients with clinical suspicion of appendicitis or only selectively to patients with equivocal findings. Some studies have demonstrated that routine use of CT scan significantly reduces the time from presentation to the operating room [12] and lowers the negative appendectomy rate [12–15], while others have failed to demonstrate that trend [16,17]. Most recent data suggest that the systematic use of abdominal

CT imaging has led to a substantial decrease in negative appendectomy rates in female patients only, from greater than 20% to less than 10% in most series [18,19]. Routine CT scanning has the disadvantage of delaying operative intervention, potentially resulting in higher perforation rates [20].

Differential Diagnosis

Acute appendicitis must be distinguished from other intra-abdominal etiologies of right lower abdominal pain, which can be broadly classified as gastrointestinal, gynecological, genitourinary, or abdominal manifestations of systemic illnesses (Table 53.1). It is important to consider the patient's age and gender and to take a thorough medical and surgical history with a focus on symptom progression. In older patients, appendicitis should be differentiated from cecal diverticulitis and obstructing or perforated cecal cancer. Crohn ileocolitis is often difficult to distinguish from acute appendicitis preoperatively.

Management

Acute Appendicitis

The standard of care consists of prompt appendectomy (Figure 53.3). Delays in surgical treatment due to delayed presentation or in-hospital delays are associated with more advanced pathology and higher morbidity [10,21]. Patients should be resuscitated with fluids and receive perioperative intravenous antibiotic prophylaxis, which reduces the risk of wound infection and intra-abdominal abscess formation [22]. A single dose of a second-generation cephalosporin (cefoxitin or cefotetan) is adequate to cover common Gram-negative (*Pseudomonas*, *Escherichia coli*), Gram-positive (*Enterococcus*, *Streptococcus*) and anaerobic (Bacteroides) organisms. Alternatively, a first-generation cephalosporin can be given in combination with metronidazole.

 Surgical options include open and laparoscopic appendectomy (Video 16). Evidence from several randomized trials have demonstrated substantial benefits of the laparoscopic approach over open appendectomy, including reduced postoperative pain, length of hospital stay, recovery time, and wound infection rates [23–25]. On the other hand, the laparoscopic approach is associated with

Table 53.1 Differential diagnosis of acute appendicitis.

Abdominal causes
  Gastrointestinal
  Appendiceal neoplasm
  Gastroenteritis (*Salmonella*, *Yersinia*, *Campylobacter*)
  Mesenteric adenitis
  Omental torsion
  Constipation
  Perforated ulcer
  Intussusception
  Small bowel obstruction
  Crohn disease
  Meckel diverticulitis
  Cecal diverticulitis
  Typhlitis
  Pancreatitis

Gynecological
  Ectopic pregnancy
  Pelvic inflammatory disease
  Ruptured ovarian follicle or cyst (Mittelschmerz)
  Ovarian torsion

Genitourinary
  Testicular torsion
  Nephritis
  Urinary tract infection
  Renal colic (stone, ureteropelvic junction obstruction)

Other
  Sickle cell crisis
  Mesenteric adenitis
  Primary peritonitis

Extra-abdominal causes
  Pneumonia
  Hemolytic uremic syndromes
  Diabetes ketoacidosis
  Henoch–Schönlein purpura
  Streptococcal pharyngitis

Reproduced with permission from: Goldberg JE, Hodin RA. Appendicitis in adults-I. In: Basow DS, ed. *UpToDate*. Waltham, MA: UpToDate, 2008. Copyright © 2008 UpToDate, Inc. http://www.uptodate.com

longer operative time and higher cost. Although most studies demonstrate no difference in morbidity following open versus laparoscopic appendectomy, a large meta-analysis concluded that laparoscopic appendectomy was associated with a higher rate of intra-abdominal abscess relative to open appendectomy [25].

Perforated Appendicitis

Based on pooled data from a recent meta-analysis, 3.8% of patients (CI 2.6–4.9) with acute appendicitis present

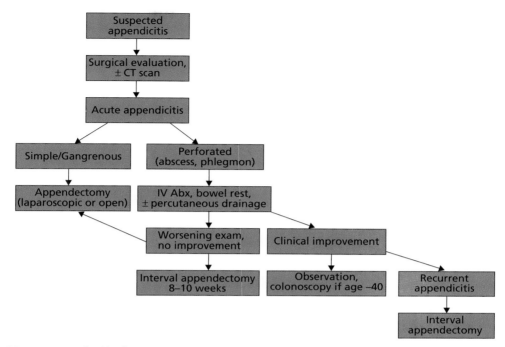

Figure 53.3 Management algorithm for acute appendicitis. IV Abx, intravenous antibiotics.

with a phlegmon or localized abscess [4]. Typically, these patients present after several days of symptoms. The most common organisms involved in perforated appendicitis are *Escherichia coli*, *Peptostreptococcus*, *Bacillus fragilis*, and *Pseudomonas*. Several antibiotic combinations can achieve broad-spectrum coverage against those pathogens including: (i) triple coverage with ampicillin, aminoglycoside, and metronidazole or clindamycin; (ii) monotherapy with a broad-spectrum agent such as piperacillin/tazobactam [26]; and (iii) combination therapy with a third-generation cephalosporin (cefotaxime or ceftriaxone) combined with metronidazole [27,28]. Duration of antibiotic treatment should be tailored to clinical response but is usually transitioned to monotherapy within 5 to 7 days. In one study in pediatric patients, antibiotics were discontinued when patients were afebrile for 24 h and had normalized their white blood cell count with less than 3% bands with a minimal risk of recurrent intra-abdominal abscess [29].

Perforated appendicitis can be managed non-operatively or with immediate appendectomy depending on the clinical presentation, time course, and CT scan find-

ings. Immediate appendectomy can be technically challenging, depending on the degree of inflammation and is associated with higher risk of laparotomy and ileocecal resection than in non-perforated appendicitis. Alternatively, patients can be managed conservatively with broad-spectrum antibiotics, bowel rest, and percutaneous drainage of any periappendiceal abscess, with subsequent observation or interval appendectomy following resolution of the acute episode. Neither approach has been demonstrated to be superior, and the choice largely depends on the clinical presentation and the surgeon's experience. Patients with generalized peritonitis should undergo immediate surgery, whereas patients with an appendiceal mass from a walled-off phlegmon or periappendiceal abscess might benefit from initial non-operative management. Several studies have found that immediate appendectomy is feasible with morbidity and length of stay comparable to conservative management [30,31]. In the majority of studies, however, conservative management with or without percutaneous drainage was associated with lower morbidity [4,32–34] and reduced length of stay relative to immediate appendectomy [33–

35]. Based on pooled data from a meta-analysis, failure of conservative management occurs in 7% of patients [4] (CI 4–10.5). With respect to operative management, perforated appendicitis is not a contraindication to laparoscopic appendectomy. In experienced hands and when technically feasible, laparoscopic appendectomy appears to significantly reduce the incidence of intra-abdominal abscess formation relative to an open approach [35–37].

Interval Appendectomy

Interval appendectomy was traditionally recommended following resolution of perforated appendicitis successfully managed non-operatively. Interval appendectomy is typically performed 8 to 10 weeks following resolution of the episode, the rationale being that acute appendicitis recurs in 5–40% of patients [30,38]. Another argument in favor of interval appendectomy is that other pathology might be missed, such as cecal malignancy or Crohn disease. The same meta-analysis found malignancy present in 1.2% of patients (CI 0.6–1.7) following non-operative treatment of perforated appendicitis, with the majority detected in patients 40 years and older [4]. There is growing debate regarding the need for interval appendectomy as multiple studies have demonstrated long-term recurrence rates as low as 5%, at follow-up as long as 4 years [39]. Therefore, after ruling out malignancy in patients 40 years or older in age with an interval colonoscopy or barium enema following resolution of the acute episode, patients may be observed with interval appendectomy reserved for those with recurrent symptoms.

Complications

The overall mortality of acute appendicitis has declined from 30% in the early 1900s to well below 1% [40] as a result of the use of broad-spectrum antibiotics, advances in diagnostic accuracy, and improvements in surgical and perioperative care. Surgery, either open or laparoscopic, is associated with a negative appendectomy rate ranging from 10 to 30% and is typically higher in female patients (11–34% vs. 5–16%) [14,18]. There is ongoing debate as to whether routine use of CT scan in the diagnosis of appendicitis reduces the negative appendectomy rate. Operative complications include bleeding, appendiceal stump leak or breakdown of the appendiceal staple line, and bowel injury. Complications specific to the laparoscopic approach include trocar-related organ and vascular injuries, trocar site hernias, and cautery-related injuries. The most common complications are wound infections and intra-abdominal abscesses, which occur in 10 to 20% of appendectomies. Factors associated with infection include the degree of appendiceal inflammation, with infection rates ranging from less than 5% in simple appendicitis to 20% in perforated appendicitis [4].

Take-home points

Diagnosis:
- The diagnosis of acute appendicitis is primarily based on careful history taking and focused physical examination.
- CT scan evaluation should be performed in equivocal cases and patients with atypical presentation, particularly in female patients.
- Delays in presentation, diagnosis, and surgical treatment are associated with increased rates of perforation and higher morbidity.

Management:
- Surgery remains the gold standard in the management of acute appendicitis. Prompt surgical treatment reduces the morbidity associated with acute appendicitis.
- Perioperative intravenous antibiotics reduce the incidence of infectious complications following surgery for acute appendicitis.
- Laparoscopic appendectomy is associated with lower wound infection rates and shorter length of hospital stay but longer operative time and higher costs than open appendectomy.
- In perforated appendicitis with localized abscess or phlegmon, initial non-operative management with intravenous antibiotics, bowel rest, and percutaneous drainage is often a safer alternative to immediate surgery.
- Following successful non-operative management of perforated appendicitis, patients can be observed or undergo interval appendectomy if symptoms recur.

References

1 Addiss DG, Shaffer N, Fowler BS, *et al.* The epidemiology of appendicitis and appendectomy in the United States. *Am J Epidemiol* 1990; **132**: 910–25.
2 Liu K, Ahanchi S, Pisaneschi M, Lin I, *et al.* Can acute appendicitis be treated by antibiotics alone? *Am Surg* 2007; **73**: 1161–5.

3 Abeş M, Petik B, Kazil S. Non-operative treatment of acute appendicitis in children. *J Pediatr Surg* 2007; **42**: 1439–42.

4 Andersson RE, Petzold MG. Nonsurgical treatment of appendiceal abscess or phlegmon. A systematic review and meta-analysis. *Ann Surg* 2007; **246**: 741–8.

5 Murphy J. Two thousand operations for appendicitis, with deductions from his personal experience. *Am J Med Sci* 1904; **128**: 187–211.

6 Hale DA, Jaques DP, Molloy M, *et al*. Appendectomy. Improving care through quality improvement. *Arch Surg* 1997; **132**: 153–7.

7 Kearney D, Cahill RA, O'Brien E, *et al*. Influence of delays on perforation risk in adults with acute appendicitis. *Dis Colon Rectum* 2008; **51**: 1823–7.

8 Pittman-Waller VA, Myers JG, Stewart RM, *et al*. Appendicitis: why so complicated? Analysis of 5755 consecutive appendectomies. *Am Surg* 2000; **66**: 548–54.

9 Wagner JM, McKinney WP, Carpenter JL. Does this patient have appendicitis? *JAMA* 1996; **276**: 1589–94.

10 Ditillo MF, Dziura JD, Rabinovici R. Is it safe to delay appendectomy in adults with acute appendicitis. *Ann Surg* 2006; **244**: 656–60.

11 Paulson EK, Kalady MF, Pappas TN. Suspected appendicitis. *N Engl J Med* 2003; **348**: 236–42.

12 Rao PM, Rhea JT, Novelline RA, *et al*. Effect of computed tomography of the appendix on treatment of patients and use of hospital resources. *N Engl J Med* 1998; **338**: 141–6.

13 Brandt MM, Wahl WL. Liberal use of CT scanning helps to diagnose appendicitis in adults. *Am Surg* 2003; **69**: 727–31.

14 Rao PM, Rhea JT, Rattner DW, *et al*. Introduction of appendiceal CT: impact on negative appendectomy and appendiceal perforation rates. *Ann Surg* 1999; **229**: 344–9.

15 Rhea JT, Halpern EF, Ptak T, *et al*. The status of appendiceal CT in an urban medical center 5 years after its introduction: experience with 753 patients. *AJR Am J Roentgenol* 2005; **184**: 1802–8.

16 McDonald GP, Pendarvis DP, Wilmoth R, *et al*. Influence of preoperative computed tomography on patients undergoing appendectomy. *Am Surg* 2001; **67**: 1017–21.

17 DeArmond GM, Dent DL, Myers JG, *et al*. Appendicitis: selective use of abdominal CT reduces negative appendectomy rate. *Surg Infect* 2003; **4**: 213–18.

18 Bendeck SE, Nino-Murcia M, Berry GJ, *et al*. Imaging for suspected appendicitis: negative appendectomy and perforation rates. *Radiology* 2002; **225**: 131–6.

19 Wagner PL, Eachempati SR, Soe K, *et al*. Defining the current negative appendectomy rate: for whom is preoperative computed tomography making an impact? *Surgery* 2008; **144**: 276–82.

20 Musunuru S, Chen H, Rikkers LF, *et al*. Computed tomography in the diagnosis of acute appendicitis: definitive or detrimental? *J Gastrointest Surg* 2007; **11**: 1417–21.

21 Eldar S, Nash E, SaboE, *et al*. Delay of surgery in acute appendicitis. *Am J Surg* 1997; **173**: 194–8.

22 Andersen BR, Kallehave FL, Andersen HK, *et al*. Antibiotics versus placebo for prevention of postoperative infection after appendicectomy. *Cochrane Database Syst Rev* 2005; **20**: CD001439.

23 Olmi S, Magnone S, Bertolini A, *et al*. Laparoscopic versus open appendectomy in acute appendicitis: a randomized prospective study. *Surg Endosc* 2005; **19**: 1193–5.

24 Pedersen AG, Petersen OB, Wara P, *et al*. Randomized clinical trial of laparoscopic versus open appndicectomy. *Br J Surg* 2001; **88**: 200–5.

25 Sauerland S, Lefering R, Neugebauer EA. Laparoscopic versus open surgery. *Cochrane Database Syst Rev* 2004; **18**(4): CD001546.

26 Nadler EP, Reblock KK, Ford HR, *et al*. Monotherapy versus multi-drug therapy for the treatment of perforated appendicitis in children. *Surg Infect* 2003; **4**: 327–33.

27 Maltezou HC, Nikolaidis P, Lebesii E, *et al*. Piperacillin/tazobactam versus cefotaxime plus metronidazole for treatment of children with intra-abdominal infections requiring surgery. *Eur J Clin Microbiol Infect Dis* 2001; **20**: 643–6.

28 St Peter SD, Tsao K, Spilde TL, *et al*. Single daily dosing ceftriaxone and metronidazole vs standard triple antibiotic regimen for perforated appendicitis in children: a prospective randomized trial. *J Pediatr Surg* 2008; **43**: 981–5.

29 Hoelzer DJ, Zabel DD, Zern JT. Determining duration of antibiotic use in children with complicated appendicitis. *Pediatr Infect Dis J* 1999; **18**: 979–82.

30 Samuel M, Hosie G, Holmes K. Prospective evaluation of nonsurgical versus surgical management of appendiceal mass. *J Pediatr Surg* 2002; **37**: 882–6.

31 De U, Ghosh S. Acute appendicectomy for appendicular mass: a study of 87 patients. *Ceylon Med J* 2002; **47**: 117–18.

32 Oliak D, Yamini D, Udani VM, *et al*. Initial non-operative management for periappendiceal abscess. *Dis Colon Rectum* 2001; **44**: 936–41.

33 Henry MC, Gollin G, Islam S, *et al*. Sylverster K, Walker A, Silverman BL, MossRL. Matched analysis of non-operative management vs immediate appendectomy for perforated appendicitis. *J Pediatr Surg* 2007; **42**: 19–23.

34 Brown CV, Abrishami M, Muller M, *et al*. Appendiceal abscess: immediate operation or percutaneous drainage? *Am Surg* 2003; **69**: 829–32.

35 Katkhouda N, Friedlander MH, Grant SW, *et al*. Intraabdominal abscess rate after laparoscopic appendectomy. *Am J Surg* 2000; **180**: 456–9.

36 Lin HF, Wu JM, Tseng LM, *et al.* Laparoscopic versus open appendectomy for perforated appendicitis. *J Gastrointest Surg* 2006; **10**: 906–10.

37 Yau KK, Siu WT, Tang CN, *et al.* Laparoscopic versus open appendectomy for complicated appendicitis. *J Am Coll Surg* 2007; **205**: 60–5.

38 Meshikhes AWN. Management of appendiceal mass: controversial issues revisited. *J Gastrointest Surg* 2008; **12**: 767–75.

39 Kaminski A, Liu IL, Applebaum H, *et al.* Routine interval appendectomy is not justified after initial non-operative treatment of acute appendicitis. *Arch Surg* 2005; **140**: 897–901.

40 Guller U, Hervey S, Purves H, *et al.* Laparoscopic versus open appendectomy: outcomes comparison based on a large administrative database. *Ann Surg* 2004; **239**: 43–52.

CHAPTER 54

Pregnancy and Luminal Gastrointestinal Disease

Nielsen Q. Fernandez-Becker[1] and Jacqueline L. Wolf[2]

[1] Division of Gastroenterology and Hepatology, Stanford University School of Medicine, Stanford, CA, USA
[2] Division of Gastroenterology, Beth Israel Deaconess Medical Center, Boston, MA, USA

Summary

Symptoms due to luminal gastrointestinal disease are among the most common complaints encountered in pregnancy. These disorders may develop *de novo* during pregnancy, be unique to pregnancy, or be an exacerbation of a pre-existing condition. The diagnosis and management of conditions such as gastroesophageal reflux disease (GERD), nausea, vomiting, constipation, irritable bowel syndrome, and inflammatory bowel disease in pregnant women pose special challenges for the clinician in balancing efficacy of therapy and safety in both mother and fetus. This chapter discusses diagnosis and management of luminal GI diseases in pregnancy.

Esophagus and Stomach

Gastroesophageal Reflux Disease and Peptic Ulcer Disease

Gastroesophageal reflux disease (GERD) is common, with women reporting reflux symptoms in 40–80% of pregnancies [1]. Onset has equal occurrence in each trimester, and usually resolves within days of delivery [2,3]. Gestational age, history of heartburn, and previous pregnancies are risk factors [3]. Pre-pregnancy body mass index (BMI), weight gained during pregnancy, and ethnicity do not correlate with GERD, while advanced maternal age seems to have a protective effect [4]. Although symptoms can be quite severe, reflux is rarely associated with serious complications. The lower esophageal sphincter (LES) pressure does not change until the second and third trimesters when it gradually decreases, returning to baseline quickly after delivery [4]. Increased progesterone and estrogen relax the LES pressure [4].

Lower LES pressures, especially in combination with increased abdominal pressure imparted by the enlarging uterus, may lead to reflux of gastric contents. Abnormal esophageal or gastric motility may also contribute to development of GERD [3].

The incidence, severity of symptoms, and frequency of complications of peptic ulcer disease (PUD) are decreased in pregnant women. Because the incidence estimate is based on case reports and retrospective studies, and diagnostic tests are often avoided during gestation the rate of PUD in pregnancy may be underestimated [5]. Esophagogastroduodenoscopy (EGD) is the test of choice when there is concern for PUD [1]. With monitoring of vital signs and careful use of conscious sedation, an EGD can be done safely in pregnancy [5].

Treatment

Lifestyle modification is the first line of treatment. Smaller more frequent meals, food abstinence 3 to 4h before bed, elevation of the head of the bed, and avoidance of known triggers usually suffice for treatment of mild symptoms [4].

For more severe symptoms medications are usually required. Benefit to the mother versus potential risk to the fetus has to be assessed. Unfortunately, prospective,

Table 54.1 FDA classification for drug use in pregnancy. From Thukral C, Wolf JL [1].

Category	Description
A	Adequate, well-controlled studies in pregnant women have not shown an increased risk of fetal abnormalities to the fetus in any trimester of pregnancy
B	Animal studies have revealed no evidence of harm to the fetus, however, there are no adequate and well-controlled studies in pregnant women OR Animal studies have shown an adverse effect, but adequate and well-controlled studies in pregnant women have failed to demonstrate a risk to the fetus in any trimester
C	Animal studies have shown an adverse effect and there are no adequate and well-controlled studies in pregnant women OR No animal studies have been conducted and there are no adequate and well-controlled studies in pregnant women
D	Adequate well-controlled or observational studies in pregnant women have demonstrated a risk to the fetus; however, the benefits of therapy may outweigh the potential risk
X	Adequate well-controlled or observational studies in animals or pregnant women have demonstrated positive evidence of fetal abnormalities or risks The use of the product is contraindicated in women who are or may become pregnant

controlled trials are lacking and thus the safety data on drugs for gastrointestinal illness are limited. The FDA has assigned categories for drug safety in pregnancy (Table 54.1).

The first-line pharmacologic treatment for GERD/PUD includes antacids and sucralfate. The second-line treatment is histamine receptor antagonists, followed by proton pump inhibitors. All are category B, except omeprazole which is category C. See Table 54.2 for a summary of GERD drugs in pregnancy.

Nausea and Vomiting of Pregnancy (NVP)

Nausea and vomiting are common in pregnancy, with the spectrum ranging from mild nausea to intractable nausea and vomiting known as hyperemesis gravidarum (HG). NVP occurs in 70–80% of all pregnancies [6]. The symptoms can occur at any time [6]. Risk factors for NVP include first pregnancy, multiple gestations, young age, obesity, and non-smoking status [6]. In a prospective study of 160 women, nausea and vomiting were most common in the first trimester and resolved by week 22 in 90% of the women [6]. Pregnancy-related factors, including human chorionic gonadotropin (βHCG), estrogen, progesterone, and prostaglandin E2, are believed to play a role in the pathogenesis [6]. Koch *et al.* found that 26 of 32 pregnant women with morning sickness exhibited gastric dysrythmias [6,7]. Delay in gastric emptying has not been documented.

Diagnosis
Nausea is a common complaint in normal pregnancies but it can also be a manifestation of a myriad of other diseases. In NVP, nausea and vomiting is present without other symptoms. Physical exam is normal and notable for lack of abdominal tenderness, distension, or masses. While a positive βHCG is necessary for the diagnosis, other tests may be needed to exclude other entities. Complete blood count (CBC), liver function tests, thyroid stimulating hormone (TSH), and thyroxine levels may be helpful [6].

Treatment
Lifestyle modification is the initial treatment. A diet with salty liquids (such as sports drinks, soups/broth), starches, and proteins and avoidance of fatty foods is recommended [6]. If tolerated, diets can be advanced to starches such as pasta and crackers, then to proteins such as fish or chicken. Eating small, frequent meals is often helpful. If this approach fails, medications with or without nutritional support via a nasojejunal tube or TPN is utilized [6].

Drug Therapy. In the US, no drugs are specifically approved for the treatment of NVP. Commonly used drugs are Vitamin B_6 (pyridoxine) and antiemetics including metoclopramide, phenothiazine antiemetics (promethazine, prochlorperazine, chlorpromazine, and trimethobenzamide), and ondansetron. In Canada, Diclectin, which contains the antihistamine, doxylamine, with or without pyridoxine, is approved for NVP but is not available in the US because of a question of increased

Table 54.2 Drugs used for gastrointestinal disease in pregnancy.

Drug	Pregnancy use category	Dosing	Comments
Gastroesophageal reflux disease			
Antacids			Quickly treated symptoms in 30–50% of pregnant women with GERD [4]
Aluminum and magnesium hydroxide	B	10–30 mL as needed	Considered safe [1]
Sucralfate	B	1 g 1 h before meals and at bedtime	An aluminum salt containing polysaccharide complex that interferes with pepsin activity Cytoprotective [1] Safe and effective in a randomized control study in pregnancy [4]
Bismuth subsalicylate	C		Chronic bismuth tartrate in lambs caused poor outcomes In humans chronic salicylate use linked to congenital defects and premature closure of ductus arteriosus *in utero* [1]
H_2RA	B	Dosing according to retail brand	Excellent safety profile in humans [1,4] No congenital abnormalities in infants exposed to H2 blockers during the 1st trimester of pregnancy in surveillance study of 200 000 Medicaid recipients (cimetidine (460), ranitidine (516), famotidine (33)) [1]
Proton pump inhibitors	B/C	Dosing according to retail brand	Proven efficacy in GERD, esophagitis, and PUD [1,4] Considered safe in pregnancy Category B except for omeprazole which is Category C due to reports of fetal toxicity, not confirmed in additional studies All studies under-powered [25]
Nausea and vomiting of pregnancy			
Vitamin B_6	A	10–25 mg three times daily	Effective in two small studies [1]
Antihistamine			
Doxylamine	A	12.5 mg twice daily	Available in Canada not in US for concern of congenital malformations
Antiemetics			
Prochlorperazine	C	5–10 mg three times daily	Effective but safety in pregnancy not proven [1]
Promethazine	C	12.5–25.0 mg four times daily	Effective but safety in pregnancy not proven [1]
Metoclopramide	B	10–20 mg four times daily	Antiemetic of choice for NVP in Europe; frequently used in US [1]
Ondansetron	B	4–8 mg three times daily	Limited experience in NVP; seems safe [1]
Erythromycin	B		Two case reports: no large studies available [1] (excludes estolate salts which cause LFT abnormalities [25])
Corticosteroids	C	Low dose	Associated with marginal increase risk of major congenital abnormalities and cleft lip [1]
Constipation			
Polyethylene glycol (PEG)	C	17 g daily	Efficacy in a prospective study of 40 pregnant women [26]
Lactulose	B	15–30 mL up to four times daily	Can cause bloating, flatulence, cramping, and exacerbate nausea [3]

Table 54.2 continued

Drug	Pregnancy use category	Dosing	Comments
Senna	C	2 tablets daily Maximum 4 tablets twice daily	Safe and effective; can be used with bulk-forming laxatives
Bisacodyl	B	5–15 mg as needed	Use limited because of induced cramping
Mineral oil	C	15–45 mL daily per manufacturer directions	Aspiration can cause pneumonia; large amount can decrease maternal absorption of fat-soluble vitamins, neonatal hypoprothrombinemia, and hemorrhage [15]
Castor oil	C	15 mL once or twice daily or as directed by manufacturer	Not recommended; can induce uterine contractions
Diarrhea			
Loperamide	B	2–4 mg after each unformed stool	No safety data in human pregnancy; in animal fetuses no abnormalities when exposed to 30 times the maximal dose recommended in humans [15]
Diphenoxylate with atropine sulfate	C	1–2 tablets four times a day	Uncertain if slightly increased risk for birth defects [25]
Irritable bowel syndrome			
Antispasmodics			Not adequately assessed in pregnancy
Dicyclomine	B	10–20 mg four times daily	Possible increase in polydactyly Considered safe [19,25]
Hyoscyamine	C	0.125–0.250 mg every 6 h as needed	Possible increase in limb defects [25]
Tricyclic antidepressants	C	Dose differs according to retail brand	Reports of limb abnormalities in animals and humans Can cause neonatal withdrawal syndrome [19]
SSRI	C/D	Dose differs according to retail brand	Paroxetine class D, others C Some implicated in congenital defects, newer ones have not [19] Exposure can cause neonatal withdrawal syndrome, possible neurobehavioral abnormalities [19]
Inflammatory bowel disease			
5-aminosalicylic acid (5-ASA)	B/C	Dose differs according to retail brand	Sulfasalazine, mesalamine, balsalazide are category B and can be safely used rectally and orally Olsalazine (category C) Folate supplementation is recommended for sulfasalazine
Corticosteroids	C	Variable	Effective for induction but not maintenance
Budesonide	C	9 mg daily	Probably safe for ileocolonic Crohn disease but no controlled studies in pregnancy [1]
Immunomodulators			
6-mercaptopurine/ azathioprine	D	Up to 1.5 mg/ kg/2.5 mg/kg	Use justified for active disease refractory to other medications [1] Possibly minimal teratogenic effects in human fetuses [25]
Cyclosporine	C	Weight based intravenous/oral form	Growth retardation, but may be disease causality
Methotrexate	X		Not to be used in pregnancy
Thalidomide	X		Not to be used in pregnancy

Table 54.2 continued

Drug	Pregnancy use category	Dosing	Comments
Biologics			
Infliximab	B	5 mg/kg IV Induction at 0, 2, 4 weeks Maintenance every 8 to 10 weeks	Chimeric mouse/human IgG1 anti-TNF crosses placenta in late 2nd/early 3rd trimester [20,25] Likely low risk in pregnancy Consider discontinuation in early 3rd trimester to decrease exposure to fetus given limited long-term safety data on fetus [20]
Adalimumab	B	Induction: 160 mg SC week 0, 80 mg SC week 2 Maintenance: 40 mg SC every other week	Humanized IgG1 anti-TNF antibody Three case reports demonstrate safe use in pregnancy [20, 25] OTIS (Organization for Teratology Information Specialists) on-going prospective study reports of 13 outcomes, 12 resulted in healthy full-term infants without birth defects [25]
Certolizumab	B	Induction: 400 mg SC at 0, 2, 4 weeks Maintenance: 400 mg SC monthly	PEGylated Fab fragment of humanized anti-TNF monoclonal antibody Not known if crosses placenta in 1st trimester [20] More human data needed to understand effects on fetus
Natalizumab	C	300 mg IV every 4 weeks	Monoclonal antibody to α-4 integrin approved for patients failing anti-TNF therapy On-going pregnancy registry for MS patients Not widely recommended in pregnancy Consideration for its use in pregnancy should be case by case basis
Antibiotics			
Metronidazole	B	250–500 mg oral/intravenous 3 times daily	Contraindicated in 1st trimester if alternative Teratogenic risk low, exposure in 2nd and 3rd trimesters may be linked to cleft lip[20]
Fluoroquinolones	C	Doses according to retail brand	Quinolones associated with cartilage damage in dogs and rats but not in humans Thought to be safe but best avoided in light of safer alternatives [20]
Rifaximin	C		Little information available in pregnancy, questionable teratogenicity in animals [20]
Bisphosphonates	C		Alendronate crosses placenta and causes anatomic changes to fetus Best avoided in pregnancy [20]

GERD, gastroesophageal reflux disease; PUD, peptic ulcer disease; NVP, nausea and vomiting of pregnancy; SSRI, serotonin reuptake inhibitors; LFT, liver function test; MS, multiple sclerosis; H_2RA, histamine receptor agonist.

fetal congenital abnormalities which was not found in a meta-analysis after FDA withdrawal [1]. See Table 54.2 for a summary on NVP drugs used in pregnancy.

Hyperemesis Gravidarum (HG)

Hyperemesis gravidarum, characterized by intractable vomiting that may result in dehydration, weight loss, and electrolyte abnormalities, is most common in the first trimester but can persist beyond it. Risk factors include teenage pregnancy, obesity, multiparity, multiple gestations, and hydatiform mole [6,7]. Patients may present with dry mouth, sialorrhea, hyperolfaction, or a metallic taste in the mouth. Physical exam is notable for signs of dehydration including poor skin turgor, dry mucous membranes, and hypotension. Labs may demonstrate electrolyte abnormalities, abnormal liver function tests (LFTs), and ketonuria. Management is primarily supportive. In severe cases thiamine 100 mg IV should be given before administering any dextrose to avoid Wernickie encephalopathy. Initial management includes intravenous fluids, repletion of sodium and potassium if necessary, and monitoring of calcium levels. If tolerated, replenishment can be oral, beginning with salty liquids, electrolyte fluid preparations, or oral rehydration solutions [6]. Once better, the patient can advance the diet as described above. In refractory cases TPN may be necessary. Acupuncture plus acupressure may be an option, with one study finding it more efficacious compared to metoclopramide plus vitamin B_{12} [1]. Ginger is another option that may be beneficial [6]. In a 2-week double blind study corticosteroids were more effective in treatment of HG than promethazine [6]. Erythromycin is rarely used [1]. See Table 54.2 for a summary on HG drugs used in pregnancy.

Abdominal Pain

Abdominal pain in pregnancy poses a clinical challenge [8]. The natural history and presentation of common diseases may be altered, leading to difficulty in diagnosis. Early in pregnancy ectopic pregnancy and miscarriage are common etiologies, whereas in late pregnancy placental abruption and uterine rupture are of concern. Leiomyomas, urolithiasis, and pyelonephritis are possible culprits of non-gastrointestinal disease. Gastrointestinal causes of pain include gall-bladder disease, PUD, GERD, acute pancreatitis, liver disease, acute appendicitis, and intestinal obstruction. The latter two entities are important causes of abdominal pain that are difficult to diagnose in pregnancy [9]. By the second trimester the uterus displaces the appendix to the right upper quadrant, making a timely diagnosis and treatment of appendicitis difficult. In late pregnancy symptoms may present as vague and diffuse pain in the right upper quadrant with infrequent rebound tenderness and guarding. Symptoms may be absent if the gravid uterus prevents the appendix from touching the peritoneum. Maternal mortality is rare, but fetal demise remains high in cases of perforation [8]. Bowel obstruction most often occurs in the third trimester and postpartum but can occur when the uterus enters the abdomen in the fourth and fifth months. The incidence of intestinal obstruction is 1

in 2500–3500 pregnancies [9]. The most common cause of bowel obstruction is adhesions from prior abdominal surgery, including C-sections [10,11] followed by volvulus (25%) [9,10]. Volvulus can involve all regions of small and large intestine, (most commonly the sigmoid colon) [12]. Intussusception, malignancies, hernias, and diverticular disease can also cause bowel obstructions.

Small Intestine and Large Bowel

Constipation

The true incidence of constipation in pregnancy is unknown. It varies from 11% of 1000 women with decreased stool frequency in a retrospective study by Levy to 51% of pregnant women at the University of Iowa in a 2007 study using Rome II criteria (16–26% incidence in each trimester) [13,14]. A Dutch prospective study of pregnant women defining constipation to be "less than three bowel movements per week and straining with 25% of bowel movements", reported constipation in only 5–9% of 487 participants [13].

Pathophysiology
Several animal and human studies have implicated high levels of progesterone in the etiology of constipation [15]. Lower levels of motilin have also been implicated [15]. Colonic transit in pregnant women has not been adequately studied, but studies in menstruating women suggest that it is not a factor causing constipation during pregnancy.

Treatment
Education and reassurance are important in treatment. First-line therapy is dietary modification through increased fluid and fiber intake. Wheat bran is highly effective but often causes abdominal bloating or flatulence. Soluble fiber such as pectin, psyllium and oat bran causes fecal water retention, while non-soluble fiber such as cellulose enhances fecal bulk. Fiber, up to 25–40 g/day, in the form of psyllium, methylcellulose, guar, calcium polycarbophil, pectin, and flaxseed are safe and effective [1]. Docusates have questionable efficacy but are well tolerated with the exception of one associated case of neonatal hypomagnesemia [15]. The next line of therapy is hyperosmolar laxatives such as polyethylene glycol (PEG), and non-absorbable sugars such as lactulose, sorbitol, and glycerin. Lubricant laxatives such as mineral

oil may be used rectally or orally and are effective for softening fecal impactions. Laxatives such as senna and bisacodyl are thought to be safe and effective. Castor oil use is not recommended since it can induce uterine contractions [1]. See Table 54.2 for a summary on constipation drugs used in pregnancy.

Acute Diarrhea

Diarrhea is much less common than constipation in pregnancy and the differential diagnosis is similar to that in non-pregnant patients [15]. Most cases of acute diarrhea are caused by viral, bacterial, or parasitic pathogens. In the case of bacterial infection, the common culprits are *Campylobacter*, *Shigella*, *E. coli*, and *Salmonella* [15]. Stool cultures are useful for diagnosis. Non-infectious causes of diarrhea include food intolerances, ingestion of osmotic agents and chronic conditions such as irritable bowel syndrome (IBS) or inflammatory bowel disease (IBD). Severe symptoms, such as bloody stool, fever, and abdominal pain, should raise concern for bacterial infections that can be detrimental to the health of mother and fetus and should trigger an immediate work up. *Campylobacter* infection during pregnancy can cause intrauterine infection of the fetus, abortion, stillbirth, or early neonatal death. In the newborn it may cause neonatal sepsis or enteritis [16]. Similarly, *Salmonella* and *Shigella* have been associated with poor pregnancy outcomes [17,18]. When bacterial infection is suspected, stool cultures should be sent. *Clostridium difficile* should always be excluded. Depending on symptom severity, empiric antibiotics may be considered. In the absence of alarm symptoms, the treatment of uncomplicated diarrhea is supportive. Symptoms lasting longer than 7 days warrant further evaluation. Chronic diarrhea with a negative work up may require empiric drug therapy. Loperamide is a commonly used and efficacious agent. Diphenoxylate with atropine (Lomotil) is likely safe with a possibility of a slight increase in limb abnormalities. Bismuth subsalicylate should be avoided in pregnancy because animal studies revealed poor fetal outcome and chronic salicylate use in human fetuses results in congenital defects, including premature closure of the ductus arteriosus *in utero* and intrauterine growth retardation [15]. Bile sequestrants such as cholestyramine may be used with caution as they can cause malabsorption of fat-soluble vitamins if used in large quantities over a long period of time [1].

Irritable Bowel Syndrome

Irritable bowel syndrome (IBS) is a clinical diagnosis and is discussed in Chapter 60. The pathophysiology of IBS is multifactorial, involving a combination of abnormal gut motor and sensory function, central nervous system dysfunction, genetic predisposition, and enteric infections [19]. There have not been studies of IBS during pregnancy, but given that pregnancy-related hormones affect gut function and IBS worsens around the menstrual period it is likely that pregnancy affects the course of IBS, but has not been reported to cause its onset. Evaluation in pregnancy is similar to that of the non-gravid woman.

Treatment

The treatment of IBS is discussed in Chapter 60. Conventional treatments include laxatives for constipation-predominant IBS, antidiarrheal agents for diarrhea-predominant IBS, antispasmodics, tricyclic antidepressants (TCA), and serotonin reuptake inhibitors (SSRI)) for pain-predominant IBS. See Table 54.2 for a summary on IBS drugs used in pregnancy.

Inflammatory Bowel Disease

The peak incidence of inflammatory bowel disease (IBD) coincides with the child-bearing period. Therefore understanding the effect of IBD on and the course of IBD in pregnancy are of great importance to gastroenterologists and obstetricians alike. Patients with IBD are often concerned with genetic transmission of IBD to their offspring and whether the disease will affect their fertility. The lifetime risk of IBD in offspring of patients with IBD has been estimated to be 2 to 12 times higher than the general population [20]. First-degree relatives of Crohn disease patients are more likely to develop IBD compared to those of ulcerative colitis. Offspring of Jewish patients are more likely to develop the IBD than non-Jewish counterparts [20].

While some older studies involving Crohn disease patients [9] found decreased fertility rates, those studies failed to consider voluntary childlessness, treatment, or surgical history. Newer studies have not shown decreased fertility. Patients with ulcerative colitis also have normal fertility rates, the exception being individuals who have undergone an ileopouch–anal anastamosis (IPAA) [20]. These patients have decreased fecundability which is believed to be due to extensive dissection during the surgery that may lead to scarring. There is a modest decreased rate of fertility among these patients (69% infertility seen postoperatively vs. 46% preoperatively P = 0.005) [20]. Given the difficulties in conception, many suggest that women with UC should consider delaying IPAA surgery until they have had all their children.

Effect of Pregnancy on IBD

There is no conclusive evidence to suggest that pregnancy alters the course of IBD. Pregnant women with IBD are as likely to experience flares as their non-pregnant counterparts with some studies actually suggesting that disease activity may be lower in pregnancy [20]. The course of IBD activity in one pregnancy is not predictive of activity in subsequent pregnancies. The most important predictor of IBD course in pregnancy is the level of disease activity at the time of conception [21]. Two-thirds of patients with active Crohn disease at conception are likely to experience the same or worsening disease activity throughout the pregnancy [22]. Therefore it is strongly recommended that the disease be in remission before attempting a pregnancy.

Effect of IBD on Pregnancy

Many studies indicate that disease activity, prior surgery, and ileal Crohn disease are predictors of adverse outcome in pregnancy [20]. In 2007, a Kaiser Permanente population study did not find disease activity to be predictive of negative outcomes. One possible explanation for this is that the majority of patients in this study had inactive or mild disease during the study period [23]. Nevertheless, it does appear that having IBD, particularly the sequelae of active disease such as malnutrition, infection, and inflammation, is likely to impart risk on pregnancy. To maximize the chance of a normal pregnancy, it is recommended to keep the disease in control as much as possible.

Drugs Used in IBD

Treatment of IBD is guided by the principle that active disease rather than medical treatment poses a greater risk to the pregnancy. Given the lack of prospective studies in the pregnant population, the safety data of medications used to treat IBD are limited [1]. The benefits of medication use must be weighed carefully against potential risk. The patient should be well informed. Most IBD drugs are

considered safe in pregnancy. Two drugs, thalidomide and methotrexate, are Category X and should never be used [1]. See Table 54.2 for a summary of IBD drugs in pregnancy.

Celiac Disease

In the past decade there has been much progress in the understanding of the pathogenesis of celiac disease. With the widely available diagnostic lab test, tissue transglutaminase antibody, celiac disease has been found to be much more prevalent than previously thought. Available studies suggest that active celiac disease is associated with modest increase in adverse pregnancy outcomes including low birth weight, very low birth weight, preterm delivery, intrauterine growth retardation, and increased frequency of C-section births [24]. Many of these adverse outcomes are related to poor nutritional status. There is no evidence that pregnancy itself modifies disease activity nor is there evidence that the celiac disease activity in the mother affects lifetime risk of celiac disease in the offspring. Most studies show that for celiac patients treated with a gluten-free diet, pregnancy outcomes are no different than the general population. It is widely recommended deferring conception until the patient is in clinical remission.

Conclusions

Luminal gastrointestinal diseases account for significant morbidity in the pregnant patient. GERD, NVP, constipation, and IBS are common and are usually treated with a combination of lifestyle modification and medications. Medication use should be guided by the principle of "do no harm." Drug therapy of IBD has limited safety data in pregnancy. However, since active disease poses the greatest risk to the growing fetus medical therapy of the mother is often needed.

Take-home points

- Luminal gastrointestinal diseases account for significant morbidity in the pregnant patient.
- Luminal GI disease can develop *de novo* during pregnancy, be unique to pregnancy, or be an exacerbation of a pre-existing condition.

- Treatment should be guided by the principle "do no harm" taking into consideration potential risks to mother and fetus.
- FDA has assigned categories for drug safety in pregnancy.
- GERD is common in pregnancy while the incidence of PUD is decreased in pregnancy.
- Appendicitis may be difficult to diagnose late in pregnancy due to the displacement of the appendix by the gravid uterus and an atypical presentation.
- Diarrhea in pregnancy is less common than constipation and the differential is similar to that of non-pregnant patients.
- The most important predictor of the IBD course in pregnancy is the level of disease activity at the time of conception.
- Treatment of IBD is guided by the principle that active disease rather than medical treatment poses a greater risk to the pregnancy.

References

1 Thukral C, Wolf JL. Therapy insight: drugs for gastrointestinal disorders in pregnant women. *Nat Clin Pract Gastroenterol Hepatol* 2006; **3**: 256–66.

2 Rey E, Rodriguez-Artalejo F, Herraiz MA, *et al*. Gastroesophageal reflux symptoms during and after pregnancy: a longitudinal study. *Am J Gastroenterol* 2007; **102**: 2395–400.

3 Richter JE. Gastroesophageal reflux disease during pregnancy. *Gastroenterol Clin North Am* 2003; **32**: 235–61.

4 Richter JE. Review article: the management of heartburn in pregnancy. *Aliment Pharmacol Ther* 2005; **22**: 749–57.

5 Cappell MS. Gastric and duodenal ulcers during pregnancy. *Gastroenterol Clin North Am* 2003; **32**: 263–308.

6 Koch KL, Frissora CL. Nausea and vomiting during pregnancy. *Gastroenterol Clin North Am* 2003; **32**: 201–34, vi.

7 Koch KL. Gastrointestinal factors in nausea and vomiting of pregnancy. *Am J Obstet Gynecol* 2002; **186** (5 Suppl.): S198–203.

8 Cappell MS, Friedel D. Abdominal pain during pregnancy. *Gastroenterol Clin North Am* 2003; **32**: 1–58.

9 Wells R, Wolf J. Gastrointestinal disease in pregnancy. In: Brandt LJ, ed. *Clinical Practice of Gastroenterology*. Philadelphia: Churchill Livingstone, 1998: 1586–97.

10 Connolly MM, Unti JA, Nora PF. Bowel obstruction in pregnancy. *Surg Clin North Am* 1995; **75**: 101–13.

11 Perdue PW, Johnson HW, Jr, Stafford PW. Intestinal obstruction complicating pregnancy. *Am J Surg* 1992; **164**: 384–8.

12 Montes H, Wolf J. Cecal volvulus in pregnancy. *Am J Gastroenterol* 1999; **94**: 2554–6.

13 Bradley CS, Kennedy CM, Turcea AM, *et al*. Constipation in pregnancy: prevalence, symptoms, and risk factors. *Obstet Gynecol* 2007; **110**: 1351–7.

14 Levy N, Lemberg E, Sharf M. Bowel habit in pregnancy. *Digestion* 1971; **4**: 216–22.

15 Wald A. Constipation, diarrhea, and symptomatic hemorrhoids during pregnancy. *Gastroenterol Clin North Am* 2003; **32**: 309–22, vii.

16 Simor AE, Ferro S. Campylobacter jejuni infection occurring during pregnancy. *Eur J Clin Microbiol Infect Dis* 1990; **9**: 142–4.

17 Rebarber A, Star Hampton B, Lewis V, Bender S. Shigellosis complicating preterm premature rupture of membranes resulting in congenital infection and preterm delivery. *Obstet Gynecol* 2002; **100**: 1063–5.

18 Scialli AR, Rarick TL. Salmonella sepsis and second-trimester pregnancy loss. *Obstet Gynecol* 1992; **79**: 820–1.

19 Hasler WL. The irritable bowel syndrome during pregnancy. *Gastroenterol Clin North Am* 2003; **32**: 385–406, viii.

20 Dubinsky M, Abraham B, Mahadevan U. Management of the pregnant IBD patient. *Inflamm Bowel Dis* 2008; **14**: 1736–50.

21 Miller JP. Inflammatory bowel disease in pregnancy: a review. *J Roy Soc Med* 1986; **79**: 221–5.

22 Keller J, Frederking D, Layer P. The spectrum and treatment of gastrointestinal disorders during pregnancy. *Nat Clin Pract Gastroenterol Hepatol* 2008; **5**: 430–43.

23 Mahadevan U, Sandborn WJ, Li DK, *et al*. Pregnancy outcomes in women with inflammatory bowel disease: a large community-based study from Northern California. *Gastroenterology* 2007; **133**: 1106–12.

24 Leffler D, Kelly C. Celiac disease: What the last few years have taught us. In: Howden CW, ed. *Advances in Digestive Diseases*. AGA Institute Press, 2007: 49–58.

25 Briggs GG, Freeman RK, Yaffe SJ. *Drugs in Pregnancy and Lactation*, 8th edn. Philadelphia: Lippincott Williams and Wilkins, 2008.

26 Neri I, Blasi I, Castro P, *et al*. Polyethylene glycol electrolyte solution (Isocolan) for constipation during pregnancy: an observational open-label study. *J Midwifery Womens Health* 2004; **49**: 355–8.

CHAPTER 55

Consequences of Human Immunodeficiency Virus (HIV) Infection

Vera P. Luther and P. Samuel Pegram

Department of Internal Medicine, Wake Forest University School of Medicine, Winston-Salem, NC, USA

Summary

HIV-infected individuals can develop gastrointestinal (GI) disorders throughout the course of HIV infection. Recent studies have demonstrated that HIV infection involves the GI tract (including the colon and rectum) from early infection with depletion of gut-associated lymphoid tissue (GALT), throughout chronic infection (when GALT may not be fully restored even with adequate antiretroviral therapy), and into full-blown acquired immunodeficiency syndrome (AIDS). HIV itself can result in a unique enteropathy. The associated progressive immunodeficiency which occurs in untreated HIV-infected patients can allow fulminant reactivation of usually benign, latent infections (e.g., cytomegalovirus (CMV) colitis or chronic, severe perirectal herpes simplex type 2 (HSV-2) infection) or the transformation of a ubiquitous pathogen into a malignant, invasive agent (e.g., *Mycobacterium avium* complex). Many sexually-transmitted infections may be more severe and more varied in presentation in HIV-infected patients, and their therapy may be more complex. These patients are also at increased risk for certain malignancies of the colon (especially Kaposi sarcoma) and rectum (human papillovirus-associated intraepithelial neoplasia).

Case

A 26-year-old gay male was diagnosed with HIV infection 5 years ago. His CD4 nadir was 140 cells/mm³ 2 years after diagnosis, but he has been on antiretroviral therapy for 3 years with excellent adherence (last CD4 = 480 cells/mm³ and HIV RNA undetectable). In addition to HIV infection, he has a history of syphilis (adequately treated with appropriate rapid plasma reagin (RPR) response), gonorrhea on two occasions (oral and rectal), and past hepatitis A and B. His glycoprotein G herpes simplex-2 serology was negative. He is otherwise healthy. Despite multiple prevention interventions by physicians and social workers, he continues to episodically have unprotected, receptive oral and anal intercourse. He attends clinic complaining of painful, blood-tinged bowel movements for 5 days associated with a low-grade fever and malaise. He denies recent travel, foreign body exposure, animal contact, or similar prior symptoms. On general physical examination the only abnormalities were mild perianal ulcerations and several tender inguinal lymph nodes; on anoscopy, there were diffuse, painful, and shallow ulcerations with overlying bloody exudates throughout the visualized anorectal field. The following studies were ordered: darkfield examination, syphilis serology, gonococcal and chlamydial DNA probes, viral culture (primarily for herpes simplex viruses in light of his good immune status), repeat glycoprotein G herpes simplex serology, *Clostridium difficile* toxin assay, and routine stool culture. Within 24h his HSV-2 culture was positive; all other studies were negative including HSV-2 serology. The patient was treated with valacyclovir 1 g three times per day for 10 days then placed on 500 mg twice per day for prophylaxis of anogenital herpes. Follow-up serologies 8 weeks later demonstrated glycoprotein G HSV-2 seroconversion—thus, the patient had primary HSV-2 anoproctitis.

Practical Gastroenterology and Hepatology: Small and Large Intestine and Pancreas, 1st edition. Edited by Nicholas J. Talley, Sunanda V. Kane and Michael B. Wallace. © 2010 Blackwell Publishing Ltd.

Definition and Epidemiology

Patients with HIV infection can experience a wide array of colonic and rectal problems. Most problems are infectious in etiology, especially as the untreated patient becomes more and more CD4 T-cell lymphopenic. The gut-associated lymphoid tissue (GALT) is the largest lymphoid organ infected by HIV. Pathologic changes, both structural and immunological, occur in the gut from the very onset of HIV infection [1,2]. Within weeks of primary infection there is an acute depletion of CD4+ T lymphocytes in the gastrointestinal tract which then leads to a cascade of events, including microbial translocation, systemic immune activation, chronic HIV replication, and immune destruction, and finally advanced AIDS with its associated opportunistic infections and malignancies [3–6].

Pathogenesis

CD4 T lymphocytes in the GI tract are rapidly and radically depleted in acute human HIV infection [7,8]. The mechanism(s) by which this GALT depletion occurs is gradually being unraveled [1,9]. There appear to be both direct and indirect systems involved. HIV preferentially replicates in activated memory CD4 T cells (which represent a majority of CD4 lymphocytes in the gut), and up to 30 to 60% of CD4 T cells are infected within 2 weeks of infection of the host.

Early HIV infection and depletion of GALT result in a damaged mucosal barrier and loss of mucosal immunity. This can lead to HIV-induced enteropathy manifested as diarrhea, increased GI inflammation and permeability, and malabsorption (particularly of bile acids and vitamin B_{12}). This occurs in the absence of enteropathogens. Histologically, there is damage to the GI epithelial layer and inflammatory infiltrates of lymphocytes [10,11].

A second consequence of GALT depletion is microbial translocation [12]. Microbial translocation leads to increased levels of plasma lipopolysaccharide (LPS) in patients chronically infected with HIV compared with uninfected patients. LPS is a potent immunostimulatory factor which can add to the systemic immune activation accompanying chronic HIV infection. Over time there is a slow but continuous decrease in gut CD4 T cells, result-ing in a progressive decline in the production of these cells from the central memory pool [13,14].

The goal of combination antiretroviral therapy (cART) is to decrease the plasma HIV RNA to undetectable levels. This is typically followed by a gradual increase in plasma CD4 T lymphocytes. Although it has been demonstrated that rectal HIV is decreased with cART, the restoration of intestinal CD4 T cells in chronically HIV-infected patients is substantially delayed and incomplete [15,16]. There is some evidence that by initiating cART early in HIV infection near complete restoration of the mucosal immune system can be achieved.

Clinical Features

The consequences of HIV infection affecting the colon and rectum are variable depending on the causative etiology, the patient's degree of immunocompromise, and the portion of the GI system involved. In general, the diseases of the colon and rectum in HIV-infected patients can be categorized into those that cause enterocolitis and those that cause proctitis. These two processes have distinct clinical characteristics and distinct causative organisms.

The disease entities of enteritis, colitis, and enterocolitis are characterized by inflammation of the small intestine, colon, or both. Clinical manifestations include diarrhea, abdominal cramps, and bloating. Patients who engage in sexual practices involving direct or indirect oral–anal contact are at higher risk for developing these illnesses. Anorectal disease is seen most commonly in patients who engage in receptive anal intercourse. Perirectal abscesses, anal fistulae, perianal herpes simplex virus infections, aphthous ulcerations, and infectious proctitis may occur in these patients.

Enterocolitis

While some pathogens cause relatively distinct clinical manifestations, there is significant overlap in clinical features between the various causes of diarrhea. Therefore, when evaluating patients with HIV infection and enterocolitis, it is often useful to classify the illness into syndromes characterized by watery diarrhea and those that cause an inflammatory diarrhea. Important causes of watery diarrhea in HIV-infected patients include: rotavirus, norovirus, *Vibrio* spp., enterotoxigenic *Escherichia coli* (ETEC), enteroaggregative *E. coli* (EAEC), enteropathogenic *E. coli* (EPEC), *Giardia lamblia*, *Cryptosporidium parvum*, *Isospora belli*, *Cyclospora cayetanensis*, and microsporidia [17,18]. Of note, *Cryptosporidium* is the most common protozoa identified in HIV-infected patients [19]. The clinical syndrome is characterized by watery diarrhea and may be accompanied by nausea, vomiting, myalgias, arthralgias, abdominal pain, and chills. If a fever is present, it is generally mild. Leukocytes and blood are notably absent from the stool. Chronic diarrhea may ensue [20].

Important causes of inflammatory diarrhea (dysentery) in HIV-infected patients include: *Shigella* spp., *Salmonella* spp., *Yersinia* spp., *Campylobacter* spp., enteroinvasive *E. coli* (EIEC), enterohemorrhagic *E. coli* (EHEC), and *Entamoeba histolytica* [17,18]. This diarrheal syndrome is caused by invasive organisms and is characterized by fever and the presence of blood, mucus, and leukocytes in the stool. Vomiting, tenesmus, and abdominal cramping may also be present. The onset of fever and diarrhea are often acute. Bacteremia is common with *Shigella* spp., *Salmonella* spp., and *Campylobacter* spp. Infections due to these organisms in HIV-infected individuals may be recurrent and severe [21]. Toxic megacolon has been described in association with *Shigella* spp. *Salmonella* enterocolitis occurs more commonly in HIV-infected patients than in the general population, and a diagnosis of *Salmonella* bacteremia in an HIV-infected individual meets the Centers for Disease Control (CDC) definition of AIDS [21,22]. Infections due to *Salmonella* spp. may present with fever alone and no localizing symptoms [21].

Cytomegalovirus (CMV) is an important cause of diarrhea in severely immunocompromised HIV-infected individuals and the clinical manifestations of colonic infection due to CMV are widely variable. Patients may be asymptomatic or experience any combination of crampy abdominal pain, diarrhea, hematochezia, urgency, tenesmus, weight loss, or fevers [23,24]. CMV is the most common viral cause of diarrhea and chronic diarrhea in AIDS patients with multiple negative stool studies [25]. Simultaneous involvement of the esophagus, stomach, or small bowel may be present as well. Bleeding or perforation may result from diffuse, ulcerating involvement of the intestine. Appendicitis due to CMV has been described [23]. Of note, concomitant CMV retinitis may be present, and all patients should undergo ophthalmologic evaluation at the time of diagnosis. CMV reactivation occurs only with advanced HIV infection (CD4 <50 cells/mm^3) [26,27].

HIV-infected individuals who develop *Clostridium difficile*-associated diarrhea (CDAD) are prone to experience more severe clinical symptoms, relapse, or chronic disease. Toxic megacolon can occur as a complication [28].

Mycobacterium avium-intracellulare complex (MAC) is the most commonly identified organism in patients with chronic diarrhea and advanced AIDS (CD4 lymphocyte counts <50 cells/mm^3) [29]. Infections may be asymptomatic, or they may be characterized by a combination of fever, night sweats, abdominal pain, malabsorption, severe weight loss, mycobacteremia, lymphadenopathy, and anemia. Involvement of the duodenum is most common and yellow mucosal nodules may be visualized on esophagogastroduodenoscopy (EGD) [29,30].

In contrast to MAC, intestinal infection due to *Mycobacterium tuberculosis* is quite rare but is always symptomatic. Involvement of the colon or ileocecal region is most common. Fistulae, intussusceptions, perforation, peritoneal, and rectal involvement have been reported [31].

While intestinal infections due to fungi are very rare, histoplasmosis is the most commonly reported fungal infection of the gastrointestinal tract in HIV-infected patients with the most highly endemic region being the Ohio and Mississippi river valleys. *Histoplasma capsulatum* usually affects the colon and is often associated with concomitant pulmonary and hepatic involvement. In addition to diarrhea and fever, patients may present with large ulcerations, mass lesions, or peritonitis [32].

The helminths *Ancylostoma duodenale* and *Strongyloides stercoralis* are very uncommon causes of diarrhea in HIV-infected patients. Clinical manifestations include abdominal pain, diarrhea, and eosinophilia [33].

Proctitis

Proctitis refers to inflammation of the rectum. Clinical manifestations include pruritis, anorectal pain, rectal bleeding, mucopurulent anal discharge, and painful defecation. Patients with severe symptoms may also experience tenesmus or constipation. Some pathogens can cause inflammation throughout segments of the colon as well (proctocolitis). These patients may experience diarrhea and abdominal cramping in addition to symptoms of proctitis.

Neisseria gonorrhoeae is the most commonly identified cause of proctitis (approximately 30%), followed by *Chlamydia trachomatis*—genital immunotypes D or K (19%). Rectal infections due to *Neisseria gonorrhoeae* are most often asymptomatic (as often as 85% of the time, according to a recent study) [34]. When symptoms occur, mild anorectal pain, mucopurulent or bloody discharge may develop 5–7 days after exposure. Rectal infections due to *Chlamydia trachomatis* are most often asymptomatic as well, but when symptoms occur, they are typically milder. Friable mucosa and mucopurulent discharge are typically seen on anoscopy, even in asymptomatic patients. In contrast to the asymptomatic or mild disease caused by immunotypes D or K, lymphogranuloma venereum (LGV) strains of *Chlamydia trachomatis* (L1, L2, or L3) often cause severe symptoms characterized by severe anorectal pain, bloody or mucopurulent discharge, ulceration, and tenesmus. A recent re-emergence of an LGV variant (L2b) has been diagnosed (and requires special specimen handling through state health departments and the CDC) in mostly HIV-infected, gay men. A characteristic presentation is a rectal ulcer with a bloody or mucoid/purulent anorectal discharge [35].

In the primary stages of syphilis, rectal infection due to *Treponema pallidum* is often asymptomatic as the initial chancre is usually painless. However, patients may experience classic symptoms of proctitis. Also, symptoms of secondary syphilis may manifest as condylomata lata lesions, which are smooth, moist-appearing, wart-like lesions and are highly contagious [36].

Perianal disease due to herpes simplex virus (HSV) infection is most often characterized by local vesicles, pustules, or ulcerations; however, involvement of the distal rectum can occur. In addition to symptoms of proctitis, inguinal lymphadenopathy may be present. Sacral nerve dysesthesias, paresthesias, urinary retention, temporary erectile dysfunction, as well as systemic symptoms such as fever, chills, malaise, headache, and meningismus have been associated with primary HSV (usually HSV-2) infection. Recurrent infections tend to be milder, and this is especially the case with HSV-1 anogenital infection [37].

Diagnosis

In patients with advanced HIV infection or AIDS, sys-temic disease may accompany a gastrointestinal illness. This is more common with *Salmonella* spp., *Shigella* spp., *Campylobacter* spp., CMV, and MAC. In this case, identification of a pathogen outside of the gut (i.e., via appropriate blood cultures) may suggest a diagnosis in conjunction with or in lieu of a directed GI evaluation.

Initial Evaluation for Diarrhea in an HIV-infected Patient. Obtain stool specimens for bacterial culture, Clostridium difficile toxin assay, ova and parasite examination, fecal leukocyte examination, and acid-fast stain.
- If diarrhea is chronic, severe or proctitis is present:
  ○ Perform flexible proctosigmoidoscopy or colonoscopy with mucosal biopsy for pathology plus virologic and parisitologic evaluation
  ○ Culture rectal tissue for bacteria and viruses in addition to above.
- If diarrhea and weight loss persists and above evaluation is negative:
  ○ EGD with small bowel biopsy

Initial Evaluation for Proctitis. Perform a careful physical examination of the skin, mucous membranes, and lymph nodes in the anogenital region. This examination should include a visual inspection of the anus for fissures, ulcerations, masses and foreign bodies, followed by digital rectal examination. Anoscopy and sigmoidoscopy with mucosal biopsy should follow if the initial examination does not yield a diagnosis. Anoscopy will often reveal rectal exudate and friability of mucus membranes. Biopsies should be evaluated for neoplasm and infection. Bacterial (including gonococcal and chlamydial), viral, and fungal cultures should be obtained as well (Table 55.1).

Gonococcal and chlamydial nucleic acid amplification testing (NAATs) may be performed on urine, rectal, and pharyngeal specimens; however, they are not currently cleared by the Food and Drug Administration (FDA) for use on rectal and pharyngeal specimens [38].

Differential Diagnosis

While most GI consequences of HIV are infectious in etiology, the availability of combination antiretroviral therapy (cART) has decreased the occurrence of GI complications. Therefore, it is important to consider drug-induced or non-infectious etiologies in the differential

Table 55.1 Diagnostic tools for specific pathogens.

Pathogen	Diagnostic tools
CMV	Viral cytopathic effect (CPE) in tissue specimens, immunostaining, *in situ* hybridization Cultures (less sensitive and specific than histopathology)
Enteric bacteria	Stool cultures, blood cultures (*Salmonella* spp., *Shigella* spp., *Campylobacter* spp.)
Clostridium difficile	Toxin assay on stool
Mycobacterium avium-intracellulare complex	Culture of mucosal biopsy specimens, acid-fast staining of biopsy specimens Acid-fast blood cultures may be positive
Histoplasmosis	Fungal smear, culture of mucosal biopsies or blood Urine or serum *Histoplasmosis* antigen assay
Cryptosporidium	Acid-fast stain of stool, small bowel or rectal biopsies; or enzyme immunoassay (EIA) of stool samples
Isospora	Acid-fast stain of stool or mucosal biopsies
Microsporidia	Gram stain or modified trichrome stain of stool or mucosal biopsies, electron microscopy
Giardia lamblia	Ova and parasite examination or stool samples or mucosal biopsies Enzyme immunoassay (EIA) of stool samples can also be used
Entamoeba histolytica	Morphologically similar to non-pathogenic *Entamoeba dispar* Enzyme-linked immunoassay (ELISA) or PCR tests are required on stool samples to distinguish the species
Neisseria gonorrhoeae	NAATs, Gram stain, culture (see comment in section Proctitis)
Chlamydia trachomatis	NAATs, Gram stain, culture (see comment in section Proctitis)
Treponema pallidum	Darkfield microscopy (rarely used in clinical practice) Physical examination and serologic tests Rapid Plasma Reagin (RPR), Venereal Disease Research Laboratories (VDRL) or toluidine red unheated serum test (TRUST) are screening tests *Treponema Pallidum* Particle Agglutination (TP-PA) assay and Fluorescent Treponemal Antibody Absorption (FTA-ABS) test are confirmatory studies
Herpes simplex virus	Viral culture, PCR testing of swabs from lesions confirm the diagnosis Serology can assist in making the diagnosis as well

NAATs, nucleic acid amplification testing.

diagnosis as well [39]. It is also important to note that in patients with advanced HIV infection or AIDS, multiple infections may be present simultaneously [40] (Table 55.2).

Therapeutics

Therapeutic management for all causes of diarrhea should include appropriate fluid and electrolyte replacement. Symptomatic therapy with antidiarrheal agents such as bismuth subsalicylate and loperamide may be used to decrease the number of stools passed per day. However, caution should be observed with the use of antimotility drugs in the treatment of invasive forms of diarrhea as the development of toxic megacolon may occur [42]. Appropriate antimicrobial therapy is generally pathogen-specific. However, if empiric therapy is necessary, ciprofloxacin 500 mg orally twice daily for 3–5 days is appropriate for adults with febrile dysenteric diarrhea. For the empiric therapy of persistent diarrhea (>14 days' duration), metronidazole 250 mg orally three times daily for 7 days may be administered to adults. For opportunistic infections due to CMV, MAC, *Cryptosporidium* and microsporidia, cART should be included in the treatment regimen [43]. Appropriate immune reconstitution is often necessary for the cure of disease caused by these pathogens.

Table 55.2 Causes of enterocolitis and proctitis in HIV-infected individuals.

	Enterocolitis	Proctitis
Viruses	Rotavirus, norovirus, adenovirus, herpes simplex virus, cytomegalovirus*, astrovirus, calcivirus, picobirnavirus, HIV	Herpes simplex virus, condyloma acuminatum (human papillomavirus infection), cytomegalovirus*
Bacteria	*Salmonella* spp., *Shigella* spp., enteroadherent *E. coli* (EAEC), enterotoxigenic *E. coli* (ETEC), enteropathogenic *E. coli* (EPEC), enteroinvasive *E. coli* (EIEC), enterohemorrhagic *E. coli* (EHEC), *Campylobacter* spp., *Yersinia* spp., *Vibrio* spp., *Clostridium difficile*, *Mycobacterium tuberculosis†*, small bowel bacterial overgrowth†, *Aeromonas hydrophila†*, *Mycobacterium avium complex**	*Neisseria gonorrhoeae, Chlamydia trachomatis, Chlamydia trachomatis* (lymphogranuloma venereum or LGV), *Treponema pallidum, Shigella flexneri†, Mycobacterium tuberculosis†*
Fungi	*Histoplasma capsulatum†, Cryptococcus neoformans*†, Coccidioides immitis†, Penicillium marneffei†*	*Histoplasma capsulatum†*
Protozoa	*Cryptosporidium parvum*, Isospora belli*, Cyclospora cayetanensis*, microsporidia** (*Enterocytozoon bienusi, Encephalitozoon intestinalis*), *Giardia lamblia, Entamoeba histolytica, Toxoplasma gondii†, Pneumocystis jiroveci†, Leishmania donovani†*	*Entamoeba histolytica, Leishmania donovani†*
Non-infectious considerations	Neoplasms: lymphoma, Kaposi sarcoma Idiopathic: "AIDS enteropathy" Drug-induced: protease inhibitors Pancreatic disease Inflammatory bowel disease	Neoplasms: lymphoma, Kaposi sarcoma, squamous cell carcinoma‡ Perirectal fistulae Aphthous ulcerations Foreign bodies

*More likely to occur in patients with CD4 lymphocyte count <100 cells/mm^3.
†Uncommon pathogens.
‡Squamous cell carcinoma of the anus and rectum is more common in men who have sex with men than in any other demographic group of HIV-infected individuals. These carcinomas are the result of HPV infection, particularly with types 16 and 18. Cytologic examinations of the anal canal, comparable to Papanicolaou smears, have been recommended [41].

For the empiric treatment of proctitis, ceftriaxone 125 mg IM once, plus doxycycline 100 mg orally twice daily for 7 days may be used. Fluoroquinolones should not be used in the treatment of gonococcal disease or suspected gonococcal disease due to the high rate of fluoroquinolone resistance [44] (Figure 55.1).

Prognosis

The prognoses of colonic and rectal complications of HIV infection are somewhat variable since they are disease specific and dependent on the patient's degree of immunocompromise. In general, HIV-infected individuals with good immune system preservation or reconstitu-

tion (due to cART) are likely to have favorable outcomes after appropriate therapy has been administered. However, patients with prolonged immunodeficiency states are likely to experience more severe disease, persistent disease, recurrences, and treatment failures.

Take-home points

- Patients with HIV infection frequently have infectious and non-infectious colonic and rectal problems.

- The first immunologic casualty of primary HIV infection is the gut-associated lymphoid tissue (GALT); this depletion occurs within the first several weeks of infection and remains throughout HIV infection (restoration may not be complete even with appropriate combination antiretroviral therapy).

- HIV itself can cause a unique enteropathy.
- With advancing CD4 lymphopenia in the untreated HIV-infected patient, latent organisms may reactivate to cause severe disease:
  - HSV-2 anorectal infection
  - CMV colitis.
- Common organisms may become invasive with advanced CD4 lymphopenia:
  - MAC infection with pan-intestinal involvement and associated mycobacteremia
  - HSV-2 primary anorectal infection
  - Cryptosporidiosis, etc.

- Genital pathogens may present atypically and be more difficult to diagnose and treat:
  - Primary (intra-anorectal chancre) and secondary (perianal condylomata lata) syphilis may be present simultaneously, and syphilis serology may be confusing with advanced HIV infection.
  - *Chlamydia trachomatis* LGV variant (L2b) can cause rectal ulcers, rectal bleeding, and mucoid/purulent anorectal discharge; diagnosis requires special specimen handling.
- HIV-associated malignancies may affect the colon and rectum:
  - Kaposi sarcoma of colon and rectum
  - HPV-associated intraepithelial neoplasia (squamous cell carcinoma) of the anorectum.

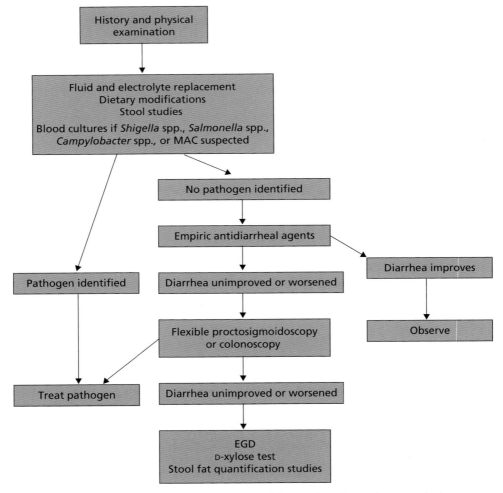

Figure 55.1 Management algorithm. MAC, *Mycobacterium avium-intracellulare* complex; EGD, esophagogastroduodenoscopy.

References

1 Johnson RP. How HIV guts the immune system. *N Engl J Med* 2008; **358**: 2287–9.

2 Dandekar S. Pathogenesis of HIV in the gastrointestinal tract. *Curr HIV/AIDS Rep* 2007; **4**: 10–15.

3 Chen TW, Nickle DC, Justement JS, *et al.* Persistence of HIV in gut-associated lymphoid tissue despite long-term antiretroviral therapy. *J Infect Dis* 2008; **197**: 640–2.

4 Guadalupe M, Reay E, Sandaran, *et al.* Severe CD4 depletion in gut lymphoid tissue during primary human immunodeficiency virus type 1 infection and substantial delay in restoration following highly active antiretroviral therapy. *J Virol* 2003; **77**: 11708–17.

5 Centlivre M, Sala M, Wain-Hobson S, Berkhout B. In HIV-1 pathogenesis the die is cast during primary infection. *AIDS* 2007; **21**: 1227–8.

6 van Marie G, Gill MJ, Kolodka D, *et al.* Compartmentization of the gut viral reservoir in HIV-1 infected patients. *Retrovirology* 2007; **4**: 87–92.

7 Mattapalil JJ, Douek DC, Hill B, *et al.* Massive infection and loss of memory CD4+ T cells in multiple tissues during acute SIV infection. *Nature* 2005; **434**: 1093–7.

8 Okoye A, Meyer-Schellersheim M, Brenchley JM, *et al.* Progressive CD4+ central memory T cell decline results in CD4+ effector memory insufficiency and overt disease in chronic SIV infection. *J Exp Med* 2007; **204**: 2171–85.

9 Read SW, Sereti I. HIV infection and the gut: scarred for life? *J Infect Dis* 2008; **198**: 453–5.

10 Kotler DP, Gaetz HP, Lange M, *et al.* Enteropathy associated with the acquired immunodeficiency syndrome. *Ann Intern Med* 1984; **101**: 421–8.

11 Douek DC, Picker LJ, Koup RA. T cell dynamics in HIV-1 infection. *Annu Rev Immunol* 2003; **21**: 265–304.

12 Brenchley JM, Price DA, Schacker TW, *et al.* Microbial translocation is a cause of systemic immune activation in chronic HIV infection. *Nat Med* 2006; **12**: 1365–71.

13 Giorgi JV, Lyles RH, Matud JL, *et al.* Predictive value of immunologic and virologic markers after long or short duration of HIV-1 infection. *J Acq Immun Def Synd* 2002; **29**: 346–55.

14 Brenchley JM, Schacker TW, Ruff LE, *et al.* CD4+ T cell depletion during all stages of HIV disease occurs predominantly in the gastrointestinal tract. *J Exp Med* 2004; **200**: 749–59.

15 Mehandru S, Poles MS, Tenner-Racz K, *et al.* Lack of mucosal immune reconstitution during prolonged treatment of acute and early HIV infection. *PLoS Med* 2006; **3**: e484.

16 Schacker TW, Reilly C, Bellman GJ, *et al.* Amount of lymphatic tissue fibrosis in HIV infection predicts magnitude of HAART-associated change in peripheral CD4 cell count. *AIDS* 2005; **19**: 2169–71.

17 Thom K, Forrest G. Gastrointestinal infections in immunocompromised hosts. *Curr Opin Gastroenterol* 2006; **22**: 18–23.

18 Wilcox CM, Saag MS. Gastrointestinal complications of HIV infection: changing priorities in the HAART era. *Gut* 2008; **57**: 861–70.

19 Weber R, Ledergerber B, Zbinden R, *et al.* Enteric infections and diarrhea in human immunodeficiency virus-infected persons: Prospective community-based cohort study. *Arch Intern Med* 1999; **159**: 1473.

20 Manabe YC, Clark DP, Moore RD, *et al.* Cryptosporidiosis in patients with AIDS: Correlates of disease and survival. *Clin Infect Dis* 1998; **27**: 536.

21 Angulo FJ, Swerdlow DL. Bacterial enteric infections in persons infected with human immunodeficiency virus. *Clin Infect Dis* 1995; **21** (Suppl. 1): S84–93.

22 Centers for Disease Control and Prevention (CDC). Revision of the CDC surveillance case definition for acquired immunodeficiency syndrome. *MMWR* 1987; **36**: 1–15S

23 Wilcox CM, Chalasani N, Lazenby A, *et al.* Cytomegalovirus colitis in AIDS: An endoscopic and clinical study. *Gastrointest Endosc* 1998; **48**: 58.

24 Monkemuller KE, Bussian AH, Lazenby AJ, *et al.* Special histologic stains are rarely beneficial for the evaluation of HIV-related gastrointestinal infections. *Am J Clin Pathol* 2000; **114**: 387.

25 Wilcox CM. Etiology and evaluation of diarrhea in AIDS: A global perspective at the millennium. *World J Gastroenterol* 2000; **6**: 177.

26 Chevret S, Scieux C, Garrait V, *et al.* Usefulness of the cytomegalovirus (CMV) antigenemia assay for predicting the occurrence of CMV disease and death in patients with AIDS. *Clin Infect Dis* 1999; **28**: 758.

27 Kirk O, Reiss P, Uberti-Foppa C, *et al.* Safe interruption of maintenance therapy against previous infection with four common HIV-associated opportunistic pathogens during potent antiretroviral therapy. *Ann Intern Med* 2002; **20**: 137–9

28 Tumbarello M, Tacconelli E, Leone F, *et al.* Clostridium difficile-associated diarrhoea in patients with human immunodeficiency virus infection: a case-control study. *Eur J Gastroenterol Hepatol* 1995; **7**: 259–63.

29 Liesenfeld O, Schneider T, Schmidt W, *et al.* Culture of intestinal biopsy specimens and stool culture for detection of bacterial enteropathogens in patients infected with human immunodeficiency virus. *J Clin Microbiol* 1995; **33**: 745.

30 Horsburgh Jr CR, Gettings J, Alexander LN, *et al.* Disseminated Mycobacterium avium complex disease among

patients infected with human immunodeficiency virus, 1986–2000. *Clin Infect Dis* 2001; **33**: 1938.

31 Van Altena R, Van Beckevoort D, Kersemans P, *et al.* Imaging of gastrointestinal and abdominal tuberculosis. *Eur Radiol* 2004; **14**: E103.

32 Lamps LW, Molina CP, West AB, *et al.* The pathologic spectrum of gastrointestinal and hepatic histoplasmosis. *Am J Clin Pathol* 2000; **113**: 64.

33 Cimerman S, Cimerman B, Lewi DS. Prevalence of intestinal parasitic infections in patients with acquired immunodeficiency syndrome in Brazil. *Int J Infect Dis* 1999; **3**: 203.

34 Kent CK, Chaw JK, Wong W, *et al.* Prevalence of rectal, urethral, and pharyngeal chlamydia and gonorrhea detected in 2 clinical settings among men who have sex with men: San Francisco, California, 2003. *Clin Infect Dis* 2005; **41**: 67–74.

35 Centers for Disease Control and Prevention (CDC). Lymphogranuloma venereum among men who have sex with men—Netherlands, 2003–2004. *MMWR* 2004; **53**: 985–88.

36 Mindel A, Tovey SJ, Timmins DJ, Williams P. Primary and secondary syphilis, 20 years' experience. 2. Clinical features. *Genitourin Med* 1989; **65**: 1–3.

37 Goodell SE, Quinn TC, Mkrtichian E, *et al.* Herpes simplex virus proctitis in homosexual men. Clinical, sigmoidoscopic, and histopathological features. *N Engl J Med* 1983; **308**: 868–71.

38 Young H, Manavi K, McMillan A. Evaluation of ligase chain reaction for the non-cultural detection of rectal and pharyngeal gonorrhoea in men who have sex with men. *Sex Transm Infect* 2003; **79**: 484–6.

39 Call SA, Heudebert G, Saag M, *et al.* The changing etiology of chronic diarrhea in HIV-infected patients with CD4 cell counts less than 200 cells/mm3. *Am J Gastroenterol* 2000; **95**: 3142.

40 Quinn TC, Stamm WE, Goodell SE, *et al.* The polymicrobial origin of intestinal infections in homosexual men. *N Engl J Med* 1983; **309**: 576–82.

41 Panther LA, Wagner K, Proper JA, *et al.* High resolution anoscopy findings for men who have sex with men: Inaccuracy of anal cytology as a predictor of histologic high-grade anal intraepithelial neoplasia and the impact of HIV serostatus. *Clin Infect Dis* 2004; **38**: 1490.

42 King CK, Glass R, Bresee JS, Duggan C; Centers for Disease Control and Prevention. Managing acute gastroenteritis among children: oral rehydration, maintenance, and nutritional therapy. *MMWR* 2003; **52** (RR-16): 1–16.

43 Gilbert DN, Moellering RC, Eliopoulos GM, Sande MA. *The Sanford Guide to Antimicrobial Therapy*, 38th edn. Antimicrobial Therapy, Inc, USA, 2008: 15–17, 123.

44 Centers for Disease Control and Prevention (CDC). Increase in fluoroquinolone-resistant Neisseria gonorrhoeae among men who have sex with men—United States, 2003, and revised recommendations for gonorrhea treatment, 2004. *MMWR* 2004; **53**: 335–8.

PART 7

Diseases of the Pancreas

CHAPTER 56

Acute Pancreatitis and Peripancreatic Fluid Collections

Peter A. Banks[1] and Koenraad J. Mortele[2]

[1] Division of Gastroenterology, Center for Pancreatic Disease, Harvard Medical School, Brigham and Women's Hospital, Boston, MA, USA
[2] Division of Abdominal Imaging and Intervention, Department of Radiology, Brigham and Women's Hospital, Boston, MA, USA

Summary

Ninety percent of patients with acute pancreatitis have interstitial disease and 10% have necrotizing disease. Contrast-enhanced computed tomography (CT) scan provides valuable information regarding the severity of the disease and complications, including peripancreatic fluid collections. Assessment of disease severity at admission and within the first 24 h is of critical importance in providing optimal care. Fluid resuscitation and careful pulmonary care are also of critical importance. The two most important markers of severity during hospitalization are persistent organ failure and pancreatic necrosis. Therapy of sterile pancreatic necrosis is medical during the first several weeks; at a later stage, when pancreatic necrosis becomes walled-off, symptoms such as fever or persistent abdominal pain are treated by either surgical or endoscopic debridement. Therapy of infected pancreatic necrosis, which can reliably be diagnosed by image-guided percutaneous aspiration, is debridement (usually surgical or endoscopic, occasionally percutaneous).

Case

A 44-year-old woman presented with severe epigastric pain requiring administration of narcotic agents. Abdominal ultrasound revealed multiple small gall stones. The common bile duct was not dilated. Serum amylase and lipase values were five times the upper limit of normal. Contrast-enhanced computed tomography (CT) scan showed an enlarged pancreas with heterogeneous enhancement and considerable fluid around the pancreas (Figure 56.1a). She was started on fluid replacement at a rate of 200 mL/h. Twenty-four hours after admission, her hematocrit was noted to be increased from 48 to 50 and blood urea and nitrogen (BUN) from 17 mg/% to 24 mg/%. Because of labored respiration and deterioration of oxygenation, she was transferred to an intensive care unit, intubated with assisted ventilation, and eventually needed dialysis for acute renal failure. She was also treated prophylactically with imipenem and received total parenteral nutrition. A CT scan

obtained weekly showed evolution from necrotizing pancreatitis to walled-off pancreatic and peripancreatic necrosis involving 85% of the pancreas (Figure 56.1b). She gradually improved, was extubated, and her renal function returned to normal. However, during the next several weeks, she developed abdominal pain each time she tried to consume a low fat diet such that her caloric intake remained unsatisfactory.

Introduction

Acute pancreatitis is an acute inflammatory condition of the pancreas [1]. At one end of the spectrum is interstitial pancreatitis with mild edema of the pancreas associated at times with inflammation of the fat in the peripancreatic area and the development of fluid collections around the pancreas. At the other end is a more severe form of the disease characterized by necrosis of the parenchyma, at times associated with considerable fat necrosis around

Practical Gastroenterology and Hepatology: Small and Large Intestine and Pancreas, 1st edition. Edited by Nicholas J. Talley, Sunanda V. Kane and Michael B. Wallace. © 2010 Blackwell Publishing Ltd.

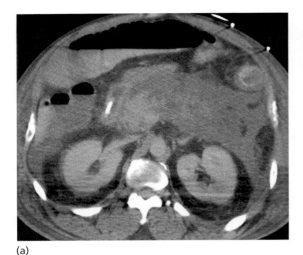

(a)

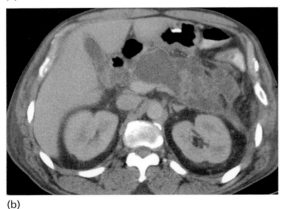

(b)

Figure 56.1 (a) Axial contrast-enhanced CT image obtained in a 44-year-old female shows subtotal necrosis of the pancreatic gland with acute fluid collections in the anterior pararenal space. (b) Axial contrast-enhanced CT image obtained 4 weeks later shows walled-off pancreatic and extrapancreatic necrosis.

the pancreas. The use of contrast-enhanced CT scan is of great help in distinguishing interstitial from necrotizing pancreatitis [2].

Definitions

Interstitial Pancreatitis

Interstitial pancreatitis is characterized by focal or diffuse enlargement of the pancreas. The parenchyma of the pancreas enhances in a homogeneous fashion when

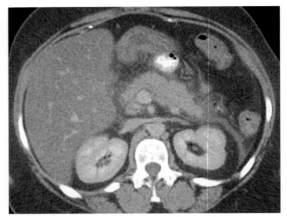

Figure 56.2 Interstitial pancreatitis. Axial contrast-enhanced CT image obtained in a 39-year-old female shows mild swelling of the pancreatic gland but normal enhancement. Note acute fluid collections in the anterior pararenal space.

imaged by contrast-enhanced CT scan or magnetic resonance imaging (MRI) (Figure 56.2).

Pancreatic Necrosis

Pancreatic necrosis is defined by the presence of diffuse or focal areas of non-viable pancreatic parenchyma with at least 30% of non-enhancement of the pancreas when imaged by contrast-enhanced CT scan or MRI. Pancreatic necrosis is usually associated with at least some peripancreatic fat necrosis (Figure 56.3) [3].

Extrapancreatic Fluid Collections

Extrapancreatic fluid collections form when pancreatic fluid extravasates out of the pancreas into the anterior pararenal space and at times elsewhere during acute pancreatitis. Extrapancreatic fluid collections may occur in either interstitial or necrotizing pancreatitis. In most instances, extrapancreatic fluid collections resolve as pancreatic inflammation resolves. In some instances, the fluid collection persists. There appear to be two possible outcomes when the fluid collection persists. In one outcome, when there is little in the way of peripancreatic fat necrosis, the fluid collection becomes a somewhat oval or rounded fluid-filled structure enclosed by a fibrous capsule, termed a pancreatic pseudocyst. In the other, when the fluid becomes associated with substantial peripancreatic fat necrosis, the collection may persist

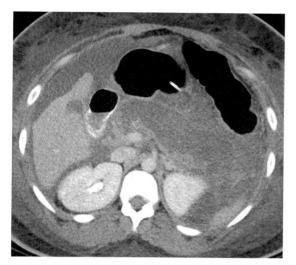

Figure 56.3 Necrotizing pancreatitis. Axial contrast-enhanced CT image obtained in a 38-year-old female shows necrosis of the pancreatic gland with acute fluid collections in the anterior pararenal space.

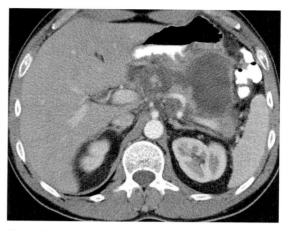

Figure 56.4 Extrapancreatic fluid collection. Axial contrast-enhanced CT image obtained in a 49-year-old male with necrotizing pancreatitis shows pancreatic necrosis and presence of extrapancreatic walled-off necrosis.

indefinitely, or may evolve into a structure enclosed by a fibrous capsule overlying the pancreas, termed peripancreatic walled-off necrosis. The CT appearance of extrapancreatic fluid collection is that of homogeneous low-density fluid, whereas peripancreatic fat necrosis is a more heterogeneous collection frequently containing globules of fat (Figure 56.4) [4–6].

Pancreatic Pseudocyst

A pancreatic pseudocyst is a collection of pancreatic juice enclosed by a wall of fibrous or granulation tissue. It occurs in association with acute pancreatitis, pancreatic trauma, or chronic pancreatitis. It requires at least 4 weeks from the onset of acute pancreatitis to form a well-defined wall. Pseudocysts may gradually enlarge, stay approximately the same size, diminish, or even resolve completely. While most pseudocysts occur as a result of loculation of an extrapancreatic fluid collection, some occur as a result of pancreatic ductal disruption leading to a localized collection of enzymes rich pancreatic fluid that loculates close to the pancreas and at times at remote sites. The appearance of a pancreatic pseudocyst on CT scan is that of an encapsulated, homogenous, non-enhancing low-density fluid collection (Figure 56.5) [7].

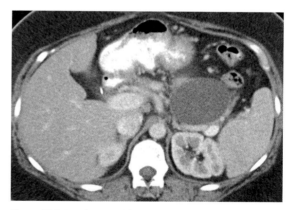

Figure 56.5 Pseudocyst. Axial contrast-enhanced CT image obtained in a 39-year-old female 6 weeks following an episode of interstitial pancreatitis shows a 6-cm well-defined homogenous low-density fluid collection.

Walled-off Peripancreatic Necrosis

On rare occasion, peripancreatic necrosis evolves into a walled-off collection involving only peripancreatic tissue with sparing of the pancreatic parenchyma. It requires 3–4 weeks from the onset of pancreatitis to develop walled-off peripancreatic necrosis. On CT scan it is a heterogeneous, non-enhancing low-density structure which may contain tiny globules of fat.

Walled-off Pancreatic Necrosis

Walled-off pancreatic necrosis occurs when the necrosis is substantial and is confined to the pancreas. It usually takes at least 3–4 weeks to form and contains solid or semisolid pancreatic necrotic debris. On CT scan it appears as a heterogeneous, non-enhancing low-density structure conforming to the expected size of the pancreas demarcated by a fibrous capsule. This entity was originally termed central cavitary necrosis. Walled-off necrosis in the absence of walled-off peripancreatic necrosis is very uncommon.

Walled-off Pancreatic and Peripancreatic Necrosis

This entity can also be recognized 3–4 weeks after severe necrotizing pancreatitis. Walled-off pancreatic and peripancreatic necrosis involves both the pancreatic tissue that has become necrotic and peripancreatic fat which has also become necrotic. The structure that is visualized on CT scan is a somewhat ovoid or rounded, non-enhancing low-density structure demarcated by a fibrous capsule (Figure 56.6). After a period of some additional weeks, the walled-off pancreatic and peripancreatic necrosis undergoes progressive liquefaction. On contrast-enhanced CT scan, it is difficult to distinguish the extent to which the necrosis liquefies since the density of fluid and necrosis as imaged on CT scan can be identical. Imaging by MRI or endoscopic ultrasound can frequently distinguish necrotic from liquefied material (Figure 56.6) [7].

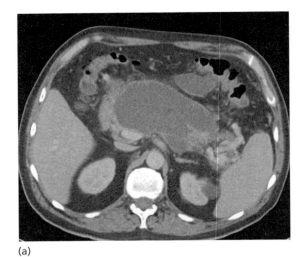

(a)

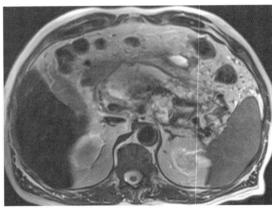

(b)

Figure 56.6 Walled-off pancreatic and peripancreatic necrosis. (a) Axial contrast-enhanced CT image obtained in a 63-year-old female with necrotizing pancreatitis shows pancreatic necrosis and presence of extrapancreatic walled-off necrosis. (b) Axial contrast-enhanced MR image obtained in the same patient 5 days later better illustrates the heterogeneous appearance of the extrapancreatic necrosis.

Epidemiology

There are recent data that the absolute number and rate of emergency ward visits for these conditions is increasing in the USA. Hospital admissions (200 000 admissions in 2002) and direct health-care costs are also increasing (annual direct costs in excess of $US2 billion) [8,9].

Pathophysiology

The initiating event appears to be inappropriate activation of trypsinogen to trypsin within pancreatic acinar cells. Activated trypsin then activates a variety of other proteases and phospholipase A-2, resulting in pancreatic injury. A variety of cytokines and chemokines are released from acinar cells that attract inflammatory cells from the circulation, including macrophages and neutrophils. Inflammatory mediators from these cells intensify the inflammatory response within the pancreas and also set in motion an amplified systemic inflammatory response that can culminate in organ failure, including refractory shock, renal failure, and respiratory failure [1].

Clinical Features

Acute Pancreatitis

Almost all patients have severe abdominal pain lasting for many hours. The pain is frequently in the epigastrium and left upper quadrant, and may radiate to the back. The intensity of the pain rarely fluctuates and is frequently intolerable. Additional symptoms are nausea and vomiting. Physical examination is noteworthy for severe upper abdominal tenderness at times with guarding.

Risk factors for increased severity of acute pancreatitis that are available at admission include older age, comorbid disease, and obesity. Markers of disease severity at admission include systemic inflammatory response syndrome (SIRS), presence of organ failure, hemoconcentration with hematocrit greater than 44%, and an increase in APACHE II score (such as >8) [2,10,11].

The SIRS is defined by two or more of the following criteria:

• Pulse greater than 90 beats/min;
• Respirations greater than 20/min or pCO_2 less than 32 mmHg;
• Rectal temperature less than 36°C or greater than 38°C;
• White blood count <4000 or >12 000/mm^3.

Further assessment of severity during the first 24 h includes follow-up values of APACHE II and additional scoring systems, such as the newly established BISAP score. The BISAP scoring system has 5 variables; BUN greater than 25 mg/dL; impaired mental status (Glasgow coma scale score <15); SIRS; age 60 years or older; and pleural infusion detected on imaging. BISAP scores range from 0 to 5 and correlate strongly with survival [12]. Patients with evidence of increased severity should be transferred to an intensive care unit for closer monitoring, improvement in fluid resuscitation, and improvement in pulmonary care.

It is now recognized that there are two phases in acute pancreatitis. In the early phase, lasting 7–10 days, the classification of severity is mainly clinical. The major component of this clinical classification is persistent organ failure (i.e. organ failure lasting >48 h).

Definition of organ failure is, as follows:
• Shock—systolic blood pressure less than 90 mmHg;
• Pulmonary insufficiency—PaO$_2$ less than or equal to 60 mmHg;
• Renal failure—creatinine greater than 2 mg/dL.

In the second phase of acute pancreatitis, which takes place after 7–10 days, the classification of severity is both clinical (persistent organ failure) and morphologic (necrotizing pancreatitis versus interstitial pancreatitis).

Peripancreatic Fluid Collections

Thirty to 50% of patients with interstitial pancreatitis have peripancreatic fluid collections. At times, a peripancreatic fluid collection causes a severe inflammatory response resulting in intractable pain, fever, and leukocytosis. Peripancreatic fluid collections rarely become infected. When infection is suspected because of prolongation of abdominal pain, leukocytosis, and fever, percutaneous aspiration with Gram stain and culture helps distinguish a sterile from an infected collection. The insertion of a transabdominal catheter by a radiologist to provide drainage of peripancreatic fluid is rarely necessary unless the fluid collection is infected or is of great size and causing intractable abdominal pain.

Pancreatic Pseudocyst

Some pancreatic pseudocysts remain asymptomatic. The most common symptom of a pancreatic pseudocyst is abdominal pain. When a pancreatic pseudocyst becomes infected, there may also be leukocytosis and fever. A pancreatic pseudocyst that is symptomatic can be drained by a variety of techniques, including surgical (such as cystogastrostomy or Roux-en-Y cystojejunostomy), endoscopic (such as endoscopic cystogastrostomy), or by radiologic method (percutaneous catheter drainage).

Peripancreatic Necrosis

Peripancreatic necrosis is frequently associated with symptoms such as intractable abdominal pain, nausea and vomiting, leukocytosis, and at times fever. After 7–10 days, peripancreatic necrosis can become secondarily infected. The distinction between sterile and infected peripancreatic necrosis can be made by guided percutaneous aspiration with Gram stain and culture. If sterile, the treatment is continuation of medical therapy [13]. If infection is documented, surgical debridement is usually required. If the patient is clinically stable and receiving appropriate antibiotic therapy, surgery can, at times, be delayed until the peripancreatic necrosis is walled-off, which offers a better target for a variety of surgical (or endoscopic) procedures [14,15].

Pancreatic Necrosis

The clinical course of pancreatic necrosis is variable, whether alone or associated with peripancreatic necrosis. It was once thought that almost all patients with pancreatic necrosis experienced organ failure. More recent information indicates that only half of patients with necrotizing pancreatitis have organ failure. Patient who die within the first 1–2 weeks do so because of refractory organ failure that cannot be overcome by intensive care. Those who survive may continue to experience organ failure or have resolution of organ failure as the necrotizing pancreatitis evolves to walled-off pancreatic necrosis. At this stage, some patients have no residual symptoms and can be fed orally without experiencing symptoms. Others continue to have symptoms including intractable pain, nausea and vomiting, persistence of low-grade temperature, and inability to maintain a satisfactory weight. Many of the symptoms are due to increased pressure within the walled-off pancreatic necrosis that increases with each attempt to eat. This increased pressure is frequently due to continuation of secretion of pancreatic juice from a viable remnant of the tail of the pancreas into the area of walled-off necrosis.

Symptomatic walled-off pancreatic necrosis can be treated surgically (with either cystogastrostomy or Roux-en-Y cystojejunostomy with finger dissection of the necrotic tissue), endoscopically (with insertion of the endoscope through the back wall of the stomach and careful debridement utilizing a snare), and rarely by percutaneous placement of a catheter [2]. The latter is more difficult to accomplish successfully because of the difficulty in irrigating and aspirating the semisolid necrotic debris. Failure to remove the necrotic debris frequently leads to secondary infection.

Diagnosis

The diagnosis of acute pancreatitis requires two of the following three features:
• Abdominal pain strongly suggestive of acute pancreatitis;
• Serum amylase and/or lipase at least three times the upper limit of normal;
• Characteristics findings of acute pancreatitis on imaging studies, such as contrast-enhanced CT scan.

Table 56.1 Differential diagnosis of acute pancreatitis.

Abdominal conditions
• Intestinal perforation
• Intestinal obstruction
• Mesenteric vascular disease
• Biliary tract disease
• Abdominal aortic aneurysm

Thoracic conditions
• Acute myocardial infarction

Case continued

In the case under consideration, the severe upper abdominal pain and markedly elevated amylase and lipase (five times the upper limit of normal) are sufficient to make a diagnosis of acute pancreatitis. CT scan in this case was not necessary to confirm the diagnosis of acute pancreatitis and did not provide additional information during the first 1–2 weeks that helped in the care of the patient, who was undergoing active treatment for multisystem organ failure. The confirmation of pancreatic necrosis based on contrast-enhanced CT scan provided important information to the clinician that recovery would be prolonged and the patient would need nutritional support.

Differential Diagnosis

The differential diagnosis of acute pancreatitis is wide (Table 56.1). Elevations of amylase and lipase (even occasionally more than three times the upper limit of normal) may occur in at least some of these diseases.

Therapeutics (Table 56.2 and Figure 56.7)

Interstitial Pancreatitis

The therapy of interstitial pancreatitis is supportive. Fluid resuscitation and careful monitoring of oxygen saturation are key. Organ failure occurs in less than 10% of cases and is usually transient.

Necrotizing Pancreatitis

Necrotizing pancreatitis is generally a more severe disease than interstitial pancreatitis [2,4,11]. One half of the patients who die do so in the first 7–14 days because of persistent organ failure. The other half die later because of complications from the necrotizing pancreatitis, such as unresolved organ failure, development of infected necrosis, or some other complication of necrotizing pancreatitis. Clinical care in the first several weeks is domi-

Table 56.2 Evidence-based therapeutics.

- Supportive care (level of evidence 3)
- Transfer to an intensive care unit (level of evidence 3)
- Nutritional support: enteral feeding (level of evidence 2)
- Use of prophylaxis antibiotics in necrotizing pancreatitis not recommended (level of evidence 3)
- Treatment of infected necrosis—surgical debridement (level of evidence 3)
- Treatment of sterile necrosis—medical (level of evidence 3)
- Role of endoscopic retrograde cholangiopancreatography (ERCP) and biliary sphincterotomy—limited role (level of evidence 1)

nated by fluid resuscitation, careful pulmonary care, and treatment of other clinical features, such as refractory shock, renal failure, and evolving pulmonary insufficiency which may require intubation. Adequacy of fluid resuscitation should be monitored every 12 h. If the BUN has increased during this interval, additional fluid resuscitation is required.

Patients who will be without oral nourishment for several weeks should be started on nasojejunal feeding. If this is ineffective, total parenteral nutritional (TPN) will be needed.

Nasojejunal feeding is currently thought to be safer and less expensive than TPN, but has not as yet been proven to reduce the severity of acute pancreatitis. ,Several recent randomized prospective placebo-con-

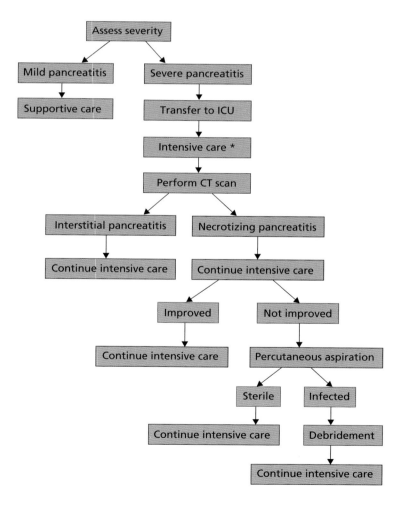

Figure 56.7 Management algorithm for treatment of acute pancreatitis. *Treat organ failure, start enteral feeding.

trolled trials have failed to establish benefit of prophylactic antibiotics to prevent the development of infected necrosis. The use of antibiotics should be restricted to those who have an infection, and at times during a prolonged hospitalization, a patient may require brief courses of antibiotics for well-documented infection, such as pneumonia, urinary or respiratory track infection. Antibiotics should be discontinued once infections are properly treated. At other times, a patient may appear septic, may be placed on broad-spectrum antibiotics for a few days while appropriate cultures are obtained. If a source of infection is not discovered, the antibiotics should be discontinued.

The role of endoscopic sphincterotomy in severe biliary pancreatitis remains somewhat controversial. In general, if there is strong suspicion of a retained stone in the common bile duct and persistent organ failure that could reflect ascending cholangitis, an endoscopic biliary sphincterotomy is recommended.

Starting at approximately day 10, patients with evidence of refractory organ failure or a sepsis-like condition manifested by high temperature and high white blood count should receive an image-guided percutaneous aspiration with Gram stain, culture and sensitivity to determine whether the necrotizing pancreatitis has secondarily become infected. Patients with infected necrosis require the use of appropriate antibiotics and debridement of the infected necrosis. The timing of debridement of the infected necrosis is dictated by the overall condition of the patient. In recent years, there has been consideration for delaying debridement until such time as the process has evolved into walled-off necrosis. Choices for debridement include traditional surgical debridement, laparoscopic surgical debridement, minimally invasive surgical debridement, radiologic debridement, or endoscopic debridement [15].

Case continued

In the case under consideration, early transfer to an intensive care unit was required when there was evidence of organ failure that required more intensive supervision. Her fluid resuscitation of only 200 mL/h was clearly inadequate in view of the increased hematocrit and increased BUN during the first 24 h of hospitalization. The patient was placed on TPN rather than nasojejunal feeding. The patient was also given imipenem as a prophylactic antibiotic. A biliary sphincterotomy was not performed because there was no evidence of ascending cholangitis, her common bile duct was not dilated, and her liver function tests returned to normal within 48 h. Because she developed severe abdominal pain each time she tried to eat, she underwent a surgical cystojejunostomy with aspiration of the fluid and debridement of necrotic pancreatic tissue and left the hospital 1 week after the surgery, receiving insulin for diabetes mellitus and pancreatic enzymes for steatorrhea.

Prognosis

Prognosis of interstitial pancreatitis is generally favorable with mortality below 3%. Mortality is usually due to unresolved organ failure, especially in a patient with co-morbidity.

Prognosis of necrotizing pancreatitis is more severe. In necrotizing pancreatitis not associated with organ failure or other complications, mortality is less than 5%. Mortality of necrotizing pancreatitis in association with multisystem organ failure is as high as 50%.

Take-home points

- The diagnosis of acute pancreatitis requires two of the following three features: abdominal pain strongly suggestive of acute pancreatitis; serum amylase and/or lipase at least three times the upper limit of normal; characteristic findings of acute pancreatic on imaging studies, such as contrast-enhanced CT scan.

- There are two phases of acute pancreatitis: in the early phase lasting 7–10 days, clinical classification of severity is based on persistent organ failure. After 7–10 days, the clinical classification of severity is persistent organ failure; morphologic classification of severity is necrotizing versus interstitial pancreatitis.

- Approximately 90% of cases of acute pancreatitis are interstitial (mortality approximately 3%); 10% are necrotizing pancreatitis (overall mortality approximately 15%).

- Risk factors of severity at admission include older age, co-morbidity, and obesity.

- Markers of severity at admission include systemic inflammatory response syndrome, organ failure, serum hematocrit, and APACHE II score.

- Severity of acute pancreatitis during hospitalization is defined primarily by persistent organ failure and pancreatic necrosis.

- Distinction of interstitial versus necrotizing pancreatitis is made by contrast-enhanced CT scan.

- There are now well-defined criteria on contrast-enhanced CT scan to define interstitial pancreatitis, necrotizing pancreatitis, extrapancreatic fluid collections, pancreatic pseudocyst, walled-off peripancreatic necrosis, and walled-off pancreatic necrosis (with or without walled-off extrapancreatic necrosis).
- Treatment guidelines include supportive care with aggressive rehydration, transfer to the intensive care unit for organ dysfunction, nutritional support by enteral feeding, and use of endoscopic retrograde cholangiopancreatography (ERCP) primarily for suspected ascending cholangitis.
- Antibiotics should be given only for proven infection.
- Treatment of sterile necrosis is generally non-surgical except for symptomatic walled-off necrosis.
- Treatment of infected necrosis is usually surgical or endoscopic debridement (rarely percutaneous debridement).

References

1 Pandol SJ, Saluja AK, Imrie CW, Banks PA. Acute pancreatitis: bench to the bedside. *Gastroenterology* 2007; **132**: 1127–51.

2 Banks, PA, Freeman ML. Practice guidelines in acute pancreatitis. *Am J Gastroenterol* 2006; **101**: 2379–400.

3 Bollen TL, van Santvoort HC, Besselink MGH, *et al.* Update on acute pancreatitis: ultrasound, computed tomography, and magnetic resonance imaging features. *Semin Ultrasound CT MRI* 2007; **28**: 371–83.

4 Lenhart DK, Balthazar EJ. MDCT of acute mild (non-necrotizing) pancreatitis: abdominal complications and fate of fluid collections. *AJR Am J Roentgenol* 2008; **190**: 643–9.

5 Morgan DE. Imaging of acute pancreatitis and its complications. *Clin Gastroenterol Hepatol* 2008; **6**: 1077–85.

6 van Santvoort HC, Bollen TL, Besselink MG, *et al.* Describing peripancreatic collections in severe acute pancreatitis using morphologic terms: an international interobserver agreement study. *Pancreatology* 2008; **8**: 593–9.

7 Takahashi N, Papachristou GI, Schmit GD, *et al.* CT findings of walled-off pancreatic necrosis (WOPN): differentiation from pseudocyst and prediction of outcome after endoscopic therapy. *Eur Radiol* 2008; **18**: 2522–9.

8 Fagenholz PJ, Fernandez-del Castillo C, Harris NS, *et al.* Direct medical costs of acute pancreatitis hospitalization in United States. *Pancreas* 2007; **35**: 302–7.

9 Fagenholz PJ, Fernandez-del Castillo C, Harris NS, *et al.* Increasing United States hospital admissions for acute pancreatitis 1988–2003. *Ann Epidemiol* 2007; **17**: 491–7.

10 Frossard JL, Steer ML, Pastor C. Acute pancreatitis. *Lancet* 2008; **371**: 143–52.

11 Forsmark CE, Baillie J. AGA Institute technical review on acute pancreatitis. *Gastroenterology* 2007; **132**: 2022–44.

12 Wu BU, Johannes RS, Sun X, Tabak Y, Conwell DL, Banks PA. The early prediction of mortality in acute pancreatitis: a large population-based study. *Gut* 2008; **57**: 1698–703.

13 Banks PA, Mortele KJ. Nonsurgical management of acute pancreatitis. In: Beger HG, Matsuno S, Cameron J (eds). *Diseases of the Pancreas—Current Surgical Therapy*. New York: Springer, 2008: 203–11.

14 Besselink MG, van Santvoort HC, Schaapherder AF, *et al.* Feasibility of minimally invasive approaches in patients with infected necrotizing pancreatitis. *Br J Surg* 2007; **94**: 604–8.

15 Berzin TM, Mortele KJ, Banks PA. The management of suspected pancreatic sepsis. *Gastroenterol Clin N Am* 2006; **35**: 393–407.

CHAPTER 57
Chronic Pancreatitis and Pancreatic Pseudocysts

Nison Badalov and Scott Tenner

Division of Gastroenterology, Department of Medicine, Maimonides Medical Center, State University of New York – Health Sciences Center, New York, NY, USA

Summary

Although chronic pancreatitis has a variety of clinical manifestations, most commonly patients present with intermittent chronic abdominal pain. The pain originates from a myriad of protean manifestations, including inflammation and increased ductal and/or parenchymal pressure. In select patients, endoscopic or surgical decompression of the pancreatic duct has been shown to decrease pain. Pancreatic duct disruption and/or increased pancreatic ductal pressure can lead to a pseudocyst formation. In patients with chronic pancreatitis, the pancreatic duct becomes obstructed by fibrous scarring, inspissated protein, or stone(s), and the ongoing pancreatic secretion proximal to the obstruction leads to a saccular dilation of the duct, filled with pancreatic juice. These pseudocysts can cause symptoms of pain, early satiety, nausea, vomiting, weight loss, and can be complicated by obstruction (biliary and or enteric), hemorrhage, and infection. In the patient with chronic pancreatitis who develops a symptomatic pseudocyst(s), a multidisciplinary approach to drain these cysts, including endoscopic, surgical, and percutaneous methods, should be considered depending on local expertise and the character and location of the pseudocyst.

Case

A 51-year-old gentleman with a history of alcohol abuse and chronic pancreatitis presents with complaints of abdominal pain. After a divorce 15 years prior, he had begun drinking heavily. After developing recurrent attacks of pain 7 years ago, he was diagnosed as having chronic pancreatitis. Endoscopic retrograde cholangiopancreaticography (ERCP) at that time had shown stricturing of the pancreatic duct and areas of dilatation diffusely to 1 cm. Endoscopic stent placement was partially effective in relieving pain. Although he had considered a lateral pancreaticojujenostomy, a conservative approach was preferred. Last month, due to increased pain, his primary care physician began oxycodone and pancreatic enzymes. A computed tomographic scan (CT) was performed which revealed classic calcification seen in patients with chronic pancreatitis (Figure 57.1a) and a 6-cm cyst in the body of the pancreas adjacent to the wall of the stomach (Figure 57.1b).

Practical Gastroenterology and Hepatology: Small and Large Intestine and Pancreas, 1st edition. Edited by Nicholas J. Talley, Sunanda V. Kane and Michael B. Wallace. © 2010 Blackwell Publishing Ltd.

Chronic Pancreatitis

Diagnosis and effective treatment of chronic pancreatitis is challenging. Chronic pancreatitis (CP) is a syndrome of progressive, irreversible destructive inflammatory changes in the pancreas that results in permanent structural damage, leading to impairment of exocrine and endocrine function. Histologic changes include irregular fibrosis, acinar cell loss, islet cell loss, and inflammatory cell infiltrates. The gold standard for the diagnosis of CP is tissue diagnosis; however, this is invasive and rarely performed. Therefore the diagnosis of CP is based upon a combination of clinical, radiographic, and functional findings.

The hallmark manifestations of CP are abdominal pain and exocrine insufficiency. Abdominal pain is the most common presenting complaint, seen in 50–90% of patients. The pain is typically epigastric, radiates to the back, worse after meals, and may be relieved by sitting upright or leaning forward (pancreatic position). Early in the course, the pain may be intermittent and occur in

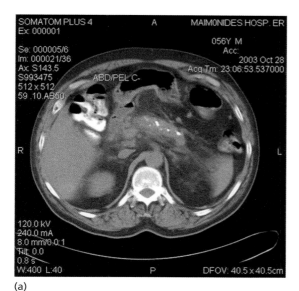

(a)

(b)

Figure 57.1 (a) Calcification in the body of the pancreas pathognomonic for chronic pancreatitis. (b) A 6 cm pseudocyst.

discrete attacks, but as the disease progresses, the pain becomes more continuous. Severe pain may decrease the appetite and limit food consumption, contributing to weight loss and malnutrition.

The mechanism of pain in CP is multifactorial, including inflammation, duct obstruction, increased pancreatic tissue pressure (compartment syndrome), fibrotic encasement of sensory nerves, and a neuropathy characterized by both increased numbers and sizes of intrapancreatic sensory nerves and by inflammatory injury to the nerve sheaths allowing exposure of the neural elements to proteolytic enzymes.

Pseudocysts—Natural History

A pancreatic pseudocyst is an amylase-rich fluid collection located within or near the pancreas. Whether occurring in a patient with acute pancreatitis or CP, a pseudocyst forms when there is direct leakage of pancreatic juice from an inflamed area of the gland into the parenchyma or to an adjacent space. Rarely, these cystic lesions can occur at significant distances from the pancreas, including the mediastinum and pelvis. Regardless, ductular disruption is the most important event in the formation of a pseudocyst. Ductular disruption allows this pancreatic enzyme-rich fluid to evoke an inflammatory response leading to the formation of granulation tissue and fibrosis. Over time, the cyst becomes lined by a fibrous, non-epithelialized wall.

Pancreatic pseudocysts are one of the most frequent complications in acute and CP, ranging between 20 and 60% of patients [1]. Most cysts are single and when multiple typically occur in patients with CP. The size varies from 1 to 30 cm [2].

Whereas most pseudocysts in patients with acute pancreatitis resolve spontaneously, in patients with CP many pseudocysts persist and become symptomatic. In some series, more than 90% of pseudocysts in CP that are larger than 6 cm, persist, and many become infected or cause pain [3,4]. Although once considered a standard of care to intervene in large pseudocysts (>6 cm), or pseudocysts that failed to resolve in 6 weeks, the management of pancreatic pseudocysts has evolved over the last decade. In general, asymptomatic pseudocysts do not warrant intervention. However, in patients with pseudocysts who have symptoms related to the cyst, such as pain, early satiety, and/or infection, obstruction of the common bile duct, or enteral tract, drainage should occur.

Diagnosis

The diagnosis of CP is generally made by detecting calcifications in the pancreas, either on plain abdominal radiograph or computed tomography (CT) scan (Figure

57.1a). Although insensitive, the finding of pancreatic stones is quite specific. In patients with early CP, the diagnosis is often difficult and is usually established by a combination of findings related to the pancreatic duct that are identified by ERCP, magnetic resonance cholangiopancreaticography (MRCP), and/or endoscopic ultrasonography (EUS). Early structural changes can be detected by endoscopic ultrasound. Early functional deficiencies can be established by a secretin stimulation test.

There is a consensus that CT or magnetic resonance imaging (MRI) scanning is mandatory for planning therapy for a pancreatic pseudocyst. CT imaging yields the highest sensitivity (82–100%) and specificity (98%; negative predictive value, 92–94%) and an overall accuracy of 88–94% [5]. Although the diagnosis of pseudocyst often seems simple based on the finding of a cystic lesion in the pancreas in the clinical setting of acute pancreatitis, less common cystic pathology of the pancreas often mimics pseudocysts and lead to inappropriate interventions. Approximately 10% of pancreatic cysts are neoplastic, including mucinous cystadenomas. It important that the clinician maintain a sense of suspicion when faced with the patient with no prior history of acute pancreatitis and found to have a "pseudocyst". A pseudocyst generally takes 3–4 weeks for the fibrous non-epithelialized wall to develop. Differentiating between pseudocysts and neoplastic cysts is important to determine the method of intervention. In general, a cystic lesion can be considered a pseudocyst if the patient had an attack of acute pancreatitis more than 3–4 weeks prior, or the patient has a history or clinical findings consistent with CP. Although cross-sectional imaging such as CT and MRI can provide detailed information on anatomic and morphologic characteristics of the neoplastic cysts and pseudocysts, there is a significant overlap in morphology of these cysts. In addition to providing high-resolution images of cyst morphology, EUS also provides the opportunity for fine needle aspiration (FNA) for fluid analysis and cytology.

EUS-guided fluid analysis can assist in differentiating cystic lesions of the pancreas. Brugge [6] showed the value of an EUS cyst fluid analysis for carcinoembryonic antigen (CEA) in guiding cyst fluid drainage. Whereas pseudocysts and serous cysts have low CEA levels, elevated pancreatic cyst CEA is associated with a mucinous cystadenoma. The Cooperative Pancreatic Cyst Study in 2004 reported on 341 patients with cystic lesions greater than 1 cm on EUS. The major finding of this large multicenter study in favor of FNA is that when CEA is found to be greater than 192 ng/mL in the cystic fluid, a malignant pancreatic lesion can be assumed with a sensitivity of 73% and a specificity of 84% [7].

Another problem is the patient with an attack of acute pancreatitis who develops pancreatic necrosis. As the pancreatic necrosis becomes walled off, on CT these necrotic pancreatic lesions appear cystic. Walled off pancreatic necrosis (WOPN) cannot be differentiated on CT from a pancreatic pseudocyst when the cystic lesion is within the pancreatic parenchyma. Although a history of acute pancreatitis can help identify the patient with a WOPN, in an alcoholic patient, who likely has underlying CP, the history may not be as helpful. Endoscopic ultrasound or MRI can assist by identifying debris within the cystic lesion. The debris would interfere with either endoscopic or radiologic drainage.

A pseudocyst is unlikely to resolve spontaneously if: (i) it persists for more than 6 weeks; (ii) chronic pancreatitis is evident; (iii) there is a pancreatic duct anomaly (except for a communication with the pseudocyst); or (iv) the pseudocyst is surrounded by a thick wall [8]. Studying 92 patients with chronic alcoholic pancreatitis, Gouyon and colleagues [9] reported a spontaneous regression rate of 25.7%. However, pseudocysts larger than 4 cm and those localized extrapancreatically were found to represent predictive factors for persistent symptoms and/or complications.

Symptoms

Pain in the upper abdomen is the most common symptom in patients with pseudocysts complicating CP. The pathophysiology is likely related to increased intraductal and/or intraparenchymal pressure in the pancreas. Drainage procedures appear to relieve pain by a reduction of pressure within the pancreas [10]. Occasionally, the pain becomes increasingly intense simulating that of pancreatic carcinoma. The pain may be referred to the left more than the right hypochondrium with radiation to the back. When there is diaphragmatic involvement, the pain may be pleuritic and even felt in the shoulder. A sudden onset of pain or exacerbation of a pre-existing pain signifies hemorrhage into the cyst or peritoneum.

Small cysts and even some moderately sized cysts may be totally asymptomatic and discovered only incidentally.

Drainage of Pseudocysts

There are multiple non-randomized, non-blinded trials demonstrating resolution of pain in patients with chronic pancreatitis when pseudocysts are drained. Usatoff and colleagues [11] evaluated 112 patients with confirmed chronic pancreatitis who underwent open operation by drainage, resection, or a combination of both. The morbidity rate was 28%, and mortality rate was 1%. In 74% of patients, pain was relieved, and pseudocyst recurrence rate was 3%. In general, studies have shown that patients with CP suffering from pain or early satiety from an obstructive effect of a pseudocyst clearly benefit from a drainage procedure (Table 57.1).

Medical Therapy

Medical therapy has a very limited role in the management of pancreatic pseudocysts. Although somatostatin, or its octopeptide synthetic analog, octreotide, have been extensively studied, there is no evidence that a symptomatic pseudocyst can be effectively treated by using these inhibitors of pancreatic secretion alone. However, as an adjuvant treatment, octreotide and/or somatostatin may be effective [12]. In a patient who had undergone a drainage procedure for a pancreatic pseudocyst, octreotide may assist in decreasing the size and drainage, if continuous.

Pancreatic enzymes also have a limited role. Only one of six of randomized controlled trials showed a statistically significant benefit and only 52% of the pooled patient population expressing a preference for enzyme

Table 57.1 Indications for drainage of a pseudocyst complicating chronic pancreatitis pain.

Weight loss and early satiety thought to be related to compression from cyst
Gastric or duodenal outlet obstruction
Infection of the pseudocyst (abscess)
Biliary obstruction

over placebo [13]. It is the opinion of the authors that pancreatic enzymes do not treat pain in patients with CP, regardless of cause. Pancreatic enzymes should be reserved for use in patients manifesting malabsorption as part of the process of CP.

Surgical Drainage

The indications for surgery, although generally defined, are not clearly established by evidence and are open to interpretation [14]. Typically, patients are referred to surgery late in the course of the disease, which implies that the inflammatory process rarely can be halted. The usual technical complexities of pancreatic surgery are made even more imposing by the inflammatory process that can affect tissue planes and extend to adjacent structures and organs. Surgical treatment of pseudocysts in patients with CP can include external or internal drainage (cystogastrostomy, cystduodenostomy, and cystojejunostomy), and resection. The specific methods of drainage used depend upon maturity of the cyst wall, location of the cyst, and whether cyst infection is present or not. In a recent series of 206 patients with CP and pseudocysts treated by surgical intervention, 94% of patients had complete pain relief or improved pain after a median follow-up of 7.3 years [1]. There was only one post operative death. There were 10 patients, 6%, who required reoperation for complications, including bleeding, fistula, and infection. Most of the patients in this series had pseudocysts in the head of the pancreas. The high rate of pain relief after resection compared to drainage may lead to fewer attacks of recurrent pain. Aside from removing the cyst, surgical therapy allows resection of the inflammatory process in the pancreas that has led to the cyst. This may have the advantage of preventing a recurrence of the cyst or development of new cysts. In general, surgeons have been performing internal drainage procedures less often and focusing on the underlying pathology of the pancreatic duct. There is a beneficial effect to identifying the source of the cyst, the defect in the duct [14].

More versatile cystojejunostomy is preferred for giant pseudocysts (>15 cm), which are predominantly inframesocolic. In pseudocysts with coexisting CP and a dilated pancreatic duct, duct drainage procedures (such as longitudinal panacreaticojejunostomy) should be preferred to cyst drainage.

Radiologic (Percutaneous) Drainage

Percutaneous drainage is typically performed by a radiologist using a 7–12 French pigtail catheter inserted in the pseudocyst over a needle-inserted guidewire. This guidewire can be placed by sonography, CT, or fluoroscopy. This method is less invasive, ideal for diagnosis, but often ineffective due to a combination of factors, including failure to collapse the wall of the pseudocyst and failure to removed the ductal communication that feeds the pancreatic cyst the pancreatic enzyme-rich fluid. Continuous catheter drainage has more impressive results, with a low failure rate of only 16%, recurrence rate of 7%, and low complication rate of 18% and mortality rate of 2% [15].

Percutaneous drainage is not the procedure of choice in the presence of a stricture of the main pancreatic duct because of the risk of a permanent external fistula. Percutaneous catheter diagnosis is less effective in multiple and loculated pseudocysts. Contraindications to percutaneous catheter diagnosis include suspicion of malignancy, intracystic hemorrhage, and presence of pancreatic ascites. Percutaneous catheter drainage should be the initial mode of treatment for high-risk patients in need of pseudocyst drainage, for patients with symptomatic or expanding immature cysts, and for patients with infected pseudocysts.

Endoscopic Drainage

An endoscopic approach to the management of pseudocysts requires careful evaluation of the patient, local expertise, and the character and location of the pseudocyst [16]. Identifying the characteristics of the collection by transabdominal ultrasound, MRI, or ideally, EUS, will help direct the appropriate approach, either through endoscopy, deferring to surgical drainage, or observation, especially in minimally asymptomatic patients. In the best hands, an endoscopic approach can result in successful resolution in as much as 92% of patients with CP [17].

Endoscopic cyst drainage can be performed by a transmural (transgastric/transduodenal) or transpapillary route. The transpapillary approach has been shown to be effective 85% of the time [18]. This approach is ideal for cysts that communicate with the main pancreatic duct.

Single-step needle drainage of pancreatic pseudocysts is associated with an unacceptably high recurrence rates. Prolonged drainage with an indwelling catheter is associated with a high drainage success rates and low recurrence rates [19].

Most pancreatic pseudocysts (>70%) communicate with the main pancreatic duct. For this reason, a transpapillary approach to drainage should be considered. If the pseudocyst communicates with the main pancreatic duct on ERCP, a 5–7 French pancreatic duct stent should be placed beyond the stricture or cyst cavity. Factors predictive of success include the presence of pancreatic duct strictures, size of the pseudocyst (6 cm or more), location in the body of the pancreas, and duration of the pseudocyst of less than 6 months [20]. A review of the published literature [19] shows that transpapillary drainage to be a safe procedure with low morbidity and no reported mortality. Hemorrhagic complications occurred in less than 1% of patients, pancreatitis in 5%, and stent migration was rare.

Endoscopic transmural drainage of a pseudocyst could be performed via a transgastric or transduodenal approach, depending on its location (Table 57.2). The technique involves the endoscopic identification of the area of maximum bulge with the use of a side-viewing endoscope, needle localization of the tract for cautery, entry into the pseudocyst using a needle-knife papillotome with radiologic verification by contrast injection, and insertion of a guidewire followed by several 7- to 10-Fr stents (Figure 57.2a,b) [19] (Video 17). Cystogastrostomies are especially prone to early closure if not stented, resulting in recurrence rates as high as 20%. Use of nasogastric catheter is optional.

Table 57.2 General requirements for a transmural approach to drainage of pseudocysts.

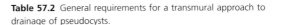

Distance of pseudocyst to gastrointestinal wall <1 cm

Location judged by bulge into the lumen of upper gastrointestinal tract (or EUS)

EUS location confirmed (or bulge noted)

Size greater than 5 cm

No debris on EUS

Neoplasm ruled out

Pseudoaneurysm ruled out

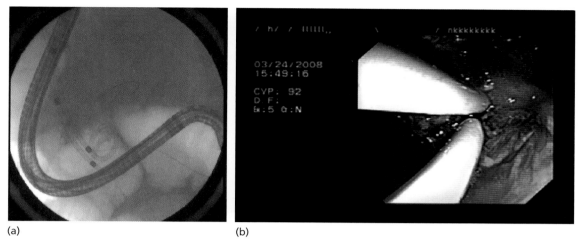

(a) (b)

Figure 57.2 (a,b) Fluoroscopic view and endoscopic view of stents allowing continuous drainage of pseudocyst.

Prior to a transenteric approach to cyst drainage (cystogastrostomy, cystoduodenostomy), an EUS should be performed. Although there is little evidence that this approach increases efficacy, EUS not only highlights approximate vascular structures, but also characterizes the cyst contents, which may contain debris. A biopsy of the pseudocyst wall could be obtained at the time of drainage to rule out malignancy or cystadenoma.

There are almost 1000 cases of endoscopic transmural drainage of pancreatic pseudocysts in the published literature. Technical success in achieving drainage was associated with location of the pseudocysts in the head or body rather than the tail of the gland, when the transmural thickness was less than 1 cm as measured on CT scan or EUS, and when the pseudocysts complicated CP compared to acute pancreatitis. Complications have been reported to occur in as many as 7% of cases, including perforation, sepsis, and bleeding. Antibiotic prophylaxis should be considered despite the absence of evidence that antibiotics are efficacious in the prevention of infectious complications in the drainage of pseudocysts.

There are currently no randomized controlled studies comparing the various minimally invasive approaches in the management of pancreatic pseudocysts. Depending on the available local expertise and technology, intervention should be applied. It remains unclear whether an ERCP is necessary to document communication with the main pancreatic duct in order to attempt a transpapillary approach compared to a transmural approach. Further study will be needed to clarify the best approach to managing pseudocysts complicating CP. Due to the minimal invasiveness of the approach, reported safety, and success rates in the literature, if expertise is available, an endoscopic approach is preferred.

Case continued

The patient presented has abdominal pain and underlying CP now complicated by the formation of a large pseudocyst. Medical therapy is not likely to be beneficial. From multiple case series, it appears that the pain will be relieved by drainage of the pseudocyst.

Take-home points

- The highest incidence of pancreatic pseudocysts can be found in patients with chronic pancreatitis due to alcohol abuse.

- The diagnosis of pseudocysts is accomplished most often by CT scanning, endoscopic ultrasound, or by endoscopic retrograde cholangiopancreaticography (ERCP); rapid progress in the improvement of diagnostic tools has enabled detection with high sensitivity and specificity.

- There are different therapeutic strategies: endoscopic transpapillary or transmural drainage, percutaneous catheter drainage, or laparoscopic and/or open surgery.

- The feasibility of endoscopic drainage is highly dependent on the anatomy and topography of the pseudocyst;

however, in general, endoscopic drainage provides high success and low complication rates.

- Internal drainage and pseudocyst resection are frequently used as surgical approaches with a good overall outcome, but a somewhat higher morbidity and mortality compared with endoscopic intervention.

References

1 Schlosser W, Siech M, Beger HG. Pseudocyst treatment in chronic pancreatitis – surgical treatment of the underlying disease increases the long term success. *Dig Surg* 2005; **22**: 340–5.

2 Pitchumoni CS, Agarwal N. Pancreatic pseudocysts: when and how should drainage be performed. *Gastroenterol Clin North Am* 1999; **28**: 610–45.

3 Warshaw AL. Pancreatic cysts and pseudocysts: new rules for a new game. *Br J Surg* 1988; **76**: 533–4.

4 Bradley EL, Clements J, Gonzales A. The natural history of pancreatic pseudocysts: a unified concept of management. *Am J Surg* 1979; **137**: 135–41.

5 Aghdassi A, Mayerle J, Kraft M, *et al*. Diagnosis and treatment of pancreatic pseudocysts in chronic pancreatitis. *Pancreas* 2008; **36**: 105–12.

6 Brugge WR. Approaches to the drainage of pancreatic pseudocysts. *Curr Opin Gastroenterol* 2004; **20**: 488–92.

7 Brugge WR, Lewandrowski K, Lee-Lewandrowski E, *et al*. Diagnosis of pancreatic cystic neoplasms: a report of the Cooperative Pancreatic Cyst Study. *Gastroenterology* 2004; **126**: 1330–6.

8 Warshaw AL, Rattner DW. Timing of surgical drainage for pancreatic pseudocyst. Clinical and chemical criteria. *Ann Surg* 1985; **202**: 720–4.

9 Gouyon B, Levy P, Ruszniewski P, *et al*. Predictive factors in the outcome of pseudocysts complicating alcoholic chronic pancreatitis. *Gut* 1997; **41**: 821–5.

10 Ebbehoj N, Borly L, Bulow J, *et al*. Pancreatic tissue fluid pressure in chronic pancreatitis. Relation to pain, morphology and function. *Scand J Gastroenterol* 1990; **25**: 1046–51.

11 Usatoff V, Brancatisano R, Williamson RC. Operative treatment of pseudocysts in patients with chronic pancreatitis. *Br J Surg* 2000; **87**: 1494–9.

12 Gullo L, Barbara L. The treatment of pancreatic pseudocysts with octreotide. *Lancet* 1991; **338**: 540–1.

13 Brown A, Hughes M, Tenner S, Banks PA. Does pancreatic enzyme supplementation reduce pain in patients with chronic pancreatitis: a meta-analysis. *Am J Gastroenterol* 1997; **92**: 2032–5.

14 Bell R. Current surgical management of chronic pancreatitis. *J Gastrointest Surg* 2005; **9**: 144–54.

15 Gumaste V, Pitchumoni CS. Pancreatic pseudocyst. *Gastroenterologist* 1996; **4**: 33–43.

16 Wilcox CM. Varadarajulu S. Endoscopic therapy for chronic pancreatitis: an evidence based review. *Curr Gastroenterol Rep* 2006; **8**: 104–10.

17 Baron TH, Harewood GC, Morgan DE, *et al*. Outcome differences after endoscopic drainage of pancreatic necrosis, acute pancreatic pseudocysts, and chronic pancreatic pseudocysts. *Gastroitnestinal Endoscopy* 2002; **56**: 7–17.

18 De Palma GD, Galloro G, Puzziello A, *et al*. Endoscopic drainage of pancreatic pseudocysts: a long-term follow-up study of 49 patients. *Hepatogastroenterology* 2002, **49**: 1113–15.

19 Bhattacharya D, Ammori BJ. Minimally invasive approaches to the management of pancreatic pseudocysts. *Surgical Lapro Endo Per* 2003; **13**: 141–8.

20 Catalano MF, Geenen JE, Schmalz MJ, *et al*. Treatment of pancreatic pseudocysts with ductal communication by Transpapillary pancreatic duct endoprosthesis. *Gastrointest Endosc* 1995; **42**: 214–8.

CHAPTER 58

Pancreatic Cancer and Cystic Pancreatic Neoplasms

Field F. Willingham and William R. Brugge

Harvard Medical School and Gastrointestinal Unit, Massachusetts General Hospital, Boston, MA, USA

Pancreatic Cancer

Summary

Pancreatic cancer is the fourth most common cause of cancer death in men and women. Patients typically present at an advanced stage with a poor prognosis. The clinical presentation may involve weight loss, abdominal discomfort, and or jaundice. Painless jaundice, depression, and new-onset diabetes can suggest the diagnosis. Cross-sectional imaging has utility in diagnosis and staging. Endoscopic ultrasound (EUS) with fine needle aspiration (FNA) is a standard approach to tissue diagnosis. Endoscopic retrograde cholangiopancreaticography (ERCP) with palliative stenting can relieve obstructive jaundice. A minority of patients are candidates for resection. Patients with metastatic disease or with contraindications to resection (e.g., invasion of the superior mesenteric artery) may be considered for chemoradiation therapy.

Case

A 59-year-old African American man presents with a history of progressive jaundice and recent-onset depression. He is a former smoker. He has a family history of pancreatic cancer. His blood sugar is elevated. Computed tomography (CT) scan of the abdomen and pelvis reveals a 2.3-cm mass in the head of the pancreas. There is regional lymphadenopathy.

Definition and Epidemiology

The majority of pancreatic cancer results from malignant transformation of the exocrine pancreas, and greater than 80% are ductal adenocarcinomas [1]. In 2007, there were an estimated 37 170 new cases of pancreatic cancer diag-

Practical Gastroenterology and Hepatology: Small and Large Intestine and Pancreas, 1st edition. Edited by Nicholas J. Talley, Sunanda V. Kane and Michael B. Wallace. © 2010 Blackwell Publishing Ltd.

nosed [2]. In terms of new diagnoses, pancreatic cancer is the tenth most common malignancy in men, but does not make the top ten in women. The poor prognosis makes pancreatic cancer the fourth most common cause of cancer death in both women and men [2].

Pathophysiology

Pancreatic ductal carcinoma is acquired through the accumulation of multiple genetic mutations [3]. More than 85% of ductal carcinomas have a mutation in the K-*ras* oncogene [4], and more than 90% have inactivation of the *p16* tumor-suppressor gene [5]. The major risk factors for pancreatic cancer include age, smoking, chronic pancreatitis, diabetes mellitus, male gender, and African American race. Less commonly, hereditary syndromes may be implicated. Hereditary chronic pancreatitis caused by a mutation in the cationic trypsinogen gene accounts for a small percentage of cases [6,7]. Cancer syndromes that increase the risk of pancreatic cancer include (in order of decreasing risk) Peutz–Jeghers syndrome, familial atypical multiple mole syndrome, and *BRCA* 1 and 2 genotypes, familial adenomatous polyposis, and hereditary non-polyposis colon cancer [8].

Clinical Features

Patients with pancreatic cancer may present with abdominal or back pain, weight loss, and/or jaundice. Weight loss may be associated with diarrhea, early satiety, and/or steatorrhea. The jaundice of pancreatic cancer is classically obstructive and is characterized by an elevated direct/conjugated bilirubin, acholic (pale) stool, and dark urine. Painless jaundice is a typical presentation concerning for underlying pancreatic cancer. Atypical diabetes mellitus, with new onset in an older thin adult, and/or depression may be observed.

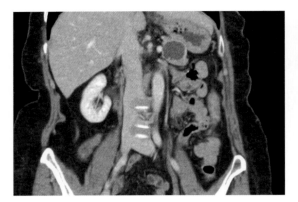

Figure 58.1 Contrast enhanced computed tomography scan of a pancreatic mass involving the stomach.

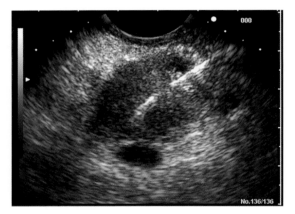

Figure 58.2 Endoscopic ultrasound guided fine needle aspiration of a hypoechoic pancreatic mass.

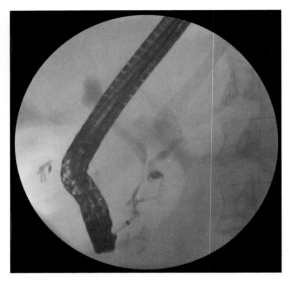

Figure 58.3 Fluoroscopic image at endoscopic retrograde cholangiopancreaticography in a patient with metastatic cancer to the pancreas demonstrating a classic double duct sign. Strictures are present in both the pancreatic and bile ducts with upstream dilatation. Incidental note is made of clips from a prior cholecystectomy.

Diagnosis

Abdominal ultrasound may reveal dilatation of the biliary tree and pancreatic duct. Laboratory testing of liver function, total and direct bilirubin, amylase, lipase, and complete blood count may direct subsequent investigations. Cross sectional imaging may reveal a pancreatic mass, biliary or pancreatic ductal dilatation, regional or distant lymphadenopathy, metastasis, or regional invasion or vessels or duodenum (Figure 58.1). In many cases, the finding of a mass in the pancreas will prompt referral for endoscopic ultrasound (EUS) guided fine needle aspiration (FNA) for a cytologic diagnosis and more detailed locoregional staging (Figure 58.2). Endo-

scopic retrograde cholangiopancreaticography (ERCP) can demonstrate ductal stricturing and is diagnostic in some cases with brushing and biopsy. The double duct sign refers to the finding of dilatation of both the common bile duct and the pancreatic duct (Figure 58.3) and is concerning for a distal obstruction (i.e., pancreatic head mass or carcinoma of the ampulla of Vater). The tumor marker CA19-9 correlates with tumor size, but is not recommended for use in screening or selecting patients for surgery.

Case continued

The patient is referred for EUS-FNA for tissue diagnosis and staging. The EUS reveals a 2.9-cm irregular, hypoechoic mass in the head of the pancreas. There is locoregional lymphadenopathy. The mass appears to invade the superior mesenteric artery. The pathologic diagnosis from the FNA is poorly differentiated adenocarcinoma.

Differential Diagnosis

See Table 58.1.

Therapeutics

Surgical resection is the only potentially curative option in the management of pancreatic cancer (Figure 58.4). Because the stage is typically advanced at presentation, surgery is only considered in a minority of cases. Approx-imately 20% of patients will be operative candidates at the time of diagnosis [9]. Even with appropriate patient selection and complete surgical resection, only a subset of resected patients will achieve a cure. Table 58.2 lists contraindications to surgical resection [10]. ERCP has a role in the palliation of obstructive jaundice. External beam radiation therapy with concomitant chemotherapy (5-fluorouracil, gemcitabine, paclitaxel) is primarily used for symptom palliation with modest improvements in mean survival.

Table 58.1 Differential diagnosis of mass lesions in the pancreas.

Pathologic diagnosis	Tumor type
Pancreatic adenocarcinoma	Malignant
Pancreatic neuroendocrine tumor	Malignant
Acinar cell carcinoma	Malignant
Metastatic tumor to the pancreas	Malignant
Lymphoma	Variable malignant grade
Cystic lesion of the pancreas	Benign, premalignant, or malignant
Focal pancreatitis	Benign
Autoimmune pancreatitis	Benign

Table 58.2 Absolute and relative contraindications to surgical resection of pancreatic cancer [10]. The range is represented from top (absolute) to bottom (relative) of the table.

Metastases to the liver, peritoneum, omentum, or any extra-abdominal site

Encasement of celiac axis, hepatic artery, or superior mesenteric artery

Involvement of splenoportal confluence

Involvement of bowel mesentery

Involvement of superior mesenteric vein or portal vein

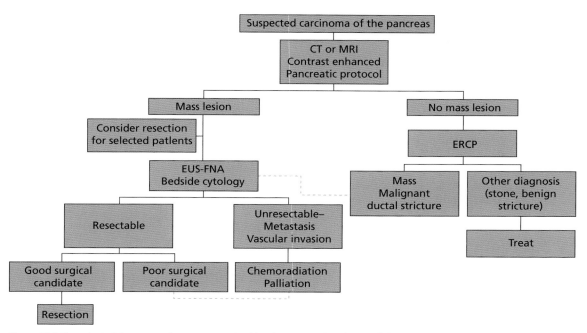

Figure 58.4 Flow chart of the proposed management algorithm for suspected carcinoma of the pancreas. EUS-FNA, endoscopic ultrasound guided fine needle aspiration; ERCP, endoscopic retrograde cholangiopancreaticography.

Case continued

The patient is not a candidate for resection due to involvement of the superior mesenteric artery (stage T4) and is referred to oncology. Oncology recommends chemoradiation therapy for palliation of symptoms. The patient undergoes chemoradiation therapy with initial improvement in his symptoms. His cancer progresses and he elects hospice care.

Prognosis

The prognosis for most patients with pancreatic adeno-carcinoma is poor. The 5-year survival is approximately 15% for patients with presumed localized disease who undergo resection [9]. Patients who do not receive cancer-directed therapy have a 5-year survival rate of 1–5% [11]. Less common pancreatic mass lesions such as neuroendocrine tumors have a much more favorable prognosis.

Take-home points

- Pancreatic cancer has a poor prognosis; however, a subset of patients may achieve a cure.
- Painless jaundice, new-onset diabetes, and weight loss with depression are concerning.
- Cross-sectional imaging is useful for diagnosis and staging.
- The double duct sign suggests a malignant obstruction.
- EUS with FNA can allow a tissue diagnosis and is highly sensitive for locoregional staging.

Cystic Pancreatic Neoplasms

Summary

Cystic neoplasms of the pancreas were thought to be relatively rare; however, the widespread use of cross-sectional imaging has dramatically increased their identification. These cystic lesions may represent true cysts or pseudocysts and may be benign, premalignant, or malignant. Although most lesions are discovered incidentally, some patients may present with jaundice, pancreatitis, or abdominal pain. Patients with a history of alcoholism or recurrent pancreatitis have a higher pretest probability of pseudocyst. Cross-sectional imaging and EUS with FNA are helpful in the stratification of patients by risk of malignancy. Resection is the definitive means of diagnosis and management. Management strategies such as observation are considered in older patients with co-morbidities and low risk features.

Case

A 76-year-old woman with congestive heart failure and hematuria undergoes a CT scan to rule out nephrolithiasis. A 2-cm cystic lesion is noted in the tail of the pancreas. She denies any history of pancreatitis or heavy alcohol consumption. She denies abdominal pain or discomfort. There is mild dilatation of the main pancreatic duct.

Definition and Epidemiology

While previously thought to be rare, the widespread use of cross-sectional imaging has revealed the presence of cystic lesions of the pancreas in a significant number of patients [12]. By autopsy, pancreatic cystic lesions may be found in 24% of patients [13]. Cystic lesions are more common in older patients, and the prevalence of neoplasia is related to age. The majority of cystic lesions are pseudocysts and do not have a true epithelial lining. Approximately 30% of lesions may represent true cysts with variable malignant potential.

Pathophysiology

The etiology of cystic lesions of the pancreas varies by cyst type, and the pathogenesis is not well understood. Pseudocysts are not true cystic lesions but represent extravasated pancreatic secretions and necrosis which has become walled off by neighboring structures and omentum. Serous cystadenoma is a benign multiloculated/multiseptated lesion lined by glycogen rich cells. Mucinous cystadenoma is a true cyst lined by columnar goblet cells and a stroma of ovarian-like epithelium. Intraductal papillary mucinous neoplasms (IPMN) may be multiple and are characterized by ductal communication and a lining of mucin-secreting cells.

Clinical Features

Patients with pseudocysts generally have a history of pancreatitis, often recurrent, and may have radiographic evidence of chronic pancreatitis (gland atrophy, duct dilatation, calcification of the parenchyma, calculi in pancreatic duct). Patients with true cysts are often asymptomatic. Symptoms attributed to cystic lesions include abdominal pain, jaundice, and weight loss, and some patients may develop recurrent pancreatitis.

Diagnosis

A history of pancreatitis or longstanding heavy alcohol use increases the pretest probability of pseudocyst. Cross-sectional imaging allows the visualization of calcifications, septa, and mural nodules, and can also suggest underlying chronic pancreatitis [14,15]; however, imaging alone is frequently insufficient for diagnosis.

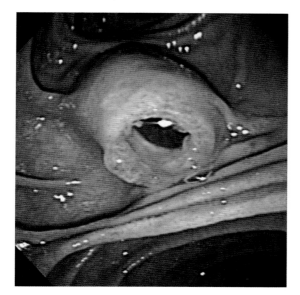

Figure 58.5 Endoscopic image of a classic fish mouth deformity, secondary to mucin overproduction and extrusion, pathognomonic for intraductal papillary mucinous neoplasm.

EUS provides a more sensitive examination and can be performed with FNA and aspiration of cyst fluid for amylase, tumor markers, cytology, and DNA analysis. High levels of carcinoembryonic antigen (CEA) are concerning for malignancy. ERCP may be useful in the evaluation of IPMN revealing a fish mouth deformity (extrusion of mucous from a widely patent ampulla (Figure 58.5)), mucinous filling defects within the pancreatogram, ductal dilatation, and/or cystic dilation of side branches. For a majority of patients, surgical resection with pathologic examination is the only definitive means of diagnosis.

Differential Diagnosis
See Table 58.3.

Therapeutics
Because of the risk of malignancy, surgical resection of suspected malignant cystic neoplasms may be indicated (Figure 58.6). A dilated main pancreatic duct, mural nodules, size greater than 3 cm, dysplasia on a biopsy, and the presence of pancreatic symptoms are indications for resection. Small incidental pancreatic cysts may enlarge over a prolonged period, and morbidity or mortality due to these cysts is low; therefore, observation may be a safe management option in some cases [16,17]. The decision to monitor high-risk patients with small (<2 cm)

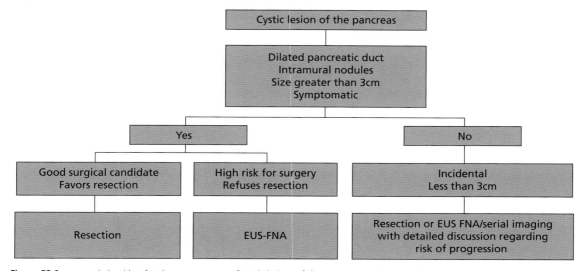

Figure 58.6 Proposed algorithm for the management of cystic lesions of the pancreas. EUS-FNA, endoscopic ultrasound guided fine needle aspiration.

Table 58.3 Features and characteristics of common cystic lesions of the pancreas. Other less common cystic lesions include cystic endocrine neoplasm, ductal adenocarcinoma with cystic degeneration, lymphoepithelial cyst, and acinar cell cystadenocarcinoma.

Cyst type	Pathology	Aspirate	CEA ng/mL	Amylase	Management
Pseudocyst: no true epithelial lining, walls are of adjacent structures Frequently associated with pain Look for gland atrophy, duct dilatation, calcification of the parenchyma, calculi in pancreatic duct	Develops as a result of pancreatic inflammation and necrosis, communicates with the ductal system Contains high concentrations of amylase Lining is fibrous with granulation tissue Lacks an epithelial lining.	Thin, dark, opaque, non-mucinous, with inflammatory cells	Low	High	No malignant potential, resection or endoscopic management indicated for symptoms
Mucinous cystadenoma: most common cystic neoplasm Typically occurs in middle-aged women Typically solitary 97% are distal (body and tail) May be malignant at time of diagnosis	Dense mesenchymal ovarian-like stroma Lack communication with pancreatic duct May have 1 or more macrocystic spaces lined by mucous-secreting cells Peripheral eggshell calcification is suggestive of malignancy	Viscous, clear, variable cellularity, positive for mucin	High >200	Low	After resection, non-invasive MCN–no recurrence
Serous cystadenoma: 2nd most common cystic tumor of the pancreas Middle-aged women Typically solitary Very LOW malignant potential Central scar highly suggestive but found in ~20%	Typically composed of multiple, small cysts lined by glycogen-rich cuboidal epithelium Chromosomal alterations of gene for von Hippel–Lindau locus 3p25 found in majority	Less viscous, thin, clear, non-mucinous, may be bloody	Low <5	Low	Resection is curative
Intraductal papillary mucinous neoplasm (side branch or main duct) Patients may have multiple cysts More common in men A dilated pancreatic duct implies a main duct IPMN Mucin extrusion from widely patent ampulla (fish mouth deformity) is pathognomonic Side branch IPMN is more common	Consists of dilated ductal segments, usually within the head of the pancreas, lined by mucous-secreting cells Main duct IPMN has greater malignant potential Mural nodules and a segmental or diffuse dilation of the pancreatic duct >15 mm are worrisome for malignancy	Viscous, clear, with mucin	High (>1000 concerning for malignancy)	High	Resection (especially for patients with nodules or symptoms) Serial imaging for high-risk patients with low-risk features

CEA, carcinoembryonic antigen; IPMN, intraductal papillary mucinous neoplasm.

incidental cystic neoplasms should follow a discussion regarding the low risk of cancer (3.5%) but high risk of progression to malignancy (50%) [12]. Most mucinous cystic neoplasms are located in the tail of the pancreas. The risk of progression can be weighed against the risk of postoperative pancreatic fistula (29%) and mortality (0.8%) with distal pancreatectomy [18]. Surveillance can be performed with CT, magnet resonance imaging (MRI), or EUS-FNA. Resection may be readdressed if imaging demonstrates a significant change in diameter or morphology.

Case continued

The patient is referred for EUS with FNA. EUS-FNA reveals a 2-cm lesion with a mural nodule and mild main pancreatic ductal dilation. A distal pancreatectomy is performed, revealing IPMN. The patient develops a postoperative pancreatic leak but recovers and is discharged home.

Prognosis

The prognosis for cystic lesions of the pancreas is much better than for pancreatic cancer. Many patients have a benign condition and many patients with a premalignant lesion will be cured with surgical resection.

Take-home points

- Cystic lesions of the pancreas may be benign or malignant.
- EUS with FNA is helpful tool in the evaluation of cystic lesions.
- A fish mouth deformity with mucin extrusion from the ampulla is pathognomonic for IPMN.
- Peripheral eggshell calcification suggests a mucinous neoplasm.
- A multicystic lesion with a central scar indicates a serous cystadenoma.

References

1 Winter JM, Maitra A, Yeo CJ. Genetics and pathology of pancreatic cancer. *HPB (Oxford)* 2006; **8**: 324–36.
2 Jemal A, Siegel R, Ward E, *et al.* Cancer statistics, 2007. *CA Cancer J Clin* 2007; **57**: 43–66.
3 Li D, Xie K, Wolff R, Abbruzzese JL. Pancreatic cancer. *Lancet* 2004; **363**: 1049–57.
4 Almoguera C, Shibata D, Forrester K, *et al.* Most human carcinomas of the exocrine pancreas contain mutant c-K-ras genes. *Cell* 1988; **53**: 549–54.
5 Schutte M, Hruban RH, Geradts J, *et al.* Abrogation of the Rb/p16 tumor-suppressive pathway in virtually all pancreatic carcinomas. *Cancer Res* 1997; **57**: 3126–30.
6 Howes N, Lerch MM, Greenhalf W, *et al.* Clinical and genetic characteristics of hereditary pancreatitis in Europe. *Clin Gastroenterol Hepatol* 2004; **2**: 252–61.
7 Lowenfels AB, Maisonneuve P, DiMagno EP, *et al.* Hereditary pancreatitis and the risk of pancreatic cancer. International Hereditary Pancreatitis Study Group. *J Natl Cancer Inst* 1997; **89**: 442–6.
8 Brentnall TA. Management strategies for patients with hereditary pancreatic cancer. *Curr Treat Options Oncol* 2005; **6**: 437–45.
9 Mulcahy MF. Adjuvant therapy for pancreas cancer: advances and controversies. *Semin Oncol* 2007; **34**: 321–6.
10 Ryan DP, Fernandez-del Castillo C, Willett CG, *et al.* Case records of the Massachusetts General Hospital. Case 20-2005. A 58-year-old man with locally advanced pancreatic cancer. *N Engl J Med* 2005; **352**: 2734–41.
11 Ujiki MB, Talamonti MS. Guidelines for the surgical management of pancreatic adenocarcinoma. *Semin Oncol* 2007; **34**: 311–20.
12 Fernandez-del Castillo C, Targarona J, Thayer SP, *et al.* Incidental pancreatic cysts: clinicopathologic characteristics and comparison with symptomatic patients. *Arch Surg* 2003; **138**: 427–3; discussion 33–4.
13 Kimura W, Nagai H, Kuroda A, *et al.* Analysis of small cystic lesions of the pancreas. *Int J Pancreatol* 1995; **18**: 197–206.
14 Curry CA, Eng J, Horton KM, *et al.* CT of primary cystic pancreatic neoplasms: can CT be used for patient triage and treatment? *AJR Am J Roentgenol* 2000; **175**: 99–103.
15 Minami M, Itai Y, Ohtomo K, *et al.* Cystic neoplasms of the pancreas: comparison of MR imaging with CT. *Radiology* 1989; **171**: 53–6.
16 Edirimanne S, Connor SJ. Incidental pancreatic cystic lesions. *World J Surg* 2008; **32**: 2028–37.
17 Garcea G, Ong SL, Rajesh A, *et al.* Cystic lesions of the pancreas. A diagnostic and management dilemma. *Pancreatology* 2008; **8**: 236–51.
18 Ferrone CR, Warshaw AL, Rattner DW, *et al.* Pancreatic fistula rates after 462 distal pancreatectomies: staplers do not decrease fistula rates. *J Gastrointest Surg* 2008; **12**: 1691–7; discussion 7–8.

CHAPTER 59

Palliation of Malignant Biliary Obstruction

Yan Zhong and Nib Soehendra

Endoscopy Practice am Glockengiesserwall, Hamburg, Germany

Summary

Obstruction due to pancreatic cancer predominantly affects the distal common bile duct (CBD) and the ductal system of the gland itself, causing jaundice, pruritus, pain, maldigestion, and malabsorption. Involvement of the duodenum is less frequent, and usually occurs in advanced stage of the disease. Palliation of these malignant obstructions is achieved with either stenting or surgical bypass. Non-surgical endoscopic or percutaneous-transhepatic biliary drainage is generally preferred because it is less invasive as compared to surgical bypass. For malignant distal CBD obstruction, endoscopic transpapillary stent placement is the treatment of choice. Percutaneous transhepatic approach may be needed in cases of failed or insufficient endoscopic drainage. In such cases, transpapillary stent placement by combined radiologic and endoscopic approach (rendezvous technique) is preferable. Gastric outlet obstruction is increasingly managed non-surgically with endoscopic stenting.

Case

A 74-year-old male presents with progressive vomiting, jaundice, and abdominal pain. CT scan revealed a 5-cm mass in the head of pancreas, compressing the second portion of the duodenum with a distended stomach and common bile duct (CBD). Multiple, small, rim-enhancing lesions were seen in the liver consistent with metastases. An endoscopic retrograde cholangiopancreatography (ERCP) was performed. After initial endoscopic balloon dilation of the duodenal narrowing, an expandable metal stent was placed across a distal common bile duct stricture. A second luminal stent was place through the endoscopic in the duodenum with the distal end just proximal to the ampulla (Figure 59.1). Brushing from the bile duct revealed adenocarcinoma. The patient's obstructive symptoms were relieved. He survived 4 months after the initial stent placement, while receiving palliative chemotherapy.

Practical Gastroenterology and Hepatology: Small and Large Intestine and Pancreas, 1st edition. Edited by Nicholas J. Talley, Sunanda V. Kane and Michael B. Wallace. © 2010 Blackwell Publishing Ltd.

Introduction

In the majority of cases, malignant biliary obstruction is caused by pancreatic cancer located mainly in the pancreatic head. Obstructive jaundice is the most frequent leading symptom and usually presents in the late stage of the disease, explaining the dismal prognosis of these patients. The 5-year survival remains less than 5% [1]. Palliative measures therefore form the mainstay of the treatment. For the most common distal CBD obstruction caused by unresectable malignant tumors, endoscopic stenting is widely accepted as the first-line palliative treatment, because it is less invasive as compared to percutaneous-transhepatic drainage (PTCD) and surgical bypass [2].

In case of failed endoscopic stenting, a 5 French catheter can be placed percutaneous-transhepatically and a hydrophilic guidewire negotiated through the papilla, enabling endoscopic transpapillary placement of a large-bore stent. This combined "rendezvous" technique, also used in patients after Whipple procedure, is associated with a lower risk as compared to PTCD alone.

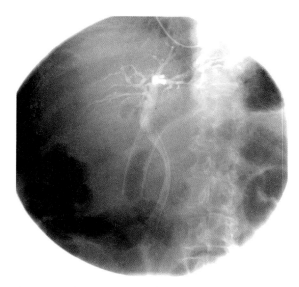

Figure 59.1 Fluoroscopic image of common bile duct and duodenal expandable metal stent. (Courtesy of Dr Todd Baron.)

In patients with proximal biliary obstruction involving the intrahepatic ducts, magnetic resonance cholangio-pancreatography (MRCP) may be helpful to assist targeted drainage, hence reducing the risk of contamination and cholangitis [3].

The indication for stenting is based on clinical evaluation which includes the patient's symptoms, condition, age, and tumor stage. The decision whether the patient will benefit more from surgery needs to be made in an interdisciplinary meeting with the oncologist and the surgeon. Patients suffering from severe jaundice and concomitant cholangitis are, apart from medical treatment, subjected to immediate endoscopic drainage.

Stenting of Distal CBD Obstructions

For palliation of malignant distal CBD obstruction, 10–11.5 French plastic stents are still commonly used, as they provide sufficient drainage in the majority of inoperable patients; the median patency durations ranging from 62 to 165 days. Self-expandable metal stents (SEMS) provide a lumen diameter of 10 mm with significantly better immediate drainage effect; the median patency durations ranging from 111 to 273 days. The median survival of stented patients usually ranges from 99 to 175 days, sug-

gesting that many of them die before either stent occludes [4]. Thus, patients with a predicted longer survival and/or cholangitis may benefit more from SEMS. However, it should be mentioned that patient survival may be prolonged with improved chemotherapy [5]; hence occlusion of SEMS appears to be seen more frequently in these patients and, in case of recurrent jaundice, placement of either a plastic stent or a covered SEMS through the occluded SEMS is required.

Choice of Stent

Plastic stents are made of radiopaque polyethylene or Teflon. Most of the plastic stents are made of polyethylene because probably it is easier to extrude as compared to Teflon. Teflon has, however, a smoother surface and is stiffer than polyethylene, and therefore preferable for tight strictures. In comparisons, however, there have been no statistical difference found between the two stent materials with regards to technical success, 30-day mortality, or patency [4].

For distal CBD strictures plastic stents should be curved, adapting to the ductal anatomy. To prevent migration in both directions and to facilitate drainage, side flaps and side holes are made at both ends of the stent. Double-pigtail stents provide the best prevention of dislocation and perforation (Figure 59.2). The Tannenbaum Teflon stent (three-layered stent) without side holes was thought to improve patency by avoiding sludge formation at the side holes and plant fibers sticking at the side flaps. However, in comparison to polyethylene stent with side holes, this type of stent did not show a statistically significant improvement of drainage [6].

Uncovered SEMS with 10 mm lumen diameter showed significantly lower recurrence rate of jaundice, as compared to plastic stents. Newer SEMS are made of more flexible nitinol wire. Covered SEMS have been developed to prevent tumor ingrowth, thus prolonging patency. However, they may be more prone to migration and associated with higher risk of cholecystitis and pancreatitis [7].

Compared to plastic stents, SEMS did not show statistically significant improvement of survival. Furthermore, no difference between these two stent types has been found with regard to technical success, therapeutic success, complication, or 30-day mortality. However, patients treated with SEMS need fewer re-interventions due to stent occlusion [4].

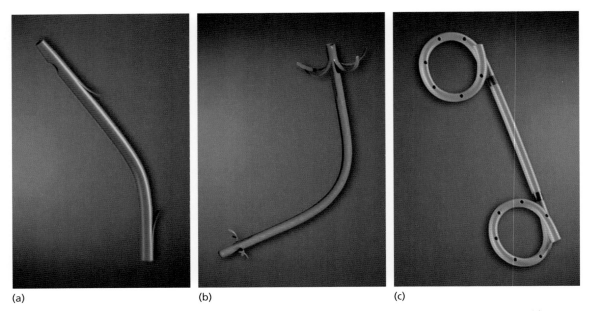

Figure 59.2 Commonly used plastic stents made of radiopaque polyethylene or Teflon. (a) Polyethylene stent with side holes and flaps at both ends. (b) Tannenbaum stent without side holes. (c) Double-pigtail stent.

There are no strict criteria for making an optimal stent choice. Patient survival appears to be one of the decisive factors. However, the life expectancy of patients with advanced pancreatic cancer is difficult to predict. According to a prospective multicenter trial, the median survival of patients with inoperable malignant distal CBD obstruction was 4.7 months, and the median survival of patients with a tumor larger than 3 cm was 3.2 months [8]. Liver metastases were found to be another independent factor related to survival. Median survival of these patients was 2.7 months [9]. When cost-effectiveness is considered, plastic stent should be sufficient for initial biliary drainage in patients with a tumor larger than 3 cm and/or hepatic metastases. Initial endoscopic placement of a SEMS is cost-effective in patients expected to survive longer than 4 months, particularly if the cost of endoscopic re-intervention is significantly higher than that of a metal stent [4].

Follow up

Since 40 to 50% of stented patients survive beyond 4 months [4], surveillance after initial endoscopic placement of a plastic stent is required. To prevent cholangitis caused by stent occlusion, scheduled follow-up after 3 months has been recommended. Most important is that the patient and the family are informed about the possibility of stent clogging. If signs of cholangitis (fever) and cholestasis (dark urine and light-colored stools) occur, patients must be immediately readmitted to the hospital for stent exchange. In case of purulent cholangitis, apart from intravenous administration of antibiotics and other conservative measures, a nasobiliary catheter may be additionally placed following stent exchange to allow irrigation of the bile duct. For patients with frank cholangitis, SEMS is the treatment of choice enabling rapid drainage of the infected bile duct and re-establishment of bile flow.

Duodenal Stenting

Around 10% of patients with malignant distal biliary obstruction eventually develop duodenal stenosis. Most patients with malignant gastric outlet obstruction can be palliatively managed by placing an uncovered SEMS. Duodenal metal stents are made of nitinol and have a diameter of 18 to 22 mm. The delivery catheter of the stent has a diameter of 10.5 French, so that it can be introduced through a therapeutic gastroscope with a working channel of 3.7 to 3.8 mm. If the stenosis cannot be traversed with the therapeutic gastroscope, a biliary hydrophilic guidewire is first placed under fluoroscopic monitor or using a slim pediatric endoscope. The through-the-scope (TTS) placement and deployment of the stent is performed under additional fluoroscopic monitor (see Video 18). A systematic review of the literature confirmed a technical success rate of 97% and a clinical success rate of 89%. Severe complications occurred in 1.2%. There was no reported procedure-related mortality. Stent occlusion occurred in 18%, and migration in 5% of the cases [10].

In patients presenting both biliary and duodenal obstruction, an uncovered duodenal stent is first placed. To enable subsequent biliary stent placement, complete expansion of the duodenal stent is achieved by using a 20 mm sized TTS dilating balloon catheter. Alternatively, a SEMS biliary stent is placed 24 to 48 h after the duode- nal stent has fully expanded (see Video 19).

Pancreatic Duct Stenting

Most of the patients with malignant jaundice do not suffer from pain. In case of "obstructive"-type pain identified by correlation with meals, endoscopic transpapillary stenting of the obstructed pancreatic duct may provide complete relief of pain in about 60% of patients and partial relief in 25% [11].

Take-home points

- Malignant obstruction due to pancreatic cancer affects distal CBD, pancreatic main duct, and the duodenum.
- Most of these obstructions can be palliated by endoscopic stenting.
- Ductal decompression is achieved using either plastic or self-expandable metal stent (SEMS). SEMS provides a better immediate drainage and a longer patency. SEMS is therefore preferable in patients with life expectancy of longer than 6 months.
- In patients with liver metastases, MRCP may be helpful to determine whether stenting is justified, and to facilitate targeted stent placement.

- Gastric outlet obstruction is treated either with surgical bypass or endoscopic placement of SEMS.
- Complex obstructions occur particularly in patients with postsurgical recurrence and may be managed by a combined endoscopic and percutaneous-transhepatic procedure (rendezvous technique).

References

1 Wray CJ, Ahmad SA, Matthews JB, Lowy AM. Surgery for pancreatic cancer: Recent controversies and current practice. *Gastroenterology* 2005; **128**: 1626–41.

2 Johnson CD. Guidelines for the management of patients with pancreatic cancer periampullary and ampullary carcinomas. *Gut* 2005; **54** (Suppl .V): v1–v16.

3 Hintze RE, Abou-Rebyeh H, Adler A, *et al.* Magnetic resonance cholangiopancreatography-guided unilateral endoscopic stent placement for Klatskin tumors. *Gastrointest Endosc* 2001; **53**: 40–6.

4 Moss AC, Morris E, MacMathuna P. Palliative biliary stents for obstructing pancreatic carcinoma (Review). *Cochrane Database Syst Rev* 2006, 2.

5 Lockhart AC, Rothenberg ML, Berlin JD. Treatment for pancreatic cancer: Current therapy and continued progress. *Gastroenterology* 2005; **128**: 1642–54.

6 England RE, Martin DF, Morris J, *et al.* A prospective randomized multicentre trial comparing 10 Fr Teflon Tannenbaum stents with 10 Fr polyethylene Cotton-Leung stents in patients with malignant common duct strictures. *Gut* 2000; **46**: 395–400.

7 Isayama H, Komatsu Y, Tsujino T, *et al.* A prospective randomised study of "covered" versus "uncovered" diamond stents for the management of distal malignant biliary obstruction. *Gut* 2004; **53**: 729–34.

8 Prat F, Chapat O, Ducot B, *et al.* Predictive factors for survival of patients with inoperable malignant distal biliary strictures: a practical management guideline. *Gut* 1998; **42**: 76–80.

9 Kaassis M, Boyer J, Dumas R, *et al.* Plastic or metal stents for malignant stricture of the common bile duct? Results of a randomized prospective study. *Gastrointest Endosc* 2003; **57**: 178–82.

10 Dormann A, Meisner S, Verin N, Wenk Lang A. Self-expanding metal stents for gastroduodenal malignancies: systematic review of their clinical effectiveness. *Endoscopy* 2004; **36**: 543–50.

11 Costamagna G, Mutignani M. Pancreatic stenting for malignant ductal obstruction. *Dig Liver Dis* 2004; **36**: 635–8.

PART 8

Functional Gastrointestinal Disorders

CHAPTER 60
Irritable Bowel Syndrome

Elizabeth J. Videlock and Lin Chang

Center for Neurobiology of Stress, Division of Digestive Diseases, David Geffen School of Medicine at UCLA, Los Angeles, CA, USA

Summary

Irritable bowel syndrome (IBS) is a prevalent chronic gastrointestinal disorder. The diagnosis is based on the presence of chronic or recurrent abdominal pain associated with altered bowel habits, although IBS is heterogeneous because symptoms can vary amongst affected individuals. While IBS can sometimes be challenging to manage, patient care should be focused on reducing costs and improving patient satisfaction and health-related quality of life. There are frequent advances in our knowledge about the clinical presentation, pathophysiology, and treatment of IBS. This chapter reviews current theories of pathophysiology as well as epidemiology, symptoms, co-morbidities, and current and evidence-based approaches to evaluation and treatment of IBS. Emphasis is placed on the importance of biopsychosocial aspects of care in addition to symptom management.

Case

A 28-year-old woman is referred to a gastroenterologist by her primary care physician for evaluation and management of abdominal pain and constipation for the past year. The patient reports having intermittent abdominal pain and bloating that are associated with feeling constipated. Her constipation symptoms include hard stools, difficulty evacuating stools, and sensation of incomplete evacuation. She has a bowel movement every 1 to 2 days. Her abdominal pain and bloating improve after having a bowel movement. She has had similar symptoms since college, which she associated with stress, but they were milder and she never sought care for them. Now her symptoms, especially the pain and bloating, make it difficult for her to concentrate on her work, and she misses work 1–2 days per month. Her sleep is sometimes disturbed, particularly when her symptoms are worse and she feels tired during the day. She has tried increasing her fluid intake and different over-the-counter laxatives and fiber supplements. While these medications help to loosen her stool, she does not like taking them. The

discomfort and urgency caused by the laxatives are very bothersome, and she still has pain and bloating which is sometimes increased with the medication. She denies unintentional weight loss, blood in the stool, and a family history of colon cancer. She has annual pelvic examinations by her gynecologist and they have been normal. Her physical examination is normal except for a mildly distended lower abdomen which is tender to palpation without rebound. A rectal examination is normal without paradoxical pelvic floor contraction during bear down command. The diagnosis of irritable bowel syndrome with constipation is discussed with the patient. She is reassured that while the symptoms can be debilitating and difficult to treat, they can be managed with appropriate care. Educational materials are given to the patient. After several regular visits with her provider, her symptoms have improved by avoiding certain food triggers and starting lubiprostone. Although her abdominal pain, bloating, and sensation of incomplete evacuation are improved, she continues to be bothered by these symptoms. A low dose of a tricyclic antidepressant as well as a probiotic are recommended.

Practical Gastroenterology and Hepatology: Small and Large Intestine and Pancreas, 1st edition. Edited by Nicholas J. Talley, Sunanda V. Kane and Michael B. Wallace. © 2010 Blackwell Publishing Ltd.

Definition and Epidemiology

Irritable bowel syndrome (IBS) is a functional gastrointestinal (GI) disorder characterized by abdominal pain that is associated with alterations in stool form and/or frequency. IBS is frequently diagnosed in both primary care and specialty practices. It has a high worldwide prevalence and is estimated to affect 7–15% of the general population in the United States. IBS accounts for significant health care costs with annual direct and indirect costs estimated at $1.35 billion and at least $200 million, respectively [1].

Pathophysiology

Our understanding of the pathogenesis of IBS has evolved over recent years but is still far from complete. A unifying theme is that the symptoms of IBS result from dysregulation of the "brain–gut axis," which manifests as enhanced visceral perception. There is not a consensus on the underlying etiology of this dysregulation, and the disorder may represent a combination of factors. Evidence suggests that the symptom constellation of IBS may arise from several etiologies which can differ within subgroups of patients. Figure 60.1 illustrates the range of vulnerability factors and pathophysiologic mechanisms within the brain–gut axis which can contribute to the onset and exacerbation of symptoms of IBS. Due to the fact that IBS is a multicomponent disorder with a complex pathophysiology, biomarkers that can reliably diagnose IBS or monitor treatment response are currently lacking.

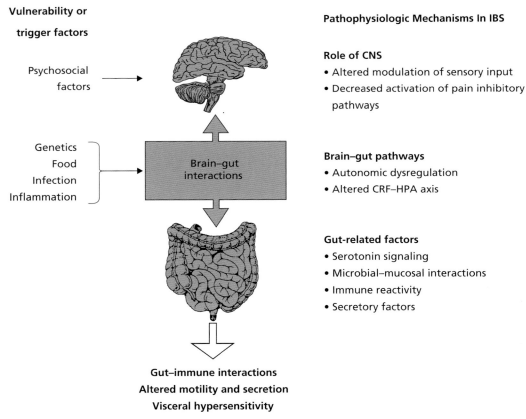

Figure 60.1 Both "brain" and "gut" related mechanisms as well as their interactions are being explored in IBS. IBS patients show an enhanced responsiveness of this system manifesting in altered modulation of gastrointestinal motility and secretion and enhanced perception of visceral events. IBS, irritable bowel syndrome; CNS, central nervous system; CRF, corticotropin releasing factor; HPA, hypothalamic–pituitary–adrenal.

Table 60.1 The symptom-based Rome III criteria for the diagnosis of irritable bowel syndrome.

These criteria should be filled for the last 3 months with symptom onset at least 6 months prior to diagnosis:

    Recurrent abdominal pain or discomfort* at least 3 days per month in the last 3 months that is associated with 2 or more of the following:
    Improvement with defecation
    Onset associated with a change in frequency of stool
    Onset associated with a change in form (appearance) of stool

Supportive symptoms (non-diagnostic)
    Abnormal stool frequency (<3 bowel movements per week or >3 bowel movements per day)
    Abnormal stool form (lumpy/hard stool or loose/watery stool)
    Defecation straining, urgency, or a feeling of incomplete evacuation
    Passing mucus
    Bloating

*Discomfort means an uncomfortable sensation not described as pain.

Table 60.2 Irritable bowel syndrome subtypes by bowel habit.

Subtype*	Percent of stools that meet the description	
	Hard or lumpy stools	Loose or watery stools
IBS with constipation (IBS-C)	≥25%	<25%
IBS with diarrhea (IBS-D)	<25%	≥25%
Mixed IBS (IBS-M)†	≥25%	≥25%
Unsubtyped IBS (IBS-U)	<25%	<25%

*The word *with* is preferred to *predominant* due to symptom instability.

†Patients with both diarrhea and constipation that may alternate within hours or days were previously classified as IBS-A according to the Rome II criteria but should now be referred to as IBS-M. The category of alternating IBS (IBS-A) should be reserved for patients with bowel habits that have changed over time, e.g., weeks to months.

Clinical Features

Gastrointestinal Symptoms

The key symptom of IBS is chronic or recurrent abdominal pain and/or discomfort associated with altered bowel habits. The Rome III criteria for the diagnosis of IBS were published in 2006 and are listed in Table 60.1 along with other supporting symptoms that are commonly present but not included in the diagnostic criteria [2]. IBS is often subgrouped by predominant bowel habit. Because stool form was found to be the best predictor of predominant bowel habit in IBS, stool form rather than frequency determines classification according to Rome III [2]. These criteria are outlined in Table 60.2. The prevalence of IBS with diarrhea (IBS-D), IBS with constipation (IBS-C), and IBS with a mixed pattern (IBS-M) are similar, but IBS-M is the subtype most frequently encountered in primary care. Patients change subtypes frequently, with the IBS-M group being the least stable with transitions to and from IBS-C and to a lesser extent with IBS-D [3].

Extraintestinal Symptoms and Co-morbid Disorders

IBS patients make more health-care visits and incur more health-care costs than individuals without IBS. More than half of additional visits and additional costs are for non-GI concerns [4]. Non-GI symptoms that are more common in IBS than controls include the following (prevalence): headache (23–45%), back pain (27–81%), fatigue (36–63%), myalgia (29–36%), dyspareunia (9–42%), urinary frequency (21–61%), other urinary symptoms, and dizziness (11–27%). IBS patients with co-morbid somatic disorders (e.g., fibromyalgia) report more severe IBS symptoms and lower health-related quality of life (HRQOL) [4]. Common co-morbid GI and somatic disorders include gastroesophageal reflux disease (GERD), functional dyspepsia, fibromyalgia, chronic fatigue syndrome, chronic pelvic pain, temporomandibular joint disorder, and interstitial cystitis [5]. There is a higher prevalence of psychiatric disorders in the IBS population than in controls, which is most evident in those with more severe symptoms and in tertiary referral clinics.

Diagnosis

The differential diagnosis for the symptoms of IBS (Table 60.3) is very broad; however, use of the symptom-based Rome III criteria and evaluation for alarm signs or symptoms, as well as excluding celiac disease in some populations, is sufficient to make the diagnosis of IBS. While the presence of "red flag" or alarm signs and symptoms (Table 60.4) may indicate a need for further diagnostic workup, it is not recommended that patients with red flag symptoms be excluded from the diagnosis of IBS. On average, IBS patients report the presence of at least 1.65 red flag symptoms but these have a low positive predictive value for organic disease [6]. Nocturnal symptoms (40%) and onset over the age of 50 (32%) are the most common alarm signs.

Historically, IBS has been a diagnosis of exclusion, but the current best evidence suggests that a battery of diagnostic tests is not necessary. The prevalence of organic disease in the population with symptoms of IBS (particularly in those without alarm features) is similar to that in the general population with the exception of celiac disease [7]. There is good evidence that serologic testing for celiac disease followed by endoscopic biopsy confirmation of positive results is a cost-effective strategy in North American IBS-D patients [8]. Additionally, a negative finding on colonoscopy is not associated with an increased sense of reassurance in patients with IBS [9]. Testing of GI motility and visceral sensation is commonly used in research settings, but their use in clinical practice is limited due to their invasive nature and small to moderate correlations with global or even specific IBS symptoms and treatment response.

Management

An approach to management of IBS is outlined in Figures 60.2 and 60.3. Assessing severity and impact of the symptoms on the patient's HRQOL is important, as this will shape a management strategy. Although IBS is characterized by altered stool frequency and/or consistency, the astute clinician will not assume that the patient seeks care primarily for the relief of these symptoms. Some patients seek care out of fear that they have a life-threatening illness such as colon cancer. These patients may find relief in receiving a positive diagnosis, reassurance, and education and may not require pharmacotherapy. However, patients with moderate to severe symptoms often require pharmacological and/or psychological therapies.

Table 60.4 Alarm features.

Recent symptom onset at age ≥50 years
Unintentional weight loss
Family history of GI malignancy
Severe, unrelenting large volume diarrhea
Fevers, chills, recent travel to endemic region
Nocturnal diarrhea
Hematochezia
Relevant findings on physical exam (arthritis, skin lesions, lymphadenopathy, abdominal mass)

Table 60.3 Differential diagnosis of irritable bowel syndrome.

Colon cancer
Inflammatory bowel disease (IBD)
Malabsorption disorders (e.g., celiac disease, chronic pancreatitis)
Parasitic infection
Dietary factors (lactose and fructose intolerance)
Carcinoid
Gynecologic conditions (e.g., endometriosis)
Psychological conditions (e.g., depression, anxiety)

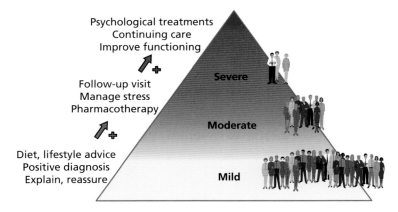

Psychological treatments
Continuing care
Improve functioning

Severe

Follow-up visit
Manage stress
Pharmacotherapy

Moderate

Diet, lifestyle advice
Positive diagnosis
Explain, reassure

Mild

Figure 60.2 Severely affected patients often suffer anxiety, depression, or panic in addition to severe GI symptoms and are those most often encountered by specialists, or in tertiary care. Often such patients are best managed by a multidisciplinary team including a primary care physician, a specialist, and psychologist and/or psychiatrist. Permission to use granted by the Rome Foundation.

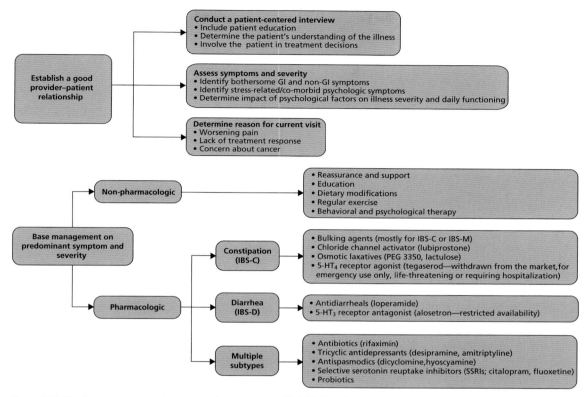

Figure 60.3 This flow-chart represents an approach to treatment of irritable bowel syndrome. A non-pharmacologic approach is recommended initially and the use of medication should not preclude trials of non-pharmacologic therapies; a combination of both may be required.

Patient-centered Care

A good health-care provider–patient relationship is the cornerstone of effective care of IBS. The quality of this relationship has been shown to improve patient outcomes [10]. Elements of a good provider–patient relationship are listed in Figure 60.3. Additionally, addressing psychosocial factors may improve health status and treatment response [11].

Non-pharmacologic Therapies

Diet. While in most patients symptoms cannot be completely relieved through diet alterations alone, including elimination diets, diet-related exacerbations can be minimized. Trigger foods may be identified if the patient keeps a food and symptom diary. Common food triggers include high-fat foods, raw fruits and vegetables, and caffeinated beverages.

Psychotherapy and Hypnotherapy. There are several psychological and behavioral treatments for which there is convincing evidence of efficacy [12]. Cognitive–behavioral therapy (CBT) is a short-term, goal-oriented form of psychotherapy that focuses on the role that thoughts play in determining behaviors and emotional responses. Gut-directed hypnotherapy (GDH) is hypnosis that is directed towards relaxation and control of intestinal motility by repeated suggestion of control over symptoms followed by ego-strengthening.

Pharmacologic Therapy

Pharmacologic therapies are summarized in Table 60.5, which is designed to be a practical clinical reference and includes recommended dosages, pertinent information, and numbers needed to treat where available.

Table 60.5 Agents available to treat irritable bowel syndrome by predominant symptom.

Drug class	Generic name	Dose	Comments	NNT [Ref.]
Constipation				
Bulking agents	Psyllium	1–3 tbsp daily	First-line for mild–moderate constipation. Start with 4 g/d; gradually increase over 2–3 weeks to 20–25 g/d	6 [30]
	Methycellulose	1–3 tbsp daily		
	Polycarbophil	2–4 tablets daily		
Osmotic laxatives	Milk of Magnesia	1–2 tbsp daily-bid		
	Magnesium citrate	6–12 oz (177–354 mL)		
	Lactulose	1–2 tbsp daily-bid		
	Polyethylene glycol	17 g in 237 mL (8 oz fluid)		
	Sorbitol	1–2 tbsp daily-bid		
Stimulant laxatives	Senna	8.6 mg tablets; 1–2 tablets qd		
	Ricinoleic acid (Castor oil)	1–2 tbsp daily		
	Diphenylmethane derivatives (e.g., bisacodyl)	10 mg 1–2 tablets qd or 1 suppository qd		
Emollient laxatives	Docusates	100 mg; 1–3 tablets qd		
	Mineral oil	1 tspn–1 tbsp qd		
5-HT$_4$ agonist	Tegaserod	6 mg bid	Emergency use only	11 [31]
Chloride channel activator	Lubiprostone	8 μg bid	Also available in 24 μg for chronic constipation	
Diarrhea				
Antidiarrheals	Loperamide	1 tablet qid	Use prophylactically (start at 1/d but can use up to 8/d)	
	Diphenoxylate	1–2 tablets tid		
Binding agents	Cholestyramine	1 g bid to qid		
5-HT$_3$ antagonist	Alosetron	0.5 mg to 1 mg daily-bid	Women with severe IBS-D, only through restricted use program	8 [32]

Category	Drug	Dose	Comments	NNT
Tricyclic antidepressants	Amitriptyline	10–150 mg qhs	Sedating	4 [22]
	Doxepin	10–150 mg qhs	Sedating	
	Imipramine	10–150 mg qhs		
	Clomipramine	25–100 mg qhs		
	Trimipramine	10–150 mg qhs		
	Desipramine	10–150 mg qhs	Most evidence for efficacy; less sedation and constipation Least sedating	
	Nortriptyline	10–150 mg qhs		
Antibiotics	Rifaximin	400 mg tid for 10–14 days		
Pain/bloating				
Antispasmodics	Hyoscamine sulfate	0.125 mg sl/po qid prn, 0.375 mg po bid	May be difficult for some patients to tolerate due to side effects	3.5 [15]
	Dicyclomine	10 mg po bid		
	Propantheline hydrocholoride	15 mg tid ac and 30 mg qhs		
	Clidinium + chlordiazepoxide	5–10 mg tid–qid		
	Hyoscamine + scopolamine + atropine + phenobarbital	1–2 tablets tid–qid		
TCAs	See above			
SSRIs	Fluoxetine	10–40 mg daily	Long half-life; less withdrawal effects	3.5 [22]
	Citalopram	20 mg daily	Less side effects and drug interactions	
	Paroxetine	20–50 mg daily	Short half-life; more withdrawal effects; more anticholinergic effect; use in IBS-D	
	Sertraline	25–100 mg daily	Less side effects and drug interactions	
	Escitalopram	10 mg daily		
SNRIs	Venlafaxine	37.5–75 mg bid–tid	Duloxetine is FDA approved for depression and diabetic neuropathy	
	Duloxetine	40–60 mg daily	Unlabeled uses include chronic pain syndromes, fibromyalgia, stress incontinence	
5 HT$_4$ agonist	Tegaserod	See above		
Antibiotics	Rifaximin	400 mg tid	Ongoing open labeled trial for IBS	
Probiotics	*Bifidobacterium infantis*	1 tablet daily		
	VSL # 3	1 packet bid		

NNT, number needed to treat; bid, twice daily; tid, three times daily; qd, once a day; qid four times daily; qhs, at night; tbsp, tablespoon; tspn, teaspoon, ac, before meals; CIC, chloride channel; sl, sublingual; po, per orally; prn, as needed.

Bulking Agents. Bulking agents include psyllium, methylcellulose, corn fiber, calcium polycarbophil, and ispaghula husk. Fiber supplementation has often been used as initial management of IBS. Fiber may increase stool frequency in IBS-C, but this may not be well-correlated with relief of pain or other symptoms. Additionally, bulking agents in quantities that are therapeutic can cause adverse effects including bloating and abdominal pain and discomfort, and therefore it may be helpful to recommend a gradual initiation of the dose to minimize side effects, particularly in those who have relatively little fiber in their diets or those with predominant bloating [13]. Soluble fiber (psyllium, ispaghula, calcium polycarbophil) is more effective than insoluble fiber (corn, wheat bran) [14].

Antidiarrheal Agents. While loperamide appears to be effective at prolonging intestinal transit time and improving stool consistency in IBS-D, the use of antidiarrheal agents has shown no benefit for global IBS symptoms or abdominal pain [13]. These agents, which can be used on a regular or an as-needed basis, may be very useful in some IBS-D patients to manage stool urgency, frequency, and fecal incontinence. It is often useful for patients to use antidiarrheals prophylactically before leaving the house, a long car trip, meal, or a stressful event. This can decrease both the diarrhea during a flare and the anticipatory anxiety often felt by IBS patients due to the unpredictable nature of symptom exacerbations.

Laxatives. Although no randomized, controlled studies evaluating the efficacy of osmotic or stimulant laxatives have been conducted in IBS, they may be useful in treating constipation symptoms in those with IBS-C. Osmotic laxatives are available over-the-counter and are widely used in the treatment of IBS-C and chronic constipation. Polyethylene glycol or magnesium-containing products are generally safe and well tolerated. Polyethylene glycol can be easily titrated by the patient under the supervision of the physician. Lactulose and sorbitol may also increase stool frequency, but are often associated with the side effects of bloating and/or cramping in IBS patients. Although there are insufficient data to determine their efficacy in IBS, stimulant laxatives such as senna, cascara, or bisacodyl may be useful on an intermittent basis for refractory constipation, though frequently cause cramping, loose stools, and urgency.

Antispasmodics. Antispasmodics work by either by a direct effect on intestinal smooth muscle (e.g., mebeverine, pinaverine) or via their anticholinergic or antimuscarinic properties (e.g., dicyclomine, hyoscamine). A recent meta-analysis suggests good efficacy for antispasmodics for global relief of IBS symptoms [15] although most of the studies are not of high quality. An unfavorable side-effect profile, including dry mouth, constipation, urinary retention, and visual disturbances, may preclude treatment at therapeutic doses in some patients [16].

Serotonergic Agents. Tegaserod is a selective $5HT_4$ partial agonist that stimulates gut transit and may also have an effect on visceral sensation [17]. Several large and well-designed trials have shown tegaserod to be more efficacious than placebo in improving symptoms of IBS-C in women. In 2007, tegaserod was suspended and subsequently withdrawn by the FDA based on a small but statistically significant increase in the incidence of cardiovascular ischemic events in patients taking tegaserod compared to those taking placebo (0.1% vs. 0.01%). All of these patients had a history of cardiac disease or risk factors [18]. It is currently only available through the FDA on an emergency basis.

Alosetron is a $5HT_3$ receptor antagonist that is currently available under a restricted use program and is approved only for women with severe IBS-D who have failed conventional therapy. This restriction is due to the occurrence of GI-related adverse events including ischemic colitis and serious complications of severe constipation. A systematic review concluded that there is a significantly increased rate of ischemic colitis among alosetron-using patients compared to placebo-using patients (0.15% vs. 0.0%), but no significant difference in the rate of serious complications of constipation. All of the alosetron-using patients with ischemic colitis had a reversible colopathy without long-term sequelae and most cases occurred within the first month of treatment [19]. The restriction notwithstanding, alosetron has been proven efficacious in multiple clinical trials for relief of abdominal pain or discomfort and urgency [19,20].

Chloride Channel Activator. In 2008, the chloride channel (ClC-2) activator lubiprostone, which is used to treat chronic idiopathic constipation at a dose of 24µg twice daily, received an FDA indication for IBS-C in women. Two 12-week, randomized, placebo-controlled trials evaluated the efficacy of lubiprostone at a dose of 8 μg twice daily in patients with IBS-C [21]. Compared to placebo, lubiprostone was found to significantly improve the secondary endpoints of stool consistency, straining, abdominal pain/discomfort, health-related quality of life (HRQOL), and constipation severity.

Antidepressants. The rationale of using antidepressants in IBS is that these agents may alter pain perception via a central modulation of visceral afferent input and decreased firing of primary sensory afferent nerve fibers, slow GI transit, and treat of co-morbid psychological symptoms. Tricyclic antidepressants (TCAs) are the best studied in IBS, and are often used at low doses, because their major impact in IBS may be more associated with analgesic and motility effects rather than treatment of psychological symptoms. Desipramine and nortriptyline are less sedating than others in the same family such as amitriptyline due to their lower antihistamine effect. If a TCA is used in IBS-C, desipramine should be considered since it has less anticholinergic effects and is therefore less constipating than the other TCAs.

A recent meta-analysis of placebo-controlled trials of selective serotonin reuptake inhibitors (SSRIs) in IBS suggests good efficacy for these agents although most studies have small sample sizes [22]. SSRIs have an effect on the physical component of HRQOL, symptom frequency and abdominal pain, and these effects appear to be independent of effects on mood [23].

Antibiotics. Small intestinal bacterial overgrowth (SIBO) has been theorized to play a role in IBS [24]. Rifaximin is an antibiotic which has very low systemic absorption and broad-spectrum activity against Gram-positive and Gram-negative aerobes and anaerobes. In a Phase IIb, multicenter, placebo-controlled study, treatment of IBS-D patients with rifaximin was associated with significantly greater adequate relief of global IBS symptoms (52% vs. 44%) and bloating (46% vs. 40%) which was maintained at the end of the 12-week follow-up period [25]. Future studies including an ongoing phase III RCT will likely provide more information on the efficacy of this antibiotic treatment in IBS-D.

Probiotics

Probiotics are hypothesized to work by several mechanisms. These include a shift from a proinflammatory to an anti-inflammatory cytokine profile and enhanced epithelial barrier function [26]. While many species of probiotics subjectively reduced flatulence and bloating, the best evidence for global improvement in IBS symptoms is for formulations containing species of *Bifidobacterium* [27,28].

Complementary and Alternative Medicine (CAM)

Because even the most effective treatments for IBS do not help all patients, many turn to CAM in search of other treatment options. Additionally, CAM treatments often provide a more holistic approach and meaningful clinician–patient relationship than western medicine. Acupuncture is popular therapy for IBS patients. The authors of a recent Cochrane review concluded that acupuncture was likely no better than sham acupuncture, but may have been better than usual care; however, more research is required to make any recommendations [29]. Other alternative or herbal medicines that have been studied are Chinese herbal medicine, peppermint oil, extract of artichoke, carmint, the herbal mixture STW 5, and melatonin.

> **Take-home points**
> - IBS is a prevalent and heterogeneous disorder and patient care should be focused on reducing costs and improving patient satisfaction and health-related quality of life (HRQOL).
> - Diagnosis is based on symptom criteria and diagnostic tests are not indicated in the majority of patients.
> - Altered GI motility and enhanced visceral perception due to altered brain–gut interactions are key pathophysiologic mechanisms of IBS.
> - Gut transit time is often normal in IBS-C and decreased in IBS-D.
> - Stool form is a better predictor of bowel habit subtype and GI transit than stool frequency in IBS.
> - The most effective treatment involves a collaborative effort of patient and clinician to find the treatments which provide the greatest relief of symptoms and management of their illness and improvement of daily functioning.

Acknowledgment
Dr Chang is supported by NIH grants # P50 DK64539, NIAMS grant AR46122, and M01-RR00865. She also reports consulting for Albireo, Forest, Ironwood, McNeil,

Prometheus, Salix, Synergy, Takeda, Ocera and Glaxo-SmithKline, and research grant support from Prometheus, and Rose Pharma and Takeda Pharmaceuticals.

References

1 Longstreth GF, Thompson WG, Chey WD, *et al.* Functional bowel disorders. *Gastroenterology* 2006; **130**: 1480–1.

2 Whitehead WE. *Development and Validation of the ROME III Diagnostic Questionaire. Rome III: The Functional Gastrointestinal Disorders.* Durham: Degnon, 2006: 835–53.

3 Drossman DA, Morris CB, Hu Y, *et al.* A prospective assessment of bowel habit in irritable bowel syndrome in women: defining an alternator. *Gastroenterology* 2005; **128**: 580–9.

4 Riedl A, Schmidtmann M, Stengel A, *et al.* Somatic comorbidities of irritable bowel syndrome: A systematic analysis. *J Psychosom Res* 2008; **64**: 573–82.

5 Whitehead WE, Palsson O, Jones KR. Systematic review of the comorbidity of irritable bowel syndrome with other disorders: what are the causes and implications? *Gastroenterology* 2002; **122**: 1140–56.

6 Whitehead WE, Palsson OS, Feld AD, *et al.* Utility of red flag symptom exclusions in the diagnosis of irritable bowel syndrome. *Aliment Pharm Therap* 2006; **24**: 137–46.

7 Cash BD, Chey WD. Irritable bowel syndrome—an evidence-based approach to diagnosis. *Aliment Pharm Therap* 2004; **19**: 1235–45.

8 Spiegel BM, DeRosa VP, Gralnek IM, *et al.* Testing for celiac sprue in irritable bowel syndrome with predominant diarrhea: a cost-effectiveness analysis. *Gastroenterology* 2004; **126**: 1721–32.

9 Spiegel BM, Gralnek IM, Bolus R, *et al.* Is a negative colonoscopy associated with reassurance or improved health-related quality of life in irritable bowel syndrome? *Gastrointest Endosc* 2005; **62**: 892–9.

10 Stewart M, Brown JB, Donner A, *et al.* The impact of patient-centered care on outcomes. *J Fam Practice* 2000; **49**: 796–804.

11 Chang L, Drossman D. Optimizing patient care: the psychological interview in irritable bowel syndrome. *Clin Perspect* 2002; **5**: 336–42.

12 Drossman DA, Toner BB, Whitehead WE, *et al.* Cognitive-behavioral therapy versus education and desipramine versus placebo for moderate to severe functional bowel disorders. *Gastroenterology* 2003; **125**: 19–31.

13 Schoenfeld P. Efficacy of current drug therapies in irritable bowel syndrome: what works and does not work. *Gastroenterol Clin North Am* 2005; **34**: 319–35, viii.

14 Bijkerk CJ, Muris JW, Knottnerus JA, *et al.* Systematic review: the role of different types of fibre in the treatment of irritable bowel syndrome. *Aliment Pharm Therap* 2004; **19**: 245–51.

15 Ford AC, Talley N, Spiegel BM, *et al.* Efficacy of antispasmodics and peppermint oil in irritable bowel syndrome: systematic review and meta-analysis. *Am J Gastroenterol* 2008; **103**: S459.

16 Page JG, Dirnberger GM. Treatment of the irritable bowel syndrome with Bentyl (dicyclomine hydrochloride). *J Clin Gastroenterol* 1981; **3**: 153–6.

17 Coffin B, Farmachidi JP, Rueegg P, *et al.* Tegaserod, a 5-HT4 receptor partial agonist, decreases sensitivity to rectal distension in healthy subjects. *Aliment Pharm Therap* 2003; **17**: 577–85.

18 Patricia P. Desperately seeking serotonin…A commentary on the withdrawal of tegaserod and the state of drug development for functional and motility disorders. *Gastroenterology* 2007; **132**: 2287–90.

19 Harris L, Chang L. Alosetron: an effective treatment for diarrhea-predominant irritable bowel syndrome. *Women's Health* 2007; **3**: 15–27.

20 Chey WD, Chey WY, Heath AT, *et al.* Long-term safety and efficacy of alosetron in women with severe diarrhea-predominant irritable bowel syndrome. *Am J Gastroenterol* 2004; **99**: 2195–203.

21 Drossman D, Chey WD, Panas R. Lubiprostone significantly improves symptom relief rates in adults with irritable bowel syndrome and constipation (IBS-C): Data from two twelve week, randomized, placebo controlled double blind trials. *Gastroenterology* 2007; **132**: 2586–7.

22 Ford AC, Talley N, Schoenfeld P, *et al.* Efficacy of antidepressants in irritable bowel syndrome: systematic review and meta-analysis. *Am J Gastroenterol* 2008; **103**: S476.

23 Tack J, Broekaert D, Fischler B, *et al.* A controlled crossover study of the selective serotonin reuptake inhibitor citalopram in irritable bowel syndrome. *Gut* 2006; **55**: 1095–103.

24 Pimentel M, Chow EJ, Lin HC. Normalization of lactulose breath testing correlates with symptom improvement in irritable bowel syndrome. a double-blind, randomized, placebo-controlled study. *Am J Gastroenterol* 2003; **98**: 412–9.

25 Lembo A, Zakko S, Ferreira N, *et al.* Rifaximin for the treatment of diarrhea-associated irritable bowel syndrome: short term treatment leading to long term sustained response. *Gastroenterology* 2008; **134**: A545.

26 Spiller P. Review article: probiotics and prebiotics in irritable bowel syndrome (IBS). *Aliment Pharmacol Ther* 2008; **28**: 385–96.

27 Whorwell PJ, Altringer L, Morel J, *et al.* Efficacy of an encap-

sulated probiotic Bifidobacterium infantis 35624 in women with irritable bowel syndrome. *Am J Gastroenterol* 2006; **101**: 1581–90.

28 Nikfar S, Rahimi R, Rahimi F, *et al.* Efficacy of probiotics in irritable bowel syndrome: a meta-analysis of randomized, controlled trials. *Dis Colon Rectum* 2008; **51**: 1775–80.

29 Lim B, Manheimer E, Lao L, *et al.* Acupuncture for treatment of irritable bowel syndrome. *Cochrane Database of Systematic Reviews* 2006; **4**: CD0051111.

30 Ford AC, Talley NJ, Spiegel BM, *et al.* Efficacy of fiber in irritable bowel syndrome: systematic review and meta-analysis. *Am J Gastroenterol* 2008; **103**: S459.

31 Ford AC, Brandt LJ, Foxx-Orenstein A, *et al.* Efficacy of 5-HT4 agonists in non-diarrhea predominant irritable bowel syndrome: systematic review and meta-analysis. *Am J Gastroenterol* 2008; **103**: S478.

32 Ford AC, Brandt LJ, Foxx-Orenstein A, *et al.* Efficacy of 5-HT3 antagonists in non-constipation predominant irritable bowel syndrome: systematic review and meta-analysis. *Am J Gastroenterol* 2008; **103**: S477.

CHAPTER 61

Functional Constipation and Pelvic Floor Dysfunction

Ernest P. Bouras

Division of Gastroenterology and Hepatology, Mayo Clinic, Jacksonville, FL, USA

Summary

Constipation is variably defined, and its diagnosis is often arbitrary. Patients with functional constipation (FC) present with difficult, infrequent, or seemingly incomplete defecation without meeting criteria for irritable bowel syndrome. There are a variety of secondary causes of constipation, including medications that slow colonic transit. A functional defecation disorder secondary to pelvic floor dysfunction (PFD) is a common, often under-appreciated abnormality in patients presenting with constipation. While fiber supplementation and osmotic laxatives are successful for many patients with FC, the treatment of choice for PFD is pelvic floor rehabilitation (biofeedback). Therefore, a stepwise diagnostic and therapeutic approach to patients with FC based on historical and physical examination features is recommended. Clinical awareness and focused testing to identify the physiologic abnormalities underlying constipation facilitate management and improve patient outcomes.

Case

A 58-year-old woman presents with over 25 years of constipation she defines as the urge to expel a bowel movement but the inability to evacuate satisfactorily. She strains excessively at hard stools and occasionally uses her finger to assist rectal emptying. Following a negative colonoscopy, she was instructed to use fiber supplements and various laxative preparations, but she has experienced minimal improvement. Her history is notable for two previous "difficult" vaginal deliveries. She has urinary dysfunction and has had surgery for urogynecologic prolapse. She wishes to consider colon resection for her refractory symptoms.

Practical Gastroenterology and Hepatology: Small and Large Intestine and Pancreas, 1st edition. Edited by Nicholas J. Talley, Sunanda V. Kane and Michael B. Wallace. © 2010 Blackwell Publishing Ltd.

Definition and Epidemiology

Constipation is variably defined, and its diagnosis is often arbitrary. Physicians tend to consider stool frequency (<3 defecations per week), whereas patients more often consider straining, stool consistency, incomplete evacuation, and non-productive urges to have a bowel movement [1]. While most studies suggest an adult prevalence for constipation of about 15%, estimates range from 2 to 27% [1–4]. Risk factors include advancing age, medications, female sex, non-white race, and low levels of physical activity, education, and income. Severe constipation is reported almost exclusively in women. There are over 4 million physician visits per year for constipation [5], the majority with primary care providers. However, it is likely that this under-represents the actual impact of constipation and subsequent medical utilization as many people undoubtedly either do not seek medical attention and/or use over-the-counter remedies, either alone or in combination with those prescribed by their physician.

Patients referred to gastroenterologists tend to represent the more refractory cases.

Functional Constipation

Functional constipation (FC) is a functional bowel disorder. Patients present with difficult, infrequent, or seemingly incomplete defecation without meeting criteria for irritable bowel syndrome [6]. Table 61.1 outlines the Rome III diagnostic criteria for FC.

Pelvic Floor Dysfunction

The functional anatomy of the pelvic floor consists of the pelvic diaphragm (levator ani and coccygeus muscles) and anal sphincters, innervated by the sacral nerve roots (S_{2-4}) and pudendal nerve (Figure 61.1). Normal func-

---

Table 61.1 Diagnostic criteria* for functional constipation [6].

1. Must include two or more of the following:
   a. Straining during at least 25% of defecations
   b. Lumpy or hard stool in at least 25% of defecations
   c. Sensation of incomplete evacuation for at least 25% of defecations
   d. Sensation of anorectal obstruction/blockage for at least 25% of defecations
   e. Manual maneuvers to facilitate at least 25% of defecations (e.g., digital evacuation, support of the pelvic floor)
   f. Fewer than three defecations per week

2. Loose stools are rarely present without the use of laxatives

3. Insufficient criteria for irritable bowel syndrome

---

*Criteria fulfilled for the last 3 months with symptom onset at least 6 months prior to diagnosis.

---

tioning of this neuromuscular unit allows the efficient elimination of stool from the rectum. Although the exact prevalence of pelvic floor dysfunction (PFD) in constipation is unknown, some studies have demonstrated a prevalence of up to 50% or more of constipation cases can be attributed to PFD [7–9]. PFD is common in both the young and elderly, and more common in women and those with a history of anorectal surgery or other pelvic floor trauma, including childbirth. In addition to defecatory dysfunction, PFD manifests with disorders of urinary and sexual function. Identifying PFD is important, as pelvic floor retraining has been shown to be most useful treatment for this type of constipation.

In patients with FC, PFD may be more appropriately termed a functional defecation disorder (FDD), which can be characterized by: (i) paradoxical contractions or inadequate relaxation of the pelvic floor muscles; or (ii) inadequate propulsive forces during attempted defecation [10]. Table 61.2 provides the Rome III diagnostic criteria for FDD, which are based on formal studies of pelvic floor function. PFD associated with fecal incontinence is covered in a separate chapter.

Pathophysiology

The major etiologies of constipation include disorders of colonic transit and pelvic floor function. Although previous colonic injury (e.g., diverticular disease, ischemia) with stricture formation or obstructing masses may present with altered bowel function, abnormalities of colonic structure rarely account for constipation. In

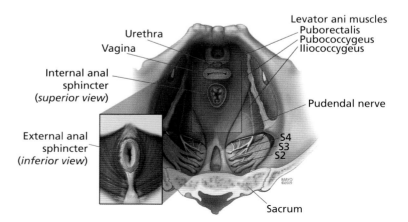

Figure 61.1 Functional anatomy of the pelvic floor. Reproduced with permission of Elsevier from Bouras EP, Tangalos EG. *Gastroenterol Clin N Am* 2009; **38**: 463–80.

addition to slow colonic transit or PFD, a variety of psychological and behavioral issues are important, and more than one mechanism may be present in a single patient. Several additional mechanisms may be present in the elderly, particularly the institutionalized.

Colonic Transit

The colon absorbs water and electrolytes from its lumen, serving both as a reservoir and conduit for fecal material. There are various secondary causes of slow colonic transit (metabolic, neurologic, endocrine, infiltrative diseases), and medication usage (opiates, anticholinergics, antihy-

---

Table 61.2 Diagnostic criteria* for functional defecation disorders [10].

---

1. The patient must satisfy diagnostic criteria for functional constipation
2. During repeated attempts to defecate must have at least two of the following:
   a. Evidence of impaired evacuation, based on balloon expulsion testing or imaging
   b. Inappropriate contraction of the pelvic floor muscles (i.e., anal sphincter or puborectalis) or less than 20% relaxation of basal resting sphincter pressure by manometry, imaging, or EMG
   c. Inadequate propulsive forces assessed by manometry or EMG

---

*Criteria fulfilled for the last 3 months with symptom onset at least 6 months prior to diagnosis.
EMG, electromyography.

---

pertensives, others) is a common, often overlooked but modifiable etiology. Primary or idiopathic slow colonic transit and global gastrointestinal motility disturbances (intestinal pseudo-obstruction) are rare. Although the terms tend to be used freely, colonic inertia and megacolon are better reserved for abnormalities identified on formal testing, such as colonic manometry. Typically, there are relatively straightforward explanations for slow transit, such as medications or PFD with secondary slowing of colonic transit via inhibitory reflexes.

Pelvic Floor Function and Dysfunction

Normal defecation is accomplished through a series of coordinated, neurologically-mediated movements of the pelvic floor and anal sphincter (Figure 61.2). Abnormalities in this complex series of actions lead to abnormal stool expulsion, or a functional outlet obstruction to defecation [11]. This may be secondary to inadequate relaxation or paradoxical contractions of the musculature or the inability to produce the effective propulsive forces needed to expel the stool. Specific anatomic abnormalities, such as rectoceles, may impact defecation. However, these findings are common and the significance is not always clear. Classically raising concerns for colorectal cancer, small-caliber stools more commonly represent patients straining to expel stool through an inadequately relaxed or open outlet.

PFD is a comprehensive phrase, and other terms relating to defecatory dysfunction include dyssynergia,

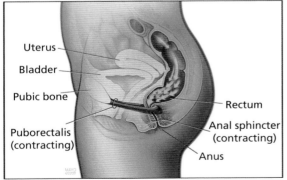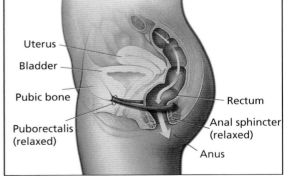

Figure 61.2 Dynamics of defecation. At rest (left panel), the puborectalis sling holds the rectum at an angle and the anal sphincters are closed. Upon normal defecation (right panel), (a) the puborectalis relaxes, (b) the anorectal angle straightens, (c) the pelvic floor descends, and (d) the anal sphincter relaxes allowing stool expulsion when accompanied by adequate propulsive force. Reproduced with permission of Elsevier from Bouras EP, Tangalos EG. *Gastroenterol Clin N Am* 2009; **38**: 463–80.

anismus, obstructed defecation, outlet delay, among others. Although there are subtle differences to the meanings, the key concept of disordered defecation secondary to abnormal pelvic floor function is the same. The Rome III working group has defined a disorder of the pelvic floor that impacts stool evacuation in patients with FC as a FDD, with specific laboratory criteria for dyssynergic defecation and inadequate defecatory propulsion [9]. Pelvic floor spasm can lead to pelvic and abdominal pain. Descending perineum syndrome, which is believed to result from repeated excessive straining, can lead to constipation, rectal prolapse, mucosal ulceration, and fecal incontinence. Appreciating pelvic floor function and dysfunction is essential to effectively manage individuals with constipation.

Psychological and Behavioral Factors

Personality factors, psychological distress, and a history of physical or sexual abuse have been associated with constipation [12–14]. PFD can be considered a behavioral disorder, as it may be learned at any age in response to specific demands and physical or mental injury. An altered psychological state can lead to muscular tension or spasticity which negatively impacts pelvic floor function. Subsequently, the defecation disorder interferes with quality of life and may alter interpersonal, intimate, and interfamily relationships. Adequate caloric intake is beneficial for development and stimulation of bowel movements, and eating disorders should be excluded.

Clinical Features

As with the definition of constipation, there is variability in patient presentation. Excessive or prolonged straining, assisting stool evacuation by assuming certain positions or with rectal or vaginal digital manipulation, and the sensation of incomplete rectal evacuation are among several features that suggest PFD [15]. Others include urinary and sexual dysfunction, previous pelvic or rectal surgery, history of anal fissures, prolapse, and a history of pelvic floor trauma, including child birthing. Although these symptoms and features do not always correlate with formal testing, they are suggestive of PFD, whereas symptoms such as a decreased urge to defecate and infrequent stools may be more suggestive of slow transit.

Fecal seepage is an underappreciated condition that is frequently misdiagnosed as fecal incontinence [16]. Patients often have a history of constipation with the sensation of poor rectal evacuation with frequent, incomplete bowel movements and excessive wiping. They commonly present with anal pruritus and staining of their undergarments. The antidiarrheals often prescribed for presumed incontinence tend to exacerbate the situation. Fecal impaction may be an associated finding. Paradoxically, the problem is one of obstructed defecation rather than true incontinence. Fecal impaction may be complicated by stercoral ulceration and bleeding. A thorough history and examination are essential.

Other factors to recognize include age, the use of constipating medications, a general decline in physical or mental health, other medical conditions (neurologic illness, collagen vascular disorders, diabetes mellitus), dietary habits, and a history of physical, mental, or sexual abuse. The presence of alarm features (e.g., rectal bleeding, weight loss) and a family or personal history of colon cancer should be ascertained. Constipated patients also have an increase in other gastrointestinal symptoms, such as dyspepsia, abdominal cramping, bloating, flatulence, heartburn, nausea, and vomiting.

Diagnosis

Most patients will present to their primary care physician for the initial evaluation and management of constipation. Various initial management strategies have been employed. Although there are limited data to support their routine use, standard diagnostic studies typically include baseline blood work and structural studies to exclude any significant metabolic or anatomic abnormalities.

Patients with normal investigations and a failed response to empiric, front-line therapies are the ones typically referred to the gastroenterologist. A stepwise, individualized approach to patients with constipation is useful. Patients with PFD frequently go undiagnosed; their constipation symptoms are often mistakenly attributed to irritable bowel syndrome secondary to associated cramping and discomfort. Pursuing relevant studies that help categorize patients as to the etiology of their constipation facilitates selection of the appropriate therapy for each specific physiologic subgroup [15,17].

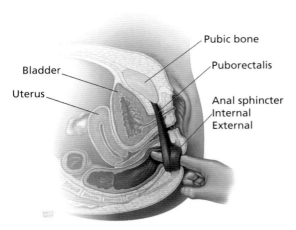

Pubic bone

Bladder

Puborectalis

Uterus

Anal sphincter
Internal
External

Figure 61.3 Anorectal examination. With the patient in the left lateral position, the examiner should assess: (a) resting sphincter tone and presence of spasm, (b) sensation, including the presence of pain, (c) the ability to squeeze, and (d) coordination of the pelvic floor and rectal muscles and extent of perineal descent during simulated defecatory straining (expelling the examiner's finger). Reproduced with permission of Elsevier from Bouras EP, Tangalos EG. *Gastroenterol Clin N Am* 2009; **38**: 463–80.

History and Physical Examination

The diagnosis of FC begins with a history, carefully assessing relevant clinical features, including a thorough medication review. The physical examination is not complete without a thorough perianal and digital rectal examination, which goes beyond looking for mass lesions, anal strictures, fissures, or stool impaction [18] (Figure 61.3).

Metabolic and Structural Evaluation

Assessing the complete blood count, electrolyte balance, calcium homeostasis, and thyroid function are common, but these investigations rarely identify the cause of FC. The yield of colonoscopy in patients with constipation is the same as the general population; however, alarm symptoms (e.g., bleeding), age, and risk factors for colon cancer should be considered. Plain abdominal radiographs can assess fecal load, impaction, and obstruction.

Colonic Transit

Radiopaque marker studies are an inexpensive and widely available way to assess colon transit [19]. In addition to total marker counts, marker distribution may also be helpful, as proximal retention suggests colonic dys-

function, whereas the retention of markers exclusively in the lower left colon is more indicative of a defecatory disorder. Scintigraphic techniques allow for shorter studies (24 to 48 h) and decreased radiation exposure; results correlate well with radiographic methods. PFD, medications, diet, and the presence of excessive stool or impaction affect transit. Some advocate bowel cleansing prior to assessment.

Pelvic Floor Function

Although experts agree on the importance of PFD, there is less agreement on which tests best identify PFD. Furthermore, the reliability and comparability of many tests are unknown. Priorities include the assessment of: (i) tone and strength of the sphincters and pelvic floor; (ii) rectal sensation; (iii) neuromuscular control, coordination, and propulsive force with defecatory straining; and (iv) anatomic abnormalities that may impact defecation. Patients who have failed initial therapy or who have symptoms suggestive of PFD should undergo formal testing. Table 61.3 outlines common diagnostic findings in patients with PFD.

1 Anorectal manometry: various measurements relay key information about the motor and sensory control of the anorectum and pelvic floor. Simulated defecation allows assessment of synergy and propulsive force [20].

2 Balloon expulsion test: the inability to expel a 50 mL balloon filled with water or air suggests PFD [9], but this test may be normal in many patients with PFD. Although some have proposed balloon expulsion as a screening tool, the study is usually performed as part of an anorectal manometry study.

3 Evacuation proctography (defecography): the goal of evacuation proctography is to identify anatomy and physiology that may contribute to outlet obstruction. It has traditionally been performed by instilling a thickened barium solution into the rectum followed by obtaining relevant measurements during rest, while squeezing, and during defecatory straining. Other techniques such as dynamic magnetic resonance imaging (MRI) and scintigraphy may be used depending on available expertise and technology [21].

These studies attempt to assess the control of the anorectal angles, presence of paradoxical contractions, extent of perineal descent, and the ability of the patient to empty the rectum. Barium and MRI studies provide the opportunity to look for anatomic abnormalities that may

Table 61.3 Diagnostic findings in patients with defecatory disorders.

History
Prolonged straining to expel stool
Unusual postures on the toilet to facilitate stool expulsion
Support of the perineum, digitation of the rectum, or posterior vaginal pressure to facilitate rectal emptying
Inability to expel enema fluid
Constipation after subtotal colectomy for constipation

Rectal examination (with patient in left lateral position)
Inspection
Anus pulled forward while the patient is bearing down
Anal verge descends <1.0 cm or >3.5 cm (or beyond the ischial tuberosities) while the patient is bearing down
Perineum balloons down while the patient is bearing down, and rectal mucosa partially prolapses through the anal canal

Palpation
High anal sphincter tone at rest
Anal sphincter pressure during voluntary contraction is only slightly higher than tone at rest
Perineum and examining finger descend <1.0 cm or >3.5 cm while patient simulates straining during defecation
Puborectalis muscle is tender on palpation through the rectal wall posteriorly, or palpation produces pain
Palpable mucosal prolapse during straining
Defect in anterior wall of the rectum, suggestive of a rectocele

Anorectal manometry and balloon expulsion (with patient in left lateral position)
Average tone of anal sphincter at rest of >80 mmHg (or >60 cm water)
Average pressure of anal sphincter during contraction of >180 mmHg (or >240 cm water)
Failure to expel balloon

Reproduced with permission from Lembo and Camilleri [15]. Copyright © 2003 Massachusetts Medical Society. All rights reserved.

impact defecation, such as rectoceles, mucosal intussusception, and prolapse. MRI offers the advantage of providing additional information on pelvic anatomy and function. The clinical significance of several findings is often unclear. Rectoceles are relatively common but may be considered clinically significant if they fill preferentially or fail to empty during simulated defecation.

Case continued

Physical examination revealed tight, spastic musculature and paradoxical contractions with defecatory straining. These findings were confirmed on anorectal manometry, where she had elevated sphincter pressures, failed relaxation during simulated defecation, and she was unable to expel a rectal balloon. Dynamic pelvic floor MRI revealed paradoxical puborectalis contraction with straining and poor rectal emptying but no significant structural abnormalities.

Therapeutics

Treatment of FC depends on the underlying physiologic etiology, being mindful of other factors influencing the presentation (e.g., medications and psychological factors). For patients who do not respond to fiber supplementation, osmotic laxatives can be titrated to clinical response. Stimulant laxatives and prokinetic agents are best reserved for patients with more refractory constipation. Throughout any treatment program, one should remain vigilant of PFD, as pelvic floor rehabilitation is the treatment of choice. Surgery is rarely indicated for constipation, and exclusion of PFD is essential. Fecal impaction should be cleared prior to beginning maintenance regimens.

Fiber and Fluids

Increasing fiber intake to 15–25 g/day may be accomplished with dietary changes, supplements, or both. Although increasing water intake on its own has not been shown to improve constipation, maintaining adequate fluid intake is sensible during fiber supplementation. A softer, bulkier stool that is easier to pass is the ultimate goal. Increasing the dose of fiber slowly over several weeks to months can lessen common side-effects (bloating, gas, and distension) and enhance compliance. Synthetic supplements may be better tolerated than other fiber preparations.

Laxatives

Osmotic laxatives work by retaining or drawing water into the gut lumen and are the agents of choice for patients not responding to fiber supplementation. There is no clearly superior osmotic agent; the choice should be based on relevant medical history (cardiac or renal status), cost, and tolerance of the various preparations. The dose should be titrated based on the clinical response. For chronic or more severe constipation, regular dosing is indicated. Although stimulant laxatives, which promote intestinal motility, do not appear to lead to tolerance or bowel injury, these drugs are better reserved for those with a failed response to osmotic agents, and may be required for the management of opioid-induced constipation.

Stool Softeners, Suppositories, and Enemas

Stool softeners are of limited overall efficacy. Suppositories, which usually work within minutes, help initiate and/or facilitate rectal evacuation. They may be used in conjunction with meals to capture the gastrocolic reflex. In general, enemas may be used judiciously on an as-needed basis, particularly for obstructed defecation with fecal impaction. Routine use is typically discouraged. Suppositories and enemas may be included as part of a standardized bowel program, particularly for the institutionalized with a history of impaction.

Prokinetics and Other Agents

Although prokinetic agents, such as tegaserod and prucalopride, appear efficacious for constipation, they are of limited availability. Metoclopramide and erythromycin are of doubtful benefit in constipation. Lubiprostone, a bicyclic fatty acid that activates chloride channels on the apical membrane of the intestinal epithelial cells, helps in constipation by moving water into the gut lumen. In light of the cost, this medication is best reserved for a lack of efficacy with less expensive alternatives.

Pelvic Floor Rehabilitation (Biofeedback)

Pelvic floor rehabilitation is the treatment of choice for PFD. Therapy concentrates on sensory and muscular retraining of the rectum and pelvic floor, with the goals of normalization of sensation, muscular relaxation and/or strengthening, and improved defecatory dynamics with resolution of any paradoxical pelvic floor contractions. Different therapeutic protocols exist, and the best approach is unclear. Uncontrolled studies suggest that biofeedback is effective in over 70% of patients [22], and these findings have been confirmed in several randomized, controlled trials [23–25]. The presence of descending perineum syndrome may limit results. Biofeedback has been shown to be superior to laxatives in patients with a FDD, and the effect was durable [23]. The key is identifying the problem and available therapeutic resources. A patient's physical and mental abilities must

be assessed. Although no physiologic, anatomic, or demographic variables clearly impact treatment outcome, many feel that psychopathology may play a role [22]. Concomitant slow colon transit frequently requires simultaneous treatment.

Surgery

Although rarely indicated, subtotal colectomy with ileorectal anastomosis is the treatment of choice for medically-refractory slow transit constipation, but only if PFD is excluded [26]. Patients with predominant bloating and pain respond poorly. Surgical indications for pelvic floor abnormalities are ill-defined. Surgery should be considered only if functional significance can be determined. Division of the puborectalis is not recommended. Anatomic abnormalities (e.g., rectoceles) are common, but they are frequently the result of PFD. Treatment of the underlying PFD first is a reasonable treatment approach, with surgery reserved for those not responding to more conservative therapy.

Additional Comments

Adjunctive therapy may be necessary for psychopathology associated with FC, and maintaining adequate caloric intake is essential. Evidence does not support the popular notion that toxins from constipation harm the body or that irrigation is needed. There is no obvious significance of an elongated colon (dolichocolon), and surgical shortening does not lead to reliable clinical improvement. Likewise, physical activity and water intake are controversial subjects, with unclear associations with colon transit and constipation [27]. Although mineral oil, colchicine, and misoprostol may improve constipation, these agents have potential side effects and complications that outweigh any benefits. Emerging therapies, such as sacral nerve stimulation, botulinum toxin injection for PFD, alteration of the bacterial milieu, and several novel medications may play more of a role in the future of constipation management.

Case continued

The patient used a daily osmotic laxative to provide stools that were soft and easy to pass. She completed a pelvic floor rehabilitation program, learning to relax her musculature and eliminate paradoxical contractions during defecation. Relieved that she avoided colectomy, she is now off of osmotic laxatives with no residual constipation.

Take-home points

Diagnosis:
- Functional constipation is common, impacting quality of life and use of health-care resources.
- Constipation is variably defined, and a careful history and physical examination is helpful in obtaining relevant clues that help direct management.
- Functional defecation disorders secondary to pelvic floor dysfunction (PFD) are common in patients presenting with constipation.
- Physiologic categorization of the etiology leading to patient presentation improves management outcomes.

Therapy:
- Fiber supplementation and osmotic laxatives are effective for many patients with functional constipation.
- Idiopathic slow transit constipation is uncommon, and surgery is rarely indicated.
- Subtotal colectomy and ileorectostomy should be considered in medically refractory patients only if PFD has been excluded.
- Pelvic floor rehabilitation (biofeedback) is the treatment of choice for PFD, with therapeutic trials demonstrating high rates of success.

References

1 Pare P, Ferrazzi S, Thompson WG, *et al*. An epidemiological survey of constipation in Canada: definitions, rates, demographics, and predictors of health care seeking. *Am J Gastroenterol* 2001; **96**: 3130–7.

2 Stewart WF, Liberman JN, Sandler RS, *et al*. Epidemiology of constipation (EPOC) study in the United States: relation of clinical subtypes to sociodemographic features. *Am J Gastroenterol* 1999; **94**: 3530–40.

3 Sonnenberg A, Koch TR. Epidemiology of constipation in the United States. *Dis Colon Rectum* 1989; **32**: 1–8.

4 Brandt LJ, Prather CM, Quigley EM, *et al*. Systematic review on the management of chronic constipation in North America. *Am J Gastroenterol* 2005; **100** (Suppl. 1): S5–S21.

5 Shah ND, Chitkara DK, Locke GR, *et al*. Ambulatory care for constipation in the United States, 1993–2004. *Am J Gastroenterol* 2008; **103**: 1746–53.

6 Longstreth GF, Thompson WG, Chey WD, *et al*. Functional bowel disorders: functional constipation. In: Drossman DA, *et al*., eds. *The Functional Gastrointestinal Disorders*, 3rd edn. Lawrence, KS: Allen Press, Inc., 2006: 515–23.

7 Surrenti E, Rath DM, Pemberton JH, Camilleri M. Audit of constipation in a tertiary referral gastroenterology practice. *Am J Gastroenterol* 1995; **90**: 1471–5.

8 Kuijpers HC. Application of the colorectal laboratory in diagnosis and treatment of functional constipation. *Dis Colon Rectum* 1990; **33**: 35–9.

9 Rao SSC, Ozturk R, Laine L. Clinical utility of diagnostic tests for constipation in adults: a systematic review. *Am J Gastroenterol* 2005; **100**: 1605–15.

10 Wald A, Bharucha AE, Enck P, Rao SS Functional anorectal disorders: functional defecation disorders. In: Drossman DA *et al*., eds. *The Functional Gastrointestinal Disorders*, 3rd edn. Lawrence, KS: Allen Press, Inc., 2006: 663–75.

11 Rao SS, Welcher KD, Leistikow JS. Obstructive defecation: a failure of rectoanal coordination. *Am J Gastroenterol* 1998; **93**: 1042–50.

12 Wald A, Hinds JP, Caruana BJ. Psychological and physiological characteristics of patients with severe idiopathic constipation. *Gastroenterology* 1989; **97**: 932–7.

13 Leroi AM, Bernier C, Watier A, *et al*. Prevalence of sexual abuse among patients with functional disorders of the lower gastrointestinal tract. *J Colorectal Dis* 1995; **10**: 200–6.

14 Nehra V, Bruce BK, Rath-Harvey DM, *et al*. Psychological disorders in patients with evacuation disorders and constipation in a tertiary practice. *Am J Gastroenterol* 2000; **95**: 1755–8.

15 Lembo A, Camilleri M. Chronic constipation. *N Engl J Med* 2003; **349**: 1360–8.

16 Rao SS. Diagnosis and management of fecal incontinence. American College of Gastroenterology Practice Parameters Committee. *Am J Gastroenterol* 2004; **99**: 1585–604.

17 Locke GR, Pemberton JH, Phillips SF. AGA technical review on constipation. American Gastroenterological Association. *Gastroenterology* 2000; **119**: 1766–78.

18 Talley NJ. How to do and interpret a rectal examination in gastroenterology. *Am J Gastroenterol* 2008; **103**: 820–2.

19 Metcalf AM, Phillips SF, Zinsmeister AR, *et al*. Simplified assessment of segmental colonic transit. *Gastroenterology* 1987; **92**: 40–7.

20 Diamant NE, Kamm MA, Wald A, Whitehead WE. AGA technical review on anorectal testing techniques. *Gastroenterology* 1999; **116**: 735–60.

21 Bharucha AE, Fletcher JG, Seide B, *et al*. Phenotypic variation in functional disorders of defecation. *Gastroenterology* 2005; **128**: 1199–210.

22 Heymen S, Jones KR, Scarlett Y, Whitehead WE. Biofeedback treatment of constipation: a critical review. *Dis Colon Rectum* 2003; **46**: 1208–17.

23 Chiaroni G, Whitehead WE, Pezza V, *et al*. Biofeedback is superior to laxatives for normal transit constipation due to

pelvic floor dyssynergia. *Gastroenterology* 2006; **130**: 657–64.

24 Heyman S, Scarlett Y, Jones K, *et al.* Randomized, controlled trials shows biofeedback to be superior to alternative treatments for patients with pelvic floor dyssynergia-type constipation. *Dis Colon Rectum* 2007; **50**: 428–41.

25 Rao SS, Seaton K, Miller M, *et al.* Randomized controlled trial of biofeedback, sham feedback, and standard therapy for dyssynergic defecation. *Clin Gastroenterol Hepatol* 2007; **5**: 331–8.

26 Hassan I, Pemberton JH, Young-Fadok TM, *et al.* Ileorectal anastomosis for slow transit constipation: long-term functional and quality of life results. *J Gastrointest Surg* 2006; **10**: 1330–6.

27 Muller-Lissner SA, Kamm MA, Scarpignato C, Wald A. Myths and misconceptions about chronic constipation. *Am J Gastroenterol* 2005; **100**: 232–42.

CHAPTER 62

Chronic Functional Abdominal Pain

Samantha A. Scanlon[1], Madhusudan Grover[2],
Amy E. Foxx-Orenstein[3], and Douglas A. Drossman[4]

[1] Department of Internal Medicine, Mayo Clinic, Rochester, MN, USA
[2] Division of Gastroenterology and Hepatology, Mayo Clinic, Rochester, MN, USA
[3] Division of Gastroenterology and Hepatology, Miles and Shirley Fiterman Center for Digestive Diseases, Mayo Clinic, Rochester, MN, USA
[4] Division of Gastroenterology and Hepatology, University of North Carolina, Chapel Hill, NC, USA

Summary

Functional abdominal pain syndrome (FAPS) is a less common functional gastrointestinal disorder characterized by abdominal pain which is not related to food intake and defecation. It accounts for significant health care impact and has a high co-morbidity with psychiatric disorders. Its etiology is incompletely understood, however, it relates primarily to dysfunction of central pain modulatory systems. The diagnosis of FAPS is primarily based on positive symptom criteria defined by Rome III; in the absence of alarm symptoms an extensive work-up is not required. Medical evaluation must include a careful physical examination, psychosocial assessment, and a cost-effective approach to rule out an alternative or co-existing diagnosis. Effective treatment approaches hinge on the principles of biopsychosocial medicine with emphasis on the doctor–patient relationship and negotiating reasonable treatment goals. These include the use of centrally acting pharmacological and psychological therapies that focus more on adaptive coping rather than complete cure. Antidepressants (tricyclic, selective serotonin reuptake inhibitors) are the mainstay of pharmacotherapy which also aims to target associated psychiatric co-morbidities. A multidisciplinary pain clinic approach and combination therapies are often helpful at the severe, refractory end of the spectrum of FAPS.

Case

Ms R is a 43-year-old female with a past medical history of asthma, dysmenorrhea, cholecystectomy, appendectomy, and an explorative laparoscopy for evaluation of dysmenorrhea. She is referred to a gastroenterology clinic by her primary care doctor for further evaluation of her abdominal pain. She describes it as "wrenching" and "squeezing", 10/10 in severity, generalized, and present nearly all the time. There does not appear to be any relation of her pain to belching, eating, defecation, or passing flatus. She has not experienced any weight loss, fever, chills, constipation, diarrhea, melena, hematochezia, nausea, or vomiting with this pain. She has been enduring this pain over the last 18 months. She is on 40 mg of oxycodone four times a day for this abdominal pain. During this time, she has undergone an extensive evaluation including colonoscopy, esophagogastroduodenoscopy, as well as CT scan of the abdomen/pelvis, all of which are normal. She is frustrated and angry that no explanation for her pain has been found. She presents to a gastroenterology clinic after becoming offended that her primary care doctor told her that there was nothing more he could do and that he recommends that she see a psychologist or psychiatrist for further treatment.

Definition

FAPS is defined as abdominal pain that is poorly related to gut function, is associated with some loss of daily functioning, and has been present for at least 6 months.

Practical Gastroenterology and Hepatology: Small and Large Intestine and Pancreas, 1st edition. Edited by Nicholas J. Talley, Sunanda V. Kane and Michael B. Wallace. © 2010 Blackwell Publishing Ltd.

Table 62.1 Rome III diagnostic criteria for functional abdominal pain.

These criteria must be fulfilled for the last 3 months with symptom onset at least 6 months prior to diagnosis:
  Continuous or nearly continuous abdominal pain
  No or only occasional relation of pain with physiological events
    (i.e., eating, defecation, menses)
  Some loss of daily functioning
  The pain is not feigned (i.e., malingering)
  Insufficient symptoms to meet criteria for another functional
    gastrointestinal disorder that would explain the pain

It is also called "chronic idiopathic abdominal pain" or "chronic functional abdominal pain" [1,2]. According to the Rome III criteria as shown in Table 62.1, the diagnostic criteria for FAPS must be fulfilled for the last 3 months with symptom onset at least 6 months prior to diagnosis [3]. It is also important to note that this pain disorder is not affected by defecation or eating, thereby specifically distinguishing it from irritable bowel syndrome (IBS) [1]. FAPS is commonly associated with other painful conditions such as fibromyalgia, and it seems to fulfill criteria for diagnosis of somatoform pain disorder under psychiatric nosology.

Epidemiology and Health Care Impact

Due to inconsistencies in the definition of "chronic abdominal pain," the epidemiology of FAPS is not entirely well known; however, its prevalence in North America has been reported from 0.5 to 2.0% [1,2]. It is a disease that is typically more common in women (F:M = 3:2) [1,3]. The prevalence peaks in the fourth decade of life and decreases thereafter. Due to high work absenteeism and utilization of considerable health-care resources in evaluating and managing FAPS, it is associated with a significant economic burden to society [1,2].

Pathophysiology

Functional gastrointestinal disorders are best conceptualized through a biopsychosocial model, where a combination of biologic, psychologic, and social factors play a role in the disease and illness presentation [2]. At this time, FAPS is a poorly understood functional gastrointestinal disorder; however, a central neuropathic pain model has been proposed as the primary pathophysiological process.

The foundation of the pathophysiology of FAPS rests upon the abnormal perception of visceral sensations to the central nervous system (CNS). Normal gut sensitivity occurs via afferent neurons which synapse in the dorsal horn of the spiral cord, ultimately synapsing in the cortex in specialized regions that include the medial thalamus, posterior thalamus, anterior cingulated cortex (ACC), and the somatosensory cortex (SSI). Cortical modulation of sensory input originates in the ACC and in the end results in "gating" of the dorsal horn. Individuals with FAPS are thought to have increased peripheral sensitization leading to increased central sensitization. This has been shown to happen when functional pain develops in patients undergoing gynecological surgeries for non-painful conditions [4]. Central sensitization is achieved via activation of the N-methyl-D-aspartate (NMDA) receptor by removal of the magnesium ion block. Activation of the NMDA receptor allows for lesser degrees of peripheral input to result in greater central activation. Ultimately, due to this central sensitization, even non-noxious stimuli may lead to inappropriate activation of central pain receptors [5]. A compromised ability to activate descending endogenous pain inhibitory systems (opioidergic, serotonergic, and noradrenergic pathways) is another proposed mechanism [6].

Recent studies of functional brain imaging in patients with IBS found an association between the anterior cingulate cortex and traumatic life events (abuse), thereby suggesting a role of how past abusive experiences may lead to altered perception and thus development of FAPS [7].

The frequent association of FAPS with psychiatric disorders and responsiveness to treatment with antidepressants suggests a prominent role of the CNS in cognitive and emotional pain modulation in this condition.

Clinical Features

Patients with FAPS usually complain of a constant, generalized pain over a large anatomical area [2,3]. This abdominal pain may occur in the setting of other painful symptoms, suggesting a concurrent somatization disorder or perhaps overlap with other functional pain conditions such as fibromyalgia [1]. A history of physical or sexual abuse is common in patients with FAPS, as high as 30% in those attending gastroenterology clinics [8]. This history of abuse may lead to increased awareness of visceral sensation, though there is no evidence that visceral pain thresholds are reduced in such people [1,9].

Diagnosis

Case continued

When examining the patient, you notice that she has multiple surgical scars, normoactive bowel sounds are present, and her abdomen is soft, diffusely tender, and negative for hepatosplenomegaly, ascites, rebound, or masses. Before you have laid hands on her, she squeezes her eyes shut and grimaces. Carnett test is positive. You order the following labs which are all within normal limits: complete blood count (CBC), electrolyte panel, liver function tests, C-reactive protein (CRP), sedimentation rate, thyroid stimulating hormone (TSH), amylase, and lipase.

The diagnosis of FAPS can be made in patients who meet the diagnostic criteria according to Rome III as detailed in Table 62.1 [3]. Evaluation proceeds using a clinical and psychosocial approach with emphasis on the physical exam and observed behaviors [1,2]. Physical examination must be thorough and by definition will not be associated with significant abnormalities, keeping in mind however that overlap with other medical conditions can occur. Presence of abdominal scars might prompt interrogation of symptoms preceding surgery exposing exploratory versus therapeutic investigations. All surgical and pathology reports should be examined.

The observation of pain behavior is also important during physical exam as FAPS patients are likely to have absence of autonomic arousal and exhibit the "closed eyes sign" (eyes closed during examination, as opposed to an eyes open, a fearful anticipation expression commonly seen in patients with an acute abdomen). These patients may also be able to be distracted during examination [2]. Abdominal wall pain should be excluded using the Carnett test. When present, abdominal wall pain increases with head raising and contracting the rectus abdominis muscle, while visceral pain decreases. However, FAPS can also produce increased pain during abdominal wall contraction probably due to central sen-

Table 62.2 Psychosocial assessment in evaluation of functional abdominal pain syndrome.

1. Life history of illness
   Evaluate if acute vs. chronic and presence of other chronic pain conditions
2. Reasons for seeking care now
   Associated concerns, triggers, worsening functional and/or psychosocial status
3. Life history of traumatic events
   Access history of abuse, personal or family losses
4. Patient's understanding of illness
   Recognizing mind–body interactions vs. looking for an organic cause
5. Impact of pain on activities and quality of life
   To plan diagnostic and treatment decisions
6. Associated psychiatric diagnosis
   Diagnosing and treating Axis I and Axis II psychiatric disorders
7. Role of family and culture
   Recognizing dysfunctional family interactions and cultural belief systems
8. Associated psychosocial impairment and available resources
   Helping seek social networks and avoiding maladaptive coping (catastrophizing)

sitization with viscerosomatic referral [1,2]. As with other functional disorders, in the absence of alarm symptoms (i.e., unexplained weight loss, abdominal mass, bloody bowel movements, anorexia), use of diagnostic tests to exclude organic disease should not be performed routinely [10]. If the examination is negative, no further diagnostic studies are indicated. Further testing only reinforces the concept that another diagnosis is being missed and invasive studies may increase the risk of aggravating the visceral hypersensitivity.

In addition to the physical examination, physicians should pay attention to psychosocial elements which can be crucial in revealing disease and illness patterns related to FAPS. Some of the key elements of psychosocial assessment are mentioned in Table 62.2.

Differential Diagnosis

Before establishing a diagnosis of FAPS, it is important to exclude structural and metabolic gastrointestinal disorders. Diagnoses to be considered include, but are not limited to, inflammatory bowel disease, pancreatitis, intestinal obstruction, ulcer disease, abdominal wall pain, and IBS. Additionally, FAPS can co-exist with these disorders or any medical condition. Features suggestive of a structural disorder include acute onset of symptoms, variable or intermittent intensity of pain, focal location of discomfort, positive diagnostic tests, response to pro-motility and/or anti-inflammatory agents, and improvement of symptoms with nasogastric suction or fasting.

Therapeutics

Case continued

She returns a week later to discuss her labs. You explain to her that the evaluation of her abdominal pain is consistent with functional abdominal pain syndrome, a disorder associated with abnormal perception/dysregulation of pain control pathways. Given this diagnosis, the treatment is a combination of medication and psychotherapy in an effort to better control her body's mechanisms of dealing with pain perception. Unfortunately, total pain relief is unlikely; however, the ultimate goal will be to reach a point where her pain no longer disrupts her daily activities. She nods in agreement but wants something to stop her pain right now, a medication like hydromorphone which has worked really well in the past. You explain to her that unfortunately, medications like Dilaudid are not effective for her type of pain and may cause other problems such as narcotic bowel syndrome which will confound her symptoms. At this time, you recommend starting a tricyclic antidepressant which at low doses has an analgesic effect on the body's nervous system and therefore more directly targets the cause of her pain. She seems somewhat apprehensive at starting this type of medication, but seems more amenable after understanding the rationale of using this medication. You agree to have her return for a short session in 2 weeks to assess her progress, need for increased dose of medication, or referral for psychotherapy.

The etiology of FAPS rests on the biopsychosocial model, as does the approach to treatment, the basis of which is founded on a strong patient–physician relationship [1,11,12] (Figure 62.1). The focus of treatment is to manage symptoms as opposed to targeting a cure [1,2]. While it is key to demonstrate empathy, educate, validate their illness, and reassure, it is equally important to negotiate treatment, thereby establishing reasonable limits of time and effort (Table 62.3) [1,2]. It is imperative the patient understand that a definitive cure is unlikely so as to set appropriate goals and avoid disappointment [2]. It is also important to engage the patient as an active participant in their therapy. Some patients with FAPS are not willing to accept that psychosocial factors are a contributing factor to their pain. In doing so, they shirk personal responsibility in the management process and place high expectations on providers to relieve their pain entirely.

Most treatment recommendations of FAPS are based on empiric evidence lacking the support of well-designed treatment trials. Current recommendations are based upon extrapolation from treatment trials of other func-

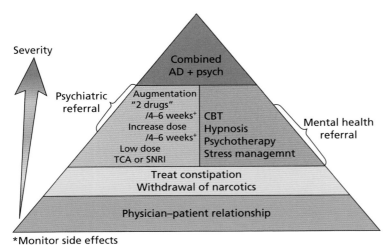

*Monitor side effects

Figure 62.1 Treatment of functional abdominal pain syndrome begins with an effective patient–physician relationship. If present, constipation should be treated and narcotics withdrawn. Low-dose tricyclic antidepressants (TCA) or serotonin norepinephrine reuptake inhibitor (SNRI), increased if necessary after 4–6 weeks is a next step, while monitoring for side effects. Alternatively, a mental health referral for psychiatric or psychological treatment may be most beneficial. For severe or refractory cases, a multidisciplinary approach combining pharmacologic and psychological interventions is used. (Reproduced from Drossman DA [14].) CBT, cognitive behavioral therapy; AD, antidepressants; psych, psychological evaluation.

tional gastrointestinal disorders and chronic pain syndromes (Table 62.4). Antidepressants are a starting point of therapy and the primary pharmacological treatment of FAPS. Low doses of tricyclic antidepressants (TCAs) are the most commonly recommended antidepressant therapy. TCAs have been found to be superior to selective serotonin reuptake inhibitors (SSRIs) for the treatment of neuropathic pain; however, superiority of one class of agents over another has not been shown in FAPS [1]. SSRIs can be considered in patients with higher levels of anxiety (general or symptom related), depression, or sleep disturbances. They may not be as successful in treating pain per se and increase coping ("The pain is still

there but it does not bother me as much"). Serotonin norepinephrine reuptake inhibitors (SNRIs), used with some success in other painful somatic conditions such as fibromyalgia, may prove beneficial in treatment of FAPS. Owing to their dual blockade of norepinephrine and 5HT receptors, agents in this class (duloxetine, venlafaxine) could potentially be as effective as the TCAs [13].

There is no role for the use of most analgesics in the treatment of FAPS. Many analgesics offer pain relief through peripheral mechanisms. Based on the theory that FAPS is a the result of abnormal central pain signaling, peripherally acting agents should have limited if any effect in providing pain relief aside from placebo effect [1]. Also, patients with chronic pain syndromes are prone to developing pain medication seeking behavior with FAPS being no exception. Thus, the use of narcotic agents for the treatment of FAPS can increase the risk of addiction as well as development of the common, yet under-recognized, narcotic bowel syndrome [15]. In narcotic bowel syndrome, persistent use of narcotics leads to progression in the frequency, duration, and intensity of pain episodes. The criteria for diagnosing narcotic bowel syndrome are listed in Table 62.5.

As with the patient described in the Case, when FAPS is complicated by narcotic bowel syndrome, the narcotics must first be discontinued (Table 62.6) [15]. Usually this can be accomplished on an outpatient basis. However, following an inpatient withdrawal protocol may be preferred if narcotic usage is high, there are secondary effects such as ileus or electrolyte imbalance, or if there is limited patient motivation or family support. The time frame of

Table 62.3 Treatment approach.

Establishing an effective patient–physician relationship
1. Empathy
2. Education
3. Validation
4. Reassurance
5. Negotiate the treatment
6. Set reasonable limits

The treatment plan
1. Set reasonable limits
2. Help the patient take responsibility
3. Base treatment on symptom severity and the degree of disability
4. Medications
5. Mental health referral
6. Specific psychological treatments
7. Multidisciplinary pain treatment center referral

Table 62.4 Medications to treat chronic functional abdominal pain‡.

TCAs*	Secondary amines (desipramine and nortriptyline)	
	Starting dose	25–50 mg po every night
	Escalating dose	Increase by 25 mg increments weekly, max daily dose 100 mg (remember that benefit may not be seen for 6 weeks after initiation)
	Additional benefits	Tends to be better tolerated than other TCAs (tertiary amines) due to lower antihistaminic and anticholinergic effects.
	Tertiary amines (imipramine and amitriptyline)	
	Starting dose	10–25 mg
	Escalating dose	Increase by 25 mg increments weekly, max. daily dose 100 mg (remember that benefit may not be seen for 6 weeks after initiation)
	Additional benefits	—
Class side effects	Sedation, constipation, tachycardia, urinary retention, dry mouth, dry eyes, weight gain, hypotension, sexual dysfunction, agitation, nightmares	
	May help depressive symptoms but dose suboptimal for treatment of major depression	
Time to action	2–6 weeks	

Table 62.4 continued

SSRIs	Short half life (paroxetine)	
	Medium half life (citalopram, escitalopram)	
	Long half life (fluoxetine)	
	Starting dose	10–20 mg po daily
	Escalating dose	Increase by 10 mg increments, up to max daily dose of 60 mg if necessary
		Often times, dose escalation is not necessary (as is the case with TCAs)
		Many patients find benefit at 20 mg daily
	Additional benefits	Anxiety reduction as well as treatment of OCD, social phobia, and agoraphobia; treatment of associated depressive disorder if present
Class side effects	Insomnia, diarrhea, night sweats, weight loss, agitation, sexual dysfunction	
Time to action	3–6 weeks	
SNRIs*	Duloxetine	
	Starting dose	20–30 mg po daily (take with meals to reduce nausea)
	Escalating dose	Increase by 30 mg increments weekly, max daily dose 90 mg
	Additional benefits	Treatment of coexisting psychiatric disorders
		Peripheral pain modulation
		Less sexual dysfunction in comparison to SSRIs
	Venlafaxine	
	Starting dose	37.5 mg po twice daily
	Escalating dose	After 1–2 weeks, increase to 50 mg po twice daily
		After 1–2 weeks, increase to 75 mg po twice daily
		Continue to increase by 25 mg increments every 1–2 weeks.
		Most people will require 150 mg total daily dose until benefit is seen
		Maximum daily dose 225 mg
	Additional benefits	Central antinociception at higher doses
		Treatment of coexisting psychiatric disorders
		Peripheral pain modulation
		Less sexual dysfunction in comparison to SSRIs
Class side effects	Nausea, agitation, dizziness, fatigue, liver dysfunction	
Time to action	3–6 weeks	
Augmenting agents†	Buspirone	
	Starting dose	7.5 mg po twice daily
	Escalating dose	After 1–2 weeks, increase to 15 mg po twice daily
		After 1–2 weeks, increase to 30 mg po twice daily
		Continue to increase in similar increments up to 30 mg po twice daily
	Additional benefits	Anxiety reduction
	Quetiapine	
	Starting dose	25 mg po daily
	Escalating dose	Increase by 25 mg increments every 1–2 weeks to max daily dose of 100 mg
	Additional benefits	Anxiety reduction, alleviates insomnia
	Side effect	Rare possibility of torsades de pointes and sudden death in high-risk individuals
		Side effects less likely given the relatively low dosage compared to 400–600 mg dose for indications of bipolar disorder and schizophrenia

*First line pharmacotherapy for the treatment of functional abdominal pain includes either a TCA or SNRI.
†These medications should not be used alone for the treatment of FAPS. They are intended to be used in conjunction with one of the above medications to augment the effect of the two medications.
‡It is important to counsel patients that side effects will typically resolve 1–2 weeks after initiation of medication or new dose. If side effects persist, try to continue same or lower dose from same class of medication before switching to another class.
TCA, tricyclic antidepressant; SSRI, selective serotonin reuptake inhibitor; SNRI, serotonin norepinephrine reuptake inhibitor; po, orally.

Table 62.5 Diagnostic criteria for narcotic bowel syndrome.

Chronic or frequently recurring abdominal pain that is treated with acute high dose or chronic narcotics and all of the following:
  The pain worsens or incompletely resolves with continued or escalating dosages of narcotics
  There is marked worsening of pain when the narcotic dose wanes and improvement when narcotics are reinstituted ("soar and crash")
  There is a progression of the frequency, duration, and intensity of pain episodes
  The nature and intensity of the pain is not explained by a current or previous gastrointestinal diagnosis

Table 62.6 Narcotic bowel syndrome treatment algorithm (over 3 days to 1–2 weeks).

1. Begin low dose TCA or SSRI
2. Consider adding medium acting benzodiazepine (e.g., lorazepam) for anxiety
3. Convert short to medium- or long-acting narcotic to achieve comfort
4. Decrease dose of medium- or long-acting narcotic 10–33.3% in equal daily dose (non-contingent)
5. Add α-2 adrenergic receptor agonist towards end of taper

Reproduced from Grunkemeier DMS *et al.* Narcotic bowel syndrome: clinical features, pathophysiology and management. *Clin Gastroenterol Hepatol* **5**: 1127 [15]. Copyright 2007, with permission from Elsevier.

the withdrawal may be over several days or weeks and is influenced by the duration of narcotic use as well as the dosage. Several days prior to narcotic withdrawal, a TCA or SNRI should be started. When instituting the withdrawal, patients should receive the maximal dose of a medium to long-acting narcotic to achieve comfort; usually the dose chronically or currently being used. This dose is then decreased by 10–33% delivered in equally divided daily dosages. Administration of therapy should be non-contingent rather than as needed to prevent acute withdrawal and to avoid the need for supplemental doses of medication. Short-acting agents (e.g., oxycodone) should be converted to equivalent dosages of longer-acting agents to avoid the "soar–crash" effect of rapid withdrawal. A medium acting benzodiazepine (e.g., lorazepam, 1 mg every 6–8 h) may be started at the time of the withdrawal initiation to reduce anxiety. In addition, clonidine, an α-2 adrenergic receptor agonist that

blocks the physiological effects of narcotic withdrawal, is added in equally divided doses of 0.1 to 0.6 mg toward the end of the taper and may be continued for several days after the withdrawal [15].

Gabapentin and pregabalin are increasingly being prescribed for chronic neuropathic pain conditions including peripheral neuropathies and more recently fibromyalgia. The benefit of these agents in treating visceral or central pain syndromes has not been established, though a few case reports have suggested a reduction in visceral pain [13]. Similar to narcotic use in FAPS, long-term treatment with benzodiazepines is not recommended due to high abuse potential and a tendency to negatively interact with medications. Patients refractory to TCA or SSRI agents or who are already receiving high-dose therapy may profit from the addition of a different class of antidepressant to achieve clinical effect by engaging different neuroreceptors. Based on clinical experience, buspirone, a non-benzodiazepine azapirone with antianxiety properties, may enhance the analgesic effect of antidepressants. Early clinical experience with quetiapine, an atypical antipsychotic agent which acts on dopamine receptors, used at low doses (25–100 mg) has demonstrated some benefit in treating patients with chronic pain syndromes.

In addition to a pharmacologic approach, there is also a role for psychological intervention in the treatment of FAPS; however, no psychological treatment has been studied in clinical trials. Psychological treatments may be instituted early on in therapy, or may be best reserved for patients with chronic or refractory abdominal symptoms. For such therapies to be most effective, it is recommended that psychological interventions be performed by a therapist or specialist with experience in treating patients with chronic abdominal pain [2]. Patients might be reluctant to see a psychologist or psychiatrist because they might feel stigmatized or see this as a failure of medical diagnosis or treatment. It is thus important for the treating physician to educate the patient, consult a mental health expert, and continue to closely follow with the patient. Recommended therapies may include cognitive behavioral therapy (CBT), dynamic or interpersonal therapy, and hypnotherapy. While no studies have examined these therapies specifically in the treatment of FAPS, studies in other functional gastrointestinal disorders suggest that psychological treatments may offer some benefit [1].

CBT aims to develop effective coping strategies to allow patients to perform their daily activities without being plagued by pain [16]. CBT employs short, medium, and long-term objectives to achieve improvement in self-management of pain, global well-being, satisfaction with treatment, pain, and quality-of-life scores [13]. Drossman *et al.* investigated CBT, education, desipramine, and placebo in the effectiveness of treatment of functional gastrointestinal syndromes. This study showed a number needed to treat (NNT) of 3.1 for CBT in contrast to desipramine which had a NNT of 8.1 in the intention to treat analysis and a NNT of 5.2 in the per-protocol analysis [16].

Dynamic or interpersonal psychotherapy has not been shown to have a considerable effect on visceral or somatic symptoms, but has been associated with improved mood, coping, quality of life, and a reduction in health-care costs. For these reasons, psychotherapy should be considered as an adjunct to other therapeutic interventions as a way of managing pain and decreasing psychological stress regarding the illness [1].

Gut-directed hypnotherapy has not been investigated in the treatment of FAPS, yet has been shown to be beneficial in the treatment of IBS [17]. This form of therapy consists of general relaxation techniques and the use of imagery or visualization in a way that the patient asserts control over their body's perception of gut sensation/function [2,5,18]. The underlying mechanism appears to be via modulation of the anterior cingulated cortex [18]. Studies have shown that rectal sensitivity to balloon distension was normalized in patients with IBS after hypnotherapy [5].

Other modalities such a multidisciplinary pain treatment center may provide a more comprehensive care plan and should be sought for more refractory patients. Combination treatments for augmenting response with two classes of antidepressants or combining psychological and pharmacological therapies can be an effective strategy for symptoms refractory to any one of these approaches.

Prognosis

The quality of life in patients with functional abdominal pain is generally poor. Ultimately, a patient's appreciation of their pain process and coping strategies are sig-
nificant predictors of quality of life and response to treatment. Patients with a history of compound traumatic life events (e.g., emotional, sexual or physical abuse, death, or divorce) tend to have a poorer prognosis [1,3].

Take-home points

- Functional abdominal pain is a chronic pain syndrome which is not explained by a structural or metabolic disorder. It relates to dysfunction of brain–gut regulatory systems.
- The etiology of functional abdominal pain rests upon the biopsychosocial model.
- The object of therapy is management of pain and improvement in coping skills. A definitive cure is unlikely.
- Therapy consists of both pharmacotherapy and psychological treatments to address the multiple etiologies as defined by the biopsychosocial model.

Acknowledgements

The authors would like to thank Lori Anderson for her assistance in preparing this manuscript.

References

1 Clouse RE, Mayer EA, Aziz Q, *et al.* Functional abdominal pain syndrome. *Gastroenterology* 2006; **130**: 1492–7.

2 Drossman DA. Functional abdominal pain syndrome. *Clin Gastroenterol Hepatol* 2004; **2**: 353–65.

3 Clouse RE, Mayer EA, Aziz Q, *et al.*. Functional abdominal pain syndrome. In: Drossman DA, *et al.*, eds. *Rome III: The Functional Gastrointestinal Disorders*, 3rd edn. McLean, VA: Degnon Associates, Inc., 2006: 557–93.

4 Sperber AD, Morris CB, Greemberg L, *et al.*. Development of abdominal pain and IBS following gynecological surgery: a prospective, controlled study. *Gastroenterology* 2008; **134**: 75–84.

5 Matthews PJ, Aziz Q. Functional abdominal pain. *Postgrad Med J* 2005; **81**: 448–55.

6 Drossman DA. Brain imaging and its implications for studying centrally targeted treatments in irritable bowel syndrome: a primer for gastroenterologists. *Gut* 2005; **54**: 569–73.

7 Ringel Y, Drossman DA, Leserman JL, *et al.* Effect of abuse history on pain reports and brain responses to aversive visceral stimulation: an FMRI study. *Gastroenterology* 2008; **134**: 396–404.

8 Drossman DA, Talley NJ, Leserman J, *et al*. Sexual and physical abuse and gastrointestinal illness. Review and recommendations. *Ann Intern Med* 1995; **123**: 782–94.

9 Ringel Y, Whitehead WE, Toner BB, *et al*. Sexual and physical abuse are not associated with rectal hypersensitivity in patients with irritable bowel syndrome. *Gut* 2004; **53**: 838–42.

10 Cash BD, Schoenfeld P, Chey WD. The utility of diagnostic tests in irritable bowel syndrome patients: a systematic review. *Am J Gastroenterol* 2002; **97**: 2812–19.

11 Chang L, Drossman DA. Optimizing patient care: The psychosocial interview in irritable bowel syndrome. *Clin Perspect Gastroenterol* 2002; **5**: 336–41.

12 Drossman DA. Biopsychosocial issues in gastroenterology. In: Feldman M, Friedman LS, Brandt LJ, eds. *Sleisenger and Fordtran's Gastrointestinal and Liver Disease*, 9th edn. Philadelphia: Elsevier, 2009.

13 Grover M, Drossman DA. Psychotropic agents in functional gastrointestinal disorders. *Curr Opin Pharmacol* 2008; **8**: 715–23.

14 Drossman DA. Severe and refractory chronic abdominal pain: treatment strategies. *Clin Gastroenterol Hepatol* 2008; **6**: 978–82.

15 Grunkemeier DM, Cassara JE, Dalton CB, Drossman DA. The narcotic bowel syndrome: clinical features, pathophysiology, and management. *Clin Gastroenterol Hepatol* 2007; **5**: 1126–39.

16 Drossman DA, Toner BB, Whitehead WE, *et al*. Cognitive behavioral therapy versus education and desipramine versus placebo for moderate to severe functional bowel disorders. *Gastroenterology* 2003; **12**: 19–31.

17 Grover M, Drossman DA. Psychopharmacologic and behavioral treatments for functional gastrointestinal disorders. *Gastrointest Endosc Clin N Am* 2008; **19**: 151–70.

18 Vlieger AM, Menko-Frankenhuis CM, Wolfkamp SC, *et al*. Hypnotherapy for children with functional abdominal pain or irritable bowel syndrome: a randomized controlled trial. *Gastroenterology* 2007; **133**: 1430–6.

CHAPTER 63

Functional Abdominal Bloating and Gas

Fernando Azpiroz

Department of Gastroenterology, University Hospital Vall d'Hebron, Barcelona, Spain

Summary

Patients complaining of intestinal gas may refer to different types of conditions: repetitive eructation, excessive or odoriferous flatus, impaired anal evacuation, or abdominal bloating/discomfort. Patients with aerophagia and excessive eructation can usually be retrained to control air swallowing but, if present, basal dyspeptic symptoms may remain. Patients with excessive or odoriferous flatus may benefit from a low-flatulogenic diet. Gas retention due to functional outlet obstruction can be resolved by biofeedback treatment, which also improves fecal evacuation and thereby reduces the time for fermentation. Other patients complaining of abdominal symptoms that they attribute to intestinal gas probably have irritable bowel syndrome or functional bloating, and they may be treated with either prokinetics or spasmolytics. There is no consistent evidence to support the use of gas-reducing substances, such as charcoal or simethicone.

Case

A 37-year-old female frequently complains of excess gas in the gut. A detailed history reveals that her complaints refer to abdominal bloating and fullness. When specifically questioned, she admits straining at stools and sensation of difficult gas evacuation, without excessive flatulence or belching. Anorectal manometry evidences functional outlet obstruction due to impaired anal relaxation during attempted evacuation. After normalization of the defecatory maneuver by biofeedback training her symptoms relieve significantly.

Definition and Epidemiology

Gas-related symptoms may refer to the following conditions:

1 Aerophagia: repetitive eructation; relatively rare

Practical Gastroenterology and Hepatology: Small and Large Intestine and Pancreas, 1st edition. Edited by Nicholas J. Talley, Sunanda V. Kane and Michael B. Wallace. © 2010 Blackwell Publishing Ltd.

2 Flatulence: voluminous or excessively odoriferous flatus; common among the general population

3 Difficult anal gas evacuation: common and frequently associated to constipation due to functional outlet obstruction

4 Abdominal bloating: sensation of abdominal distension; present in 10–30% of the general population and 90% of patients with irritable bowel syndrome (IBS).

Pathophysiology and Clinical Features

The pathophysiology of gas-related symptoms depends on their specific clinical complaint (Figure 63.1).

Aerophagia. In the absence of thoracoabdominal pathology excessive gas production within the stomach cannot be justified. These patients inadvertently swallow air that accumulates in the hypopharynx, and is then released by belching with the patients' satisfaction [1]. Frequently, the process is triggered by emotional distress or a basal

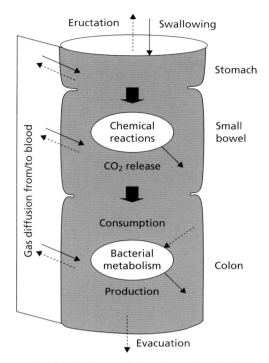

Eructation · Swallowing

Stomach

Gas diffusion from/to blood

Chemical reactions — Small bowel

CO_2 release

Consumption

Bacterial metabolism — Colon

Production

Evacuation

Figure 63.1 Intestinal gas metabolism. Gas input results from swallowing, chemical reactions, diffusion from blood, and bacterial fermentation. Gas output is achieved by eructation, absorption, bacterial consumption, and anal evacuation.

dyspeptic-type symptom of epigastric fullness, which the patients misinterpret as excessive gas in the stomach.

Flatulence. Some patients complain of voluminous or excessive flatus, which may become socially disabling. Odor depends on trace elements, such as sulfur-containing gases (H_2S, methanethiol, and dimethyl sulfide) that are produced by sulfate-reducing bacteria in the colon [2]. The frequency of anal gas evacuation in healthy subjects varies depending on the diet, but is usually around 20 evacuations per day, and the volume of daily gas evacuated ranges between 200 and 700 mL. The volume and smell of gas evacuated is determined primarily by the action of colonic microflora on unabsorbed, fermentable food residues entering the colon. Gas-producing substrates include some types of fiber, starch, oligosaccharides, and sugars. Excessive or odoriferous anal gas evacuation depends both on the composition of colonic flora and on the diet. Excessive gas production on a

normal diet is related to a highly flatulogenic colonic flora due to an increase in gas-producing bacteria, or more likely a deficit of gas-consuming microorganism. Excessive gas production may be also the consequence of diseases that affect the normal absorption of nutrients within the small bowel (i.e., intestinal malabsorption), but due to their clinical manifestations these cases are readily recognized.

Difficult anal Gas Evacuation. In contrast to the patients with excessive flatus, some patients complain of impaired anal evacuation and abdominal gas retention. Normally, rectal evacuation is achieved by a mild abdominal compression coupled to anal relaxation. Some patients have a dyscoordination with inadequate anal relaxation during straining and impaired evacuation [3]. This type of functional outlet obstruction may produce a sensation of difficult gas evacuation and gas retention, which is frequently associated with constipation. Fecal retention in these patients would prolong the process of colonic fermentation of residues and increase gas production.

Abdominal Bloating. Patients with functional gut disorders, irritable bowel and related syndromes, frequently attribute their abdominal symptoms to intestinal gas. Probably these patients represent a heterogeneous group in which bloating is produced by different combinations of pathophysiological mechanisms, that in most cases are subtle and undetectable by conventional methods [4]. Recent studies have consistently shown that IBS patients who attribute their symptoms to intestinal gas have impaired handling of intestinal content due to abnormal gut reflexes, which may result in segmental pooling and focal gut distension. Additional evidence indicates that these patients also have intestinal hypersensitivity with increased perception of intraluminal stimuli. Bloating may be associated with abdominophrenic dyscoordination. In these patients, segmental pooling within the gut releases abnormal viscerosomatic reflexes leading to paradoxical diaphragmatic contraction, relaxation of the anterior abdominal wall, and distension [5].

Diagnosis and Differential Diagnosis

Diagnosis is based on a careful clinical history. Anorectal manometry may demonstrate a functional outlet obstruction in case of anal gas retention. Other clinical tests are rarely needed to rule out thoracic or abdominal pathology (endoscopic or radiological tests) in belching, malabsorption (breath tests) in flatulence or abdominal bloating, and intestinal dysmotility (intestinal manometry) in case of severe distension.

Therapeutics

Treatment depends on the pathophysiological mechanisms involved (Figure 63.2). The level of evidence is low.

Aerophagia usually resolves, or at least improves, with a clear pathophysiological explanation of the symptoms. If present, dyspeptic symptoms may also be treated. Some patients present psychological problems that may require specific therapy [1].

Patients complaining of excessive and/or odoriferous gas evacuation may benefit from a low-flatulogenic diet that includes: meat, fowl, fish, and eggs; gluten-free bread, rice bread, and rice; some vegetables, such as lettuce and tomatoes; and some fruits, such as cherries and grapes. On the contrary, high-flatulogenic foodstuffs should be avoided including beans, Brussels' sprouts, onions, celery, carrots, raisins, bananas, wheat germ, and fermentable fiber [6]. After a 1-week gas-free diet these patients usually experience significant symptom relief. By

an orderly reintroduction of other foodstuffs, they should be able to identify the offending meal components. If strict diet fails, malabsorption may be investigated and treated accordingly.

In patients with gas retention due to impaired anal evacuation, anal dyscoordination can be resolved with biofeedback treatment [3], which also resolves fecal retention, and thereby the time for fermentation and gas production are also reduced.

Bloating and abdominal symptoms may improve with the treatment of the underlying functional gut disorder [7]. Since patients with bloating and distension seemingly suffer from a common variant of IBS, the basic approach to treatment should be similar to that prescribed for IBS. However, these patients may have mixed syndromes resulting from several altered mechanisms. A hypersensitive gut may be associated with impaired anal evacuation, particularly in constipation- predominant IBS patients, and symptoms will worsen if gas production is increased. In these patients a combined treatment strategy should be considered. Recent experimental studies suggest that mild exercise, a traditional recommendation, facilitates intestinal gas clearance [8]. Avoiding high flatulogenic foodstuffs and fiber overload usually helps, but strict exclusion diets cannot be recommended. The effect of spasmolytics, prokinetics, antibiotics, and gas-reducing substances has not been clearly established [9].

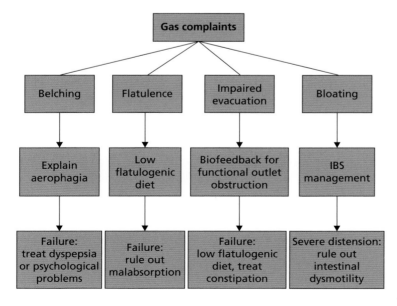

Figure 63.2 Management algorithm for gas complaints.

Prognosis

Prognosis is good, as in most functional gut disorders.

Take-home points

- Patients complaining of intestinal gas may refer to different types of conditions.
- Identify the specific clinical complaint: repetitive eructation, excessive/odoriferous flatus, impaired anal evacuation, or abdominal bloating/discomfort.
- Understand the mechanism of symptoms: aerophagia, bacterial fermentation of food residues, functional outlet obstruction, or intestinal sensory/reflex dysfunction.
- Plan the treatment strategy depending on the pathophysiology.

References

1 Bredenoord AJ, Smout AJ. Physiologic and pathologic belching. *Clin Gastroenterol Hepatol* 2007; **5**: 772–5.

2 Suarez FL, Springfield J, Levitt MD. Identification of gases responsible for the odour of human flatus and evaluation of a device purported to reduce this odour. *Gut* 1998; **43**: 100–4.

3 Azpiroz F, Enck P, Whitehead WE. Anorectal functional testing. Review of a collective experience. *Am J Gastroenterol* 2002; **97**: 232–40.

4 Accarino A, Perez F, Azpiroz F, *et al*. Intestinal gas and bloating: effect of prokinetic stimulation. *Am J Gastroenterol* 2008; **103**: 2036–42.

5 Tremolaterra F, Villoria A, Azpiroz F, *et al*. Impaired viscerosomatic reflexes and abdominal wall dystony associated with bloating. *Gastroenterology* 2006; **130**: 1062–8.

6 Suarez FL, Levitt MD. Intestinal gas. In: Feldman M, Friedman LS, Sleisenger MH, eds. *Gastrointestinal and Liver Diseases: Pathophysiology/Diagnosis/Management*. Philadelphia, PA: WB Sanders Co, 2002: 155–63.

7 Azpiroz F, Malagelada J-R. Abdominal bloating. *Gastroenterology* 2005; **129**: 1060–78.

8 Villoria A, Serra J, Azpiroz F, *et al*. Physical activity and intestinal gas clearance in patients with bloating. *Am J Gastroenterol* 2006; **101**: 2552–7.

9 Azpiroz F, Serra J. Treatment of excessive intestinal gas. *Curr Treat Option Gastroenterol* 2004; **7**: 299–305.

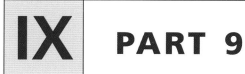

PART 9

Transplantation

CHAPTER 64
Small Bowel Transplantation

Juan P. Rocca[1] and Jonathan P. Fryer[2]

[1] Mount Sinai School of Medicine, New York, NY, USA
[2] Department of Surgery, Feinberg School of Medicine, Northwestern University, Chicago, IL, USA

Summary

Parenteral nutrition (PN) is the primary therapeutic option for intestinal failure (IF) patients and intestinal transplant (ITx) has a potential life saving role for those patients with PN failure. Most IF patients are not referred for ITx until irreversible PN-associated liver disease (PNALD) has developed and they need a liver transplant also, leading to inferior outcomes compared to patients referred earlier for isolated ITx. Intestinal rehabilitation attempts to optimize the function of the intestine with the goal of subsequently weaning PN completely or partially while expediting the identification of cases not weanable from PN and at highest risk of PN failure, where early ITx needs to be considered. Collaboration with intestinal rehabilitation centers should be initiated for IF patients if PN requirements are anticipated to be 50% or more at 3 months from the initiation of therapy. Outcomes with intestinal transplantation are steadily improving, with 1-year patient survival rates for isolated ITx being similar to liver transplant.

Case

A 29-year-old previously healthy female presented to the Emergency Department with persistent abdominal pain, nausea, and vomiting. She was taken to the Operating Room and found to have necrotic small bowel and colon as the result of a volvulus. Following resection with this surgery and after second-look procedure 24 h later she was left with 20 cm of jejunum distal to the ligament of Treitz and the colon distal to the mid-transverse colon. GI continuity was re-established at this time via jejunal–colic anastomosis. She was stabilized and started on PN and was discharged 2 weeks later with home PN. Within 3 months she developed progressive jaundice. She was referred to a center with expertise in intestinal failure management and PN-associated liver disease (PNALD). PN was cycled and lipids were minimized. Endoscopic retrograde cholangiopancreatography (ERCP) revealed normal biliary tree with possible gall stones. The patient underwent cholecystectomy and a STEP procedure was performed on her dilated jejunum. Following recovery her jaundice continued to progress and the patient was administered recombinant human growth hormone for 1 month and following this her enteral intake was

maximized and an attempt was made to wean her PN. This was unsuccessful. She was treated on speculation for bacterial overgrowth, with no improvement. Repeat liver biopsy was consistent with severe PN-associated cholestatis with periportal fibrosis. The patient was listed for isolated intestinal transplant and was successfully transplanted after 6 weeks on the list. She was discharged in 4 days and managed as an outpatient. As diet was advanced, PN was gradually weaned and eliminated by 1 month post-transplant. Liver function tests including total bilirubin were completely normal by 3 months post-transplant.

Introduction and Definitions

Intestinal failure (IF) results from a variety of disease entities [1,2] and the resultant inability to maintain protein-energy, fluid, electrolyte, or micronutrient balance despite maximal delivery of enteral nutrients [3]. Home parenteral nutrition (HPN) has allowed patients with IF an opportunity to live and it is considered the primary therapeutic option [4]. However, long-term HPN is associated with potentially life-threatening complications in high-risk patient subsets, including PN-associated liver disease (PNALD) [5], where intestinal transplantation (ITx) has a potential life-saving role if timely indicated [1,4].

Practical Gastroenterology and Hepatology: Small and Large Intestine and Pancreas, 1st edition. Edited by Nicholas J. Talley, Sunanda V. Kane and Michael B. Wallace. © 2010 Blackwell Publishing Ltd.

Classically, the role for ITx has been largely based on the development of PN failure on patients with irreversible IF, as defined by the Medicare criteria (Table 64.1). However, recent analyses of international data show that current referral practices result in patients being considered for transplantation late [6], when the finding of irreversible PNALD often mandates a combined liver–intestine transplant that is associated with inferior outcomes when compared to those patients that are referred earlier and need only an isolated ITx [4,6–8].

Intestinal rehabilitation is an active and time-sensitive process that attempts to optimize the function of the intestine using medical, surgical, and nutritional strategies with the goal of subsequently weaning PN completely or partially. This process expedites the identification of those patients that are not weanable from PN

Table 64.1 Medicare criteria for parenteral nutrition failure.

Impending liver failure (total bilirubin >3–6 mg/dL, progressive thrombocytopenia, and progressive splenomegaly) or overt liver failure (portal hypertension, hepatosplenomegaly, hepatic fibrosis, or cirrhosis)

Central venous catheter related thrombosis of ≥2 central veins

Frequent central line sepsis: ≥2 episodes/year of systemic sepsis secondary to line infections requiring hospitalization; a single episode of line-related fungemia; septic shock or adult respiratory distress syndrome (ARDS)

Frequent episodes of severe dehydration despite IV fluids resuscitation in addition to PN.

and are at highest risk of developing PN failure and who therefore need to be considered for intestinal transplantation early [8].

Indications: When to Refer for Intestinal Transplant

Intestinal transplantation is indicated for patients with irreversible intestinal failure [9]. Unfortunately, significant differences in opinion still exist regarding when patients should be considered for intestinal transplantation. Increasing attention has been directed toward the development of a more global strategy for IF patients that emphasizes early intestinal rehabilitation to eliminate PN dependence and more timely consideration of intestinal transplant in those that remain at high risk of PN-related complications as they have increased mortality before receiving a transplant (Figure 64.1) [7,10,11]. The risk factors differ in the pediatric and adult population. The high-risk group in adults include those hospitalized, those with poor quality of life because of narcotic dependency, central venous access complications, and those with deteriorating liver disease (moderate PNALD or more) [8].

PNALD may be the most controversial complication associated with long-term PN use. If the risk of PNALD is not appreciated early when preventive measures can be initiated it can rapidly progress to irreversibility, mandating the addition of a liver transplant. In the United

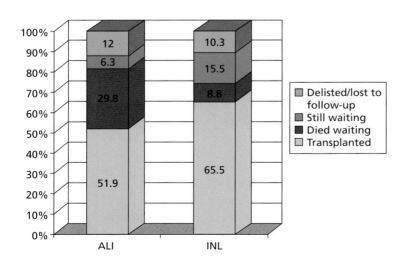

Figure 64.1 Outcomes of candidates on the intestinal transplant waiting list based on their need for a liver transplant also. ALI, all patients listed for liver/intestine; INL, listed for intestine but never for liver. (Based on Organ Procurement and Transplantation Network (OPTN) data as of Jan 2008.)

Network for Organ Sharing (UNOS) experience, approximately 75% of candidates listed for intestinal transplant have needed to be listed for a liver transplant also. This also has resulted in the need to use donor livers from an already inadequate supply [7,12].

Indications: Types of Intestinal Transplant

Ideally, IF patients should be considered for isolated ITx (small bowel ± colon) before irreversible PNALD develop. However, if PNALD has caused irreversible liver injury a combined liver-intestine transplant must be performed. The indications for liver transplant with lesser degrees of PNALD remain controversial and vary between transplant centers, as there is some evidence that even advanced PNALD is reversible following isolated ITx [13]. To maintain the anatomical continuity of the portal venous system and bile duct most combined liver–intestine transplants also include the pancreas.

Multivisceral transplants (MVTx) represent an inconsistently defined third type of intestinal transplant, and are usually indicated for diffuse gastrointestinal disorders such as motility disorders, extensive portal venous thrombosis, or benign neoplasms, where the type and number of organs to be replaced are dictated by the extent of the abdominal pathology. UNOS defines a MVTx as one that includes intestine, liver, and either pancreas or kidney [14]. The international Intestinal Transplant Registry (ITR) defines a MVTx as one that includes the stomach [6]. Others define a MVTx as one that involves replacement of all organs dependent on the celiac and superior mesenteric arteries (i.e., stomach, duodenum, liver, pancreas, small bowel ± proximal large bowel) [11] and the term "modified" multivisceral is used if the liver is excluded. A lack of consistency in the definition of and indications for a multivisceral transplant has impaired efforts to fully evaluate its role in the management of intestinal failure.

Outcomes

Intestinal transplant outcomes data from the international ITR [2,6], and US data from UNOS are updated

Table 64.2 Graft and patient survival after transplantation. (Data from 2007 UNOS Annual Report.)

		Survival (%)		
		1 Year	**3 Years**	**5 Years**
Liver only (deceased donor only)	Graft	82.3	73.7	67.6
	Patient	86.9	78.9	73.6
Intestine only	Graft	73.4	54.3	36.9
	Patient	81.0	67.4	53.6
Liver/intestine	Graft	75.0	68.2	55.7
	Patient	76.3	70.1	58.1

regularly (biannually and annually, respectively) and are available for online review [6,12].

Recent data demonstrated a significant difference in patient survival for the 2005–2007 period when isolated ITx was compared to combined liver–intestine or MVTx transplants (Figure 64.2). Accordingly, the average postoperative length of stay was also shorter for isolated ITx: 30 days versus 45 to 60 days on MVTx or combined liver–intestine transplants. Six months after transplantation 70% of the recipients had full intestinal graft function (PN independent) and modified Karnofsky performance scores of 90–100%. Interestingly, patients who received a segment of donor colon are more likely to be completely independent of all parenteral supplementation than those patients who did not receive a colon segment. Table 64.2 outlines the UNOS outcome data updated to 2007 [12]. Both registries' data analysis display an outstanding improvement in the short-term graft and patient survival when compared with the 1990s decade (Figure 64.3), possibly heralding similar improvements in long-term outcomes [15]. Modifications that clearly contributed to this were better patient selection, refinements in the surgical technique, advances on immunosuppressive strategies with antilymphocyte antibody induction and maintenance drugs such as tacrolimus and sirolimus, management of viral infectious complications such as CMV enteritis and post-transplant lymphoproliferative disease (Epstein–Barr virus), as well as the implementation of surveillance endoscopies–biopsies for the management of acute rejection episodes [16–20]. However, long-term outcomes with ITx still remain inferior to those of most other organs transplants, where problems such as chronic graft rejection, late-

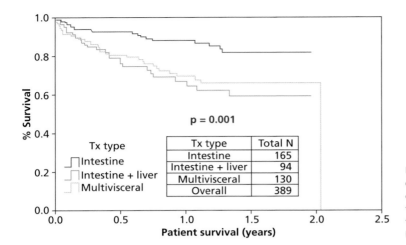

Figure 64.2 Comparative patient survival on isolated intestinal transplant versus combined liver–intestine or multivisceral transplant, period 2005–2007. Tx, transplant. (Intestine Transplant Registry, http://www.intestinetransplant.org)

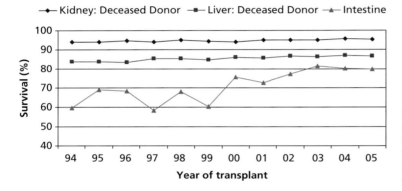

Figure 64.3 Relative improvement in 1-year patient survival for intestine transplant recipients comparing to kidney and liver transplant recipients. (2007 OPTN/Scientific Registry for Transplant Recipients (SRTR) Annual Report 1997–2006.)

onset acute rejection, and enteropathy still need to be resolved [16].

Overall, the most significant cause of morbidity and mortality has been infectious complications. Up to 60% of the deaths in intestinal transplant patients have been attributed to multiorgan failure, to which sepsis was likely the most contributing factor. Other causes of death have included rejection (10%), PTLD (6–8%), and graft thrombosis (5%). The most common causes of graft loss is rejection (56.3%), followed by ischemia/bleeding/thrombosis (20.6%), and sepsis (8.8%) [2,6].

Conclusion

Although intestinal transplantation continues to be one of the more challenging transplants, outcomes have improved dramatically in the last 10 years, becoming a viable option for individuals who are otherwise committed to a life of HPN because of intestinal failure. As with kidney transplantation and dialysis decades earlier, intestinal transplantation must prove to be superior to the established, default strategy of long-term HPN before it can be considered the treatment of choice. Existing data clearly support earlier consideration of intestinal transplantation in high-risk intestinal failure patient populations and only randomized controlled trials in this patient population will determine which therapy is associated with better outcomes. While several individual strategies have shown promise to further improve outcomes with intestinal transplantation, focused collaborative multi-center trials will be needed to move the field forward.

Take-home points

- Parenteral nutrition (PN) is the primary therapeutic option for intestinal failure (IF) patients and intestinal transplant (ITx) has a potential life-saving role for those patients with PN failure.

- Most IF patients are not referred for ITx until irreversible PN-associated liver disease (PNALD) has developed and they need a liver transplant also.

- Compared with those listed for ITx only, candidates needing both an intestine and a liver transplant have worse outcomes.

- Collaboration with intestinal rehabilitation centers should be initiated for IF patients if PN requirements are anticipated to be 50% or more at 3 months from the initiation of therapy.

- IF programs need to include intestinal rehabilitation and transplantation, or to have an active collaborative relationship with centers that perform ITx.

- Until an updated, evidence-based consensus emerges, it is recommended that the criteria for proceeding to list for ITx should be defined at the individual IF rehabilitation centers who will normally be guided by the Medicare criteria for PN failure.

References

1 Kaufman SS, Tzakis AG, *et al.* Indications for pediatric intensplantation: a position paper of the American Society of Transplantation. *Pediatr Transplant* 2001; **5**: 80–7.

2 Grant D, Farmer D, *et al.* 2003 report of the Intestine Transplant Registry. A new era has dawned. *Ann Surg* 2005; **241**: 607–13.

3 O'Keefe SJ, Shaffer J, *et al.* Short bowel syndrome and intestinal failure: consensus definitions and overview. *Clin Gastroenterol Hepatol* 2006; **4**: 6–10.

4 Pironi L, Goulet O, *et al.* Survival of patients identified as candidates for intestinal transplantation: a 3-year prospective follow up. *Gastroenterology* 2008; **135**: 61–71.

5 Buchman AL, Fryer J. Parenteral nutrition associated liver disease and the role for isolated intestine and intestine / liver transplantation. *Hepatology* 2006; **43**: 9–19.

6 http://www.intestinetransplant.org. Intestinal Transplant Registry.

7 Chungfat N, Fryer JP, *et al.* Impact of parenteral nutrition-associated liver disease on intestinal transplant waitlist dynamics. *J Am Coll Surg* 2007; **205**: 755–61.

8 Beath S, Fryer J, *et al.* Collaborative strategies to reduce mortality and morbidity in patients with chronic intestinal failure including those who are referred for small bowel transplantation. *Transplantation* 2008; **85**: 1378–84.

9 Sudan DL. Treatment of intestinal failure: intestinal transplantation. *Nat Clin Pract Gastroenterol Hepatol* 2007; **4**: 503–10.

10 Middleton SJ. Is intestinal transplantation now an alternative to home parenteral nutrition? *Proc Nutr Soc* 2007; **66**: 316–20.

11 Lopushinsky SR, Wales PW, *et al.* The optimal timing of intestinal transplantation for children with intestinal failure: a Markov analysis. *Ann Surg* 2007; **246**: 1092–9.

12 http://www.UNOS.org. United Network for Organ Sharing.

13 Fiel MI, Schiano TD, *et al.* Regression of hepatic fibrosis after intestinal transplantation in total parenteral nutrition liver disease. *Clin Gastroenterol Hepatol* 2008; **6**: 926–33.

14 Tzakis AG, Ruiz P, *et al.* 100 multivisceral transplants at a single center. *Ann Surg* 2005; **242**: 480–90.

15 Lacaille G, Goulet O, *et al.* Long-term outcome, growth and digestive function in children 2 to 18 years after intestinal transplantation. *Gut* 2008; **57**: 455–61.

16 Pascher A, *et al.* Present status and future perspectives of intestinal transplantation. *Transpl Int* 2008; **21**: 401–14.

17 Selvaggi G, Tzakis AG, *et al.* Analysis of acute cellular rejection episodes in recipients to primary intestinal transplantation: a single center, 11-year experience. *Am J Transplant* 2007; **7**: 1249–57.

18 Bond GJ, Reyes J, *et al.* Evolutionary experience with immunosuppression in pediatric intestinal transplantation. *J Pediatr Surg* 2005; **40**: 274–9.

19 Fishbein TM, Kaufman S, *et al.* Intestinal transplantation before and after the introduction of sirolimus. *Transplantation* 2002; **73**: 1538–42.

20 Ruiz P, Reyes J, *et al.* Histological criteria for the identification of acute cellular rejection in human small bowel allografts: results of the pathology workshop at the VIII international small bowel transplant symposium. *Trans Proc* 2004; **36**: 335–7.

CHAPTER 65

Gastrointestinal Complications of Solid Organ and Hematopoietic Cell Transplantation

Natasha Chandok[1] and Kymberly D.S. Watt[2]

[1] Division of Gastroenterology and Hepatology, University of Western Ontario, London, ON, Canada
[2] Division of Gastroenterology and Hepatology, William J. von Liebig Transplant Center, Mayo Clinic, Rochester, MN, USA

Summary

Solid organ transplantation (SOT) and hematopoietic cell transplantation (HCT) have dramatically improved the survival and quality of life in patients with a variety of malignancies and chronic end-organ disease. Gastrointestinal (GI) complications occur in almost 40% of solid organ recipients, and similarly account for many of the non-allograft-related adverse outcomes in the HCT population. GI disorders are frequently present prior to transplant and immunosuppression may augment symptoms. Immunosuppressive drugs also have notable GI side effects, and immunosuppression predisposes patients to infections and malignancies of the liver and GI tract. Graft-versus-host disease presents with GI manifestations and can occur following SOT but is more frequently seen after HCT. Sinusoidal obstruction syndrome (SOS), also known as veno-occlusive disease (VOD), an immunosuppression regimen-related toxicity, has been reported in SOT, but is also more often seen in the HCT population. GI complications are a prevailing source of morbidity and mortality in solid organ and bone marrow transplant recipients. The gastroenterologist should have a broad clinical approach to these complex patients with a low threshold for endoscopy as histopathology is often necessary for diagnosis and management of these patients

Case

A 56-year-old man underwent a cadaveric liver transplant 4 years ago for primary sclerosing cholangitis (PSC) and cholangiocarcinoma. He has a 12-year history of pan-ulcerative colitis, and his last surveillance colonoscopy 9 months ago showed no dysplasia and mild disease activity. Aside from mild acute rejection which was successfully treated with corticosteroids, his post-transplant course has been unremarkable. Two weeks ago, he developed a new onset of bloody diarrhea with crampy abdominal pain and intermittent fevers. He is having 10 bloody bowel movements daily, urgency and tenesmus. He has not been hospitalized nor has he received antibiotics for over a year.

He is on tacrolimus, alendronate, simvastatin, nifedipine, and mesalamine.

Physical exam is significant for normal vital signs and moderate tenderness in the left lower quadrant but no peritonitis. Laboratory studies show a leukocytosis and thrombocytosis of 1.5 times the upper limit of normal, therapeutic tacrolimus level, and normal liver function and transaminases. Stool cultures and stool for *C. difficile* toxin are pending. A colonoscopy is performed showing pan-colitis with deep ulcerations. Multiple biopsies were performed.

Introduction

Solid organ transplantation (SOT) and hematopoietic cell transplantation (HCT) are complex treatments which have dramatically improved the survival and quality of life in patients with a variety of malignancies

Practical Gastroenterology and Hepatology: Small and Large Intestine and Pancreas, 1st edition. Edited by Nicholas J. Talley, Sunanda V. Kane and Michael B. Wallace. © 2010 Blackwell Publishing Ltd.

and organ failures. The celebrated success of transplantation is in large part due to the effectiveness of immunosuppressive medications in extending graft survival, but this success is not without a heavy price.

Gastrointestinal (GI) complications occur in almost 40% of solid organ recipients, and similarly account for most of the non-allograft-related adverse outcomes in the HCT population [1,2]. GI disorders are frequently present prior to transplant and immunosuppression may augment symptoms. Immunosuppressive drugs also have notable GI side effects, and immunosuppression predisposes patients to infections and malignancies of the liver and GI tract.

In comparison to SOT, patients with HCT are at greater risk for organ toxicities and severe infections because the preparation for HCT requires aggressive myeloablative therapy or immunosuppression. As such, HCT patients are also much more susceptible to graft-versus-host disease (GVHD). In addition, sinusoidal obstruction syndrome (SOS), also known as veno-occlusive disease (VOD), an immunosuppression regimen-related toxicity, has been reported in SOT, but is more often seen in the HCT population [3].

In this chapter, we will review the important GI complications that impact transplant recipients. These complications include infections, malignancies, adverse drug events, and generalized GI disorders. We will also highlight the salient features of GVHD and SOS.

Infections in the GI System Following SOT or HCT

Infections, sometimes life-threatening, are common in patients following a solid organ or bone marrow transplant, and they can present with various GI manifestations (Table 65.1). The risk of infection depends on the surgery performed, the level of the immunosuppression, the use of antibiotic medications, infectious exposures, and prophylactic measures used to prevent infection [1,4].

The infectious etiologies can be categorized by the time from transplantation—perioperative, early (1 to 6 months), and late (beyond 6 months) [1]. Early in the perioperative period, infections can be derived from pre-existing pathogens in the recipient, donor-derived infections, or infections as a consequence of the transplant

Table 65.1 Common causes of diarrhea post transplant.

Infection	*Clostridium difficile*
	Campylobacter, Salmonella, Shigella, E. coli
	Yersinia, Vibrio parahemolyticus
	Bacterial overgrowth
	Cytomegalovirus
	Rotavirus, Adenovirus, Norwalk virus
	Giardia
	Cryptosporidium, Cyclospora
	Entamoeba histolytica
Medication	Antibiotics
	Mycophenolate mofetil
	Sirolimus
	Cyclosporine
	Tacrolimus
Other	Ischemia
	IBD, celiac, IBS recurrence
	Graft-versus-host disease
	Post-transplant lymphoproliferative disease
	Overflow diarrhea
	Colorectal cancer

IBD, inflammatory bowel disease; IBS, irritable bowel syndrome.

operation. During the first 6 months, viral and opportunistic infections prevail, although the epidemiology of infections in this period has changed considerably with the use of routine chemoprophylaxis for opportunistic microbes [4]. After 6 months, if there is good graft function, the infections in the post-transplant host are generally community-acquired, although opportunistic infections can occur at any time, particularly when chemoprophylaxis has stopped. Risk factors for infections, particularly opportunistic ones, include poor graft function, hospitalizations, and more intense immunosuppression. Frequently, it is clinically challenging to diagnose infections in patients who are immunocompromised because these patients may not mount a typical response with fever and leukocytosis. GI symptoms are sometimes the only clinical clue to an underlying infection. Broadly speaking, a therapeutic strategy for treating infections in the post-transplant setting involves potent antimicrobial medications in conjunction with reducing immunosuppressive medications.

Viral Infections

The most significant viruses infecting the transplant patient are cytomegalovirus (CMV), herpes virus (HSV) and Epstein–Barr virus (EBV), and all can produce a variety of GI symptoms.

CMV is the most common viral infection causing symptoms after any transplant. CMV should be high on the differential diagnosis for any patient at all stages post-transplantation, particularly if the patient is not receiving CMV prophylaxis. Although CMV infection in the immunocompetent host is pervasive and usually asymptomatic, transplant patients typically present with constitutional symptoms such as fever, malaise, and anorexia. CMV infection can be localized to virtually any organ, including any portion of the GI tract. The GI tract is involved in up to one-third of patients with CMV [5]. GI symptoms include dysphagia, nausea, emesis, abdominal pain, diarrhea, and GI bleeding. CMV causes oral ulcers, mucositis, esophagitis, gastritis, duodenitis, small intestinal enteritis, colitis, and even bowel perforation on rare occasion. CMV hepatitis, usually more severe in liver transplant recipients, requires a liver biopsy to confirm the diagnosis as it can be easily mistaken for rejection.

After a transplant, CMV infection can originate from infected leukocytes within the allograft transplanted into the CMV naïve recipient, cause super-infection in a CMV-positive recipient, or be reactivated by immunosuppression [1]. The risk for CMV not only depends on the severity of immunosuppression and the CMV status of the recipient prior to transplant, but also on the type of solid organ transplanted [6]. It is more common in patients with small bowel, pancreas, and lung transplantation than liver, heart, and kidney recipients [6]. The diagnosis of CMV requires confirmation by polymerase chain reaction (PCR) of CMV DNA and/or biopsy confirmation of the involved organ.

Lowance and colleagues have demonstrated that routine anti-CMV therapy has reduced the occurrence of CMV in transplant recipients [7] and thus prophylaxis is usually prescribed for the initial 3 months after transplant. CMV prophylaxis should be re-started whenever rejection of allograft is being treated, particularly if antilymphocyte drugs are used. CMV is treated with gancyclovir or valgancyclovir (dosed according to renal function), with duration dependent on end-organ involvement.

HSV is the second most common viral infection seen following transplantation and, like CMV, it has many GI manifestations. HSV can be re-activated from the latent phase during intense immunosuppression, as occurs during the first month after transplantation. HSV in the immunocompromised host usually presents as oral ulcers and odynophagia or anorectal/genitourinary ulcers, but it can involve the intestine and liver in patients not on acyclovir. Transplant patients with odynophagia or dysphagia should be evaluated with an endoscopy to determine the etiology. Oral infection from HSV can be treated with oral acyclovir, but disseminated infection requires intravenous treatment.

Other herpesviruses—EBV, varicella zoster virus (VZV), and human herpesvirus 6 or 7 (HHV-6 or 7)—are less common than CMV and HSV following transplantation. EBV is nearly ubiquitous, affecting more than 90% of the human population. EBV persists in memory B cells [8]. With immunosuppression, transplant patients develop faulty T-cell immunity and cannot contain the growth of EBV in B-cells laden with the virus. EBV, in addition to producing an infectious mononucleosis picture with adenopathy and fever, can have a variety of GI manifestations. EBV can cause oral hairy leukoplakia, a pale adherent lesion on lateral aspect of the tongue, as well as numerous malignancies. EBV-associated lymphoproliferative disorder is the most significant of these malignancies, and it will be discussed later in the chapter.

Hepatitis C virus (HCV) and hepatitis B virus (HBV), common indications for liver transplantation, are notable co-morbid diseases in other transplant patients, particularly in kidney and pancreas transplant recipients, occurring in 10–15% [1]. These patients have a much higher liver-related mortality than matched controls [9]. Treatment with antiviral medications for hepatitis B is warranted in most cases to prevent liver disease progression. Treatment of hepatitis C may be attempted prior to transplant of non-liver organs, if the side-effect profile is tolerable and no clear organ-specific contraindication exists. Anti-HCV therapy can be attempted after transplantation but requires diligent follow-up because of the significant side effects in the already immunosuppressed patient. This therapy is also associated with a risk for allograft rejection which can be minimized by careful immunosuppression monitoring.

Fungal Infections

The most common fungal infection in the transplant population is candidiasis, most notably affecting the oral cavity and esophagus. Common GI presentations include dysphagia, odynophagia, gastroesophageal reflux disease

(GERD), and, rarely, GI bleeding. *Candida* is usually seen in the first 6 months after transplantation, with increased risk associated with high-dose steroids or antibiotic use. Endoscopy reveals superficial erosions, ulcers, white nodules or plaques, and the diagnosis is confirmed by histopathology and fungal cultures. *Candida* is usually treated with topical nystatin or oral fluconazole. In cases of resistance, caspofungin, posaconazole, or voriconazole can be given.

Hepatosplenic candidiasis occurs only in HCT patients and should be considered in the HCT patient with high fever and right or left upper quadrant pain, nausea, and vomiting. The frequency of this complication is decreased with prophylactic use of antifungal agents.

Parasitic Infections

Immunosuppressed transplant patients are at risk for protozoal infections with organisms such as *Microsporidium*, *Cryptosporidium*, *Isospora belli*, and *Giardia lamblia*. These parasitic infections usually cause diarrhea, and the diagnosis can be established with stool testing for ova and parasites. Microscopic examination of small bowel or colonic biopsies may be necessary to document organisms such as *Cryptosporidium*.

Treatment of parasitic infections involves antimicrobial drugs and a reduction in immunosuppression. Interestingly, cyclosporine possesses antihelminthic properties that may suppress the parasite *Strongyloides stercoralis*.

Bacterial Infections

Infectious diarrhea is also the most common GI presentation of a variety of bacterial organisms. Notable examples of these bacteria include *Clostridium difficile*, *Yersinia enterocolitica*, *Campylobacter jejuni*, *Salmonella*, and *Listeria monocytogenes*. Half of transplant patients getting antibiotics acquire *Clostridium difficile* colitis, so the clinician should maintain a high index of suspicion for this entity.

GI Malignancies after SOT and HCT

Transplant outcomes in the United States continue to improve, with the 1-year survival better than 85% and the 3-year survival better than 75% in solid organ recipients [10]. With longer life expectancy, post-transplant malignancies are an important cause of morbidity and mortality, with increased probability of GI malignancy over longer follow-up duration. The overall risk of malignancy following SOT is elevated compared with the general population. Epidemiological studies reveal that the length of exposure to immunosuppressive therapy and the intensity of the regimen are clearly related to the post-transplant risk of malignancy. Immunosuppression facilitates post-transplant malignancy by impairing cancer surveillance mechanisms and creating an environment for oncogenic viruses to thrive. Immunosuppressive medications, such as calcineurin inhibitors, could also play a role, having pro-oncogenic effects [11], where other agents such as sirolimus are thought to have antiproliferative properties. Once cancer has established, aggressive immunosuppression can result in increased proliferation of the tumor with worse clinical outcomes [11].

Transplant patients are at risk for tumors of infectious origin as well. Examples of oncogenic infections causing malignancies that may involve the GI tract include EBV causing lymphoproliferative diseases; HHV8 causing Kaposi sarcoma; HCV and HBV causing HCC; and *Helicobacter pylori* causing gastric cancer. EBV is also linked to nasopharyngeal and oral cancer, and transplant recipients have a sixfold higher risk for oral cancer. Anal cancer, linked to HPV, also occurs at a 10 to 20-fold higher frequency in transplant recipients [1]. A large retrospective study of 73 076 patients with heart and kidney transplant found a small increased risk for colon cancer, but a curious reduction in the incidence of rectal cancer [12]. Patients who drink alcohol to excess or smoke cigarettes are at higher risk of oral/pharyngeal and GI malignancies in the transplant population, more so than in the general population.

Malignancies following HCT can be categorized as early (less than 1 year after HCT) and late (occurring beyond 1 year after HCT). Early malignancies include acute leukemia, myelodysplastic syndrome (MDS), and PTLD. Late malignancies include a variety of solid tumors.

Post-transplant Lymphoproliferative Disorder

Post-transplant lymphoproliferative disorder (PTLD) is a well known complication of chronic immunosuppression in solid organ and bone marrow transplant recipients. Aside from skin and cervical cancer, PTLD is one of the most common malignancies after transplant [13]. PTLD can involve the GI tract because the gut is endowed with an abundance of lymphoid tissue. The overall incidence of PTLD is approximately 1–3% in recipients of HCT and SOT, 30 to 50 times higher than in the general population, with a recent trend toward increased frequency [14,15]. There is some variability with the incidence based on the type of solid organ transplant, with the highest occurrence seen in intestinal or multiorgan transplant at 11–33% [16]. The intensity of the immunosuppressive regimen is directly associated with the risk for PTLD.

The pathogenesis is partly related to B-cell proliferation induced by EBV, but EBV-negative disease can also occur. In the majority of cases, PTLD cells are of host origin. Patients are at higher risk for PTLD if they receive T-cell-depleted or HLA mismatched bone marrow, antilymphocyte antibodies, have CMV, or get primary EBV after transplantation. Transplant recipients without previous exposure to EBV are at increased risk (which is why younger children tend to be at highest risk).

Patients with PTLD can present with symptoms of infectious mononucleosis or localized lymphoproliferation involving a variety of organs. GI involvement may cause obstruction, bleeding, or perforation. A biopsy is needed for a definitive diagnosis. An early detection strategy—a rise in the titer of EBV DNA after periodic measurements—should trigger a reduction in immunosuppression and careful surveillance. Imaging modalities with CT scan and positron emission tomography (PET scan) aid in the diagnosis and staging of disease.

The treatment of PTLD is partly based on the histopathologic characteristics of the tumor. Reduction of immunosuppressive drugs is the first line therapy for all PTLD, and may be all that is required in less advanced disease. There may be a potential role for antiviral treatment in the management of EBV-associated lymphoproliferation [8]. Rituximab, an anti CD20 (B cell) antibody, in conjunction with reduction of immunosuppression is evolving into the standard of care for many of these patients. Monoclonal disease not responding to therapy may require more intensive chemotherapy regimens. Surgical removal or irradiation of localized lymphoproliferative tumors in the GI tract may occasionally be considered.

Gastrointestinal Adverse Drug Events

After transplantation, recipients are exposed to a number of immunosuppressive agents to help ensure graft survival. Several of these medications have significant GI side effects.

Cyclosporine, a calcineurin inhibitor derived from a fungus, causes gingival hyperplasia by inducing collagenolytic activity in gums [1]. Gingival hyperplasia may necessitate a substitution with tacrolimus or sirolimus. Tacrolimus, another calcineurin inhibitor, as well as cyclosporine, can cause nausea, abdominal pain, diarrhea, anorexia, and weight loss. The side effects appear dose dependent. At high levels, both cyclosporine and tacrolimus can cause cholestasis and cyclosporine increases cholesterol saturation in bile, a potential risk for gall stone formation.

Sirolimus blocks IL-2 receptor signal activation of T and B lymphocytes. It can produce a dose-dependent elevation in serum aminotransferases. A black box warning exists in the liver transplant setting for association with hepatic artery thrombosis. Specific GI side effects include mouth ulceration, incisional hernias (impairs wound healing), and diarrhea.

Mycophenolate mofetil (MMF) is an immunosuppressive agent often used in combination with a calcineurin inhibitor and prednisone. It inhibits inosine monophosphate dehydrogenase, impairing purine synthesis and proliferation of B and T lymphocytes. MMF has a number of GI side effects, including oral ulcerations, nausea, vomiting, and diarrhea. Dose reduction often improves symptoms.

Myeloablative conditioning therapy, used in HCT candidates to prevent the recipient from rejecting donor hematopoietic cells and for tumor cell ablation, makes most patients nauseated and anorexic. They can also get debilitating mucositis.

General GI Complications

Mucositis is a significant problem after HCT, and it is the most common complication of myeloablative preparative regimens [2]. Severe mucositis involves extensive oral and esophageal ulceration which can take many months to heal. Patients can develop excruciating pain with swallowing, nausea, cramping, and diarrhea. Patients may even require TPN for nutritional support in severe cases. For the majority, mucositis is self-limited. A recombinant human keratinocyte growth factor, palifermin, reduces the incidence of oral mucositis after autologous transplantation [17].

Pill-induced esophagitis is another common cause of morbidity in the transplant population. Antibiotics, antivirals, potassium tablets, bisphosphonates, and non-steroidal anti-inflammatory drugs (NSAIDs) are among the most common medications causing esophagitis. The incidence of pill-induced esophageal injury can be reduced by instructing patients to remain upright for at least 30 min following their pills and to consume plenty of water with ingested tablets. Proton pump inhibitors (PPI) can be useful in preventing esophageal injury.

GERD is extremely common in Western societies, with an estimated prevalence of 10 to 20% [18]. Not surprisingly, there is a high incidence of GERD following transplantation, possibly precipitated by medications and/or vagal nerve injury during the operation.

Peptic ulcer disease (PUD) is very common in the transplant population, particularly in kidney recipients [19]. In a large retrospective study from Missouri of 254 renal transplant patients who had endoscopies before and after their transplantation, 10% developed new PUD following transplant [19]. When complications of PUD arise, renal recipients can especially have dire outcomes, with 20% experiencing significant bleeding. The high incidence of *Helicobacter pylori* in patients with chronic renal failure contributes to the magnitude of this problem [19]. Fortunately, the risk for severe PUD can be reduced through active pretransplant screening endoscopies, PPI therapy, and antimicrobials to eradicate *H. pylori* [1]. A high incidence of large gastric ulcers has also been reported in liver transplant patients. Generally speaking, transplant patients should avoid NSAIDs as much for the gastric toxicities as for the renal ones.

Acute biliary tract disease is a complication in the transplant recipient, with a mortality as high as 29% in some series [1]. Following orthotopic liver transplantation (OLT), there is particular concern over hepatic artery stenosis or thrombosis as the biliary tree receives its blood supply from the hepatic artery. This can result in significant biliary complications with multiple strictures. A gradual loss of hepatic artery blood flow can cause ductopenia, and this entity can be difficult to distinguish from ductopenic rejection. Hepatic artery thrombosis (HAT) can have a variety of presentations, ranging from mildly elevated liver enzymes to fulminant liver failure in the acute setting after OLT. In the late post-OLT setting, HAT presents as biliary stricturing with cholangitis and intrahepatic abscesses. An anastomotic stricture is the most common biliary tract abnormality after OLT, and it typically develops 2–6 months after transplant, but it can occur sooner. Strictures at the duct-to-duct anastomosis can usually be fixed with endoscopic therapy, whereas strictures with choledochojejunostomies might need percutaneous or surgical repair. Acute portal vein thrombosis (PVT) can also cause hepatic ischemia and severe graft dysfunction if it occurs early.

Another potentially life-threatening GI complication after transplant is colonic perforation, which has an incidence after transplantation of 1–2%, and a mortality rate of 20–38% [20]. Possible etiologies to colonic perforation include diverticular disease, ischemia, and CMV colitis. Kidney transplant recipients are at particularly high risk for ischemic gut because they often possess underlying vascular disease.

Diarrhea in transplant recipients is very common, with a variety of etiologies. Many of the possible causes have already been discussed including the most common infectious etiologies, and drug side effects specific to the transplant patient. The physician should actively look for organisms such as *C. difficile*, standard bacterial infections as discussed and organisms such as *E. histolytica*, *Strongyloides*, *G. lamblia*, *Cryptosporidium*, *Clostridium*, CMV, rotavirus, and adenovirus in the right setting. Exacerbations of underlying diseases such as inflammatory bowel disease, celiac disease, or even irritable bowel syndrome (IBS) should be considered once infection is ruled out. It is important to remember post surgical issues such as overflow diarrhea from constipation (possibly narcotic related), or stasis and bacterial overgrowth in the setting of Roux limb anastomosis.

Perianal pain is also common in transplant recipients, particularly after bone marrow transplantation. The pain usually originates near the anus in granulocytopenic patients and is due to bacterial infection. There may be an abscess in the supralevator and intersphincteric region without being obvious on physical exam. Ideally, a perianal abscess should be drained and treated with antibiotics before HCT. HSV2 and HPV exacerbations can result in herpes flares and condylomata growth.

Special Topics

Graft-versus-host Disease (GVHD)

GVHD is a rare complication in SOT, but it is more often encountered following HCT [21–23]. Acute GVHD occurs between day 15 and 100, and chronic GVHD occurs beyond 100 days after HCT.

Both acute and chronic GVHD affect predominantly the skin, liver, and GI tract. Patients present with fevers, skin rash, and non-specific GI symptoms such as nausea, vomiting, anorexia, and diarrhea. GVHD can also affect other organs, including the kidneys and hematopoietic system.

Acute GVHD occurs in up to 50% of patients who receive allogeneic hematopoietic cell transplantation from an HLA-identical sibling despite intensive prophylaxis with immunosuppressive medications [22]. It is also common in matched unrelated donors and in haploidentical related donors. In acute GVHD, mismatches in histocompatibility between the donor and recipient lead to activation of donor T cells which cause damage to various epithelial tissues through dysregulated cytokine production and recruitment of additional effector cells. The pathogenesis of chronic GVHD is not as well understood and further research is needed in this area [23]. Risk factors for GVHD include HLA disparity, older age, donor and recipient gender discordance, previous GVHD, amount of radiation and intensity of the transplant conditioning regimen, and the use of immunosuppression such as methotrexate, cyclosporine, or tacrolimus [23,24].

Although the skin is classically the first organ involved, the liver is the second most common organ affected. GVHD damages the bile canaliculi leading to cholestasis, and patients develop elevated conjugated bilirubin and alkaline phosphatase. The differential diagnosis to the cholestatic liver enzyme picture in the acute post HCT setting would also include SOS, infection, and drug toxicity.

GI tract involvement in GVHD can often be severe. Patients can present with extreme diarrhea of more than 10 liters per day. The stool can be watery or bloody, and patients generally require intravenous fluids, and/or blood transfusions. As diarrhea is very common after HCT, particularly from infections such as *Clostridium difficile* and CMV, diagnosing GVHD can be challenging without rectal biopsy. On biopsy, crypt cell necrosis with accumulation of degenerative material in the dead crypts is characteristic of GVHD. In severe cases, GVHD can obliterate the entire mucosa of the gut.

Patients with upper GI tract GVHD present with anorexia, dyspepsia, nausea, and vomiting. Endoscopy shows edema of the gastric antral and duodenal mucosa, and patchy erythema. Interestingly, GVHD in the upper GI tract is more responsive to immunosuppressive therapy than in other areas of the gut.

Prophylaxis for GVHD with methotrexate and cyclosporine is routinely prescribed for several months after HCT. Patients with GVHD should be managed by transplant physicians with expertise in GVHD. A variety of immunosuppressive agents can be employed, including corticosteroids, cyclosporine, tacrolimus, rapamycin, mycophenolate mofetil, and thalidomide [22,23].

Sinusoidal Obstruction Syndrome (SOS)

SOS or veno-occlusive disease (VOD) can occur after both allogenic and autologous hematopoietic stem cell transplantation. It has also been described with the use of high dose azathioprine or with various other chemotherapeutic agents and radiation treatments for a number of malignancies. SOS is uncommonly seen after liver transplantation, mostly in the context of azathioprine use [25]. In HCT recipients, depending on the study population and diagnostic criteria used, the incidence of SOS ranges from 5 to 70%, and the overall mortality also varies from 20 to 50% [3].

In SOS, damaged sinusoidal endothelium sloughs off and obstructs the hepatic circulation, destroying centrilobular hepatocytes. A number of mediators, including 5-hydroxytryptamine, prostaglandins, leukotrienes, and free radicals contribute to endothelial damage culminating in liver cell ischemic injury and death. In the later stages of the disease, intense fibrogenesis occurs in the sinusoids, ultimately causing obliteration of the venules and chronic venous outflow obstruction.

A number of risk factors for SOS have been identified. A few of the notable risk factors include chronic liver disease, C282Y allele of the HFE gene, advanced age, hepatic metastases, previous radiation treatment to the liver, high-dose conditioning regimens, busulfan or gemtuzumab ozogamicin exposure, cyclophosphamide, and possibly infections such as CMV and HCV [3,26].

The clinical manifestations of SOS usually surface around 7 to 10 days after transplant. The primary symptoms are weight gain and jaundice. Patients develop ascites, right upper quadrant tenderness, hepatomegaly, and conjugated hyperbilirubinemia. In severe cases, renal, cardiac, and respiratory failure can occur.

The diagnosis of SOS can be a difficult one to make, as so many other syndromes can have a similar presentation. Although the gold standard for diagnosis is a liver biopsy, this is seldom done because of potential complications of bleeding in the setting of thrombocytopenia. An ultrasound with Doppler flow will show portal hypertension late in the course.

The majority of patients with mild disease will improve over a few weeks. Unfortunately, there are no effective treatments to offer aside from supportive care, so prevention is critically important. Prevention strategies may involve the use of reduced intensity chemotherapy regimens, ursodiol, or a fibrinolytic agent such as defibrotide [26].

- Drugs, including immunosuppressive medications, can cause GI complications after transplant and gastroenterologists should be familiar with these medications and their side effects.
- Graft-versus-host disease and sinusoidal obstruction syndrome are more common after HCT than SOT and have significant morbidity and mortality requiring timely diagnosis and management.

References

1 Gautam A. Gastrointestinal complications following transplantation. *Surg Clin North Am* 2006; **86**: 1195–206.

2 Copelan EA. Hematopoietic stem-cell transplantation. *N Eng J Med* 2006; **354**: 1813–26.

3 Kumar S, DeLeve LD, Kamath PS, *et al.* Hepatic veno-occlusive disease (sinusoidal obstruction syndrome) after hematopoietic stem cell transplantation. *Mayo Clin Proc* 2003; **78**: 589–98.

4 Fischer SA. Infections complicating solid organ transplantation. *Surg Clin North Am* 2006; **86**: 1127–45.

5 Rubin RH. Impact of cytomegalovirus infection on organ transplant recipients. *Rev Infect Dis* 1990; **12**: S754–66.

6 Syndman DR. Infection in solid organ transplantation. *Transplant Infect Dis* 1999; **1**: 21–9.

7 Lowance D, Neumayer HH, Legendre CM, *et al.* Valacylovir for the prevention of cytomegalovirus disease after renal transplantation. International Valacylovir Cytomegalovirus Prophylaxis Transplantation Study Group. *N Engl J Med* 1999; **340**: 1462–70.

8 Cohen JI. Epstein-Barr virus infection. *N Eng J Med* 2000; **343**: 481–92.

9 Yu JTHT, Lau GKK. Treatment of hepatitis B and C following nonliver organ transplants. *Curr Hepatitis Rep* 2003; **2**: 82–7.

10 United Network for Organ Sharing, 2008. www.unos.org

11 Gutierrez-Dalmau A, Campistol JM. Immunosuppressive therapy and malignancy in organ transplant recipients. a systematic review. *Drugs* 2007; **67**: 1167–98.

12 Stewart T, Henderson R, Grayson H, *et al.* Reduced incidence of rectal cancer, compared to gastric and colonic cancer, in a population of 73,076 men and women chronically immunosuppressed. *Clin Cancer Rev* 1997; **3**: 51–5.

13 Penn, I. Cancers complicating organ transplantation. *N Engl J Med* 1990; **323**: 1767–9.

14 Andreone P, Gramenzi A, Lorenzini S, *et al.* Posttransplantation lymphoproliferative disorders. *Arch Intern Med* 2003; **163**: 1997–2004.

Case continued

The most likely diagnosis is either a flare of ulcerative colitis or an infection. Although a number of organisms can cause bloody diarrhea, the two most common entities are *C. difficile* and CMV. Histopathology is essential to establish a diagnosis in an immunocompromised host. The clinician should avoid empiric treatment for ulcerative colitis flares as corticosteroids will exacerbate most infections.

Stool for *C. difficile* toxin is negative and CMV antigenemia and PCV are strongly positive. Colonic biopsies contain severe inflammation, crypt distortion, giant cells, and intranuclear inclusion bodies, confirming CMV colitis.

The patient responded to treatment with ganciclovir.

Take-home points

- GI complications are a prevailing source of morbidity and mortality in solid organ and bone marrow transplant recipients.
- Immunosuppression predisposes patients to infections and malignancies of the liver and GI tract.

15 Caillard S, Lelong C, Pessione F, *et al.* Post-transplant lymphoproliferative disorders occurring after renal transplantation in adults: report of 230 cases from the French registry. *Am J Transplant* 2006; **6**: 2735–42.

16 Cockfield SM. Identifying the patient at risk for post-transplant lymphoproliferative disorder. *Tranpl Infect Dis* 2001; **3**: 70–78.

17 Spielberger R, Stiff P, Bensinger W, *et al.* Palifermin for oral mucositis after intensive therapy for hematologic cancers. *N Engl J Med* 2004; **351**: 2590–8.

18 Armstrong D. Systematic review: persistence and severity in gastro-oesophageal reflux disease. *Aliment Pharmacol Ther* 2008; **28**: 841–53.

19 Reece J, Burton F, Lingle D, *et al.* Peptic ulcer disease following renal transplantation in the cyclosporine era. *Am J Surg* 1991; **162**: 558–62.

20 Stelzner M, Vlahakos DV, Milford EL, *et al.* Colonic perforations after renal transplantation. *J Am Coll Surg* 1997; **184**: 63–9.

21 Smith DM, Agura E, Netto G, *et al.* Liver transplantation associated graft-versus-host disease. *Transplantation* 2003; **75**: 118–26.

22 Couriel D, Caldera H, Champlin R, *et al.* Acute graft-versus-host disease: pathophysiology, clinical manifestations, and management. *Cancer* 2004; **101**: 1936.

23 Bhushan V, Collins RH. Chronic graft-vs-host disease. *JAMA* 2003; **290**: 2599–03.

24 Cutler C, Giri S, Jeyapalan S, *et al.* Acute and chronic graft-versus-host disease after allogeneic peripheral-blood stem-cell and bone marrow transplantation: a meta-analysis. *J Clin Oncol* 2001; **19**: 3685–91.

25 Sebagh M, Debette M, Samuel D, *et al.* "Silent" presentation of SOS after liver transplantation as part of the process of cellular rejection with endothelial predilection. *Hepatology* 1999; **30**: 1144–50.

26 Wadleigh M, Ho V, Momtaz P, Richardson P. Hepatic veno-occlusive disease: pathogenesis, diagnosis and treatment. *Curr Opin Hematol* 2003; **10**: 451–62.

PART 10

Peritoneal and Other Abdominal Disease

CHAPTER 66

Peritonitis

Robert R. Cima

Department of Surgery, Mayo Clinic, Rochester, MN, USA

Summary

Peritonitis is a clinical syndrome associated with a high risk of morbidity and mortality. While there are numerous medical and pharmacologic induced conditions that share the same clinical signs of peritonitis, it is most commonly associated with either a localized or generalized bacterial infection involving the peritoneal cavity. Peritonitis is a clinical diagnosis since there are no pathagnomic laboratory or radiologic findings. The primary finding on physical examination is severe abdominal pain characterized by evidence of peritoneal irritation as manifested by abdominal wall rigidity and rebound tenderness. Treatment is directed at the underlying source of the peritoneal contamination. Surgical intervention to control or remove the source of the infection is almost always required in cases of generalized peritonitis while causes of localized peritonitis may be approached with percutaneous drainage procedures. Failure to quickly and decisively address a patient with peritonitis is associated with a high mortality rate.

Case

A 47-year-old man undergoes surgery for reversal of a sigmoid colostomy 6 months after emergency surgery for perforated sigmoid diverticulitis. He is above his ideal body weight and a Type 1 diabetic. His postoperative course is notable for an ileus that resolves with conservative management. He is dismissed to home on postoperative day 9, tolerating a regular diet and having bowel movements. Four days after dismissal, he reports a fever overnight to 102°F and some lower midline pelvic pain. He continues to tolerate a diet and is passing flatus and stool. He is seen in the office where he is afebrile, heart rate (HR) 95 bpm, blood pressure (BP) 130/78 mmHg. His wound is clean with no drainage or erythema. His exam is notable for some left flank and suprapubic discomfort on deep palpation. He has no guarding or rebound. His white blood cell (WBC) count is 13.5 cells/μL and his urine analysis shows many WBC and a few bacteria. He is started on oral antibiotics for a presumed urinary tract infection. Three days later he presents to the emergency room confused, complaining of 1 day of left lower abdominal pain which became acutely worse about 2 h before presentation. He has a heart rate of 132, BP of 87/62, and is febrile to 102.5°F. On exam he is lying

extremely still. His abdomen is distended, diffusely tender, with rebound tenderness across the lower abdomen. A computed tomography (CT) scan obtained in the Emergency Room demonstrates free air and fluid throughout the abdomen, a large pelvic extraluminal collection consistent with stool, and complete disruption of the colorectal anastomosis (Figure 66.1). He is taken directly to the operating room for exploration. The prior anastomosis is disrupted and there is feculent material throughout the abdomen. A new colostomy is brought up and the rectum oversewn. The abdomen is left open with a temporary dressing after extensive irrigation. He is sent to the ICU. He remains ventilated for 7 days suffering from acute respiratory distress syndrome (ARDS). He is returned to the operating room three times for abdominal washout and eventual closure of the abdomen with Vicryl™ mesh. He is dismissed from the hospital 33 days later.

Anatomy and Definitions

The peritoneum is the lining of the abdominal cavity and exposed surfaces of the intra-abdominal organs. It consists of a sheet of squamous epithelium originating from the mesoderm. Although it might seem that the peritoneal cavity is simply a space within which the abdominal viscera are contained, it actually is a complex compart-

Practical Gastroenterology and Hepatology: Small and Large Intestine and Pancreas, 1st edition. Edited by Nicholas J. Talley, Sunanda V. Kane and Michael B. Wallace. © 2010 Blackwell Publishing Ltd.

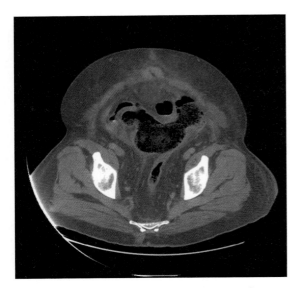

Figure 66.1 Pelvic CT scan image without oral contrast of a patient 17 days after colostomy reversal who presented with fever and peritonitis. In the lower abdomen, there is evidence of free air and a large stool-filled cavity which is outside of the large bowel lumen.

Table 66.1 Common causes of secondary peritonitis.

Primary infectious processes	Appendicitis
	Diverticulitis
	Gangrenous cholecystitis
	Toxic *C. difficile* colitis
	Pelvic inflammatory disease
	Tube–ovarian abscess
Spontaneous intestinal perforation	Gastric ulcer
	Duodenal ulcer
	Crohn disease
	Toxic ulcerative colitis
Iatrogenic intestinal perforation	Endoscopic intervention (i.e., polypectomy)
	Dislodged gastrostomy or enterostomy tube
Intestinal ischemia	Intestinal low flow state
	Arterial embolic event
	Mesenteric venous thrombosis
	Internal hernia/closed loop obstruction
	Incarcerated intestinal hernia
	Volvulus
Postsurgical complications	Anastomotic leak
	Inadvertent/unrecognized intestinal injury
	Intra-abdominal abscess
	Infected hematoma

ment [1]. The parietal peritoneum covers the abdominal wall and retroperitoneal surfaces while the visceral peritoneum envelopes the intra-abdominal organs. The surface area of the peritoneum is between 1 and 2 m². This arrangement leads to distinctly different sensory capabilities of the peritoneal lining, with the visceral peritoneum being innervated by the visceral nervous system and the innervation of the parietal peritoneum from the segmental nerve roots of the peripheral nervous system. The differential innervation results in vague, poorly localized pain from visceral peritoneal irritation while parietal peritoneal irritation is sharp, well localized pain. While the peritoneum is closed to the environment in men, it is open to the environment in women via the fallopian tubes which means that the differential diagnosis of peritonitis in women includes processes related to the gynecologic organs or infectious agents transmitted into the abdominal cavity via those organs. Furthermore, the peritoneal cavity is not just an open cavity. Rather, it is divided into numerous compartments that can transmit irritants or infectious agents to other areas of the abdomen or contain these agents in a specific area. This compartmentalization within the abdomen can influence

the course and presentation of a disease process resulting in peritonitis.

Pathophysiology

While there are a number of metabolic and toxic conditions that may induce severe abdominal pain and clinical signs worrisome for peritonitis, the majority of patients presenting with localized or diffuse peritonitis have an intra-abdominal infection. Most often this is the result of an abdominal organ infection or intestinal perforation (Table 66.1). The release of intraluminal contents into the peritoneal cavity induces an intense inflammatory response by the peritoneal lining [2]. This inflammatory stimulus promotes a rapid transudate of a protein rich fluid into the peritoneal cavity which normally only has approximately 50–100 cc of serous fluid. Resident macrophages respond to the inflammatory process by releasing strong chemoattractants that promote an influx of neutrophils and lymphocytes into the peritoneal cavity which subsequently release numerous chemokines and cytokines that coordinate the immune response [3]. Additionally, a number of factors are released that locally activate the clotting cascade, resulting in the deposition of fibrin around the inflammatory stimuli. This is the body's attempt to wall off the inflammatory process to form an abscess.

Secondary effects resulting from the inflammation cause the clinical syndrome associated with peritonitis [4]. The sympathetic nervous system is activated by the inflammatory process which inhibits intestinal peristalsis resulting in an ileus. There is impairment of intestinal fluid absorption and translocation of fluid into the intestinal lumen contributing to the ileus and abdominal distension. This shift of fluid causes systemic hypovolemia which lead to the clinical signs of peritonitis: tachycardia, hypotension, and oliguria or anuria. Persistence and progression of the inciting intra-abdominal infection will induce a systemic inflammatory response that can profoundly alter distant organ function or death.

Clinical Syndrome

As previously noted, peritonitis is a clinical diagnosis. The primary finding is severe abdominal pain characterized by evidence of peritoneal irritation on examination [5]. Classically, peritoneal irritation causes abdominal wall rigidity and severe pain with palpation, which frequently is made worse by the rapid removal of the examining hand—rebound tenderness. Early in the process, palpation may induce localized voluntary abdominal wall muscular rigidity, which is known as voluntary guarding. As the intra-abdominal process evolves, this rigidity becomes involuntary. The patient with peritonitis will avoid any movement as this makes the peritoneal irritation worse. Often, they lay perfectly still, avoiding deep breaths. They might find some relief in pulling their legs upward, thus decreasing the stretch on the abdominal wall muscles and parietal peritoneum. This is in contrast to patients with colicky pain who often move frequently, attempting to find a comfortable position or can only find comfort while ambulating.

While peritoneal irritation may be associated with a multitude of systemic and other intra-abdominal processes, such as pancreatitis, intestinal ischemia, and inflammatory bowel disease, peritonitis for the purposes of this chapter is the result of an intra-abdominal infec-

tion. Peritonitis is classified as primary or secondary [6]. Primary peritonitis is a bacterial infection of the peritoneum without a discrete intestinal perforation or organ infection. This is most commonly known as spontaneous bacterial peritonitis (SBP) [7]. Secondary peritonitis, the most common form, is associated with blunt or penetrating trauma, perforation of the intestine, localized infectious processes (appendicitis, diverticulitis, cholecystitis/cholangitis), or a complication after intra-abdominal surgery.

For the majority of patients with secondary peritonitis, there will be some type of radiologic imaging or laboratory data that supports the diagnosis. Laboratory data are perhaps the least reliable as the duration of the inciting process and the patient's underlying physiologic state can have a profound impact on key values such as the WBC, which can be suppressed, normal, or markedly elevated. Radiologic studies are extremely helpful in identifying the possible cause of peritonitis, although frequently a good history can also lead to the same diagnosis. Plain radiographs demonstrating free intra-abdominal air are suggestive of an intestinal perforation. However, in postoperative patients free air may be see for up to 7–10 days on plain films and up to 3 week on CT scans. Overall, an abdominal CT is the most sensitive radiologic study for identifying inflammatory changes associated with a local infectious process such as diverticulitis or in cases of postoperative complications [8]. Although there might be evidence of highly worrisome findings on CT scan, it must be remembered that these findings may not always be associated with clinical peritonitis and visa versa.

Spontaneous Bacterial Peritonitis (SBP)

The infection of ascitic fluid in the absence of any intra-abdominal, surgically treatable source of infection was termed spontaneous bacterial peritonitis by Harold Conn in 1971 [9]. With increasing clinical experience, improved diagnostics, and more effective antibiotics, the inhospital mortality rate associated with SBP has steadily declined from nearly 90% to less than 20% [10]. However, patients who do not receive appropriate or delayed treatment have a mortality rate approaching 50%. In patients with chronic ascites, the annual incidence of SBP ranges between 7 and 30% [10].

In the 1970s, the pathophysiology of SBP was unknown. However, intensive study has demonstrated that translocation of intestinal bacteria into the ascitic fluid is the primary cause of SBP. While low levels of bacterial translocation into mesenteric lymph nodes occur constantly in healthy individuals, in patients with cirrhosis there is baseline bacterial overgrowth due to poor intestinal motility and impairment in intestinal barrier function which predisposes to increased rates of bacterial translocation.

Patients with SBP present with fever, vomiting, diffuse abdominal pain, ileus, and decreased urine output and not uncommonly mental status changes. The only definitive way to diagnose SBP is by analysis of the ascitic fluid after an abdominal paracentesis. A number of different ascitic fluid markers are associated with SBP. Perhaps the two most sensitive diagnostic findings of SBP are a fluid WBC count above 500 cells/μL or a polymorphonuclear leukocyte (PMN) count above 250 PMN/μL [11]. The diagnostic accuracy of these tests is 95%, with a sensitivity of greater than 90%, and a specificity of 95–98%. Often, cultures of ascitic fluid are negative. However, the most common organisms cultured are Gram-negative bacteria, with the majority being *E. coli*, and *Klebsiella pneumoniae* [10].

Early initiation of antibiotic treatment is essential to avoid serious morbidity. If the ascitic fluid cell count is elevated, empiric therapy with a third-generation cephalosporin or a quinolone should be started [10]. Cephalosporins are highly effective in treating SBP, with a 75–90% resolution rate. Aminoglycosides should be avoided because of potential renal toxicity. Most patients respond rapidly after antibiotics are initiated. The difficult clinic issue is when to discontinue treatment. Most recommend continuing treatment until a repeat paracentesis demonstrates a return to a normal cell count [7].

Secondary Peritonitis

Secondary peritonitis is the most common form of peritonitis. It is related to an intra-abdominal infection either from an organ infection, perforation of the intestine, or a complication of intra-abdominal surgery. The cornerstones of treatment are source control and antibiotic therapy. According to Pieracci and Barie, source control is any physical means necessary to eradicate a focus of infection as well as modify factors that would continue the infection, such as preventing on-going leaking of intestinal contents [12]. Inadequate source control at the initial operation is associated with worse outcomes.

For specific organ infections such as appendicitis or diverticulitis, surgical intervention is directed at removing the infected organ and as much of the peritoneal contamination as possible. In some cases, particularly in diverticulitis, the fecal stream is often diverted with a proximal stoma to avoid continued contamination of the peritoneum or the risk of a leak from an anastomosis constructed in the setting of peritonitis. In severe cases of peritoneal contamination, planned reoperations, continuous peritoneal irrigation, or leaving the abdomen open may be required in order to control the source of the peritonitis. This approach has become known as "damage control" surgery [13]. There have been no trials comparing the best approach to source control in cases of advanced peritonitis. Many surgeons advocate leaving the abdomen open as it decreases intra-abdominal pressure, avoiding a compartment syndrome, improves drainage of the abdomen and early detection of on-going contamination, and facilitates repeat explorations. The abdomen is temporarily closed with a "Bogota bag" (Figure 66.2). However, the disadvantages are numerous including significant fluid and protein loss, loss of abdominal domain, prolonged recovery, and need for future operations to address the abdominal wall defect. A new technology in the form of the vacuum-assisted closure (VAC) has helped mitigate many of these problems while maintaining the advantages of an open abdominal approach [14]. Planned reoperation either as "on-demand" or "scheduled" are well recognized surgical approaches to intra-abdominal catastrophes. The "on-demand" approach is a conservative tact where the patient is re-explored only if there is evidence of on-going intra-abdominal infection while the "scheduled" re-operation is one in which the patient is returned to the operating room in planned timeframe regardless of clinical condition. In a meta-analysis of the non-randomized reports of these two different approaches, there seemed to be a slight decrease although not significant in mortality associated with the "on-demand" approach [15].

After source control, initiation of systemic antibiotics is a vital component of treatment [6]. Similar to source control, there are very few well-controlled trials to guide therapy. According to the Surgical Infection Society (SIS), high-risk patients with advanced peritoneal contamination should be treated with extended-range β-lactam/anti-β-lactamase compounds, carbapenems, and

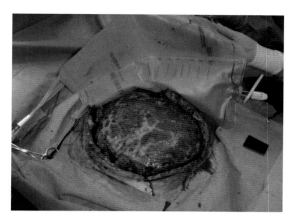

Figure 66.2 Damage control surgery performed for a patient with peritonitis from a perforated duodenal ulcer. The patient has been left with an open abdomen and returned to the operating room multiple times. A sterile plastic "Bogota" bag was used as a temporary abdominal closure. Once the peritoneal sepsis is resolved and the patient's condition improves, the abdominal cavity contents are covered with a skin graft. (Courtesy of Dr Stephen J. Ferzoco, Brigham and Women's Hospital, Harvard Medical School.)

third or fourth-generation cephalosporin plus metronidazole [16]. An increasingly important problem is the emergence of multidrug resistant Gram-negative organisms. A study from Germany has reported that 25% of isolates from patients with peritonitis demonstrate resistance to one or more commonly used advanced antibiotics [17]. An outstanding issue in the treatment of peritonitis is the duration of antibiotic therapy after the source of the intra-abdominal infection has been controlled. A current recommendation is that antibiotics are continued until the all signs of clinical infection have resolved, the WBC is normal, and gastrointestinal function has returned to normal. This typically will involve approximately a week of therapy although a survey of institutions have shown that they typically continue antibiotic therapy for over 14 days.

Obtaining accurate survival data for patients with secondary peritonitis is very difficult given the variety of etiologies. Mortality from perforated appendicitis is now extremely rare in developed countries but is not unheard of in perforated diverticulitis. The patient's overall condition and comorbidities at the time of presentation with peritonitis are risk factors for increased morbidity and mortality. Koperna and Schulz reviewed a 3-year experi-

ence with secondary peritonitis at a tertiary referral center [18]. Using the APACHE II score for stratification, patients with a score less than 15 had a mortality rate of 4.8% while the mortality rose to 46.7% in those with scores of 15 or higher. The average total mortality rate was 18.5%.

Conclusions

Primary and secondary peritonitis are life-threatening clinical conditions that require rapid recognition and treatment to avoid significant morbidity and a high mortality rate. The hallmark of peritonitis is evidence of peritoneal irritation. Most commonly, peritonitis is the result of either a localized or diffuse intra-abdominal infection. In cases of secondary peritonitis, the mainstays of treatment are source control and systemic broad-spectrum antibiotics. Source control involves surgical intervention to remove or repair the cause of the bacterial contamination within the peritoneal cavity. Even with aggressive treatment the in-hospital mortality rate for peritonitis remains very high.

Take-home points

Diagnosis:
- Peritonitis is a clinical diagnosis with few reliable laboratory or radiologic findings.
- Most often it is associated with an intra-abdominal catastrophe or a rapidly progressing infectious process within the abdominal cavity.
- A thorough history and physical examination assist in narrowing the possible causes of peritonitis.
- Peritonitis can be a localized or a diffuse abdominal process.
- The classic clinical findings of peritonitis may not be present in all patient populations including immunosuppressed, elderly, and obese patients.
- While most cases of peritonitis are classified as "surgical diseases," there are a number of medical conditions that can present with symptoms and signs suggestive of peritonitis.

Therapy:
- In patients with localized peritonitis, expeditious diagnostic evaluation can direct initiation of appropriate medical or surgical intervention.

- Diffuse peritonitis requires surgical intervention in nearly all cases although in certain patient populations medical treatment may be appropriate.

- Surgical therapy is directed at resection of part or the entire organ(s) responsible for causing the clinical syndrome and removing the agent (toxins, irritants, or infectious) that is irritating the peritoneal surface.

- While antibiotic therapy may be an appropriate initial or primary therapeutic option for localized peritonitis, it has only a supporting role for diffuse peritonitis in nearly all cases.

References

1 Turnage RH, Richardson KA, *et al*. Peritoneum and peritoneal cavity. In: Townsend CM, Beauchamps RD, *et al.*, eds. *Sabiston Textbook of Surgery: The Biological Basis of Modern Surgical Practice*, 18th edn. Philadelphia, PA: Saunders Elsevier, 2008: 1129–54.

2 Heel KA, Hall JC. Peritoneal defences and peritoneum-associated lymphoid tissue. *Br J Surg* 1996; **83**: 1031–6.

3 Cavillon JM, Annane D. Compartmentalization of the inflammatory response in sepsis and SIRS. *J Endotoxin Res* 2006; **12**: 151–70.

4 Sawyer RG, Barkun JS, *et al*. Critical care: intra-abdominal infection. In: Souba WW, Fink MP, *et al. ACS Surgery: Principles and Practice*. New York: WebMD, 2006: 1592–620.

5 Delcore R., Cheung LY. Gastrointestinal tract and abdomen: acute abdominal pain. In: Souba WW, Fink MP, *et al. ACS Surgery: Principles and Practice*. New York: WebMD, 2006: 397–412.

6 Dupont H. The empiric treatment of nosocomial intra-abdominal infections. *Int J Infect Dis* 2007; **11**: S1–S6.

7 Jansen PLM. Spontaneous bacterial peritonitis: Detection, treatment, and prophylaxis in patients with liver cirrhosis. *Neth J Med* 1997; **51**: 123–8.

8 Velmahos GC, Kamel E, Berne TV, *et al*. Abdominal computed tomography for the diagnosis of intra-abdominal sepsis in critically injured patients: fishing in murky waters. *Arch Surg* 1999; **134**: 831–8.

9 Conn HO, Fessel JM. Spontaneous bacterial peritonitis in cirrhosis: variations on a theme. *Medicine* 1971; **50**: 161–97.

10 Koulaouzidis A, Bhat S, Karagiannidis A, *et al*. Spontaneous bacterial peritonitis. *Postgrad Med* 2007; **83**: 379–83.

11 Wong CL, Holroyd-Leduc J, Thorpe KE, *et al*. Does this patient have bacterial peritonitis or portal hypertension? How do I perform a paracentesis and analyze the results. *JAMA* 2008; **299**: 1166–78.

12 Pieracci FM, Barie PS. Intra-abdominal infections. *Curr Opin Cri Care* 2007; **13**: 440–9.

13 Sagraves SG, Toschlog EA, Rotondo MF. Damage control surgery: the intensivits's role. *J Intensive Care Med* 2006; **21**: 5–16.

14 Perez D, Wildi S, Demartines N, *et al*. Prospective evaluation of vacuum-assisted closure in the abdominal compartment syndrome and severe abdominal sepsis. *J Am Coll Surg* 2007; **205**: 586–92.

15 Lamme B, Boermeester MA, Reitsma JB, *et al*. Meta-analysis of relaparotomy for secondary peritonitis. *Br J Surg* 2002; **89**: 1516–24.

16 Mazuski JE, Sawyer RG, Nathens AB, *et al*. The surgical infection society guidelines on antimicrobial therapy for intra-abdominal infections: an executive summary. *Surg Infect* 2002; **3**: 161–73.

17 Krobot K, Yin D, Zhang Q, *et al*. Effect of inappropriate initial empiric antibiotic therapy on outcome of patients with community-acquired intra-abdominal infections requiring surgery. *Eur J Clin Microbiol Infect Dis* 2004; **23**: 682–7.

18 Koperna T, Schulz, F. Prognosis and treatment of peritonitis: do we need a new scoring system. *Arch Surg* 1996; **131**: 180–6.

CHAPTER 67
Abdominal Hernia

Michael Cox

Department of Surgery, University of Sydney, Nepean Hospital, Penrith, NSW, Australia

Summary

An abdominal hernia is the protrusion of a viscus or tissue through a defect in the muscular wall of the abdomen. The hernia may present as a lump that increases with elevation of abdominal pressure or acutely with pain and symptoms of obstruction. Most hernias are diagnosed with clinical history and examination. An ultrasound or computed tomography (CT) scan may augment the clinical assessment. Symptomatic hernias need to be surgically repaired.

Case

An 83-year-old woman presented with colicky central abdominal pain and vomiting large amounts of bile-stained fluid. She had not passed flatus since the onset of the pain. There was no previous abdominal surgery and was otherwise well. She did not complain of any other symptoms, in particular had not noticed any hernias.

Clinical examination revealed she was mildly dehydrated with a pulse of 92 but was afebrile. Abdominal examination revealed moderate abdominal distension and a painful lump in the left groin (Figure 67.1a). This was tender, but not warm, and was located below and lateral to the pubic tubercle. An abdominal X-ray confirmed a small bowel obstruction (Figure 67.2).

She received intravenous fluid resuscitation, deep vein thrombosis prophylaxis, antibiotic prophylaxis, and had an emergency operation 2 h after admission. A superior, preperitoneal approach was performed and the sac delivered (Figure 67.1b). This was opened and contained a loop of small bowel that was strangulated and clearly not viable (Figure 67.1c). A small bowel resection with a primary anastomosis was performed. The hernia was repaired with three interrupted 0 prolene sutures approximating the inguinal ligament to the pectineal fascia. She had an uneventful recovery and was discharged well 5 days later.

Practical Gastroenterology and Hepatology: Small and Large Intestine and Pancreas, 1st edition. Edited by Nicholas J. Talley, Sunanda V. Kane and Michael B. Wallace. © 2010 Blackwell Publishing Ltd.

Definitions and Epidemiology

Abdominal Hernia

An abdominal hernia is the protrusion of a viscus or tissue through a defect in the muscular wall of the abdomen. The defect occurs through the fascia of the abdominal wall. The sites of hernias are related to either anatomic points of weakness in the abdominal fascia (Table 67.1) or at the sites of previous surgical incisions, such as incisional or parastomal hernias. Once the defect has developed, the abdominal contents are, over time, forced through the defect and the hernia becomes larger.

Sac

The sac is the peritoneal lining of the hernia. This is peritoneum that is pushed through the defect.

Neck

The neck of a hernia is the defect in the fascia and usually has a dense fibrotic ring. It is at the neck where obstruction may occur.

Reducible

A hernia is reducible when the visceral contents can easily be pushed back into the abdominal cavity.

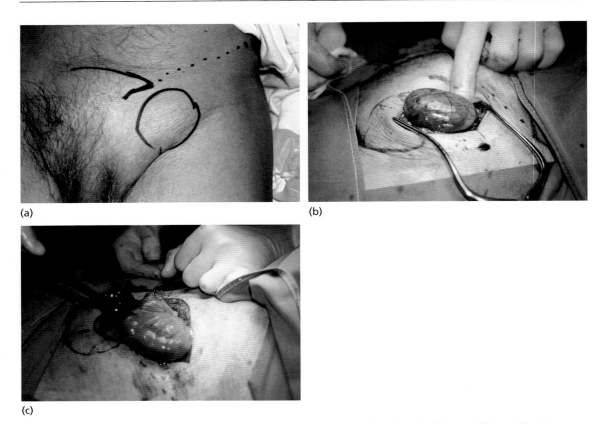

Figure 67.1 (a) Obstructed femoral hernia below and lateral to pubic tubercle. Dashed line is inguinal ligament. (b) Femoral hernia sac reduced through a superior, preperitoneal approach. (c) Reduced ischemic small bowel through a preparietal approach. This bowel required resection.

Irreducible

A hernia is irreducible when the contents are not able to be pushed back into the abdominal cavity with gentle pressure. This may be due to adhesions between the viscera and the wall of the sac, the hernia is usually a chronic long-standing hernia, or there may be excessive intra-abdominal pressure preventing easy reduction of the hernia contents. In the presence of an irreducible hernia, if there is no pain and no symptoms or signs of intestinal obstruction, this sign of irreducibility is not an indication for urgent surgery.

Obstructed

A hernia is obstructed when the intra-abdominal viscera has been pushed into the sac and the contents become trapped at the neck. There is associated edema

and swelling of the contents, which will then produce pain. This will present as acute pain, tenderness, and an irreducible lump and symptoms of small or large bowel obstruction. An obstructed hernia may become strangulated.

Strangulation

The hernia is strangulated when the obstructed viscus becomes ischemic. This is venous ischemia, due to the pressure at the neck on the viscera occluding the venous return from the viscera within the sac. This results in congestion and subsequent impairment of arterial flow and ischemia with venous infarction occurs (Figure 67.1c). Viscera that may become strangulated include small intestine, colon, omentum, or intra-abdominal fat.

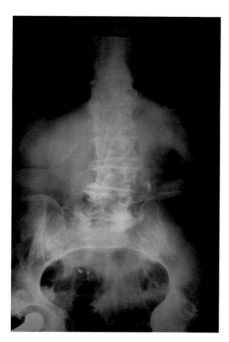

Figure 67.2 Plain erect abdominal X-ray in an 83-year-old woman that presented with vomiting and an obstructed left femoral hernia. Note the evidence of small bowel obstruction and the gas-filled bowel down to the femoral canal region.

Clinical Features

Hernias may present with a variety of clinical symptoms (Table 67.2). A hernia may be asymptomatic and found on clinical examination. The most common asymptomatic hernias are small umbilical hernias and small incisional hernias.

Hernias most frequently present as a lump that has become more prominent and increases with intra-abdominal pressure such as lifting, coughing, walking, or straining. The presence of the lump may be associated with a dull ache or some chronic discomfort. Occasionally, hernias will present with discomfort, without noting a lump. This is most commonly associated with indirect inguinal and direct inguinal hernias. A small incisional hernia may present with pain in the wound. In patients with morbid obesity the lump may not be palpable through the excess subcutaneous fat. In this setting, ultrasound may be helpful.

A hernia that has become obstructed will present with a sudden onset of severe pain in the region of the hernia. The patient will note that the hernia has become swollen, tender, and irreducible. If there is bowel present within the hernia they may present with symptoms of intestinal obstruction. Examination of the hernia may reveal it to be prominent, tender, with edema and redness of the skin. It is difficult to distinguish clinically between an obstructed and strangulated hernia.

Patients may present with intermittent intestinal obstructive symptoms. This is particularly common with large inguinal and incisional hernias. They will present with some discomfort in the hernia, associated with some abdominal bloating, colicky pain, or symptoms of constipation. They may note the reduction of the hernia will resolve these symptoms.

Patients may present with a small bowel obstruction with acute abdominal pain, nausea, vomiting, abdominal distension, obstipation, and constipation, without having noticed the hernia. This is most commonly associated with elderly women with a femoral hernia but can also occur with an incisional hernia which is large, with multiple defects where one of the defects becomes obstructed.

Clinical Signs

The clinical signs are dependent on the site of the hernia (Table 67.1). The lump shall be seen at the relevant site (Figures 67.1a, 67.3, 67.4, 67.5, 67.6a, and 67.7). The lump usually becomes more prominent with activities that increase the intra-abdominal pressure: cough, elevation of the head off the bed, standing or straining.

Once found, the type of hernia needs to be defined. The clinical signs defining the type of hernia are summarized in Table 67.1.

A hernia is irreducible when gentle pressure does not push the contents into the abdominal cavity. Not all irreducible hernias are obstructed. If a hernia is large and long-standing (particularly umbilical, large inguinal, or incisional) there may be adhesion between the herniated viscera and the hernia sac that prevents the reduction of the hernia.

An obstructed hernia will be irreducible. There may be swelling or redness. Overlying redness may indicate strangulation has occurred. The obstructed hernia shall

Table 67.1 Description, diagnosis, and treatment of abdominal hernia.

Name	Anatomical defect	Site/signs	Specific characteristics	Imaging	Treatment
Indirect inguinal hernia	Through the internal ring of the inguinal canal (Figure 67.3)	Inguinal, may descend into the scrotum above and medial to pubic tubercle (Figure 67.4a,b) Prevented with pressure over the mid-inguinal point	Common in males Occurs in females Narrow neck, may obstruct and strangulate	If suspected, ultrasound of the inguinal region is the investigation of choice Ultrasound is dynamic CT scan will define larger hernias but may miss small hernias CT is static	Open mesh hernia repair (Linctiensien) or laparoscopic mesh repair
Direct inguinal hernia	Through the posterior wall of the inguinal canal The defect is in the transversalis fascia between the conjoint tendon and inguinal ligament (Figure 67.3)	Inguinal, bulges forward; does not descend into scrotum Above and medial to pubic tubercle and prevented with pressure on the mid-inguinal point	Common in males Direct: indirect ~1:2 Rare in females Wide neck, unusual to strangulate	Ultrasound is the best imaging, as this can be done as a dynamic study CT scanning may not demonstrate the direct hernia if there is no increase in intra-abdominal pressure	Open mesh repair (Linctiensien) or laparoscopic mesh repair
Femoral hernia	Femoral canal bounded by the inguinal ligament anteriorly, the pectineal fascia posteriorly and the femoral vein laterally (Figure 67.3)	Inguinal Below and lateral to the pubic tubercle (Figures 67.3 and 1a)	Rare in males Usually older females Often presents with obstruction and strangulation	Ultrasound is the preferred imaging technique	1 Open, suprapubic, preperitoneal repair for obstructive hernia (Figure 67.1b) 2 Inferior external approach for elective repair 3 Laparoscopic repair with mesh
Umbilical hernia	Anatomical defect through the linear alba at the site of the umbilicus This may be superior or inferior to the umbilicus (para-umbilical) but is always in the midline (Figure 67.3)	Umbilical May protrude through the umbilicus or superior or inferior to the umbilicus The latter may be called paraumbilical	Common in both male and female If obstructed usually contains omentum or preperitoneal fat	Seldom required for diagnosis Ultrasound is preferred imaging CT scan will define the defect (Figure 67.6b)	Open mesh hernia repair
Epigastric hernia	The defect is in the linear alba between the xiphisternum and the umbilicus (Figures 67.3 and 67.7)	Midline between the xiphisternum and umbilicus (Figure 67.7)	Often small (3 to 5 mL defect) usually contains preperitoneal fat, rarely has bowel within it May present as epigastric pain	Ultrasound is the preferred technique Defect may not be seen on CT scan	Open mesh or sutured repair

Spigelian hernia	The defect is at the point of fusion of the transversalis and internal oblique fascia at the edge of the rectus muscle. There is no defect through the external oblique. This is a ventral hernia where the sac is deep to the external oblique aponeurosis (Figure 67.4)	Infraumbilical along the mid-inguinal line above the inguinal ligament (Figure 67.3)	Rare. May not have a palpable lump due to being deep to external oblique fascia. May present with left or right iliac fossa pain	Ultrasound is the preferred imaging, where the external oblique is noted to be intact but there is a defect with the sac through the deeper layers. CT scanning may define this but ultrasound is the preferred technique	Open mesh repair or laparoscopic mesh repair
Lumbar hernia	The defect is through the posterior fascia at the lumbar triangle	Posterior above the bony pelvis	Extremely rare. Presents with posterior pain and mass	Ultrasound or CT	Open mesh repair
Obturator hernia	The defect is through the obturator foramen of the bony pelvis. There is no palpable or external component to this hernia	There are no external landmarks for this hernia	Extremely rare. Usually female. Will present with small bowel obstruction. Consider in small bowel obstruction where there is pain radiating down the medial thigh due to compression of the obturator nerve	CT scan for acute small bowel obstruction will define the small bowel through the obturator foramen. May be seen on plain X-ray	Laparotomy and mesh repair of defect
Incisional/anatomical hernia	Defect is through an abdominal muscle wound from previous surgery. This can occur with any wound at any site. It is more common in the region of the linear alba	Along or in the proximity of a previous abdominal scar (Figure 67.5a,b)	Previous abdominal surgery. Multiple defects in the fascia may occur. May present with obstruction or strangulation	Ultrasound and CT to define the defect and the site of the defect	Open mesh repair with abdominoplasty. Laparoscopic repair
Parastomal hernia	Adjacent to an intestinal stoma through the abdominal wall. Specific form of incisional hernia	Adjacent to stoma	May present as stomal pain	CT scan is preferred as ultrasound assessment adjacent to a stoma may be difficult	Mesh repair may be performed. Resiting of the stoma may be necessary with a mesh repair of the old site

Table 67.2 Symptoms of abdominal wall hernia.

Symptom	Characteristics
Lump	Increase site with increase in intra-abdominal pressure; may be absent at times
Chronic pain	Usually low grade in morbidly obese; may be the only symptom if the lump is not detectable
Ache/discomfort	May have intermittent ache or discomfort; worse after physical activity or at the end of the day
Acute pain	Associated with obstruction and becomes irreducible; consider strangulation a possibility
Intermittent intestinal obstruction	Some hernias may cause intermitted small or large bowel obstruction and be associated with symptoms accordingly
Acute intestinal obstruction	Small bowel—colicky pain, distension, nausea, and vomiting Large bowel—colicky pain, distension, reduced bowel activity

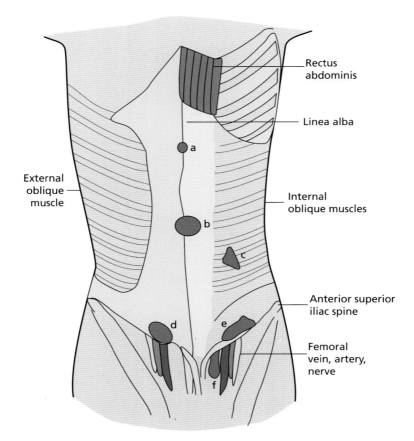

Figure 67.3 Sketch of the anterior abdominal wall musculature and hernia orifices. On the right side is the intact external oblique, on the left is with the external oblique removed. The orifices are: (a) epigastric hernia in the linea alba; (b) umbilical at the umbilical defect in the linea alba; (c) spigelian hernia at the edge of the rectus (note this is through the transverocites and internal oblique but not through the external oblique); (d) direct inguinal hernia through the posterior wall of the inguinal canal defect; (e) indirect inguinal hernia through the internal inguinal ring descending along the cord; (f) femoral hernia beneath the inguinal ligament.

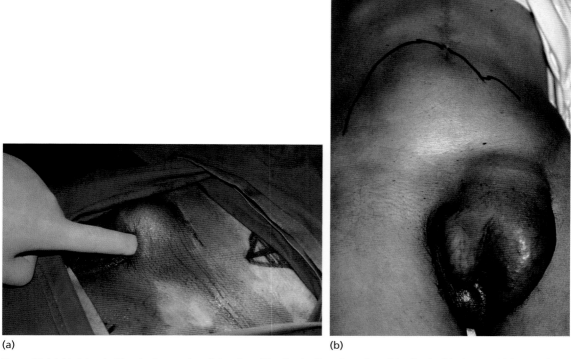

(a)   (b)

Figure 67.4 (a) Left inguinal hernia above and medial to the pubic tubercle. Finger is on the pubic tubercle. (b) Obstructed left inguinal scrotal (indirect) hernia.

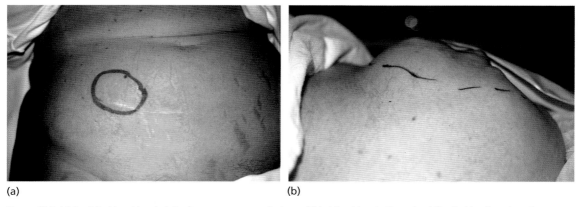

(a)   (b)

Figure 67.5 (a) Small incisional hernia following an open appendectomy. (b) Incisional hernia through midline incision for a bowel resection. Note the large area with an associated large neck.

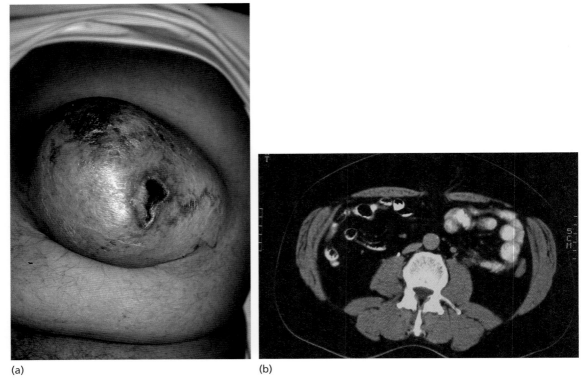

(a)   (b)

Figure 67.6 (a) Large, obstructed umbilical hernia associated with skin ulceration. (b) CT scan of umbilical hernia. Note the gap in the muscle with the protruding fat.

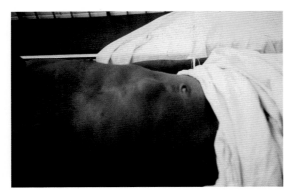

Figure 67.7 Epigastric hernia in the midline, 5 cm above the umbilicus.

be tender, the more tender the more likely there is associated strangulation.

Occasionally, large umbilical or incisional hernias may have ulcerated skin due to chronic ischemia and/or local trauma (Figure 67.6a).

Investigations

The majority of hernias are diagnosed on clinical symptoms and signs and require no further investigation. Such hernias can be treated on clinical grounds alone. Where there is suspicion of a hernia on clinical grounds, imaging with either ultrasound or computed tomography (CT) scan may be performed. For the majority of abdominal wall hernias ultrasound is the preferred technique (Table 67.1). Incisional hernias, particularly recurrent incisional hernias, require CT scanning to define the extent of the defects in order to better plan surgical intervention.

A plain abdominal X-ray should be performed in an obstructed hernia (Figure 67.2), even in the absence of clinical signs of bowel obstruction.

Treatment

Once diagnosed, the majority of symptomatic hernias require surgical repair. The type of repair most frequently uses some form of prosthetic material to repair the defect (Table 67.1).

Inguinal hernias may be repaired with either an open or laparoscopic technique. Laparoscopic inguinal hernia repair is associated with a more rapid recovery but may be associated with a higher incidence of recurrence [1].

Laparoscopic bilateral inguinal hernia repair has a much shorter recovery time and is the preferred method of treatment for bilateral inguinal hernias [2].

Recurrent inguinal hernias may be repaired with an open or laparoscopic approach. The risk of damage to the spermatic cord structures is less with a laparoscopic approach [3].

An obstructed femoral hernia needs to be repaired with a suprainguinal, preperitoneal approach in order to both reduce the hernia and, if necessary, perform a bowel resection. A femoral hernia that is being repaired as an elective operation can be repaired through an infrainguinal anterior approach as a sutured repair.

Traditionally, umbilical hernias were repaired with a sutured Mayo repair. Recent trials have clearly demonstrated that mesh repair is superior to a sutured repair [3].

Obstructed hernias require urgent surgical repair after a brief period of fluid resuscitation. If there is an ischemic bowel, this is resected. In the majority of occasions it will be the small intestine which is ischemic and can be resected with a primary anastomosis.

Take-home points

- An abdominal wall hernia usually presents with a reducible lump and is a simple clinical diagnosis.
- Hernia may present with acute obstruction, with associated bowel obstruction and ischemia.
- Where symptoms are suggestive of a hernia but no hernia is detectable, ultrasound or abdominal CT scan are the investigations of choice.
- All symptomatic hernias require surgical repair.
- Acute obstruction requires urgent surgical repair.

References

1 Takata MC, Duh QY. Laparoscopic inguinal hernia repair. *Surg Clin North Am* 2008; **88**: 157–78.

2 Bisgaard T, Bay-Nielson M, Kehlet H. Re-recurrence after operation for recurrent inguinal hernia; A nationwide 8 year follow up study on the role of type of repair. *Ann Surg* 2008; **247**: 707–11.

3 Chang H, Tsai P, Kingsworth A. Randomised clinical trial comparing suture and mesh repair of umbilical hernia in adults. *Br J Surg* 2001; **88**: 1321–3.

Index

Page numbers in *italic* refer to figures and tables.

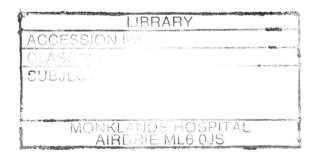